D1560949

CLINICAL MEDICAL ASSISTING
An Introduction to the Fundamentals of Practice

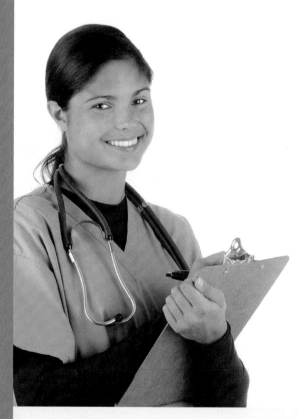

Jennifer L. Gibson, PharmD
President
Excalibur Scientific, LLC

Brinda M. Shah, PharmD
President
Advanced Knowledge Concepts, Inc.

Rebecca Umberger, CMA (AAMA), CPM
Adjunct Instructor, Health Division/
Medical Assisting Department
Stark State College, North Canton, Ohio

Vice President of Development
Family Care Centers of Ohio

JONES & BARTLETT
LEARNING

World Headquarters
Jones & Bartlett Learning
5 Wall Street
Burlington, MA 01803
978-443-5000
info@jblearning.com
www.jblearning.com

Jones & Bartlett Learning books and products are available through most bookstores and online booksellers. To contact Jones & Bartlett Learning directly, call 800-832-0034, fax 978-443-8000, or visit our website, www.jblearning.com.

Substantial discounts on bulk quantities of Jones & Bartlett Learning publications are available to corporations, professional associations, and other qualified organizations. For details and specific discount information, contact the special sales department at Jones & Bartlett Learning via the above contact information or send an email to specialsales@jblearning.com.

Production Credits

Chief Executive Officer: Ty Field
President: James Homer
SVP, Editor-in-Chief: Michael Johnson
SVP, Chief Marketing Officer: Alison M. Pendergast
SVP, Curriculum Solutions: Christopher Will
VP, Business Development: Todd Giorza
VP, Design and Production: Anne Spencer
VP, Manufacturing and Inventory Control: Therese Connell
Editorial Management: High Stakes Writing, LLC, Editor and Publisher: Lawrence J. Goodrich
Copy and Development Editor, HSW: Kate Shoup

Senior Editorial Assistant: Rainna Erikson
Production Manager: Susan Schultz
Production Assistant: Kristen Rogers
Marketing Manager: Grace Richards
Manufacturing and Inventory Control Supervisor: Amy Bacus
Director of Photo Research and Permissions: Amy Wrynn
Rights & Photo Research Assistant: Joseph Veiga
Composition: Publishers' Design and Production Services, Inc.
Cover Design: Kristin E. Parker
Cover Image: © Steve Cukrov/ShutterStock, Inc.
Printing and Binding: Courier Companies
Cover Printing: Courier Companies

Library of Congress Cataloging-in-Publication Data
Gibson, Jennifer L.
    Clinical medical assisting : an introduction to the fundamentals of practice / Jennifer L. Gibson, Brinda Shah, Rebecca Umberger.
        p. ; cm.
    Includes index.
    Summary: "The purpose of this book is to offer a complete resource for clinical medical assistant training by providing a thorough education to prepare medical assistant students for clinical practice"--Provided by publisher.
    ISBN 978-1-4496-8524-9 (hardcover)
    I. Shah, Brinda M. II. Umberger, Rebecca. III. Title.
    [DNLM: 1.   Physician Assistants. 2.   Clinical Competence. 3.   Clinical Medicine--methods.   W 21.5]

    610.73'72069--dc23

        2012035549

6048
Printed in the United States of America
16 15 14 13 12   10 9 8 7 6 5 4 3 2 1

Contents

CHAPTER 7   **Dosage Calculations** **185**

CHAPTER 8   **Integumentary System** **203**

Introduction

Health care is changing; however, your role as the most versatile member of the healthcare team is an important part of the successful physician practice, and will continue to be integral as health care changes. Although the skills you perform may vary among medical offices, our education and training in the exciting field of clinical medical assisting will prepare you with a wide variety of skills, making you an essential part of the healthcare team.

How This Book Is Organized

After an introduction to the basics of clinical medical assisting, *Clinical Medical Assisting: An Introduction to the Fundamentals of Practice* utilizes a body-systems approach to present the information a clinical medical assistant needs to know to be effective in practice. These chapters include the structure and the function of each body system, diseases and disorders of that system, treatment modalities, discussion of the common diagnostic examinations, and the skills a clinical medical assistant would use in caring for a patient.

Special Features

What Would You Do?—These scenarios show you how the content is applied to real-life situations in the classroom and in practice.

Key Terms—Terms and ideas are presented in a list at the beginning of every chapter.

Chapter Summary—In bulleted format, these summaries recall the main knowledge-base objectives within the chapter.

Learning Assessment Questions—These certification-style review questions help solidify your understanding of the chapter.

In summary, this textbook contains an organized approach to learning the roles and responsibilities of the clinical medical assistant. It encompasses all areas of practice from the very basic to the most complicated, with the intention of guiding the student to mastery of all concepts.

Acknowledgments

To ensure the accuracy of the material presented throughout this textbook, an extensive review and development process was used. This included evaluation by a variety of knowledgeable healthcare professionals. We are deeply grateful to the numerous people who have shared their comments and suggestions. The quality of this body of work is a testament to the feedback we have received.

Reviewing a book or supplement takes an incredible amount of energy, time, and attention, and we recognize the sacrifices our colleagues made to help ensure the validity and appropriateness of content in this edition. The reviewers provided us with additional viewpoints and opinions to combine to make this text an incredible learning tool.

We wish to thank the following editorial and technical review team:

Reviewers

Dana Bernard, RN, MS
President, Boston Reed

Theresa Capitonoff, LVN
Boston Reed

Christine Gaither, RN
Instructor, Boston Reed

Dianna Pledger
Instructor, Boston Reed

Tammy Fletcher, RN
Instructor, Boston Reed

Dianne Doerfer, CCMA, CPT, LPN
Instructor, Boston Reed

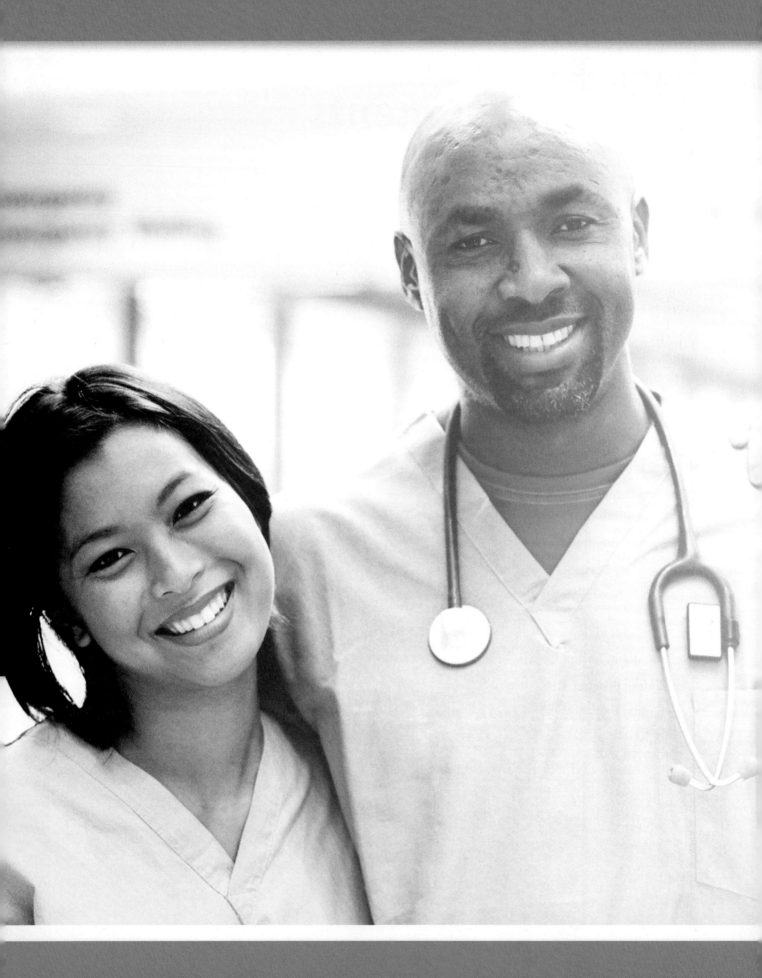

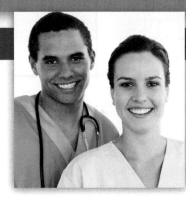

The Medical Assistant and the Healthcare Team

OBJECTIVES

After reading this chapter, you will be able to:

- Discuss the history of medical assisting.
- Describe the profession of medical assisting.
- Understand the scope of practice for the medical assistant.
- Describe the function of the healthcare team.
- Compare/contrast civil and criminal law.
- Identify the three major areas of civil law that directly affect the medical profession.
- Describe the measures to take for disposal of controlled substances.
- Recall the three main goals of HIPAA.
- Explain the differences between expressed and implied contracts.
- Discuss what constitutes battery in the ambulatory care setting.
- Describe the two forms of defamation of character and how it might occur.
- Recall how medical assistants can help to maintain a patient's privacy.
- Discuss informed consent and its importance.
- Identify various forms of advance directives.
- Identify two reasons for a code of ethics.
- Discuss the ethical guidelines for healthcare providers, giving at least four examples.
- Learn to recognize, prepare for, and respond to emergencies in the ambulatory care setting.
- Understand the legal and disease-transmission considerations in emergency caregiving.
- Perform the primary assessment in emergency situations.

KEY TERMS

Accreditation
Accrediting Bureau of
    Health Education
    Schools (ABHES)
Act
Administrative laws
Advance directives
American Association of
    Medical Assistants
    (AAMA)
American Medical
    Technologist (AMT)
Assault
Autonomy
Basic cardiac life
    support (BCLS) skills
Battery
Beneficence
Business associate
Certified Clinical Medical
    Assistant (CCMA)
Certified Medical
    Assistant (CMA-
    AAMA)
Civil laws
Commission on
    Accreditation
    of Allied Health
    Education Programs
    (CAAHEP)
Continuing education
    units (CEUs)
Contract
Contributory negligence

Covered entity
Criminal law
Damages
Defendant
Doctors of osteopathy
    (DOs)
Do-not-resuscitate
    (DNR) order
Emergency
Ethics
Expressed contract
Felony
Four Ds of negligence
Good Samaritan laws
Health Insurance
    Portability and
    Accountability Act
    (HIPAA)
Implied consent
Implied contract
Informed consent
Intentional tort
Justice
Laws
Libel
Licensed practical nurse
    (LPN)
Licensed vocational
    nurse (LVN)
Living will
Medical assistant
Medical doctors
    (MDs)
Medical liability

Medical power of
    attorney
Misdemeanor
Moral values
National Healthcareer
    Association (NHA)
Negligence
Nonmaleficence
Nurse practitioners
    (NPs)
Ordinance
Patient confidentiality
Personal protective
    equipment (PPE)
Pharmacist (PharmD)
Phlebotomist
Physician assistants
    (PAs)
Plaintiff
Precedent
Protected health
    information (PHI)
Registered medical
    assistant (RMA)
Registered nurse (RN)
Respondeat superior
Risk management
Scope of practice
Slander
Statute of limitations
Tort
Treason
Unauthorized disclosure
Unintentional tort

Chapter Overview

In the United States, approximately 10 percent of all workers are involved in the field of health care. With an ever-increasing senior population, a basic need for healthcare services by the public will demand more trained healthcare workers.

The U.S. Department of Labors' *Outlook Handbook, 2010–2011 Edition*, projects that the medical assisting field will grow much faster than the average for employment in the 2008–2018 decade. Growth is expected to be approximately 34 percent or higher. The job market for medical assistants is expected to be excellent, with approximately 62 percent of medical assistants working in physician offices.

The field of medicine has many changes and challenges, of which the medical assistant should be aware when entering the workforce. Medical assistants will be faced with many moral, ethical, and legal dilemmas throughout their careers that will test not only themselves, but the patients for whom they are caring.

Medical assistants in the field will most certainly become exposed to medical law on a daily basis. Medicine is intertwined with the legal system, making it very important to understand how laws guide us through and function in society. One way is making sure that you are practicing within the scope of your training. It is one of the most important legal considerations in your training and will help you navigate the complicated days of working in the field of medicine and avoiding a potential lawsuit.

Students considering a career in medical assisting will find it to be a very challenging, yet rewarding career. You must have strong dedication with a disciplined approach to always put the patient first as well as have patience with some who may not be feeling their best. In matters of medical emergencies in and out of the workplace, the medical assistant may be called on for immediate assistance or to assess the situation as a first responder. Knowledge, training, and use of proper basic life-support techniques, first-aid procedures, and established protocols will increase the likelihood of a positive outcome for the patient. As a medical assistant, self-discipline and professionalism will be tested on an ongoing basis. Keep in mind that the *patient* always comes first.

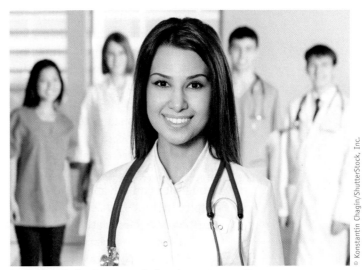

Medical assisting is a very challenging, yet rewarding career.

© Konstantin Chagin/ShutterStock, Inc.

Medical assistants can perform both administrative and clinical duties, making them one of the most versatile health professionals in the medical field. Their duties vary with the location, specialty, and size of the practice. A well-trained medical assistant who has these versatile qualities and skills will find many opportunities in his or her profession. Some may find that they want to advance their careers by seeking a higher degree in the field, working in research, or teaching other medical-assisting students by applying their years of experience and knowledge in a medical-assisting program, or becoming practice managers for a medical office. There are many paths of discovery awaiting each medical assistant to explore.

The History of Medical Assisting

Medical assisting is a relatively new profession in medicine. With the constant change in medicine and the practice of medicine becoming more organized and complicated, a need for individuals who are trained both clinically and administratively to assist physicians in their offices and clinics has grown. The first professional training college of medical assistants on record was in 1934 by Dr. M. Mandl, who felt that there was a demand for assistants. By the mid-1950s, standards for medical-assisting programs were being developed. In 1978, the U.S. Department of Health Education and Welfare formally recognized the medical assistant as an allied health professional.

Medical Assisting in Health Care Today

Medical assistants today can practice in varied healthcare settings, although the majority of them work in outpatient practices. Standards of training and education for medical assistants have evolved due to the ever-changing legal and ethical landscape and the advancement of medicine. **Accreditation** is a principle that establishes creditability through formal education with a determined standard. Each program may have varied requirements for its students, ranging from a two-year associate degree of applied science from an accredited college or university to an award of a diploma in a program through a state department of education. It is important for prospective medical assistants to recognize the need for proper training and education and to choose a program that fits their lifestyles. The chosen program should prepare them by providing the standards to function in their chosen profession. **Continuing education units (CEUs)** are awarded to medical assistants who attend educational conferences and seminars to maintain their training and credentials throughout their careers. It is very important that learning is continued past the formal training and education that the medical assistant achieves while in school. Changes and advances in medicine as well as in procedures occur constantly. A medical assistant who does not embrace the need for these updates may find himself or herself left behind and unemployable.

Medical assistants may practice in the United States without a certification, although it is an advantage to have at least one certification or registration. Some examples include the **Certified Clinical Medical Assistant (CCMA)** through the **National Healthcareer Association (NHA)**, the **Certified Medical Assistant (CMA-AAMA)** through the **American Association of Medical Assistants (AAMA)**, and the **Registered Medical Assistant (RMA)** through the **American Medical Technologists (AMT)**.

The NHA certification examination requires that a person graduate from an NHA-approved healthcare program or have one or more years of full-time experience with a high-school diploma or a General Education Diploma (GED). There are testing sites across the country where you may sit for the exam. Recertification occurs every two years, at which point the medical assistant may sit for an exam or demonstrate the accumulation of the required 10 CEUs. The official website for the NHA is www.nhanow.com.

Candidates choosing to sit for the Certified Medical Assistant CMA-AAMA certification must graduate from programs accredited through the **Commission on Accreditation of Allied Health Education Programs (CAAHEP)** or the **Accrediting Bureau of Health Education Schools (ABHES)**. CAAHEP and ABHES are both acknowledged under the U.S. Department of Education. Recertification for CMAs is required every five years, during which time the medical assistant must accumulate at least 60 CEU credits with half in specialized areas (administrative, clinical, or general) or re-sit for the examination. The website for the AAMA is www.ama-ntl.org.

The American Medical Technologists (AMT) (www.amt1.com) recognize registered medical assistants (RMAs), which requires testing candidates to meet one of the following requirements: attending accredited programs through ABHES and/or CAAHEP; attending a program that is accredited through the U.S. Department of Education with a minimum of 720 hours of training; gaining formal medical service training in the U.S. Armed Forces; or working for at least five years as a medical assistant. RMAs must recertify every three years by obtaining CEUs.

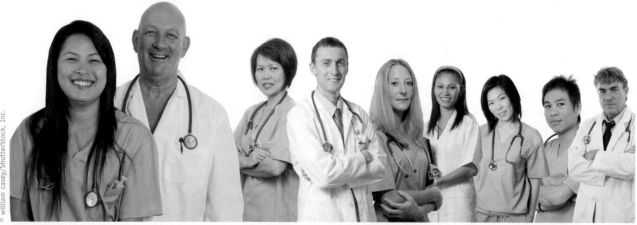

© william casey/ShutterStock, Inc.

In medicine, a team of highly skilled individuals with different levels of training and education works for the patient.

There is no current licensure for medical assistants. Medical assistants may graduate from a diploma program at a local technical college or hold a two-year associate degree in applied science (AAS) through a state college. With experience, medical assistants may advance their skills to work in the role of practice or office manager, medical assisting instructor, research assistant, author, and other careers in the allied health field.

The Healthcare Team

As in any field, a team working together collaboratively with the same goals and focus works best. In medicine, a team of highly skilled individuals with different levels of training and education is working for its biggest "customer," the patient. A centered focus on patient care with effective communication between all healthcare professionals involved increases the likelihood for a positive clinical outcome and patient satisfaction. The medical assistant plays a large role in the healthcare team and must always be aware of his or her actions with others. The medical assistant must be an effective communicator, have excellent organizational skills, possess a professional presence, and remain calm. Following concise orders sometimes under stressful situations and/ or while performing multiple duties can prove challenging at times. Other members of the healthcare team are discussed here.

Physicians

Medical doctors (MDs) are physicians who complete four years of undergraduate (pre-med) classes in college. After graduation, they undergo another four years of medical school with an additional three to eight years of internships and residency programs, depending on their chosen specialty. MDs are sometimes called allopathic physicians, and are the most recognized. Allopathic physicians are mainstream doctors who treat disease using drugs, surgery, and modern technology.

Doctors of osteopathy (DOs) are physicians who complete their training requirements very similarly to an MD, with four years of undergraduate and four years of school of osteopathic medicine with residencies lasting between two and six years. In addition to using the tools of modern medicine, DOs also offer a system of hands-on treatment known as osteopathic manipulative medicine.

Physician Assistants

Physician assistants (PAs) are trained to diagnose and treat patients as directed by a physician. They are licensed individuals and have the authority to write prescriptions in most states and possess advanced degrees in medicine. As of 2008, there are more than 74,800 physician assistants practicing in the United States according to the *United States Occupational Outlook Handbook*.

Registered Nurses

A **registered nurse (RN)** is a graduate of a school of nursing, and in most scenarios, will have an associate degree, a bachelor's degree, or a baccalaureate degree. Registered nurses must pass a state licensing exam. Most RNs work in hospitals or clinics but they may also work alongside other healthcare professionals in ambulatory settings, research, education, and home health.

Nurse Practitioners

Nurse practitioners (NPs) are registered nurses with advanced academic training who have obtained a master's degree in nursing. Nurse practitioners can diagnose and prescribe medications to patients and focus on preventive care and prevention of disease.

As of 2011, there were approximately 155,000 nurse practitioners practicing in the United States, according to the American Association of Nurse Practitioners (AANP).

Licensed Practical and Vocational Nurses

Both **licensed practical nurses (LPNs)** and **licensed vocational nurses (LVNs)** can offer bedside and personal care for patients during hospitalization. They can administer drugs, assess patients, and chart patient progress when allowed by state law. These nurses usually work in hospitals or nursing homes, but also may be found in physician offices.

Phlebotomist

A **phlebotomist** is someone who draws blood. These healthcare professionals are not only trained to draw blood from a vein (venipuncture), but process the specimen by labeling it correctly and making sure it is prepared properly for the test ordered. Many medical assistants are trained in the art of phlebotomy and become great phlebotomists, among their other varied skills. There are certifications for phlebotomists under several major accrediting agencies. You are not required to attain these certifications in most states to perform phlebotomy, although it is preferred in most hospital settings.

Pharmacist

A **pharmacist (PharmD)** distributes drugs prescribed by licensed individuals with prescribing authority (such as physicians, NPs, and PAs), and advises patients, physicians, and other healthcare professionals on dosages, interactions, and side effects of the prescribed medication. A pharmacist obtains a PharmD degree in a college of pharmacy and requires extensive training before his or her license becomes valid. The physician and medical assistant sometimes work closely with a pharmacist due to the daily interaction required for their patients and their prescribed medications.

Scope of Practice

The medical assistant should *never* perform or be asked to perform a duty outside the scope of his or her practice. **Scope of practice** can be defined as a boundary that determines what a medical professional may and may not do based on his or her training, experience, and competency. States vary in laws and regulations as to what the medical assistant is and is not allowed to perform. These tasks are delegated by the physician, which makes that physician responsible for his or her agent's actions. The applied legal term for this is **respondeat superior,** meaning, "Let the master answer." In this example, the physician can be liable for the wrongful acts of his employee while the employee is under the physician's immediate supervision, as long as the employee is performing under his or her scope of practice. Medical assistants need to have an understanding of how law is applied to medicine, not only to stay abreast of new rules, standards, and regulations, but to also protect themselves and their right to practice.

Medicine and Law

Issues of patient confidentiality and performing duties legally and ethically within standard boundaries are just some considerations the healthcare professional must keep in mind at all times. Regulations, which change frequently, are rules to make sure that risks are kept to the minimum with employees' and patients' safety in mind. A working knowledge of medicine, the relationship it has with the law, and how these interact with each other will help the healthcare team deliver excellent care to its patients while complying with legal requirements.

What Would You Do?

As a practicing medical assistant, you are allowed to perform tasks that are delegated by the physician within the scope of your practice. What would you do in a situation where you were asked to perform a procedure on a patient that you were not qualified or trained on, or was out of the scope of your practice? What if the physician requested you to do this?

© NorthGeorgiaMedia/ShutterStock, Inc.

Legal Considerations for the Medical Assistant

Medicine can be a very complicated profession, not to mention the legal aspects and considerations that the physicians and their medical assistants face on a daily basis. In a general sense, the legal system holds each and every person liable for the consequences of his or her actions and decisions. **Ethics** is a standard of behavior as well as a personal sense of right and wrong above what is considered legal. Ethical conduct is based on a person's sense of **moral values**, which are learned traits in society, the family, and the culture in which the person lives.

Basic Principles of Medical Ethics

Law and medical ethics are both intertwined and are constantly changing with new legislation, court decisions, and medical ethic issues created by laws; new technologies; new discoveries; as well as other influences. Physicians and healthcare providers should always respect and maintain the four basic principles of medical ethics when challenged with difficult decisions and procedures in health care. The main principles are as follows:

- **Autonomy** in medical ethics allows the patient to self-govern and choose his or her course of action, making informed decisions regarding his or her health care and making free and unforced choices. An example of this would be a treatment or procedure that may be recommended by the physician, but the patient does not want to pursue any further treatment or testing for his or her disease. The patient has the right to make his or her own decisions.
- **Justice** is when the physician has considered all of the benefits and burdens to the patient when weighing new or experimental treatments while helping the patient make informed healthcare decisions. The physician must consider whether the patient has had access to and been given an adequate level of health care, regardless of his or her ability to pay. The physician must also consider to what degree the patient will benefit with or without the treatment, the actual likelihood of the benefit, how long the benefit is expected to last, as well as the cost. An example of this type of dilemma might be the use of newer reproductive technologies that are currently available for patients. They are very costly, more than likely not covered by most health insurance policies, and the general public would not normally be able to afford these procedures on their own.
- **Beneficence** is achieved for the patient when the procedure or test being recommended has focused the intent on what is *best* for the patient. This is achieved by demanding that physicians and healthcare providers develop and maintain skills and knowledge with updated training and having the ability to give individual consideration to the patient as a person.
- **Nonmaleficence** is not harming the patient. This is a main factor of retaining the patient's trust of the physician and integrity to the patient. Physicians have a duty to act to prevent harm to individuals as well as not engaging in acts that

risk harm to others. A very controversial example of an ethics challenge for a physician is physician-assisted suicide. Even though the patient may desire to end his or her life, the physician has a duty to uphold this principle.

When a professional or his agent does not act in accordance to the standards of his or her profession or makes mistakes and causes injury or damages, those actions are considered negligent and the professional can be legally responsible for those damages. **Damages** are defined as a harm or injury to property or a person resulting in loss of value or the impairment of usefulness. **Negligence** is the act of being inclined to neglect, especially habitually, and/or careless ease or informality.

In law, there are three levels at which these rules of society are determined. The U.S. Constitution holds the highest level of laws over any federal, state, or local laws that have been passed. At the federal level through Congress, a law that is passed is called an **act**. An example of an act is the most recent and much debated Patient Protection and Affordable Care Act, which was passed by Congress and signed by President Obama in 2010.

At the state level, laws passed through the legislature and local governments are called **ordinances**. A required seat belt and/or child restraint ordinance is one example of an ordinance that may vary from state to state.

Many laws are based on legal decisions from the past. These decisions are called **precedents**. Precedents are followed in the courtroom by the judges and juries that are appointed when a case is presented to them for a decision. A very well-known precedent decided by the Supreme Court in 1973 is *Roe v. Wade*, which gave pregnant women the right to abort an early-term pregnancy. This precedent remains very controversial today and has been much debated in law and medicine for many years.

Criminal and Civil Laws

Laws are rules of conduct that require everyone to behave the same way or face punishment. In law, there are two basic categories: criminal law and civil law. It is important for the medical assistant to be aware of the differences and how they may affect his or her rights and responsibilities as a professional in the medical field.

A **criminal law** pertains to a crime made against the state or government. These types of crimes can harm the public's safety and welfare. There are three basic offenses in criminal law:

- A **misdemeanor** is a minor or small crime. Misdemeanors are crimes that can be punishable either with fines or imprisonment for less than one year. An example of a misdemeanor could be as minor as a traffic violation or disturbance of peace or as severe as assault and battery.
- A **felony** is a more serious crime and involves punishment of fines and imprisonment for more than one year, and can involve more severe crimes such as homicide.
- **Treason** is considered an attempt to overthrow the nation's government or in the case of high treason, an attempt or involvement in a plan to assassinate the president of the United States.

In case law, a **plaintiff** is the person who brings suit and initiates a complaint requesting damages, and who has a burden to prove the allegation brought against the defendant. A **defendant** is the person who is being charged with the complaint.

Civil laws are laws that do not pertain to criminal behavior, but involve acts against a person, a business, or the government. Most laws that affect medicine are civil, which include torts, contracts, and administrative law. **Administrative laws** are laws and legal rules that govern the administration and regulation of both state and federal agencies. A **tort** is a civil wrong or a wrongful act; it can be intentional or accidental (unintentional) when an injury occurs to another person. The most common torts in the healthcare system are known as **unintentional torts**. One example of an unintentional tort is medical negligence—when a healthcare provider injures a patient either by not using the ordinary care that another provider would have given in the same circumstance or by performing or failing to perform an act that a reasonable healthcare provider would have performed. Each healthcare provider is held to a standard of care based on his or her own profession.

For a tort to have been committed, four elements must be satisfied:

- Duty of care
- Breach of duty to perform
- Injury caused by the breach of duty
- Damages, injury, or loss suffered

If one component is missing, the tort will not be met and no negligence has occurred.

Consent

A person has the right to agree or refuse medical treatment as well as the services and procedures that are suggested by the physician and carried out by the physician and his or her staff. It is important for healthcare professionals to understand not only how laws apply to medicine, their patients, and their staff, but also the exposure for a legal loss if not performed properly. By the healthcare staff taking measures to inform the patient properly, the patient becomes informed on why the procedure is necessary, but also can ask questions, learn about the risks of the procedure, learn about the possible outcomes, and make judgments prior to the act being completed.

A physician who does not obtain consent from the patient prior to a gynecological exam and without the presence of a chaperone may be putting himself or herself at risk for a claim of battery from the patient. The same holds true if the medical assistant performs a venipuncture on a patient and does not obtain consent.

There are two basic types of consent in medicine:

- **Implied consent** is presumed consent, normally in a nonwritten fashion, such as a patient putting his or her arm down and rolling his or her sleeve up when informed by the medical assistant that he or she needs to perform venipuncture.
- **Informed consent** is achieved when the patient has an understanding of what is going to be involved in the procedure, consents to the treatment, and is advised of the risks involved, expected outcomes, alternative treatments, and the risk if no procedure is performed. Informed consent is usually in written form, signed by the patient and the physician and/or staff as witnesses.

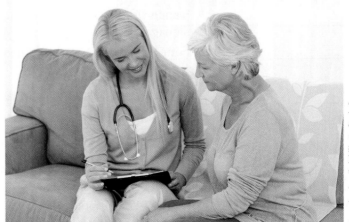

Healthcare staff must take measures to inform patients properly.

What Would You Do?

You and your coworker are friends on a large social network outside the office. Your friend writes about a patient who was recently seen in the office. She tells a detailed story relating to an indiscretion by the patient with a person other than his spouse, which caused him to contract a sexually transmitted disease. Without naming names, she says the person "deserved it." Is this professional?

© NorthGeorgiaMedia/ShutterStock, Inc.

Intentional Torts

In medicine, assault and battery are **intentional torts** and are civil offenses in general but can be criminal as well. **Battery** can be any willful or intentional touching by one person against another person's will or using an object or anything put in motion by the aggressor. It is an act that causes bodily harm. In the ambulatory care setting, a battery charge could be leveled against a medical assistant for an unauthorized touch of a patient while giving an injection or drawing blood. You must keep in mind that there are established procedures in place to avoid this type of legal issue, such as identifying the patient and explaining the procedure prior to touching the patient and starting the act. This gives the patient the courtesy and time to object if he or she does not agree to continue with the procedure.

To establish a battery case, three major elements must be proven:

- The unauthorized touch or use of an object must happen in action with the defendant.
- It must include an intentional cause of harm or offensive contact by unauthorized touching or use of object.
- There has been unauthorized touch or harmful or offensive contact with the person.

Assault is the intentional act by a person who threatens bodily harm or attempts to create injury through force, strike, or harm. An example of an assault is a threat of potential danger along with the person's apprehension for harm, such as raising a fist or flashing a knife at the intended victim. The person must be aware of the threat and have reason to fear that the threat will be carried out. Assault and battery is committed when the person threatens and then touches or uses the object put in motion (fist, knife, etc.).

Another example of an intentional tort in civil law is defamation of character. Defamation of character involves an intentional, false, or defamatory statement about another person that results in damages. There are two types of defamation of character:

- **Libel** is a false or defamatory statement in written words.
- **Slander** is a defamatory statement that is spoken in words that are intended to damage a persons' reputation, profession, or means of living.

Four legal requirements are needed to establish the tort of defamation:

- It must be intentional.
- It must be a false or defamatory statement.
- It must be said about another person.
- It must have caused some damage to another person.

With the popularity of social media sites such as Facebook, Twitter, and LinkedIn, you must be very careful of not only about whom you are writing, but also any comments, pictures, and postings for public viewing. Many corporations and physician practices have adopted human-resource policies and procedures to protect themselves from unwarranted written statements and postings from unmindful and disgruntled staff members as well as the use of social media while at work.

As a medical assistant, caution should be used when friends or patients ask your opinions of physicians and healthcare providers and your thoughts about them. You should never give a personal opinion, only a professional response. Saying "I wouldn't take my worst enemy to Dr. Peters" may be viewed as a slanderous comment and could put you at risk of a lawsuit.

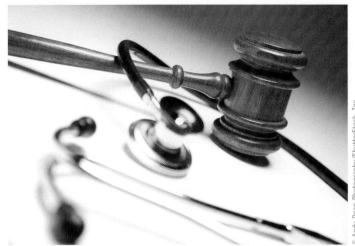

You should be aware of major legal issues that may affect you as a medical assistant and a healthcare professional.

Contracts

A **contract** exists when two parties meet in agreement and can be between two parties, an individual, or a corporation. Contracts must have four elements to be binding:

- There must be an agreement. It must not be made under duress. It must be made in good faith.
- There must be consideration. There must be something of value for the part of the agreement. In medicine, the patient is paying for the physician's services.
- The contract must be of legal subject matter. If the physician is offering his services to the patient and the patient is paying, he must hold a legal license.
- There must be a contractual capacity. The patient must be of age and capable of understanding all terms and conditions.

Contracts can be expressed or implied. An **expressed contract** between the physician and the patient is in writing and will contain a date and signature. An example of this type of contract may be when the patient first registers and is asked to sign the provided demographic form stating that he or she agrees to pay for services and that his or her assignment has been given to the physician to process the proper paperwork necessary to file with his or her insurance. An **implied contract** is created and formed when the physician agrees to see the patient and acts in good faith to the best of his or her abilities to treat the patient. The patient then agrees in the implied contract that he or she will follow the physician's directions and treatment.

One consideration that the medical assistant must remember is to never make promises or statements to patients guaranteeing results. Also, avoid making statements such as, "Dr. Brown will have you feeling better in no time." Even though this may be with good intentions, it exposes the physician and the medical assistant to potential legal complications.

Three Major Areas of Civil Law That Directly Affect Medical Professionals

It is important to be aware of major legal issues that may affect you as a medical assistant and a healthcare professional. Standards of care were developed as a basis of malpractice. Each health professional is held to a standard of care that others in the same profession with the same training and expertise would use. As previously discussed, there are three main legal issues in medicine under the civil laws in medicine. Those areas that are most affected are as follows:

- Medical liability/negligence
- Confidentiality
- Consent

Medical Liability/Negligence

Medical liability is also known as malpractice. The relationship that exists between the patient and the physician is very important. The study of medical liability and the prevention of malpractice are known as **risk management**. Many hospitals have a specific department that deals with this issue. Numerous studies over the years in risk management have shown that a patient is less likely to sue the physician if the patient has a positive relationship with the physician and the physician's support staff. A relationship that has become negative in nature may have an impact on whether the patient will sue, even if the patient has incurred no injury or basis for legal action.

For the physician to have representation for these cases, he or she must first purchase medical liability/malpractice insurance, which is much like an automobile insurance policy. Medical malpractice is very costly for physicians and increases if/when the physician is faced with a claim and a payment is made to a defendant. All hospitals and most insurance companies working with physicians under contract require the physician to hold a valid and current liability policy. It is said that all physicians will encounter at least one lawsuit in their career.

Liability is also determined by the physician's specialty. For example, if the physician is in the specialty of dermatology, the likelihood of a claim will be much less than if that same physician practiced in the specialty of neurology, performing brain surgeries on a regular basis. In comparing this with the automobile insurance analogy, if you drive an expensive automobile with a larger, faster engine, like a Porsche, your premiums will be much higher than if you drive a less-expensive, slower car, such as a Chevy Volt. Similarly, the cost of malpractice policies is determined by the number of years the physician has practiced along with any past claims the physician might have incurred throughout his or her career. Many medical malpractice insurance companies offer physicians a discount each year if they or their staff attends continuing medical education classes focused on risk management sponsored by the company each year. Some may also offer an additional discount if the practice has converted to an electronic health record (EHR) government-certified program.

If a physician has a claim in which he or she was found at fault, the claim is then considered a loss for the insurance agency covering the physician. A loss follows that physician's record for 10 years when considered for premium payments. If a physician is found to have had too many claims in his or her career, just as with car insurance, the physician can be put on a "high risk" policy in which his or her premiums are dramatically raised. In some cases, the physician's policy may be canceled by the insurance company.

Medical negligence falls under the category of a tort. Most claims in medicine fall into the category of an unintentional tort, which translates to a mistake or an accident that has caused the patient to suffer an injury or death. If the physician did not act reasonably in the situation in which the patient suffered a loss, then that physician is responsible for his or her conduct; this would be a case of negligence.

According to the American Medical Association, in order for a malpractice suit to proceed in court, the **four Ds of negligence** must occur:

- **Duty**—There must be a relationship documented between the physician and patient for the physician to owe the patient any duty.
- **Derelict**—There must be proof given that the physician did not comply with the standards of the profession (Standard of Care).
- **Direct cause**—It must be proven that any damages were a direct cause of the physician's actions with a breach of duty.
- **Damages**—There must be proof that the patient suffered an injury or loss.

There are some defenses that can be used in malpractice cases. These defenses can reduce or eliminate the defendant's liability altogether in the case, depending on the specific claim and nature of the defense used in each case. These are as follows:

- **Contributory negligence** is negligence in which the plaintiff contributed to the injury or loss. An example of contributory negligence may be in the case of failure to diagnose, in which the physician examines the patient and suggests that the patient undergo cancer screening but the patient does not schedule the suggested screening. The patient then later is found to have cancer, which the suggested screening would have detected and helped to avoid delayed treatment or death.

- There is a time limit in which a person can file a claim of medical malpractice in most states. This is called a **statute of limitations**. Most states' rulings hold that two years from the date of the injury is long enough time to file suit. Many lawyers for the plaintiff will hold the claim until close to the limitation date, hoping that details and information of the loss become cloudy, forgotten, or misplaced. Although this is not a very ethical practice, it is allowable.

- Broadly speaking, an **emergency** is an unforeseen combination of circumstances or the resulting state that calls for immediate action. Most emergencies in which a healthcare professional or physician respond or assist in are covered by **Good Samaritan laws**. These statutes can vary from state to state, but they have the intent to protect the healthcare professional during an emergency. Good Samaritan laws are only applicable in emergencies and do not cover emergencies that occur in the workplace.

Confidentiality

With **patient confidentiality** held as one of the most sacred ethical aspects of health care, the medical assistant must remember that the medical record is confidential and private documentation of healthcare information between the physician and the patient and should never be violated. Patient confidentiality pertains to the patient's rights to privacy and freedom from public release of information that the patient regards as being of a personal nature.

Special care should be taken when discussing patients' information even within the office setting by limiting access to staff who are involved in the direct care of the patient, protecting physical aspects by limiting access to monitors and other confidential areas, as well as never discussing any confidential patient information outside the office in casual conversation or with friends in social settings.

Consent

As mentioned previously in this chapter, consent is an important aspect of law for the medical assistant and other healthcare professionals to understand and cover with their patients very carefully. If proper consent is not obtained, the patient may have a

It is very important for a physician and/or healthcare professional to document detailed information on each and every encounter with a patient. The phrase "If it isn't written, it didn't happen," used commonly when reviewing documentation, comes directly from risk-management training. Trying to remember years later under oath what happened would be impossible if no records existed, and the defendant would surely forget the details of what occurred.

legitimate case of being uninformed and unable to make proper healthcare decisions or having his or her rights violated by the physician or healthcare professional.

HIPAA Standards and Goals

The **Health Insurance Portability and Accountability Act (HIPAA)** was introduced in the 1990s and became effective in April 1996. Initially, when the new laws came into effect, there was much apprehension and confusion throughout the medical community with regard to communicating with patients in spoken and written forms under the new privacy laws.

The primary goals of HIPAA were as follows:

- To improve the "portability" of a person's health care from one employer to another when changing jobs
- To simplify the administration of health insurance by standardizing transaction and code sets
- To protect and improve patients' rights by setting guidelines on how health information is disclosed
- To enhance patients' access to their own records
- To control inappropriate disclosures of patients' information.

A minimum necessary standard was developed for the covered entities to develop safeguards as necessary to limit the access of unnecessary or inappropriate access to **protected health information (PHI)**. PHI is any information about a person's health, healthcare treatment, or the payment for that person's health care. Under HIPAA's definition, a **covered entity** is a physician, a healthcare provider, a nursing home, a hospital, an insurance company, or other organization that uses electronic transmissions during a transaction. Examples of these transactions could be an electronic claim, a digital electronic funds transfer for payment to a provider, or a typed dictation from the physician for the patient's medical record transmitted to the office for the patient's file. Under the privacy rule, protected health information (PHI) is protected under HIPAA standards, yet communication and flow of that healthcare information is still allowed between covered entities if the use is for treatment, payment, or operations of the patient's health care.

A **business associate** is someone who works with a covered entity that might receive this protected health information to help with the operation of the entity. A signed agreement (called a business associate agreement) between the business associate and the covered entity must exist to ensure that the business associate is practicing standardized HIPAA policy and procedures in his or her work as well as taking care of PHI as the covered entity would. Most business associates affiliated with covered entities are on the consultant level and are not employees of the physician, healthcare provider, or hospital. In private practice, for example, a business associate could be a transcriptionist, a billing service for the practice, an accountant, an attorney, or anyone who may have the need and access to PHI to conduct business with the covered entity.

The privacy rule protects PHI from unauthorized disclosures. An **unauthorized disclosure** is defined as the unauthorized use of protected

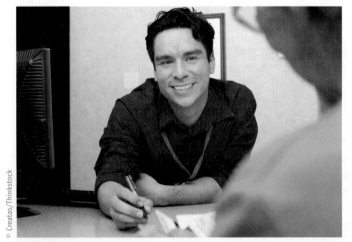

New patients must sign a form indicating that they have read and understand the provider's privacy policy.

health information that compromises the security and privacy of the PHI. An example of this may be a lab report that contains a patient's HIV status that is inadvertently faxed to the patient's employer rather than to the infectious disease specialist to whom the patient was referred. The privacy rule is also sanctioned and monitored by the Office of Civil Rights, which enforces and protects patients from discrimination and breaches of privacy and takes action legally to correct the problem.

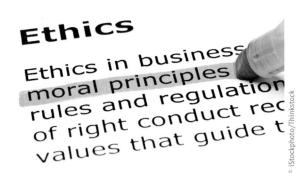

Medical professionals face new dilemmas in medical ethics and standards of care.

Advance Directives

Advance directives were developed to inform patients of their rights to refuse treatment, choose their advance directives under the state law, and choose the discontinuation of life-sustaining equipment or the refusal of it altogether. The provider is required to ask patients whether they have any wishes regarding their decision on life-sustaining measures and make note of them for future emergency treatment.

States vary in the laws of advance directives, but living wills and medical power of attorney documents are prevalent in most every state. **Living wills** express the patient's wishes regarding medical treatment and life-sustaining efforts. A living will is a document that speaks for the patient when the patient cannot speak for himself or herself. In comparison, a **medical power of attorney** is a document that gives the right of making medical decisions to another person who is responsible for carrying out the patient's wishes if the patient is mentally or physically unable to make decisions himself or herself.

A **do-not-resuscitate (DNR) order** is another example of an advance directive. The patient who chooses this advance directive wishes not to undergo CPR if found to be in cardiac or respiratory arrest. Many patients wear a bracelet or have a tattoo placed near their chest to communicate this directive in case of emergency. The DNR order should be honored and documented in the patient's chart as soon as it is communicated to the physician and carried out whether as an inpatient or outpatient. The DNR does not affect any other treatment such as chemotherapy, dialysis, antibiotics, or any other appropriate treatments the patient may be currently under for his or her condition.

It is important for the medial assistant to be aware of advance directives and their impact on patients' rights and respect their life decisions.

Codes of Ethics and Their Impact in Medicine

With the increase of medical discoveries and technologies that advance life and extend the quality of it on an almost daily basis, medical professionals face new dilemmas in medical ethics and standards of care—even more than those faced by their peers just 10 or 20 years ago. Challenged with controversial subjects such as human cloning, genetic testing, euthanasia, physician-assisted suicide, and other ethical issues, the medical assistant and other medical professionals may be questioned many times in their careers with what they have formed in their own beliefs against what they have been taught is best for the patient.

The Hippocratic Oath is one of the oldest medical teaching documents in history, formed by the "Father of Medicine," Hippocrates, in the era of 400 BCE (BC). It is still sacred to this day among physicians around the world. Physicians may swear this oath upon graduation from medical school, promising to uphold ethical and moral values such as treating patients who are ill to the best of their ability, protecting and preserving patients' confidentiality, putting in practice steps to prevent disease, and other standards and practices to place patients first in the hands of their physician. This "do no harm" mentality puts respect for the patient first. The physician will do his or her best for the patient, even if treating the patient isn't in the best interest of the physician.

Ethical Guidelines for Healthcare Providers

Medical ethics isn't just about avoiding harm; it is also a standard or a set of values, principles, and norms of the profession. These ethical standards also promote the values that are essential for good communication and enhance trust, accountability, mutual respect, and fair medical care. Ethical decisions may have more than one answer; it is your decision and up to you how you approach each issue. Making ethical decisions sometimes comes very naturally to the healthcare professional and doesn't require much thought; other times, decisions are based on the information that you have on hand at the time or on the condition of the person in consideration when you have to make the decision.

Medical Emergencies in the Office

Medical assistants as well as other healthcare professionals in the outpatient setting should be prepared for a medical emergency should it occur any time in or out of the office. A medical emergency can be any circumstance in which a person becomes ill or has an injury or an episode that requires an immediate action and/or decision. By knowing and having a clear understanding of how and when to respond to an emergency, the medical assistant will be ready to react, allowing essential assistance in an emergency situation.

At the minimum, most employers require that their clinical staff have **basic cardiac life support (BCLS) skills**, a standard training in case of an emergency. Having basic cardiac life support training enables a caregiver to recognize several life-threatening emergencies; provide CPR to victims of all ages; use an automated external defibrillator (AED); and relieve choking in a safe, timely, and effective manner. Basic cardiac life support classes are taught by trained individuals through the American Heart Association and the American Red Cross. When an emergency occurs, the medical assistant must keep in mind that his or her expertise and training allow him or her to perform certain tasks, but to not perform other tasks outside his or her scope of practice.

Offices should be prepared for emergencies by having basic supplies available and ready at all times in case such a circumstance arises. Varying by practice specialties, the contents may differ in the emergency supplies and what level of emergency care can be provided.

Most offices will have a crash cart or emergency kit. In many instances, the medical assistant may be asked to keep inventory on these supplies and may be responsible for ordering and restocking them for the office. All staff should be aware where first aid kits and emergency crash carts are located. Any equipment, medication, or supplies need to be monitored and checked carefully on a regular basis so that the item will be available immediately when an emergency occurs.

Following are supplies commonly found in most office emergency kits and/or crash carts:

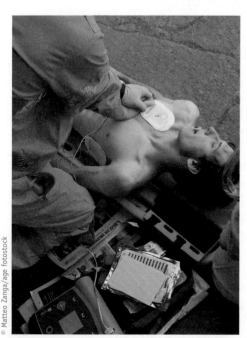

Offices should be prepared for emergencies by having basic supplies available and ready.

© Matteo Zanga/age fotostock

- AED device
- Oxygen tank with flow meter and wrench for opening

- Tubing, nasal cannulas, and adult and pediatric masks
- Ambubag
- Nasal and oral airways in various sizes
- Suction machine
- Spirits of ammonia (aromatic)
- Gloves
- Alcohol wipes
- Betadine wipes
- Penlight
- Tourniquets
- IV supplies, including tubing and needles, fluids (D5W, NS, D10W, and lactated Ringer's solution), butterflies, and angiocaths
- Protective eyeware
- Stethoscope
- Blood-pressure cuff (various sizes)
- Resuscitation masks in various sizes
- Bandages (sterile dressing)
- Adhesive tape
- Bandage scissors
- Ice and heat packages
- Bee-sting kit
- Common medications, including the following:
  - Activated charcoal
  - Atropine
  - Diphenhydramine
  - Epinephrine
  - Furosemide
  - Instant glucose
  - Insulin
  - Lidocaine
  - Nitroglycerine (sublingual)
  - Phenobarbital and diazepam
  - Saline solution
  - Sodium bicarbonate
  - Solu Cortef
  - Aspirin (81mg)

A checklist with the medications should be kept in the emergency cart and contain the name of the medication, the dosage, the amount of vials or syringes to be kept on hand, and their expiration dates. This list should be checked on a monthly basis and replenished when outdated or directly after each emergency use. The supplies on the emergency cart should *never* be borrowed from. A logbook should be kept with the emergency cart for documentation purposes.

As a medical assistant, having the ability to recognize an emergency while remaining calm during care to the patient is very important. You will not help the patient or the patient's family if you become unraveled or show fear during stressful situations. To alleviate this, practice conduct-specific site training procedures based on medi-

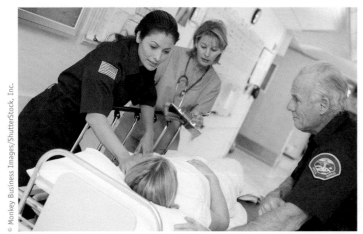

During the care of the patient, a scribe is normally assigned to write down the events of the emergency.

cal, fire, weather, or other types of disasters so that staff and physicians are prepared to move quickly, designate roles, and handle patients safely and securely during an emergency. Staff members who are designated to respond to emergencies in the office must remember their emergency training and any supplies or equipment assigned to their task during an emergency.

Upon learning of and arriving at an emergency, you must first assess the situation. The second step is to call 911 and begin to administer CPR and/or give basic first aid depending on the situation.

The physician or licensed professional will normally lead the emergency care when in office, giving orders and direction. If 911 calls are required, the communication between the office and dispatch is very important so that medical emergency personnel can assess the situation prior to and upon arrival of the scene. Depending on the size of the practice, the receptionist or medical assistant may be assigned to handle any communication and keep patients and emergency personnel apprised of any information. If the patient needs to be transported to a hospital, demographic and medical information will need to be readily available to the squad prior to departure.

During the care of the patient, either without or prior to emergency medical personnel arriving, a scribe is normally assigned to write down the events of the emergency, such as vitals, time/date, medications given, and any other procedures or orders used during the emergency. This will be used as documentation for the provider and will assist any medical care of the patient afterward. While one assistant may be assigned as the scribe, another may have been assigned to bring items such as oxygen and assist with procedures or clinically with the nurse or physician during the emergency. Medical personnel should monitor the patient and watch for any signs of unusual behavior, such as being unable to focus or follow directions.

Not all emergencies will require an ambulance or the hospitalization of the patient (such as a patient fainting after having blood drawn), but there should still be well-defined procedures for such incidents. Overhead paging systems along with telephones strategically placed where patients are regularly located can increase the likelihood of immediate assistance if necessary.

Of course, emergencies can happen in the office, but also in public. As a professional with education and training, how you respond in an emergent situation might make a real difference in someone's life.

Caregiving Obligations and Disease Transmission in Emergency Situations

As a healthcare professional, being properly trained in recognizing emergencies and initially assessing a patient's condition during an emergency is truly an asset to the physician and others in the healthcare team. Even though most emergencies do not normally occur in outpatient facilities, the importance of knowing how to assess, react, and respond is the same.

By applying the basic principles of proper aseptic techniques (infection control) along with taking proper safety measures for the patient and yourself, the medical assistant can improve the likelihood of minimizing disease transmission during emergency caregiving. Proper assessment of the situation is required to make decisions on how to proceed. Emergency situations are very stressful. The medical assistant is expected to assist or perform immediate life-saving care while remaining calm.

Priority should always be given based on injuries that are life threatening or critical threats to the individual. Conditions that involve respiratory, circulatory, cardiac, bleeding, burning, poisoning, or allergic reactions should come above others.

Control of Bleeding in Emergencies

In some instances, there may be severe or uncontrolled bleeding that the medical assistant may need to assist with or monitor for the physician. It is important to understand that there are different sources of blood loss as well as how to apply principles to control it. In any emergency setting where bodily fluids are present, wearing your personal protective equipment (PPE), described shortly, is always highly suggested.

In general terms, the word hemorrhage means there is excessive, uncontrolled bleeding. There are three major types of bleeding that can occur:

- **Arterial bleeding**—With arterial bleeding, bright red blood is produced in spurts. If there is a ruptured artery or large branch, death can occur within the first three minutes. The smaller the artery, the better chance the person has for survival. Large arteries that need immediate attention are the carotid artery, the femoral artery, and most importantly, the aortic artery in the heart. If at all possible, a constriction, such as a tourniquet, should be used to stop the flow of blood in the affected site. Any piece of cloth or rubber may suffice if it is tight enough to stem the flow of blood during an emergency. It is imperative that the patient have emergency care even if you are able to control the bleeding from the artery. You may also need to apply pressure at the point of the wound to stop the flow of blood to that area.
- **Venous bleeding**—Bleeding from a vein produces a steady flow of dark red blood. It is important to control this bleeding as quickly as possible. Cover the wound as much as possible with a clean cloth or pad and apply pressure. You may also need to elevate the area to stop the bleeding.
- **Capillary bleeding**—With bleeding in the capillaries, a steady ooze of blood normally accumulates around the wound area. Sometimes, this bleeding stops without first-aid measures, but it may require additional pressure and time to make it stop.

Nosebleeds (epistaxis) are common among patients who have an injury, have hypertension, have blown the nose too hard, or are taking medication that thins their blood, such as Coumadin or Pradaxa. In the event of a nosebleed, the patient's head should be elevated with the nostrils closed for approximately six minutes. The patient should then be instructed to keep his or her head tilted forward (so that the blood will not drip down the patient's throat) while using an ice pack or a cold compress over the nasal area.

Having **personal protective equipment (PPE)**—gloves, gowns, masks, eye protection, etc.—available at all times for emergencies would be the ultimate goal, although it may not be completely practical. For instance, if you were outside in the public and faced with a situation of an individual experiencing chest pain and more than likely having a heart

What Would You Do?

You are in the supermarket when an individual falls to the ground, clutching his chest. You check for breathing and a pulse, neither of which exist. Do you immediately start to perform CPR even without any PPE devices?

© NorthGeorgiaMedia/ShutterStock, Inc.

attack, you would not withhold CPR or refuse to assist in the procedure of CPR if you did not have a mask available during the emergency. Many healthcare providers carry their own personal PPE equipment for when this type of situation occurs.

Using standard transmission-based precautions during emergency situations will decrease the chances of spreading infectious disease between the healthcare provider and the patient. You should always assume that every patient is potentially infectious. As a healthcare professional, if you are trained to respond and assess emergency situations, *it is your duty to the patient and yourself to be prepared.* You will learn more about these precautions in Chapter 5.

WRAP UP

Chapter Summary

- In the United States, 10 percent of all workers are involved in the field of health care. According to the U.S. Department of Labor, the need for medical assistants will grow approximately 34 percent between the years of 2008 and 2018.

- Medical assistants can perform both administrative and clinical duties, making them one of the most versatile health professionals in the medical field. Advanced medical assistants may seek higher degrees, work in research, teach, or perform other advanced duties such as act as practice managers while exploring different paths in their careers.

- Today's medical assistant has evolved in formal training, education, and accreditation from their origins in the 20th century. Medical assistants must maintain their skills and education by obtaining continuing education credits to keep abreast of changes and advances of medicine after graduation. Medical assistants may practice in the United States without a certification, although it is advantageous to obtain one. There are various accreditation agencies that promote certifications and registries. There is no current license for medical assistants. There are varied educational programs in medical assisting, ranging from diploma programs to a two-year associate's degree in applied science.

- There are many different levels of health professionals working together as a team. Communication needs to be the focus for the team to effectively provide positive outcomes and patient satisfaction.

- The medical assistant should never perform duties outside the scope of his or her training or practice. When tasks are assigned by the physician, "respondeat superior" applies. Even with this, however, the employer is responsible for the employee's actions only if the employee is performing within his or her scope. Performing any duty out of the scope of practice jeopardizes this coverage and may place the medical assistant at risk.

- Ethics refers to a standard of behavior as well as a personal sense of right and wrong above what is considered legal. Physicians and other healthcare professionals should respect and maintain the four basic principles of medical ethics when confronted with a difficult decision.

- Contracts can be expressed or implied. Expressed contracts are in writing, while implied contracts can be when an agreement is made in good faith.

- Three major areas of law that affect medical professionals are medical liability, confidentiality, and consent. These can be greatly improved, increasing the likelihood of avoiding lawsuits by practicing professional communication, performing proper documentation, and following medical standards and guidelines. The Health Insurance Portability and Accountability Act (HIPAA) was a federal act passed in the 1990s to improve the portability of health care from one employer to another, simplify administration of health insurance using standardized formats, protect and improve patients' rights by establishing guidelines and enhancing patients' access to records, among other standards.

- Minimal standards were developed under HIPAA for covered entities as a safeguard to limit the access of patient information to only those who have a need to access information in treatment of the patient, including business associates who work for and alongside covered entities in healthcare operations. A business associate may need protected health information to operate daily business with the covered entity. A business associate agreement ensures that the business associate will adhere to the standards and policies that HIPAA developed and conduct business appropriately.

- New medical discoveries and technologies that advance life complicate medical ethics and the standard of care for healthcare professionals. Human cloning, genetic testing, euthanasia, and physician-assisted suicide are just a few examples of what the medical assistant and his or her team of healthcare professionals may be faced with. Ethical guidelines include standards of set values, principles, and norms of the profession. These essentials enhance and invoke trust, accountability, and mutual respect with a patient-first focus on medical care.

- Professionals are held to a standard of their profession and are responsible for their actions when negligence or damage occurs.

- A law that is passed at the federal level is called an act. At the state and local levels, laws passed through state legislatures and local governments are called ordinances.

- Many laws are based on legal decisions from the past called precedents. A well-known precedent decided by the U.S. Supreme Court in 1973 was *Roe v. Wade*, allowing women the right to abort pregnancy. Criminal laws are crimes against the state of government. Misdemeanors, felonies, and treason are considered crimes against the public, jeopardizing the safety and security of the public. Misdemeanors are crimes that are punishable by imprisonment for less than one year.

- Civil laws do not pertain to criminal behavior, but involve acts against a person, a business, or the government. Most medical lawsuits are civil in nature. When a wrongful act or a civil wrong has occurred, it is referred to as a tort. For a tort to have been committed, four elements must exist: duty of care, breach of duty to perform, injury caused by the breach of duty, and damages that incurred an injury or a loss suffered.

- A patient has the right to refuse medical treatment by the laws of consent. There are two basic types of consent in medicine: implied and informed. Implied consent is based on unwritten consent, usually something such as rolling up a sleeve when the medical assistant explains that the physician has ordered a lab test to be performed. Informed consent is a more formal, written consent, when the patient has the opportunity and understanding to be aware of what is involved with the procedure, consents to the treatment, is advised of risks involved, is aware of expected outcomes, is aware of alternative treatments, and under-

stands the risk if no procedure is performed. Informed consents are signed both by the patient and physician.

- Contracts exist when two or more parties, be they individuals or corporations, meet in agreement. Four elements of a contract must be met in order for it to be valid: An agreement must be met, a consideration must be given (something of value), the contract must contain legal subject matter, and the person in the contract must be capable of understanding all the legal terms and conditions.

- Medical assistants as well as other healthcare professionals in the outpatient setting should be prepared for a medical emergency should it occur in or out of the office. Offices should prepare for emergencies by having basic supplies available and ready at all times in case such a circumstance arises. A crash cart is a way to make emergency supplies, medications, and equipment easily accessible and ready to use immediately when an emergency occurs.

- During an emergency, there may be severe or uncontrolled bleeding that the medical assistant may need to assist with or monitor for the physician. The three major types of bleeding that may need to be controlled are arterial, venous, and capillary. It is important to understand the different sources of blood loss as well as how to apply basic first-aid principles to control it.

- A properly trained health professional who can recognize an emergency and assess the patient's condition is a true asset to the physician and others on the healthcare team. By using and adhering to proper infection control or aseptic techniques, the healthcare professional can reduce the risk of transmission of disease during caregiving emergencies. Although not all emergencies will involve the use of personal protective equipment (PPE), this would be the ultimate goal.

- You should always assume every patient is potentially infectious during emergency care. As a healthcare professional, if you are trained to respond to and assess emergency situations, it is your duty to the patient and yourself to be prepared.

Learning Assessment Questions

1. What type of training do medical assistants receive during their formal education?
   A. Administrative procedures
   B. Clinical procedures
   C. Driving procedures
   D. A and B

2. Which correctly defines accreditation?
   A. Principle that establishes creditability through formal education with a determined standard
   B. Units awarded to medical assistants who attend educational conferences and seminars
   C. A license for a medical assistant
   D. None of the above

3. A phlebotomist is defined as which of the following?
   A. A person who distributes drugs prescribed by a licensed individual
   B. A person who draws bloods
   C. A person who has an advanced degree in medicine
   D. A graduate from a school of nursing

4. A boundary that determines what a medical professional may and may not do based on his or her training, experience, and competency is called what?
   A. Respondeat superior
   B. Scope of practice
   C. Ethics
   D. Moral values

5. A precedent is which of the following?
   A. Law enacted by the federal government
   B. A case that serves as a model for future cases
   C. A rule of protocol
   D. None of the above

6. Which of the following was a Greek physician who is known as the Father of Medicine?
   A. Hippocrates
   B. Percival
   C. Hammurabi
   D. Socrates

7. Bioethics is concerned with which of the following?
   A. Healthcare laws
   B. Etiquette in medical facilities
   C. Ethical implications of biological research and results
   D. None of the above

8. Which of the following are considered members of the healthcare team?
   A. Medical assistants
   B. Pharmacists
   C. Physician assistants
   D. All of the above

9. Which of the following pertains to physicians being legally responsible for the negligent acts of their employees?
   A. Respondeat superior
   B. Good Samaritan laws
   C. Informed consent
   D. Nonmaleficence

10. HIPAA was designed to do which of the following?
    A. Reduce healthcare fraud
    B. Allow for portability of health insurance
    C. Improve accuracy and reliability of shared data
    D. All of the above

11. Which of the following is the complaining party in a court case?
    A. Bailiff
    B. Court clerk
    C. Defendant
    D. Plaintiff

12. Which of the following crimes are punishable by imprisonment in jail for less than one year?
    A. Felonies
    B. Civil crimes
    C. Military crimes
    D. Misdemeanors

13. Which type of law governs certain activities between and among persons, or between persons and the government?
    A. Military
    B. Supremes
    C. Criminal
    D. Civil

14. Which is *not* true of a tort?
    A. It is a civil wrong.
    B. It is committed against a person or property.
    C. It includes a breach of contract.
    D. It may be intentional.

15. Criminal laws do which of the following?
    A. Protect members of society from harmful acts of others
    B. Include both state and federal offenses
    C. Provide for charges to be brought by the government against a person
    D. All of the above

16. Battery involves which of the following?
    A. Publicly damaging another's reputation
    B. The open threat of bodily harm to someone
    C. The action that causes bodily harm
    D. Needless or willful damage or violence

17. A felony is which of the following?
    A. A more serious crime with imprisonment for more than one year
    B. A less serious criminal act with imprisonment for less than one year
    C. A federal violation of the law
    D. None of the above

18. Assault is an example of which of the following?
    A. An intentional tort
    B. An unintentional tort
    C. A breach of contract
    D. Fraud

19. An unintentional tort alleging that a healthcare practitioner has failed to exercise ordinary care is called which of the following?
    A. Negligence
    B. Precedent
    C. Mistaken
    D. Criminal

20. Law may be defined as which of the following?
    A. A moral code
    B. Good manners
    C. Rules of conduct
    D. Rules of behavior

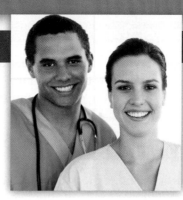

Mathematical Calculations and Conversions

OBJECTIVES

After reading this chapter, you will be able to:

- Identify whole numbers.
- Perform basic calculations using addition and subtraction.
- Perform basic calculations using multiplication and division.
- Set up problems using fractions.
- Compare fractions, express them as decimals, and find common denominators.
- Perform basic mathematical calculations that use fractions and decimals.
- Perform basic mathematical calculations using percentages.

KEY TERMS

Addition	Improper fraction	Percentage
Common denominator	Lowest common	Product
Decimal number	denominator	Proper fraction
Denominator	Mixed number	Quotient
Difference	Multiplication	Ratio
Division	Number	Subtraction
Factor	Numeral	Sum
Fractions	Numerator	Whole numbers

Chapter Overview

This chapter reviews basic mathematical skills needed to perform more complex calculations. Calculations performed in the clinical setting require a basic understanding of addition, subtraction, division, multiplication, fractions, percentages, and decimals.

Numbers

A **number** is a value expressed by a word or symbol that represents a particular quantity. There are different kinds of numbers: whole numbers, fractions, and decimal numbers. Examples of whole numbers include 3, 10, 100, 1,000, 20,000, and 3,000,000. Examples of fractions include ½, ⅗, and ⁷⁄₁₀. Examples of decimals include 0.1, 0.5, and 2.5.

A number is represented by one or more **numerals**.

Whole Numbers

The number system is a base-10 number system. That means it is based on the number 10. Any combination of the 10 digits (0, 1, 2, 3, 4, 5, 6, 7, 8, and 9) can be used to represent whole numbers. **Whole numbers** are counting numbers.

We use whole numbers to count.

Addition and Subtraction

Many calculations involve addition and subtraction. With **addition**, you add or increase the quantity by a given number **FIGURE 2.1**. The **sum** is the amount obtained when adding numbers **TABLE 2.1**. With **subtraction**, you take something away or reduce the quantity by a given number **FIGURE 2.2**. The **difference** is the amount obtained when subtracting numbers **TABLE 2.2**. Addition and subtraction are inverse operations.

Adding 0 to a number does not change the value of the original number. The value of 0 is nothing.
Examples: 0 + 2 = 2; 20 + 0 = 20; 100 + 0 = 100.
© auremar/ShutterStock, Inc.

Subtracting 0 from a number does not change the value of the original number. The value of 0 is nothing.
Examples: 2 – 0 = 2; 20 – 0 = 20; 100 – 0 = 100.
© auremar/ShutterStock, Inc.

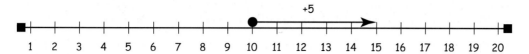

FIGURE 2.1 Using a number line for addition.
© Jones & Bartlett Learning

Table 2.1 Addition Strategy		
Addition Fact	**Example**	**Answer (Sum)**
Plus 0	4 + 0	4
Plus 1	4 + 1	5
Plus 2	4 + 2	6
Plus 3	4 + 3	7
Plus 4	4 + 4	8
Plus 5	4 + 5	9
Plus 6	4 + 6	10
Plus 7	4 + 7	11
Plus 8	4 + 8	12
Plus 9	4 + 9	13
Plus 10	4 + 10	14

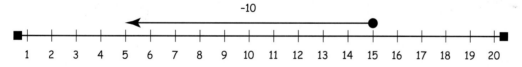

FIGURE 2.2 Using a number line for subtraction.
© Jones & Bartlett Learning

Table 2.2 Subtraction Strategy		
Subtraction Fact	**Example**	**Answer (Difference)**
Minus 0	10 – 0	10
Minus 1	10 – 1	9
Minus 2	10 – 2	8
Minus 3	10 – 3	7
Minus 4	10 – 4	6
Minus 5	10 – 5	5
Minus 6	10 – 6	4
Minus 7	10 – 7	3
Minus 8	10 – 8	2
Minus 9	10 – 9	1
Minus 10	10 – 10	0

Multiplication and Division

Multiplication and **division** are used constantly in performing calculations in the clinical setting. The **product** is the amount obtained by multiplying numbers. The **quotient** is the amount obtained by dividing one number by another number FIGURE 2.3 . TABLE 2.3 shows a multiplication table.

Division and multiplication are inverse operations.

Example: $8 \times 6 = 48$

$48 \div 6 = 8$

$48 \div 8 = 6$

Example: $12 \times 7 = 84$

$84 \div 12 = 7$

$84 \div 7 = 12$

When multiplying numbers, any number multiplied by zero always equals zero.

Example: $2 \times 0 = 0$
Example: $12 \times 0 = 0$
Example: $398 \times 0 = 0$

When dividing numbers, any number divided by one always equals the same number.

Example: $546 \div 1 = 546$
Example: $9 \div 1 = 9$
Example: $89 \div 1 = 89$

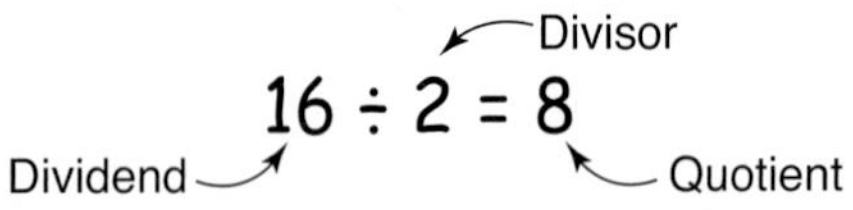

$$16 \div 2 = 8$$

Divisor — (pointing to 2)
Dividend — (pointing to 16)
Quotient — (pointing to 8)

FIGURE 2.3 Dividing with whole numbers.
© Jones & Bartlett Learning

Table 2.3		Multiplication Table										
×	1	2	3	4	5	6	7	8	9	10	11	12
1	1	2	3	4	5	6	7	8	9	10	11	12
2	2	4	6	8	10	12	14	16	18	20	22	24
3	3	6	9	12	15	18	21	24	27	30	33	36
4	4	8	12	16	20	24	28	32	36	40	44	48
5	5	10	15	20	25	30	35	40	45	50	55	60
6	6	12	18	24	30	36	42	48	54	60	66	72
7	7	14	21	28	35	42	49	56	63	70	77	84
8	8	16	24	32	40	48	56	64	72	80	88	96
9	9	18	27	36	45	54	63	72	81	90	99	108
10	10	20	30	40	50	60	70	80	90	100	110	120
11	11	22	33	44	55	66	77	88	99	110	121	132
12	12	24	36	48	60	72	84	96	108	120	132	144

Fractions

Many calculations use values other than whole numbers. Medical assistants work with these values to perform calculations. They must be able to recognize fractions and understand what values they represent.

Fractions express a portion that is a part of a whole number **FIGURE 2.4**. It is a ratio of a part to the whole. A **ratio** is a comparison of two numbers or quantities. The number above the fraction line is called the **numerator**. The number below the fraction line is called the **denominator**. The numerator tells you how many parts of the whole you are expressing and the denominator tells you how many equal parts are in the whole.

Fractions express a quantity or portion that is part of a whole number.

Another way to think about a fraction is by dividing a pie into parts. For example, imagine a pie that has been divided into eight parts or pieces. Each piece of that pie represents a fraction, or ⅛ of the whole pie **FIGURE 2.5**.

A number line can also be used to think about fractions **FIGURE 2.6**.

A **proper fraction** has a value that is always less than 1. The numerator in a proper fraction is always smaller than the denominator. Examples of a proper fraction include ¼, ½, and ¾.

The value of a proper fraction is always less than 1.

An **improper fraction** has a value that is always equal to or greater than 1. The numerator in an improper fraction is always equal to or larger than the denominator. When the numerator and the denominator are the same, the value of the fraction is 1 because any number divided by itself always equals 1. Examples of an improper fraction include ⁴⁄₄, ⁵⁄₃, and ¹¹⁄₉.

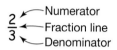

FIGURE 2.4 Defining a fraction.
© Jones & Bartlett Learning

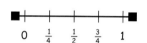

FIGURE 2.6 Using a number line to define a fraction.
© Jones & Bartlett Learning

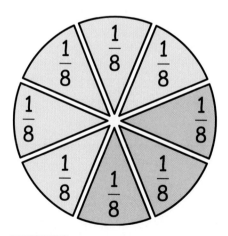

FIGURE 2.5 Using a pie to define a fraction.
© Jones & Bartlett Learning

The numerator is the number above the fraction line. It tells you how many parts of the whole you are expressing.
The denominator is the number below the fraction line. It tells you how many equal parts are in the whole.
© auremar/ShutterStock, Inc.

The value of an improper fraction is always equal to or more than 1.

A **mixed number** has whole numbers and fractions. Examples of mixed numbers include $1\frac{1}{2}$ and $2\frac{3}{4}$.

A mixed number has both whole numbers and fractions.

You can convert a mixed number to an improper fraction by multiplying the denominator by the whole number and adding the numerator to this amount. This amount is then placed over the same denominator **FIGURE 2.7**.

You can rewrite a fraction greater than 1 as a mixed number or as a whole number **FIGURE 2.8**. For example, to write $\frac{7}{3}$ as a mixed number, follow these steps:

1. Divide the numerator by the denominator.
2. Use the remainder to write the fraction part of the quotient.

A fraction in its simplest form is when the numerator and denominator have no common factor other than 1 **FIGURE 2.9**. When you divide the numerator and denominator of a fraction by a common factor until the only common factor is 1, the fraction is then in its simplest form. A **factor** is a number that you multiply by another number, which is also a factor, to make another number. Examples of a fraction in its simplest form include $\frac{3}{4}$, $\frac{1}{2}$, and $\frac{7}{9}$. You can divide the numerator and denominator by common factors until the only common factor remaining is 1.

A fraction is in its simplest form when the numerator and denominator have no common factor other than 1.

Comparing Fractions

Fractions can easily be compared when the denominators are the same. Fractions can also be compared when the denominators are different, as well as when the numerators are the same or different **FIGURE 2.10**.

$$2\frac{3}{4} = \frac{(4 \times 2) + 3}{4} = \frac{11}{4}$$

FIGURE 2.7 Converting a mixed number to an improper fraction.
© Jones & Bartlett Learning

$$\frac{7}{3} = \frac{(7 \div 3)}{3} = 2\frac{1}{3}$$

3 goes into 7 two times with a remainder of 1.

Use the remainder to write the fraction part of the quotient.

FIGURE 2.8 Converting an improper fraction to a mixed number.
© Jones & Bartlett Learning

$$\frac{6}{18} = \frac{6 \div 6}{18 \div 6} = \frac{1}{3}$$

FIGURE 2.9 Reducing a fraction.
© Jones & Bartlett Learning

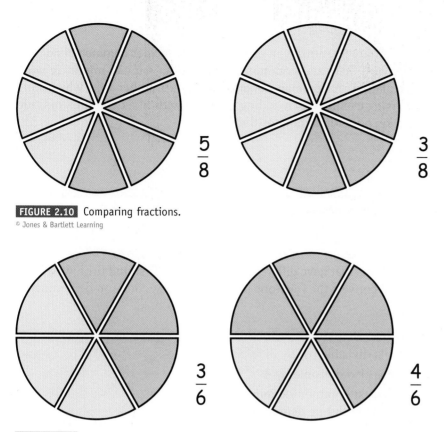

FIGURE 2.10 Comparing fractions.
© Jones & Bartlett Learning

$\frac{5}{8}$

$\frac{3}{8}$

FIGURE 2.11 Comparing fractions with the same denominator.
© Jones & Bartlett Learning

$\frac{3}{6}$

$\frac{4}{6}$

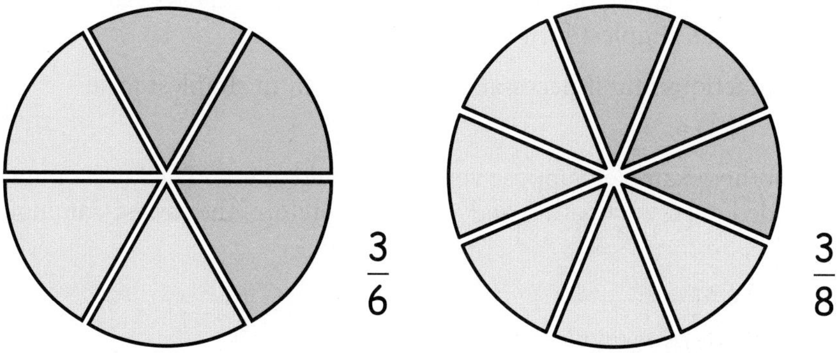

FIGURE 2.12 Comparing fractions with the same numerator. The fraction with the smaller denominator has the larger value.
© Jones & Bartlett Learning

$\frac{3}{6}$

$\frac{3}{8}$

Fractions With Like Denominators

When two fractions have the same denominator, the fraction with the smaller numerator has the smaller value FIGURE 2.11. Comparing fractions with the same denominator is similar to comparing whole numbers. If the denominator is the same, the smaller the numerator, the smaller the value.

> When two fractions have the same denominator, the fraction with the larger numerator has the larger value.

When two fractions have the same numerator, the fraction with the smaller denominator has the larger value FIGURE 2.12.

Adding and Subtracting Fractions

When you add and subtract fractions, you need to find the **lowest common denominator**. By finding the lowest or (least) common denominator, you can minimize work at the end of a calculation. A **common denominator** is a number into which both denominators can divide evenly. When adding fractions with like denominators, add the numerators and keep the denominator the same.

Example: $\frac{1}{6} + \frac{2}{6} = \frac{3}{6}$
Example: $\frac{1}{7} + \frac{3}{7} = \frac{4}{7}$

> When adding fractions with like denominators, add the numerators and keep the denominator the same.

When adding fractions that have different denominators, first find the lowest common denominator and convert the fractions using this lowest common denominator.

Example: $\frac{1}{2} + \frac{1}{4}$
Step 1: Find the lowest common denominator:
4 is divisible by 2
4 is also divisible by 4
Lowest common denominator→ 4
Rewrite the fractions with like denominators.
$\frac{1}{2} \rightarrow \frac{1}{2} \times \frac{2}{2} = \frac{2}{4}$
$\frac{1}{4} \rightarrow \frac{1}{4} \times \frac{1}{1} = \frac{1}{4}$

Next, add the numerators, placing the sum over the denominator. If necessary, reduce the resulting fraction to its simplest form.

Step 2: Add the fractions and if necessary, write the sum in simplest form.
Answer: $\frac{2}{4} + \frac{1}{4} = \frac{3}{4}$

Now, let's try another example. Suppose you want to add $\frac{1}{3} + \frac{2}{5}$. The lowest number that can be divided evenly by both 3 and 5 is 15. Therefore, the lowest common denominator is 15.

Example: $\frac{1}{3} + \frac{2}{5}$
Step 1: Rewrite the fractions with like denominators.
$\frac{1}{3} \rightarrow \frac{1}{3} \times \frac{5}{5} = \frac{5}{15}$
$\frac{2}{5} \rightarrow \frac{2}{5} \times \frac{3}{3} = \frac{6}{15}$

Step 2: Add the fractions and if necessary, write the sum in simplest form.

Answer: $\frac{5}{15} + \frac{6}{15} = \frac{11}{15}$

> When adding fractions with different denominators, find the lowest common denominator first.

When subtracting fractions that have the same denominator, subtract the numerators and keep the denominator the same.

Example: $\frac{7}{9} - \frac{2}{9} = \frac{5}{9}$
Example: $\frac{4}{5} - \frac{2}{5} = \frac{2}{5}$

When subtracting fractions that have the same denominator, subtract the numerators and keep the denominator the same.

To subtract fractions with different denominators, you must first find the lowest common denominator. For example, suppose you want to subtract $\frac{7}{8} - \frac{2}{4}$. The lowest number that can be divided evenly by both 8 and 4 is 8. Therefore, the lowest common denominator is 8.

When subtracting fractions that have different denominators, first find the lowest common denominator and convert the fractions using this lowest common denominator.

Example: $\frac{7}{8} - \frac{2}{4}$

Step 1: Rewrite the fractions with like denominators.

$$\frac{7}{8} \rightarrow \frac{7}{8} \times \frac{1}{1} = \frac{7}{8}$$
$$\frac{2}{4} \rightarrow \frac{2}{4} \times \frac{2}{2} = \frac{4}{8}$$

Next, subtract the numerators, placing the difference over the denominator. If necessary, reduce the resulting fraction to its simplest form.

Step 2: Subtract the fractions and if necessary, write the sum in simplest form.

Answer: $\frac{7}{8} - \frac{4}{8} = \frac{3}{8}$

Multiplying and Dividing Fractions

It is important to understand the mathematical concepts used in multiplying and dividing fractions. Many calculations will require the medical assistant to calculate the amount of a drug or dosage needed using multiplication and division with fractions.

To multiply fractions, simply multiply the numerators of each fraction and the denominators of each fraction.

Example: $\frac{3}{4} \times \frac{1}{2}$

$$3 \times 1 = 3$$
$$4 \times 2 = 8$$

Answer: $\frac{3}{8}$

When multiplying fractions, first convert any mixed numbers into improper fractions. Then multiply the numerators of each fraction and the denominators of each fraction. Always remember to reduce the resulting fraction to its simplest form.

Example: $1\frac{1}{2} \times \frac{3}{5}$

Step 1: Convert the mixed number into an improper fraction.

$$1\frac{1}{2} = \frac{2}{2} + \frac{1}{2}$$

Add the numerators: $2 + 1 = 3$

$$\frac{2}{2} + \frac{1}{2} = \frac{3}{2}$$

When subtracting fractions that have different denominators, first find the lowest common denominator. Suppose you want to subtract $\frac{15}{16} - \frac{3}{8}$. First, find the lowest number that all denominators divide evenly into. For the numbers 8 and 16, the lowest number is 16. Therefore, the lowest common denominator is 16.

Step 2: Multiply the numerators and multiply the denominators. If necessary, write the product in simplest form.

$$3/2 \times 3/5$$
$$3 \times 3 = 9$$
$$2 \times 5 = 10$$

Answer: $9/10$

To divide fractions, first convert any mixed numbers into improper fractions. Then invert or reverse the numbers of the second fraction (this is referred to as a reciprocal) in the equation. Next, multiply the numerators of each fraction and the denominators of each fraction and reduce the resulting equation to its simplest form, if needed. This is known as "invert and multiply."

Example: $1/3 \div 1/7$

Step 1: Multiply the dividend by the reciprocal of the divisor.

$$1/3 \times 7/1$$
$$1/3 \times 7 = 7/3$$

Step 2: Write the product in simplest form.

Answer: $7/3$, which simplifies to $2\frac{1}{3}$ **FIGURE 2.13**

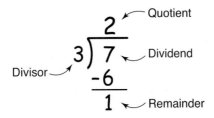

FIGURE 2.13 Reducing a fraction to its simplest form.
© Jones & Bartlett Learning

Decimals

Decimal numbers are numbers that are written using place value. The decimal system includes 10 numerals (0, 1, 2, 3, 4, 5, 6, 7, 8, and 9). Using these numerals, you can express values of all kinds using a decimal point. The decimal point, which looks like a period, is the center of the decimal system. Any value can be expressed using a combination of these numerals. Numbers to the left of the decimal point indicate whole numbers, and numbers to the right indicate fractions of a whole. The value of a number increases by a multiple of 10 each time it moves one space to the left. The value of a number decreases by a multiple of 10 each time it moves one space to the right **FIGURE 2.14**.

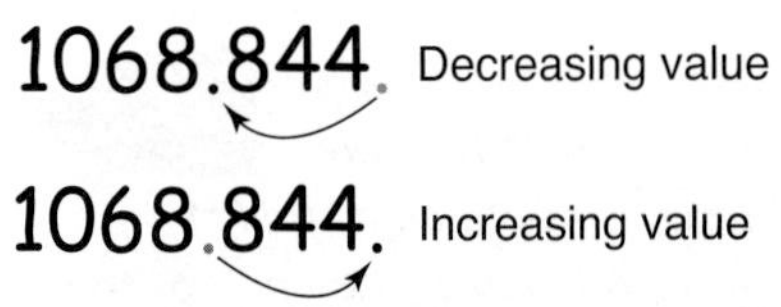

1068.844. Decreasing value

1068.844. Increasing value

FIGURE 2.14 Whole numbers and decimals.
© Jones & Bartlett Learning

Value	Ten-thousands	Thousands	Hundreds	Tens	Ones	Decimal Point	Tenths	Hundredths	Thousandths	Ten-thousandths
Table 2.4 Decimal System Notation										
Sample number	9	8	7	6	5	.	4	3	2	1

The decimal system is depicted in **TABLE 2.4**. In this case, the number 98,765.4321 is used to demonstrate decimal-system notation.

The total value of a number expressed by the decimal system is the sum of all its digits according to their place value. Therefore, the sample number, 98,765.4321 is equal to the following:

- 90,000.0000 (9 ten-thousands)
- +08,000.0000 (8 thousands)
- +00700.0000 (7 hundreds)
- +00060.0000 (6 tens)
- +00,005.0000 (5 ones)
- +00000.4000 (4 tenths)
- +00000.0300 (3 hundredths)
- +00000.0020 (2 thousandths)
- +00000.0001 (1 ten-thousandths)

When using the decimal system to express a number less than 1, a leading zero (0) is placed to the left of the decimal point. Trailing zeros, or zeros that are placed to the right of the final digit, are not used during practice, unless the zero is considered significant to the dose or calculation. Examples of trailing zeros include the zeros in 1.790, 2.80, 3.0, and 49.10. Many medication errors have been caused by the confusion of using trailing zeros. For example, 0.399 rounded to the nearest hundredth is 0.40 (written with a trailing zero). These techniques can help eliminate errors when reading decimals.

There are many ways to write the same decimal, as shown in **TABLE 2.5**.

Adding and Subtracting Decimals

When adding and subtracting decimals, the numbers should be placed in columns so that the decimal points are all aligned.

Table 2.5	Different Ways to Express a Decimal
Form	**Example**
Standard	32.67
Word	Thirty-two and sixty-seven hundredths
Expanded	$(3 \times 10) + (2 \times 1) + (6 \times 0.1) + (7 \times 0.01)$

Example: 4.7
              2.32
            +1.789
            ‾‾‾‾‾‾
              8.809

Align the decimal points before adding and subtracting decimal numbers.

Multiplying Decimals

When multiplying decimals, first multiply them as whole numbers, and then move the decimal the total number of places that were in the two numbers being multiplied, as shown in **FIGURE 2.15**. For example, to multiply 29.24×43.67, you first multiply $2924 \times 4367 = 12{,}769{,}108$.

There is an implied decimal point for all whole numbers, which is placed at the end of the last digit in the number. For example, the whole number 29 is also the same as 29.0, with the decimal point and zero being the implied decimal. Thus, when multiplying decimals, the starting point for moving the decimal begins with the implied decimal point at the end of the whole number.

For example, the product of 29.24×43.67 is $12{,}769{,}108$ (before we move the decimal point). The implied decimal point is $12{,}769{,}108.0$.

The movement of the decimal point begins after the number 8 in the ones digit place.

Next, count from right to left four decimal places (because there are four total decimal places in 29.24 and 43.67) and put the decimal point there: $1{,}276.9108$ **FIGURE 2.16**.

Multiply the decimals as whole numbers first and then move the decimal over the total number of places.

Dividing Decimals

When dividing decimals, first change each decimal to a whole number by multiplying each number by the same factor of 10. Then proceed with the division operation.

Example: $1.97 \div 2.2$
Step 1: Multiply $1.97 \times 100 = 197$
Step 2: Multiply $2.2 \times 100 = 220$
Step 3: Divide $197 \div 220$
Answer: $197 \div 220 = 0.895$

Change each decimal to a whole number by multiplying each number by the same factor of 10 before dividing decimals.

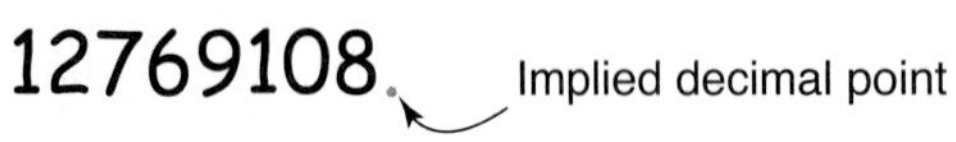

12769108. Implied decimal point

FIGURE 2.15 Implied decimal point.

1276.9108.

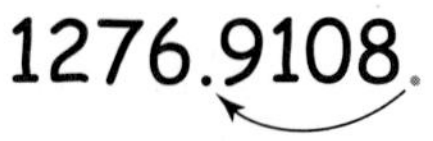

FIGURE 2.16 Moving decimals.

Percentages

A **percentage** is represented by the % symbol and is used to express a value that is part of 100. It represents the same number as a fraction whose denominator is 100.

Example: $0.9\% = {}^{0.9}\!/_{100}$

Example: $5\% = {}^{5}\!/_{100}$

Example: $10\% = {}^{10}\!/_{100}$

When converting decimals to percentages, simply move the decimal point over two places to the right.

Example: Write ¼ as a percent.

Step 1: To write ¼ as a percent, first find the equivalent fraction with a denominator of 100.

$${}^{1}\!/_{4} = {}^{?}\!/_{100}$$
$${}^{1}\!/_{4} \times {}^{25}\!/_{25} = {}^{25}\!/_{100}$$

Answer: ¼ = 25%

Example: Write ⅖ as a percent.

Step 1: To write ⅖ as a percent, first find the equivalent fraction with a denominator of 100.

$${}^{2}\!/_{5} \times {}^{20}\!/_{20} = {}^{40}\!/_{100}$$

Answer: ⅖ = 40%

Math Practice

Question: What is the sum of 179 + 216?

Answer: 395

Question: What is the sum of 47 + 85?

Answer: 132

Question: What is the difference of 198 – 63?

Answer: 135

Question: What is the difference of 278 – 129?

Answer: 149

Question: What is 7 × 6?

Answer: 42

Question: What is 14 × 13?

Answer: 182

Question: **What is 88 ÷ 11?**

Answer: 8

Question: **What is 156 ÷ 13?**

Answer: 12

Question: **What type of fraction is $\frac{9}{7}$?**

Answer: Improper fraction

Question: **What type of fraction is $\frac{3}{5}$?**

Answer: Proper fraction

Question: **What type of fraction is $1\frac{1}{2}$?**

Answer: Mixed number

Question: **What is the simplest form of the fraction $\frac{30}{60}$?**

Answer: $\frac{30}{60} \div \frac{30}{30} = \frac{1}{2}$

Question: **What is the simplest form of the fraction $\frac{12}{16}$?**

Answer: $\frac{12}{16} \div \frac{4}{4} = \frac{3}{4}$

Question: **What is the sum of $\frac{1}{5} + \frac{2}{5}$?**

Answer: $\frac{3}{5}$

Question: **What is the sum of $\frac{3}{8} + \frac{2}{8}$?**

Answer: $\frac{5}{8}$

Question: **What is the sum of $\frac{1}{5} + \frac{1}{10}$?**

Answer:

Step 1: To obtain the sum, first determine the lowest common denominator: $\frac{1}{5} \times \frac{2}{2} = \frac{2}{10}$ and $\frac{1}{10} \times \frac{1}{1} = \frac{1}{10}$

Step 2: Complete the addition operation: $\frac{2}{10} + \frac{1}{10} = \frac{3}{10}$

Question: **What is the sum of $\frac{2}{3} + \frac{2}{7}$?**

Answer:

Step 1: To obtain the sum, first determine the lowest common denominator: $\frac{2}{3} \times \frac{7}{7} = \frac{14}{21}$ and $\frac{2}{7} \times \frac{3}{3} = \frac{6}{21}$

Step 2: Complete the addition operation: $\frac{14}{21} + \frac{6}{21} = \frac{20}{21}$

Question: **What is the difference of $\frac{9}{12}$ – $\frac{2}{12}$?**

Answer: $\frac{7}{12}$

Question: **What is the difference of $\frac{9}{10}$ – $\frac{2}{10}$?**

Answer: $\frac{7}{10}$

Question: **What is the difference of $\frac{11}{12}$ – $\frac{2}{6}$?**

Answer:

Step 1: To obtain the difference, first determine the lowest common denominator: $\frac{11}{12} \times \frac{1}{1}$ = $\frac{11}{12}$ and $\frac{2}{6} \times \frac{2}{2} = \frac{4}{12}$

Step 2: Complete the subtraction operation: $\frac{11}{12}$ – $\frac{4}{12} = \frac{7}{12}$

Question: **What is the product of $\frac{2}{3} \times \frac{3}{5}$?**

Answer: $\frac{6}{15}$

Question: **What is the product of $\frac{3}{5} \times \frac{4}{6}$?**

Answer: $\frac{12}{30}$, which simplifies to $\frac{2}{5}$

Question: **What is the quotient of $\frac{4}{7} \div \frac{2}{7}$?**

Answer: $\frac{28}{14}$, which simplifies to 2

Question: **What is the quotient of $\frac{5}{8} \div \frac{3}{4}$?**

Answer: $\frac{20}{24}$, which simplifies to $\frac{5}{6}$

Question: **What is the value of the digit 7 in 982.357?**

Answer: The digit 7 is in the thousandths place. It has a value of 0.007, or 7 thousandths

---

Question: **What is the value of the digit 4 in 983.345?**

Answer: The digit 4 is in the hundredths place. It has a value of 0.04, or 4 hundredths

---

Question: **What is the sum of 3.6 + 2.35 + 2.69?**

Answer: 8.64

Question: **What is the sum of 2.45 + 1.98 + 34.678?**

Answer: 39.108

Question: **What is the difference of 9.68 – 2.69?**

Answer: 6.99

Question: **What is the quotient of 8.8 ÷ 4.4?**

Answer:

Step 1: To determine the quotient, first multiply the dividend (the first number) by 10: 8.8 × 10 = 88

Step 2: Multiply the divisor (the second number) by 10: 4.4 × 10 = 44

Step 3: Solve the problem: 88 ÷ 44 = 2

$$44\overline{)88}\;\;^{2}$$

Question: **What is the quotient of 6.4 ÷ 0.8?**

Answer:

Step 1: To determine the quotient, first multiply the dividend (the first number) by 10: 6.4 × 10 = 64

Step 2: Multiply the divisor (the second number) by 10: 0.8 × 10 = 8

Step 3: Solve the problem: 64 ÷ 8 = 8

$$8\overline{)64}\;\;^{8}$$

Question: **How do you write $\frac{5}{20}$ as a percent?**

Answer:

Step 1: To write $\frac{5}{20}$ as a percent, first find the equivalent fraction with a denominator of 100: $\frac{5}{20} \times \frac{5}{5} = [5 \times 5] \div [20 \times 5] = \frac{25}{100}$

Step 2: $\frac{25}{100} = 25\%$

Question: **How do you write $\frac{1}{10}$ as a percent?**

Answer:

Step 1: To write $\frac{1}{10}$ as a percent, first find the equivalent fraction with a denominator of 100: $\frac{1}{10} \times \frac{10}{10} = [1 \times 10] \div [10 \times 10] = \frac{10}{100}$

Step 2: $\frac{10}{100} = 10\%$

WRAP UP

Chapter Summary

- Numbers can be represented as whole numbers, fractions, and decimals.
- Each type of number can be used in addition, subtraction, multiplication, and division.
- Addition and subtraction involve adding numbers to each other or taking numbers away from each other, respectively.
- Multiplication involves changing the quantity of a number by multiplying a number by another number.
- Division involves changing the quantity of a number to determine a part or portion of a quantity needed.
- Fractions are used to express a portion that is a part of a whole number. A fraction is a ratio of a part to the whole. The numerator is the number above the fraction line, whereas the denominator is the number below the fraction line. The denominator tells you how many equal parts are in the whole or set. The numerator tells you the number of those parts you are expressing.
- Decimals are numbers that are written using place value. Any fraction can be expressed as a decimal.
- Percentages are used to express the number of parts of 100. A percentage represents the same number as a fraction whose denominator is 100, and is denoted by the % symbol.

- Fractions, decimals, and percentages can be converted to each other and used in addition, subtraction, multiplication, and division operations.
- When adding fractions, if needed, first convert the fractions to the lowest common denominator. Then add the numerators, placing the sum over the denominator. Finally, reduce the resulting fraction to its simplest form.
- When subtracting fractions, if needed, first convert the fractions to the lowest common denominator. Next, subtract the numerators, placing the difference over the denominator. Finally, reduce the resulting fraction to its simplest form.
- When multiplying fractions, if needed, first convert any mixed numbers into improper fractions. Next, multiply the numerators of each fraction and the denominators of each fraction. Finally, reduce the resulting fraction to its simplest form.
- When dividing fractions, first convert any mixed numbers into improper fractions. Next, find the reciprocal of the divisor (the second fraction). Then, multiply the first number by the reciprocal. Finally, reduce the resulting fraction to its simplest form.

Learning Assessment Questions

1. Which of the following fractions has the greatest value?
   A. $\frac{1}{2}$
   B. $1\frac{1}{2}$
   C. $\frac{6}{9}$
   D. $\frac{3}{8}$

2. What is a fraction with a value of less than 1 called?
   A. Proper fraction
   B. Mixed fraction
   C. Whole number
   D. Improper fraction

3. What is a fraction with a value greater than 1 called?
   A. Proper fraction
   B. Mixed fraction
   C. Whole number
   D. Improper fraction

4. What is $\frac{5}{15}$, simplified to its final form?
   A. $\frac{1}{2}$
   B. $\frac{2}{3}$
   C. $\frac{1}{3}$
   D. $\frac{3}{4}$

5. What is the sum of 212 + 14?
   A. 206
   B. 226
   C. 198
   D. 244

6. What is the difference of 18.6 − 14.8?
   A. 8.3
   B. 2.6
   C. 3.4
   D. 3.8

7. What is the value of the digit 6 in 2,679,325?
   A. 600,000
   B. 6,000
   C. 60
   D. 6

8. What is the value of the digit 2 in 987.632?
   A. 0.2
   B. 0.02
   C. 2
   D. 0.002

9. A percentage represents the same number as a fraction whose denominator is which of the following?
   A. 10
   B. 100
   C. 50
   D. 1,000

10. What is the value of the digit 3 in the number 3725.89?
    A. 30
    B. 300
    C. 3,000
    D. 3

11. Convert 0.7 to a fraction.
    A. $\frac{3}{7}$
    B. $\frac{2}{7}$
    C. $\frac{7}{100}$
    D. $\frac{7}{10}$

12. $\frac{2}{5}$ is the same as what percent?
    A. 40 percent
    B. 50 percent
    C. 60 percent
    D. 15 percent

13. What is the product of 8 × 6?
    A. 54
    B. 48
    C. 56
    D. 42

14. $\frac{16}{20}$ is the same as what percent?
    A. 60 percent
    B. 40 percent
    C. 80 percent
    D. 25 percent

15. What is the difference between 26.7 − 14.8?
    A. 11.9
    B. 11.7
    C. 12.1
    D. 11.8

16. What is the sum of 685 + 0?
    A. 0
    B. 658
    C. 685
    D. 865

17. What is the quotient of 6735 ÷ 1?
    A. 0
    B. 6735
    C. 6375
    D. 6573

18. What is the product of 0.65 × 3.1?
    A. 2.15
    B. 2.51
    C. 2.105
    D. 2.015

19. Convert 0.30 to a fraction.
    A. $\frac{30}{10}$
    B. $\frac{3}{10}$
    C. $\frac{10}{3}$
    D. $\frac{3}{5}$

20. $\frac{8}{10}$ is the same as what percent?

    A. 800 percent

    B. 80 percent

    C. 8 percent

    D. 85 percent

21. A physician asks his medical assistant to give a patient $\frac{1}{4}$ of a 12 oz bottle of milk of magnesia. How many ounces should this patient receive?

    A. 2 oz

    B. 3 oz

    C. 4 oz

    D. 6 oz

22. A physician gives his medical assistant a 1mL vial of solution and asks him to prepare an injection using $\frac{1}{4}$ of the solution in the vial. How much solution should the medical assistant draw into the syringe?

    A. 0.33mL

    B. 0.2mL

    C. 0.25mL

    D. 0.4mL

23. A patient receives $4\frac{1}{8}$ ounces of a nutritional supplement in the morning and $3\frac{1}{4}$ ounces of nutritional supplement in the evening. How many ounces does this patient receive in one day?

    A. $5\frac{3}{8}$

    B. $7\frac{3}{8}$

    C. $6\frac{4}{8}$

    D. $7\frac{1}{8}$

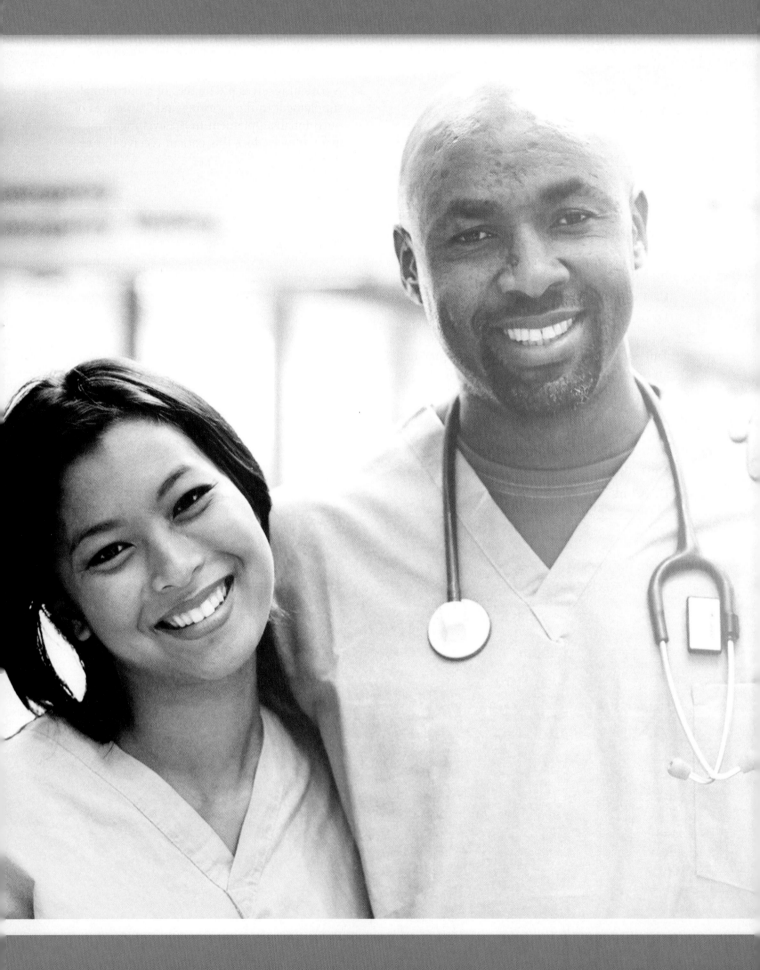

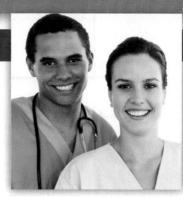

Introduction to Medical Terminology

OBJECTIVES

After reading this chapter, you will be able to:

- Identify word parts and their roles in the formation of medical terms.
- Apply word-part knowledge to new medical terms.
- Identify prefixes, suffixes, word roots, and combining forms.
- Identify medical terms and how to define and spell them.
- Define the process used to identify and locate medical terms in a dictionary.
- Define basic anatomy and physiology and know how to use anatomic reference systems to identify the anatomic position, body planes, directions, and cavities.
- Identify the abdominal cavity and peritoneum and how to recognize, define, and spell related terms.
- Recognize the structure and function of the human body and recognize, define, and spell related terms.
- Discuss body systems, the organs that make up these systems, and their functions.

KEY TERMS

Adrenal glands
Anatomic position
Anatomy
Anterior (ventral)
Antibody
Antigen

Axial plane (transverse plane)
Cardiac cycle
Cardiac muscle
Cardiovascular system
Cartilaginous joints

Cell
Central nervous system (CNS)
Cilia
Combining form
Conjunctiva

Cornea	Joint	Reproductive system
Coronal plane (frontal plane)	Keratin	Respiratory system
Dermis	Lateral	Retina
Diastole	Medial	Sagittal plane (lateral plane)
Distal	Median plane	Sclera
Endocardium	Meninges	Sebaceous glands
Endocrine system	Musculoskeletal system	Sebum
Epicardium	Myocardium	Septum
Epidermis	Orbit	Skeletal muscle
Extensor	Ovaries	Smooth muscle
Fibrous joint	Pancreas	Subcutaneous tissue
Flexor	Parathyroid gland	Suffix
Gastrointestinal (GI) system	Pathophysiology	Superior (cranial)
Homeostasis	Pericardium	Sweat glands
Hormone	Peripheral nervous system (PNS)	Synovial joints
Hypodermis	Physiology	Systole
Hypothalamus	Pineal body	Target
Immune system	Pituitary gland	Tendon
Inferior (caudal)	Posterior (dorsal)	Testes
Integumentary system	Prefix	Thyroid gland
Iris	Proximal	Word root
	Renal system	

Chapter Overview

This chapter covers the basics of medical terminology. A description of the segments of medical terms along with terms associated with anatomy, physiology, body systems, and diseases are covered.

Medical Terminology

One aspect of working with patients is the ability to understand medical terminology. As a medical assistant, you must have a strong working knowledge of medical terminology. You must be able to define and build medical terms and apply these terms when working with patients and other healthcare professionals. These terms serve as a universal language that all medical doctors, nurses, pharmacists, medical assistants, and other medical personnel can understand.

Most medical terms are derived from the Greek and Latin languages. Other cultures have also influenced medical terminology, but the Greek and Latin languages have had the greatest impact on medical language. Medical terms consist of segments or word parts. In combination, they describe all conditions and anatomy.

It is important to know the fundamentals of how medical terminology applies to various conditions. Terms fit together like a lock and key. Medical terms are formed with one or more of the following word parts:

- **The prefix**—This is placed before the combining form.
- **The suffix**—This is placed after the combining form.

- **The word root**—This is the foundation of the word that identifies the structure or anatomy being described. The suffix or prefix is added to the word root.
- **The combining form**—This is the word that results when the prefix, suffix, and word root are combined. Note: If the combining form has two vowels and the suffix begins with a vowel, drop the o.

Medical terminology is a universal language that all medical personnel understand.
© auremar/ShutterStock, Inc.

Here's an example of how a word is formed:

- **Prefix**—peri (around)
- **Word root**—cardia (heart)
- **Combining form**—cardi/o
- **Suffix**—itis (inflammation)

Now read the term from left to right, putting the segments together. The result is pericarditis, which means inflammation around the heart **FIGURE 3.1**.

A medical term may contain up to four word parts: the prefix, word root, combining form, and suffix.

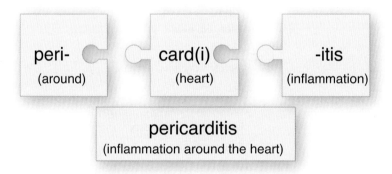

peri-
(around)

card(i)
(heart)

-itis
(inflammation)

pericarditis
(inflammation around the heart)

FIGURE 3.1 Many medical terms contain a prefix, a word root, and a suffix that result in a combining form.
© Jones & Bartlett Learning

Prefixes

A **prefix** is a word part that is found at the beginning of the medical term. It modifies the word root. It often indicates location, presence or absence, size, frequency, quantity, or position. Not every word will contain a prefix.

The prefix of a medical term often indicates location, presence or absence, size, frequency, quantity, or position.
© auremar/ShutterStock, Inc.

Not every word will contain a prefix.

When a prefix is separated from the term, it is usually followed by a hyphen. Prefixes are generally not altered when added to a word root or combining form. A basic rule is that if the combining form or word root begins with a vowel, you select the applicable prefix that ends in a consonant. Common prefixes are listed in **TABLE 3.1**.

Table 3.1 Common Prefixes	
Prefix	**Meaning**
a-, an-	Without
ante-, pre-, pro-	Before
anti-, contra-	Against
bi-, diplo-	Two
brady-	Slow
circum-	Around
de-	Away from
dia-, trans-	Through
dys-	Bad, difficult, painful
ecto-	Outside
end-, endo-	Within
epi-	Upon, on, over
eu-	Normal
ex-, exo-, extra-	Out of, away from, outside
hemi-, semi-	Half
hyper-, supra-	Above, elevated
hypo-, sub-	Below, slow, underneath
inter-	Between
intra-	Within
isch-	To hold back, suppress
iso-	Same
lipid-	Fat
mal-	Bad
megalo-, mega-, macro-	Large, big
micro-	Small
mono-	One
multi-, pluri-	Many
oligo-	Scant, few
oxy-	Rapid, sharp
pan-	All
peri-	Around, surrounding
poly-	Many
post-	After, following
pre-	Before
quadra-, quadri-	Four

Table 3.1 Common Prefixes (Continued)	
Prefix	**Meaning**
re-	Again
sub-	Below
super-, supr-	Above, superior
tachy-	Fast, rapid
tetra-	Four
ultra-	Beyond
uni-	Single

Suffixes

A **suffix** is a word part that is found at the end of the medical term. It completes the word root. It often indicates a procedure, disease, condition, or disorder. Some suffixes are also words that stand alone but when attached to a word root provide more specificity. When a suffix is separated from the term, it begins with a hyphen followed by the suffix. Common suffixes are listed in TABLE 3.2 .

> *The suffix of a medical term often indicates a procedure, disease, condition, or disorder.*
> © auremar/ShutterStock, Inc.

Table 3.2 Common Suffixes	
Suffix	**Meaning**
-ac, - al, -ar, -ary	Pertaining to
-ad	Toward
-algia, -dynia	Pain
-ase	Enzyme
-asthenia	Weakness
-blast	Immature
-cele	Hernia
-cide, -cidal	Killing, destroying
-crine	To secrete
-cyte	Cell
-derma	Skin
-eal, -ia, -ic, -ory, -ous, -tic	Condition of
-ectasia, -ectasis	Stretching, dilating
-ectomy	Surgical removal
-edema	Swelling, fluid accumulation
-ema, -iasis, -ism, -lepsy, -osis	Condition, abnormal condition
-emesis	Vomiting
-emia	Blood
-esthesia	Feeling, sensation
-gen, -genesis, -genic	Production or formation of
-globulin, -globin	Protein

(Continues)

Table 3.2 Common Suffixes (Continued)	
Suffix	**Meaning**
-gram	Recording
-graph	Instrument used to record
-graphy	Process of recording
-ic	Pertaining to
-itis	Inflammation
-kinesia, -kinesis	Movement
-lithiasis	Presence of stones
-logist	One who studies
-logy	The study of
-lysis, -lytic	Destruction
-malacia	Softening
-manic, -mania	Abnormal preoccupation or obsession
-megaly	Enlargement
-meter	Measuring device
-necrosis	Tissue death
-oid	Resembling
-oma	Tumor
-opia	Vision
-ose	Sugar
-ostomy	Formation of a new opening
-para, -parous	Bearing, producing a child
-pathy	Disease
-penia	Deficiency
-pepsia	Digestion
-phage, -phagy	To eat or digest
-phasia	Speaking
-phil, -philia	To love
-phobia	Abnormal fear
-phonia	Sound
-phrenia, -phrenic	Mind
-plasty	Surgical repair
-plegia, -plegic	Paralysis
-pnea	Breathing
-poiesis	Formation
-ptosis	Drooping
-rrhage, -rrhagia	Heavy discharge
-rrhea	Discharge, flowing
-scope, -scopy	Instrument, process of using the instrument
-sclerosis	Hardening
-somnia	Sleep
-stasis	Stopping
-stenosis	Narrowing

Table 3.2 Common Suffixes (Continued)	
Suffix	**Meaning**
-stomy	Opening
-tome	Instrument for cutting
-tomy	Process of cutting
-trophy, -trophic	Nutrition
-uresis	Urination
-uria	Urine
-version	Turning

Word Roots and Combining Forms

A **word root** usually identifies a structure or anatomy and is the foundation of the word to which the suffix or prefix is added. Word roots can also indicate color. A **combining form** is a word root that has a vowel added to the end to help connecting suffixes or other word roots and combining forms. Most often, the combing form ends in the vowel a, o, or i. Some common word roots and combining forms are listed in TABLE 3.3 .

Making flashcards is a good way to learn prefixes, suffixes, word roots, and combining forms and their meanings.

Table 3.3 Common Word Roots and Combining Forms		
Combining Form	**Word Root**	**Meaning**
Colors		
cyan/o	cyan	Blue
leuk/o	leuk	White
melan/o	melan	Black
rub/o	rub	Red
Cardiovascular System		
aort/o	aort	Aorta
angi/o, vas/o	angi, vas	Blood vessel
arteri/o	arteri	Artery
ather/o	ather	Fatty plaque
capill/o	capill	Capillary
cardi/o	cardi	Heart
erythr/o	erythr	Red
hem/o, hemat/o	hem, hemat	Blood
lymph/o	lymph	Lymph
phleb/o, ven/o	phleb, ven	Vein
thromb/o	thromb	Clot
Gastrointestinal System		
an/o	an	Anus

(Continues)

Table 3.3   Common Word Roots and Combining Forms (Continued)

Combining Form	Word Root	Meaning
append/o	append	Appendix
bucc/o	bucc	Cheek
cholecyst/o	cholecyst	Gall bladder
col/o, colon/o	col, colon	Large intestine
diverticul/o	diverticul	Diverticulum
duoden/o	duoden	Duodenum
enter/o	enter	Intestine
esophag/o	esophag	Esophagus
gastr/o	gastr	Stomach
hepat/o	hepat	Liver
ile/i	ile	Ileum
jejun/o	jejun	Jejunum
pept/o	pept	Digest
proct/o, rect/o	proct, rect	Anus or rectum
or/o	or	Mouth
pancreat/o	pancreat	Pancreas
stomat/o	stomat	Mouth
Sensory Systems (Eye/Ear)		
acous/o, ot/o	acous, ot	Ears or hearing
blephar/o	blephar	Eyelid
conjunctiv/o	conjuctiv	Conjuctiva
kerat/o	kerat	Cornea
ir/i, ir/o, irid/o	ir, irid	Iris
labyrinth/o	labyrinth	Inner ear
macul/o	macul	Spot
myring/o	myring	Middle ear
ocul/o	ocul	Eye
opt/i, opthalm/o	opt, opthalm	Eye
phac/o, phak/o	phac, phak	Lens
scler/o	scler	White of the eye
tympan/o	tympan	Membrane of middle ear
Endocrine System		
adren/o	adren	Adrenal glands
andr/o	andr	Male
calc/o, calci/o	calc, calci	Calcium
cortic/o	cortic	Cortex
dips/o	dips	Thirst
gluc/o, glyc/o	gluc, glyc	Sugar, sweet
gonad/o	gonad	Glands
home/o	home	Sameness
lact/o	lact	Milk
parathyroid/o	parathyroid	Parathyroid glands

Table 3.3 Common Word Roots and Combining Forms (Continued)

Combining Form	Word Root	Meaning
pinea/o	pinea	Pineal gland
pituit/o	pituit	Pituitary gland
thym/o	thym	Thymus
thyr/o, thyroid/o	thyr, thyroid	Thyroid gland
toxic/o	toxic	Poison
Integumentary System		
adip/o, lip/o	adip, lip	Fat
cutan/o	cutan	Skin
dermat/o, derm/o	dermat, derm	Skin
hidr/o	hidr	Sweat glands
onych/o	onych	Nails
pil/i, pil/o	pil	Hair
scler/o	scler	Hard, hardening
seb/o	seb	Sebaceous glands
xer/o	xer	Dry
Nervous System		
encephal/o	encephal	Brain
mening/o	mening	Membranes covering brain and spinal cord
myel/o	myel	Spinal cord
neur/o	neur	Nerves
Reproductive System		
amni/o	amni	Amnion
cervic/o	cervic	Cervix
embry/o	embry	Embryo
gravida	gravida	Pregnancy
hyster/o	hyster	Uterus
lact/o	lact	Milk
mammo/o	mammo	Breast
mast/o	mast	Breast
men/o	men	Month, menstruation
nat/o	nat	Birth
oophor/o, ovari/o	oophor, ovari	Ovaries
orcho/o, test/i, orchi/o	orcho, test, orchi	Testicles
ov/o	ov	Egg
pen/i, phall/i	pen, phall	Penis
placent/o	placent	Placenta
salping/o	salping	Fallopian tubes
sperm/o, spermat/o	sperm, spermato	Sperm
vagin/o	vagin	Vagina
vas/o	vas	Vas deferens
vulv/o	vulv	Vulva

(Continues)

Table 3.3   Common Word Roots and Combining Forms (Continued)

Combining Form	Word Root	Meaning
Respiratory System		
aer/o	aer	Air
aveol/o	aveol	Alveoli
bronchi/o, bronch/o	bronchi, broncho	Bronchi
laryng/o	laryng	Larynx
lob/o	lob	Lobes
nas/o	nas	Nose
pharyng/o	pharyng	Pharynx
pleur/o	pleur	Pleura
pneum/o, pnemon/o	pneum, pneumon	Lung, air
pulmon/o	pulmon	Lung
rhin/o	rhin	Nose
sinus/o	sinus	Sinus
spir/o	spir	To breathe
trache/o	trache	Trachea
Musculoskeletal System		
arthr/o	arthr	Joint
burs/o	burs	Bursa
carp/o	carp	Wrist
cost/o	cost	Ribs
crani/o	crani	Skull, head
chondr/o	chondr	Cartilage
fibul/o	fibul	Fibula
humer/o	humer	Humerus
ili/o	ili	Ilium
ligament/o	ligament	Ligament
mandibul/o	mandibul	Mandible
myel/o	myel	Bone marrow
myo	myo	Muscle
oste/o	oste	Bones
Urinary System		
cyst/o	cyst	Bladder
glomerul/o	glomerul	Glomeruli
nephr/o	nephr	Kidney
noct/o	noct	Night
pyel/o	pyel	Pelvis, kidney
ren/o	ren	Kidney
ur/o, urin/o	ur, urin	Urine
ureter/o	ureter	Ureter
urethr/o	urethr	Urethra

Breaking a Medical Term Apart

Dissecting a term into its word parts is a good way to learn about its meaning. Follow these steps to break a medical term apart:

1. Identify the suffix. A suffix can be found at the end of a word. It usually indicates a procedure, condition, disorder, or disease. It is denoted with a hyphen to the left (for example, -stasis, -uria, -itis).
2. Identify the prefix. A prefix can be found at the beginning of a word. It often indicates location, quantity, size, frequency, position, or presence or absence. It is denoted with a hyphen to the right (for example, pre-, poly-, micro-). It is important to note that not every medical term will contain a prefix.
3. Identify the word root and combining form. The word root or combining form defines a part of the body or a color. A medical term may contain more than one word root or combining form.

When you put all the word components together, you have a basic definition of the medical term **FIGURE 3.2**.

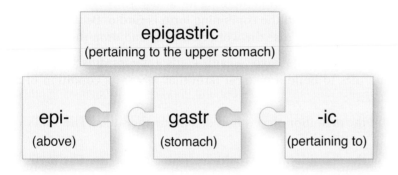

FIGURE 3.2 Breaking apart a medical term can help you determine its meaning.
© Jones & Bartlett Learning

There are several prefixes that mean the same thing, suffixes that mean the same thing, and word roots and combining forms that are similar. Through memorization, constant review, and practice, you can master this new language.

Breaking apart a medical term into word parts can help you determine its meaning.

Building a Medical Term

The same rules that apply to breaking a medical term apart also apply to building a medical term:

1. Start with the suffix and identify its meaning.
2. Identify the prefix.
3. Identify the word root and combining form. The word root or combining form defines the part of anatomy or a color. A medical term may contain more than one word root or combining form.

Let's use these rules to build a medical term that means "inflammation of the heart muscle":

1. Identify the part of the definition that denotes the suffix "inflammation." The suffix for "inflammation" is -itis.

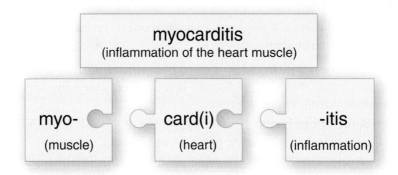

FIGURE 3.3 Building a medical term for "inflammation of the heart muscle."
© Jones & Bartlett Learning

2. Identify the part of the definition that denotes the prefix "muscle." The prefix for "muscle" is myo-.
3. Identify the part of the word root or combining form that denotes "heart." The word root for "heart" is cardi and the combining form is cardio. Because the suffix begins with the vowel "i," use the word root cardi and drop the extra "i."

Combine all the various components: myo- + cardi + -itis = myocarditis **FIGURE 3.3**.
   Let's use the same rules to build a medical term that means "a condition of an abnormally fast heart rate":

1. Identify the part of the definition that would determine the suffix. The suffix for "a condition of" is -ia.
2. Identify the part of the definition that would determine the prefix. The prefix for "abnormally fast" is tachy-.
3. Identify the word root or combining form. The word root or combining form for "heart" is cardi/o. Because the suffix begins with the vowel "i," choose the word root cardi.

Combine all the components together: tachy- + cardi + -ia = tachycardia **FIGURE 3.4**.

When combining word components to make a medical term, if the suffix begins with a vowel, drop the vowel of the combining form to make the correct medical term. If the suffix starts with a consonant, then the combining form is kept.

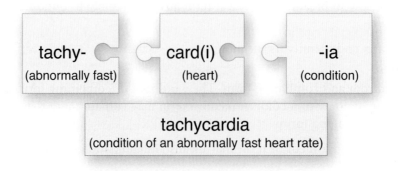

FIGURE 3.4 Building a medical term to describe "a condition of an abnormally fast heart rate."
© Jones & Bartlett Learning

Table 3.4 Singular and Plural Forms	
Singular Ending	**Plural Ending**
-a	-ae
-en	-ina
-ex, -ix	-ices
-is	-es
-nx	-nges
-on	-a
-um	-a
-us	-i

Singular and Plural Terms

The rules for making a plural form of a singular term are more complex for terms derived from foreign languages. In the English language, adding "s" or "es" to the singular term makes it plural. **TABLE 3.4** lists the basic rules for changing medical terms from their singular to plural form.

Anatomy and Physiology

The study of the human body can be divided into two parts: anatomy and physiology. **Anatomy** is the study of the structures of the human body and its organs. **Physiology** is the study of the function and physical and chemical processes that take place in cells, tissues, and organs.

Anatomy is the study of the structures of the human body and its organs. Physiology is the study of the processes that take place in the human body.

The structures and organs of the human body must all work together. When the body functions properly, the body is said to be in homeostasis. **Homeostasis** is the state of equilibrium that produces a constant internal environment throughout the body. When the normal state of the body is disrupted, it may result in the development of an illness or disease. **Pathophysiology** is the study of the processes or mechanisms by which an illness or disease occurs, the body's response to this state, and the effects of these processes on normal bodily function.

Anatomic Directional Terms

Certain directional terms for describing body structure are used universally by health-care professionals. A body is in **anatomic position** when standing erect, with arms down at the sides and the palms of hands facing forward. Anatomic directional terms describe the positions of structures relative to other structures or locations in the body **FIGURE 3.5** :

- Superior (cranial)—**Superior (cranial)** means toward the head of the body or upper.
- Inferior (caudal)—**Inferior (caudal)** means away from the head or lower.
- Anterior (ventral)—**Anterior (ventral)** means front.
- Posterior (dorsal)—**Posterior (dorsal)** means back.

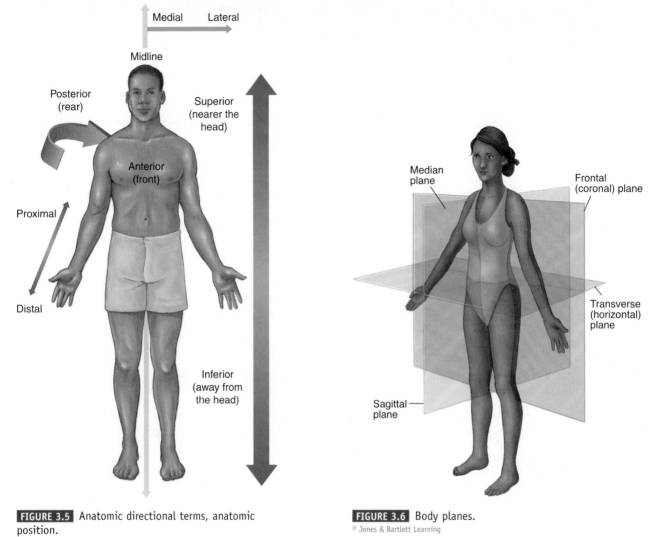

FIGURE 3.5 Anatomic directional terms, anatomic position.
© Jones & Bartlett Learning

FIGURE 3.6 Body planes.
© Jones & Bartlett Learning

- **Medial**—**Medial** means toward the midline of the body.
- **Lateral**—**Lateral** means away from the midline of the body.
- **Proximal**—**Proximal** means toward or nearest the trunk or the point of origin of a part.
- **Distal**—**Distal** means away from or farthest from the trunk or the point of origin of a part.

Anatomic directional terms describe the positions of structures relative to other structures or locations in the body.

Body Planes

You can divide a body into four planes by drawing an imaginary line through the side of the body from the top of the head to the feet and by drawing a horizontal line across the body. The resulting planes are as follows **FIGURE 3.6**:

- **Coronal plane (frontal plane)**—The **coronal plane (frontal plane)** is a vertical plane running from side to side that divides the body or any of its parts into anterior and posterior portions.

- **Sagittal plane (lateral plane)**—The **sagittal plane (lateral plane)** is a vertical plane running from front to back that divides the body or any of its parts into right and left sides.
- **Axial plane (transverse plane)**—The **axial plane (transverse plane)** is a horizontal plane that divides the body or any of its parts into upper and lower parts.
- **Median plane**—The **median plane** is a sagittal plane through the midline of the body that divides the body or any of its parts into right and left halves.

Body Cavities

The body is divided into cavities or spaces that contain the internal organs or viscera. The two main cavities are the posterior (dorsal) cavity and the anterior (ventral) cavity. The ventral cavity is the larger cavity and is subdivided into two parts—thoracic and abdominopelvic—by the diaphragm, a dome-shaped respiratory muscle.

> The human body is divided into two main cavities: the posterior (dorsal) cavity and the anterior (ventral) cavity.

The thoracic cavity, also called the chest or upper ventral cavity, contains the heart, lungs, trachea, esophagus, large blood vessels, and nerves. The thoracic cavity is bound laterally by the ribs.

The lower part of the ventral (abdominopelvic) cavity can be further subdivided into two parts: an upper abdominal portion and a lower pelvic portion. The abdominal cavity extends from the diaphragm to the top of the pelvic bones and contains most of the gastrointestinal tract, as well as the kidneys and adrenal glands. The abdominal cavity can also be further divided into four quadrants or nine regions **FIGURE 3.7** and **FIGURE 3.8**. The pelvic cavity is surrounded by the pelvic bones and contains most of the urinary system, reproductive organs, as well as the rectum.

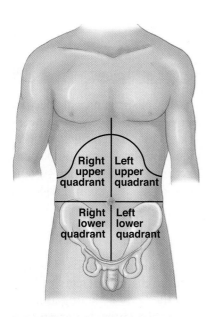

FIGURE 3.7 The abdominal cavity can be divided into four quadrants.
© Jones & Bartlett Learning

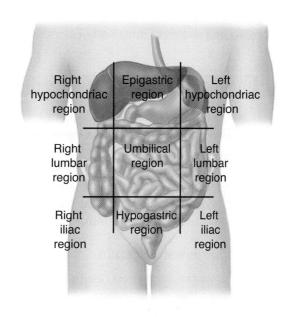

FIGURE 3.8 The abdominal cavity can be divided into nine regions.
© Jones & Bartlett Learning

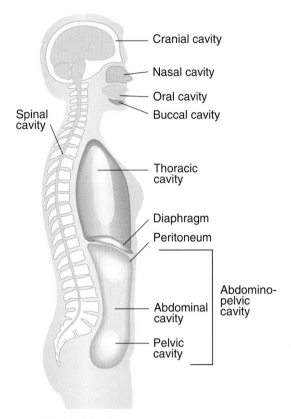

FIGURE 3.9 Body cavities.
© Jones & Bartlett Learning

The smaller of the two main cavities is the dorsal cavity. It contains organs lying more posterior in the body. The dorsal cavity, again, can be divided into two portions. The upper portion, or the cranial cavity, houses the brain, and the lower portion, or vertebral canal, houses the spinal cord. There are three other smaller cavities: the orbital cavity for the eyes, the nasal cavity for the structures of the nose, and the buccal cavity, or mouth.

FIGURE 3.9 shows various body cavities.

Body Systems

The basic building block of the human body is the **cell**. Cells organize to become tissues and tissues form organs. Organs work together and collectively form organ systems. Each organ system works to carry out specific and complex bodily functions. Systems are the most complex components of the human body. The systems of the body include the integumentary system, musculoskeletal system, cardiovascular system, respiratory system, gastrointestinal system, renal system, nervous system, endocrine system, reproductive system, immune system, and sensory system.

The Integumentary System

The **integumentary system** is composed of the skin, hair, nails, and glands. The skin is the largest organ of the human body. It accounts for more than 10 percent of body weight. The skin is our first line of defense and protects the body by acting as a barrier, protecting the body from chemical, physical, and microbial injury. It also protects the body by regulating body temperature. The nerves allow the skin to detect pain, heat, and cold.

Skin is the human body's primary defense mechanism. Healthy skin is imperative for maintaining a
healthy body and lifestyle. Like other organs, it must
be nourished and maintained. The skin is divided
into three layers that contain nerves, glands, hair,
and blood vessels **FIGURE 3.10** :

*The integumentary system is composed of
skin, hair, nails, and glands.*
© auremar/ShutterStock, Inc.

- **Epidermis**—The **epidermis** is the outermost layer of skin and protects the layers below it. The epidermis contains melanocytes, which produce skin pigment.
  The epidermis lacks blood supply. The epidermis continually sheds dead, dry
  cells and produces new, healthy cells. The epidermis produces glands, nails, and
  hair. Beneath the epidermis are the dermis and subcutaneous layer.
- **Dermis**—The **dermis** is the second layer of skin. It is 40 times thicker than the
  epidermis. The dermis supports the epidermis and separates it from the lower
  layers of skin. The dermis is composed of elastic and connective tissue that
  contains collagen. Collagen helps support blood vessels, glands, and nerves.
  The dermis is responsible for sensory input.
- **Hypodermis**—The **hypodermis**, also known as **subcutaneous tissue**, is the innermost layer of skin. It contains loose connective tissue and fatty tissue firmly
  anchored to the dermis. The fatty component of the hypodermis facilitates temperature control, maintains food reserves, and provides cushioning for the body.

Hair is made up of proteins called **keratin**. Hair has roots that are embedded in
the skin's dermis. Nails are also composed of keratin. The nail root is embedded into
the epidermis and provides protection to the surface of the toes and fingers.

There are two types of glands within the layers of skin: sebaceous glands and sweat
glands. **Sebaceous glands** are located within the dermal layer of the skin and secrete
an oily substance called sebum. **Sebum** lubricates the skin, retains water, and helps
keep skin and hair soft and supple. Sebaceous glands can be found everywhere in the
skin except the palms of the hands and soles of the feet. **Sweat glands** (also called
sudoriferous glands) allow sweat to flow through pores of the skin.

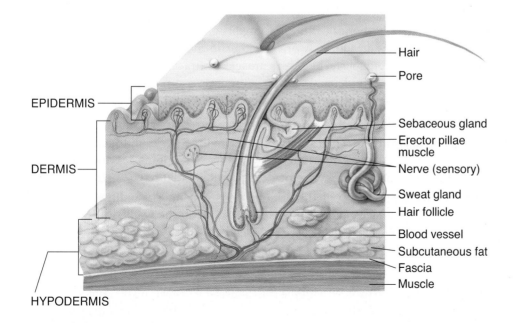

FIGURE 3.10 Anatomy of human skin.
© Jones & Bartlett Learning

Practice defining a word associated with the integumentary system. Try breaking down the term hypodermic. Start with the suffix, -ic, meaning "pertaining to." Then identify the prefix, hypo-, meaning "under." Finally, identify the combining form, derm, meaning "skin." Putting it all together, the definition is "pertaining to under the skin."

The Musculoskeletal System

Underneath the integumentary system is the **musculoskeletal system**. This system consists of bones and the tissues that connect them, such as tendons, ligaments, and cartilage. The skeletal system provides support for the human body. Bones provide a rigid framework, known as the skeleton, that supports and protects the organs of the body. There are 206 bones and 646 muscles in the human body.

The musculoskeletal system is composed of bones and the tissues that connect them, such as tendons, ligaments, and cartilage.
© auremar/ShutterStock, Inc.

Bones are connected to each other at joints. A **joint** is the place where two or more bones meet **FIGURE 3.11**. Joints allow the body to move in many ways and make the skeleton flexible. Joints can be classified according to structure, function, or region. Joints classified by their structure can be divided into the following types:

- **Fibrous joints** connect bones without allowing any movement. The bones of your skull and pelvis are held together by fibrous joints. The union of the spinous processes and vertebrae are fibrous joints.
- **Cartilaginous joints** are joints in which the bones are attached by cartilage. These joints allow for only a little movement, such as in the spine or ribs.
- **Synovial joints** allow for much more movement than cartilaginous joint. Cavities between bones in synovial joints are filled with synovial fluid. This fluid helps lubricate and protect the bones.

Muscles, attached to bones or internal organs and blood vessels, are responsible for movement. Muscles and joints work together to move body parts by working in pairs of **flexors** and **extensors**. The flexor muscle contracts to bend a limb at a joint. When the movement is completed, the extensor muscle contracts to straighten the limb at the same joint. Muscles are connected to bones by cordlike tissues called **tendons**. Muscles can be grouped into the following three types **FIGURE 3.12**:

- **Skeletal muscles** are attached to bones and hold the skeleton together, give the body its shape, and allow voluntary movements. These muscles are also called striated muscles because they are made up of fibers that have horizontal stripes.
- **Smooth muscles** are controlled by the nervous system. The contraction of these muscles is involuntary. Smooth muscles are found in the walls of the stomach and intestines and the walls of blood vessels.
- **Cardiac muscles** are involuntary muscles found in the heart.

Practice defining a word associated with the musculoskeletal system. Try breaking down the term polymyalgia. Start with the suffix, -algia, meaning "pain." Then identify the prefix, poly-, meaning "many." Finally, identify the word root or combining form, my, meaning "muscle." Putting it all together, the definition is "pain of many muscles."

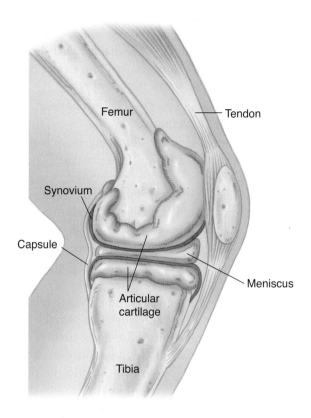

FIGURE 3.11 Anatomy of a joint.
© Jones & Bartlett Learning

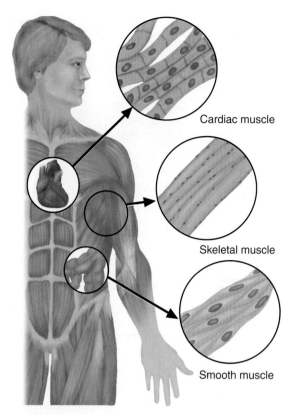

FIGURE 3.12 The three types of muscle tissue.
© Jones & Bartlett Learning

The Cardiovascular System

The **cardiovascular system**, sometimes called the circulatory system, includes the heart and blood vessels. The cardiovascular system plays a vital role in maintaining homeostasis. The heart is located in the chest cavity between the lungs. The heart is a large muscle that consists of two pumps (the right heart and the left heart) that drive the unidirectional flow of blood through the blood vessels of the pulmonary system, where the exchange of oxygen, nutrients, and hormones takes place. Each side of the heart has one ventricle and one atrium. The heart is divided into right and left sections by tissue called the **septum**. The left side of the heart pumps oxygen and nutrient-rich blood out through the aorta and ultimately to the cells. The right side of the heart receives oxygen-poor, waste-rich blood, which is pumped back through the lungs for oxygenation. Each beat of the heart, or **cardiac cycle**, involves several coordinated events, including the electrical activation of the atria and ventricles and the contraction (**systole**) and relaxation (**diastole**) of the atria and ventricles. Also, cardiac valves open and close to allow the atria and ventricles to fill with blood and then empty as the heart pumps blood to the rest of the body. The electrical activation of the heart begins in the sinoatrial node (located in the upper-right atrium wall) and spreads rapidly to the atrial muscle. Next, the atrioventricular node (located in the septum between the right atrium and right ventricle) is activated, followed by the ventricular muscle. The entire process takes about 0.2 seconds. The rate of activation can be affected by nerves in the sinoatrial node, hormones, calcium concentration in the heart muscle cells, and body temperature. A normal heart beats between 60 and 100 times per minute.

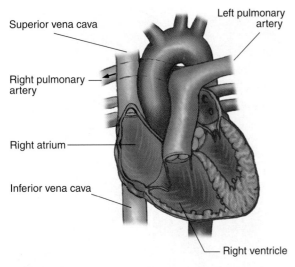

Superior vena cava

Left pulmonary artery

Right pulmonary artery

Right atrium

Inferior vena cava

Right ventricle

The heart wall is composed of three main layers:

- **Endocardium (inner layer)**—The **endocardium** has a smooth pleatlike surface that allows the heart wall to collapse when it contracts.
- **Myocardium (middle layer)**—The **myocardium** is the heart muscle that contracts.
- **Epicardium (outer layer)**—The **epicardium** is the outer layer of the heart tissue. The coronary arteries that supply the heart with oxygenated blood and the coronary veins that return deoxygenated blood to the heart are located in the epicardium.

The heart is surrounded by connective tissue called the **pericardium**, which is anchored by ligaments to the chest wall and diaphragm.

The heart receives oxygen-poor blood via two large veins called the superior and inferior venae cavae. The superior vena cava transports blood from the upper portion of the body such as the head and neck and the inferior vena cava carries blood from the lower portion of the body such as the legs and abdomen. Blood travels from the vena cavae into the right atrium. The blood passes through the tricuspid valve to the right ventricle, and then flows through the pulmonary arteries to the lungs to receive oxygen. Oxygen-rich blood returns to the heart through the pulmonary veins into the left atrium. Blood then flows through the mitral valve into the left ventricle, then through the aortic valve. The blood enters the aorta, and then flows to the rest of the body **FIGURE 3.13**.

The lymphatic system, circulatory system, and immune system are also included with the cardiovascular system.

Practice defining a word associated with the cardiovascular system. Try breaking down the term thrombophlebitis. Start with the suffix, -itis, meaning "inflammation." Then identify the prefix, thrombo-, meaning "clot." Finally, identify the word root or combining form, phleb, meaning "vein." Putting it all together, the definition is "inflammation of a vein due to a blood clot."

The Respiratory System

When the **respiratory system** is mentioned, people generally think of breathing, but breathing is only one of the activities of the respiratory system. The body's cells need a continuous supply of oxygen for the metabolic processes that are necessary to maintain life. The respiratory system works with the circulatory system to provide oxygen and to remove the waste products of metabolism. It also helps to regulate pH of the blood.

The respiratory system is composed of the nose and nasal cavities, pharynx, larynx, trachea, bronchial tree, and lungs. The function of the respiratory system is to oxygenate the blood and remove carbon dioxide. The respiratory system can be divided into the upper respiratory and lower respiratory systems. The upper respiratory tract filters, warms, and moistens the air before it enters the lower respiratory tract.

The upper respiratory system is composed of the nose and nasal cavities, pharynx, and larynx. A mucosal lining forms a protective cover over the respiratory tract and helps trap irritants such as dust and pollen. The nasal septum separates the nasal cavity into two distinct cavities. The cavities are also lined by a mucous membrane with hairlike structures called cilia. The **cilia** filter the air by catching small dust particles from the air that we breathe in. The pharynx is also part of the digestive system. The tonsils are also located in the pharynx. The larynx is also known as the voice box because it contains the vocal cords. They provide air distribution and voice production.

The lower respiratory system is composed of the trachea, bronchial tree, and lungs. The trachea (windpipe) is lined with mucous membranes with cilia. The trachea branches into the right bronchus and left bronchus, each leading to the right and left lungs, respectively. Each bronchus branches into smaller bronchi and then into smaller bronchioles. The bronchioles provide oxygen and a passageway for air to reach the alveoli. The bronchioles end in alveolar sacs deep in the lungs. Respiration—the exchange of oxygen and carbon dioxide in the capillaries surrounding the alveoli—occurs in the alveolar sacs. The lungs are divided into lobes: three in the right lung and two in the left. The lungs are located in the pleural cavity and are separated from each other by the mediastinum. The main function of the lungs is breathing. The diaphragm, a large dome-shaped muscle, separates the chest cavity from the abdominal cavity. It helps with inhalation and exhalation **FIGURE 3.14**.

Practice defining a word associated with the respiratory system. Try breaking down the term rhinitis. Start with the suffix, -itis, meaning "inflammation." Then identify the prefix. In this case, there is no prefix. (Remember, not every medical term has a prefix.) Finally, identify the word root or combining form, rhin, meaning "nose." Putting it all together, the definition is "inflammation of the nose."

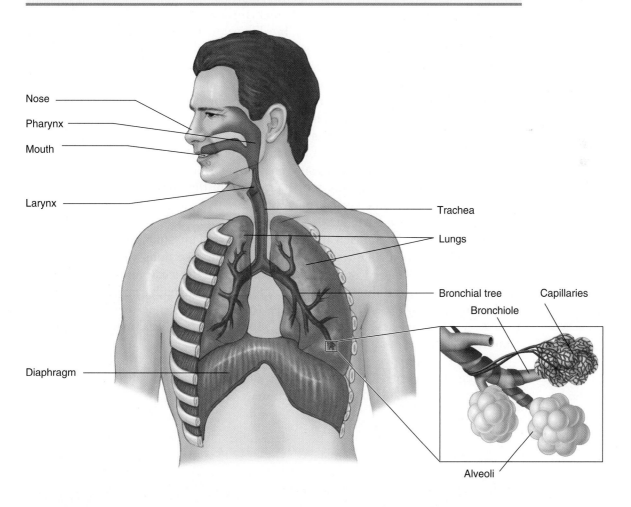

FIGURE 3.14 The respiratory system.

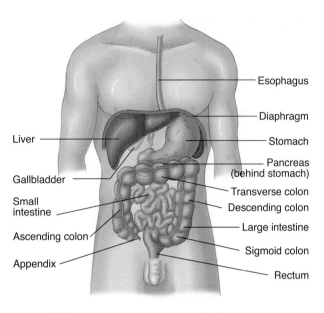

Esophagus

Diaphragm

Liver

Stomach

Pancreas
(behind stomach)

Gallbladder

Transverse colon

Small
intestine

Descending colon

Large intestine

Ascending colon

Sigmoid colon

Appendix

Rectum

FIGURE 3.15 The gastrointestinal system.
© Jones & Bartlett Learning

The Gastrointestinal (Digestive) System

The **gastrointestinal (GI) system** breaks down food and fluids into small compounds that can be readily absorbed into the bloodstream and used by the body for energy production, for protein synthesis, and as enzymes for essential metabolic reactions **FIGURE 3.15**. The four main functions of the GI system are digestion, absorption, metabolism, and excretion. Primarily controlled by the autonomic nervous system, the specialized part of the peripheral nervous system that controls the internal organs and other self-regulated body functions, and hormones present in saliva, the stomach, the pancreas, and the liver, the GI system is responsible for eliminating solid waste products from the body.

The GI tract is made up of a long tube that begins in the mouth, travels through the pharynx, esophagus, stomach, and small and large intestines, and ends at the anus. Peristalsis (propulsive movements and contractions of the GI tract) moves food in one direction.

When food is taken into the body, it enters through the mouth. The mouth begins the process of digestion by physically breaking down food into smaller pieces via chewing. Within the mouth, several structures such as the tongue, teeth, and salivary glands help break the food into smaller parts. As the food is chewed, it is moistened and mixed with saliva, which contains the enzyme ptyalin. Ptyalin changes some of the starches in the food to sugar. With the help of the tongue, the food is swallowed and makes its way into the pharynx. The pharynx connects the mouth to the esophagus. Peristalsis in the esophagus propels food downward into the stomach. The stomach secretes enzymes and gastric juices, which liquefy and degrade it into smaller compounds. The pancreas produces digestive enzymes and bicarbonate to neutralize gastric acid. The liver produces bile salts, which promote the digestion and absorption of fat. The GI tract also contains normal microbial flora that aid in digestion and prevent the overgrowth of fecal bacteria.

The food leaves the stomach and travels to the small intestine, where most absorption takes place. The small intestine is divided into three sections: the duodenum, the jejunum, and the ileum. Most digestion occurs within the small intestine. Nutrients, vitamins, minerals, and fluids are absorbed for use by the body's cells. Products that are not absorbed by the small intestine pass to the large intestine. The large intestine removes water from these waste products, producing a firm fecal mass. This mass is eliminated from the body through defecation.

Within the digestive system are auxiliary organs that assist the GI tract in the processing of nutrients. These include the pancreas, liver, and gallbladder. All three organs have ducts that lead to the duodenum.

The GI tract is lined with a mucous membrane that protects it from damage from harsh enzymes and an acidic environment.
© auremar/ShutterStock, Inc.

Practice defining a word associated with the gastrointestinal system. Try breaking down the term appendectomy. Start with the suffix, -ectomy, meaning "surgical removal." Next, identify the prefix. In this case, there is no prefix. (Remember, not every medical term has a prefix.) Finally, identify the word root or combining form, append, meaning "appendix." Putting it all together, the definition is "surgical removal of the appendix."

The Renal (Urinary) System

The **renal system**, or urinary system, performs many functions that maintain homeostasis, a state of equilibrium that produces a constant internal environment throughout the body. The renal system is composed of two kidneys, two ureters, one bladder, and one urethra **FIGURE 3.16**. The renal system:

- Maintains the body's balance of water, salts, and acids by removing excess fluids from the body or reabsorbing water as needed
- Filters the blood to remove urea and other waste products from the bloodstream
- Converts these waste products and excess fluids into urine and excretes them from the body via the bladder

The kidneys are found inside the upper abdominal cavity, between the 12th thoracic and 3rd lumbar vertebrae. The kidneys are responsible for maintaining the chemical compositions of the electrolytes, fluids, and tissues within the body, including acid-base balance, preservation of normal blood pressure, and production of some hormones. The ureters are tubes that connect the kidney to the bladder. Urine produced in the kidney passes through the ureters to the bladder. The bladder is a muscular sac found in the pelvis just above and behind the pubic bone. The bladder is lined with muscles that allow it to expand to hold urine. During urination, the bladder muscles contract, allowing urine to flow out into the urethra, which carries the urine out of the body.

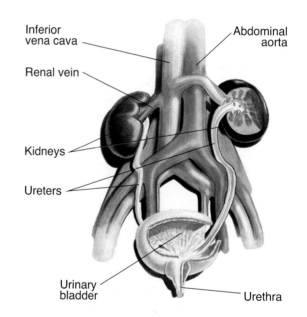

Practice defining a word associated with the renal system. Try breaking down the term cystoscopy. Start with the suffix, -scopy, meaning "process of using a lighted instrument." Then identify the prefix. In this case, there is no prefix. Finally, identify the word root or combining form, cyst/o, meaning "bladder." Putting it all together, the definition is "process of viewing the bladder with a lighted instrument."

The Nervous System

The **central nervous system (CNS)** includes the brain and spinal cord. Both the brain and spinal cord are covered by **meninges**. The spinal cord and parts of the brain are filled with cerebrospinal fluid, which helps the brain maintain its normal pressure. The brain is divided into right and left hemispheres. Each hemisphere has different functions. The left hemisphere controls language, math, and logic. The right hemisphere controls spatial abilities, facial recognition, visual imagery, and music. Each hemisphere

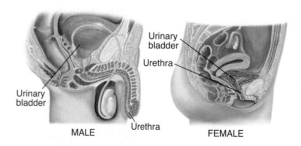

FIGURE 3.16 The renal system (upper) and the male (lower left) and female (lower right) urinary tracts.
© Jones & Bartlett Learning

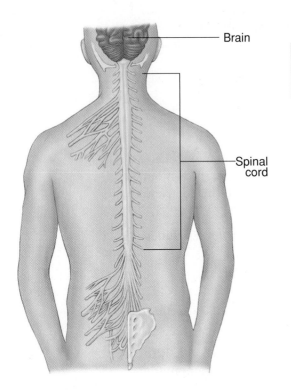

— Brain

—Spinal
cord

FIGURE 3.17 The central nervous system.
© Jones & Bartlett Learning

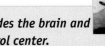

The central nervous system includes the brain and spinal cord. It is the body's control center.
© auremar/ShutterStock, Inc.

is essential to the other. The CNS is the body's control center. The spinal cord contains nerve pathways called tracts that send signals from sensors in the body to the brain. The brain interprets these signals and sends signals to the body organs telling them what to do **FIGURE 3.17**.

The signals that are sent to and from the brain are electrical signals. These electrical signals stimulate the release of neurotransmitters or chemicals at many nerve endings. These neurotransmitters allow the electrical signal to continue to the next nerve. Neurotransmitters can either stimulate or inhibit these signals. Lack or incorrect amounts of these neurotransmitters can cause many different physical, emotional, and mental disorders.

The **peripheral nervous system (PNS)** includes all the nerves throughout the body except those in the CNS. The PNS is divided into the afferent system and the efferent system. The afferent system includes all the nerves and sense organs. These nerves and organs take in information and send it to the CNS. The efferent system includes all the nerves and pathways that send information from the CNS to other organs and body systems. The efferent system is further divided into the autonomic nervous system, parasympathetic nervous system, and somatic nervous system. The autonomic nervous system controls organs and body systems automatically. The parasympathetic nervous system returns the body to a normal state. The somatic nervous system controls all the skeletal muscles in the body.

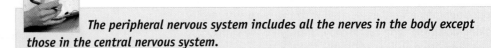

The peripheral nervous system includes all the nerves in the body except those in the central nervous system.
© auremar/ShutterStock, Inc.

Practice defining a word associated with the nervous system. Try breaking down the term neuromuscular. Start with the suffix, -ar, meaning "pertaining to." Next, identify the prefix. In this case, there is no prefix. Finally, identify the word root or combining form, neur/o and muscul/o, meaning "nerves" and "muscles." Putting it all together, the definition is "pertaining to the nerves and muscles."

The Endocrine System

The **endocrine system** is a system of glands that produce and secrete hormones. These **hormones**, or chemical messengers, are released directly into the bloodstream. They regulate mood, growth and development, tissue function, metabolism, sexual function, and reproduction. The hormones that regulate these activities are also used to treat hormonal disorders. Laboratory tests can measure the level of hormones in the bloodstream. These blood tests are frequently drawn in healthcare providers' offices.

The organs of the endocrine system are very specific in the way they function. The endocrine system is composed of the following **FIGURE 3.18** :

> *Hormones regulate mood, growth and development, tissue function, metabolism, sexual function, and reproduction.*
> © auremar/ShutterStock, Inc.

- **Thyroid gland**—The **thyroid gland** is located at the base of the neck. It produces and secretes three hormones, thyroxine (T4), triiodothyronine (T3), and calcitonin, that stimulate metabolic activity, growth, and the activity of the nervous system.

- **Hypothalamus**—The **hypothalamus** is located below the thalamus. It is an area of the brain that produces hormones that control body temperature, appetite, mood, sex drive, and the release of hormones.

- **Pituitary gland**—The **pituitary gland** produces hormones that affect the activity of other endocrine glands and specific organs of the body. In essence, it is the control tower of the endocrine system. The gland is composed of two portions: the anterior and posterior lobes.

- **Parathyroid gland**—The **parathyroid gland**, also known as the master gland, is located slightly behind and above the thyroid gland. It produces parathyroid hormone, which helps maintain calcium levels.

- **Adrenal glands**—The **adrenal glands** are located on top of the kidneys. They are composed of two layers of tissue: the medulla and the cortex. The medulla synthesizes and secretes the catecholamines, epinephrine and norepinephrine. These hormones are stored in the adrenal medulla until activated by the sympathetic nervous system. The sympathetic nervous system is the part of the autonomic nervous system that increases the activity of the smooth, involuntary muscles of the body's organs. The cortex of the adrenal gland produces glucocorticoids, mineralocorticoids, and sex hormones. Glucocorticoids affect the metabolism of lipids, carbohydrates, and proteins. Mineralocorticoids regulate the secretion of water and sodium by the kidneys.

- **Pineal body**—The **pineal body** is a gland that produces and secretes melatonin, a hormone that regulates the sleep-wake cycle. The target tissue of melatonin is the hypothalamus.

- **Ovaries**—The **ovaries** are female organs responsible for hormones that regulate the menstrual cycle and pregnancy. The ovaries sit above the uterus and are attached to the fallopian tubes, which connect the two organs. The ovaries secrete the hormones estrogen and progesterone. Estrogen is responsible for the development of breasts and genitals and the regulation of the menstrual cycle, which prepares the female for pregnancy.

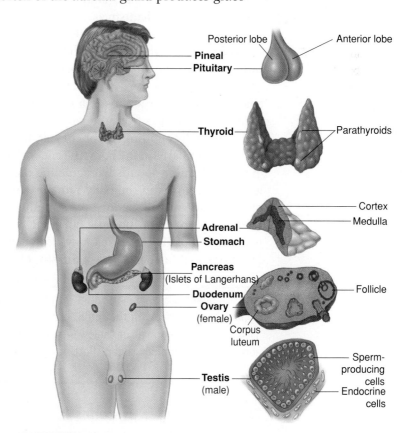

FIGURE 3.18 The endocrine system.
© Jones & Bartlett Learning

- **Testes**—**Testes** are male sex glands that produce testosterone, which is responsible for the growth of adjacent organs: the prostate gland, seminal vesicles, vas deferens, and others. It is also responsible for secondary sex characteristics such as changes in voice pitch as a boy enters puberty. The two testes in men are responsible for the production and secretion of sperm. The testes are located within the scrotum.
- **Pancreas**—The **pancreas** is located behind the left kidney at the back of the abdominal wall. It aids in digestion and is responsible for the production and secretion of hormones from cells called islets of Langerhans. These cells contain alpha cells that produce glucagon and beta cells that produce insulin.

The endocrine system glands secrete hormones that maintain homeostasis by regulating physiological processes. Hormones in general can be considered specialized keys that unlock specific doors. The tissue or organ that these hormones affect is called its **target**. Each hormone secreted by an endocrine organ targets a specific organ. The same hormone will not affect any other organ within the body. Hormones perform many functions throughout the body, including the following:

- **Maintaining homeostasis**—Maintaining normal physiological limits by increasing and decreasing blood glucose levels for energy use
- **Preparing the body for an emergency situation**—Instigating the "fight or flight" reaction
- **Developing the reproductive system**—Causing sexual maturity and reproductive functions, such as menstruation and pregnancy

The endocrine system is regulated by an intricate negative feedback mechanism that involves a particular gland, the hypothalamic-pituitary axis, and autoregulation. This feedback mechanism is the primary regulatory mechanism used to maintain homeostasis. The hormone levels in the endocrine system are regulated by a negative feedback mechanism in almost the same way that a thermostat regulates the temperature in a room. That is, the endocrine system senses levels of hormones in the body just as a thermostat senses the temperature of a room. In the case of a thermostat, it communicates instructions to a furnace or air conditioner so that if the temperature of the room changes from the temperature at which the thermostat is set, the system will respond by emitting hot or cold air. In this way, the temperature in the room stays constant. Similarly, in the body, the endocrine system senses the levels of the hormones in the body and responds by regulating the production of these hormones so that the level of hormones in the body remains constant. In negative feedback, the stimulus results in actions that reduce the stimulus. If a gland stops producing a hormone or secretes too much or too little hormone, various conditions of the endocrine system may result. Positive feedback may also occur. In positive feedback, a stimulus results in actions that further increase the stimulus.

> Practice defining a word associated with the endocrine system. Try breaking down the term hypoglycemia. Start with the suffix, -emia, meaning "blood." Next, identify the prefix, hypo-, meaning "below normal" or "below or under." Finally, identify the word root or combining form, glyc/o, meaning "sugar." Putting it all together, the definition is "below normal blood sugar."

The Reproductive System

The function of the **reproductive system** is to ensure survival of the species. The reproductive system has four main functions: to produce egg and sperm cells, to transport these cells, to develop off-spring, and to produce hormones. These functions are divided between the primary and secondary, or accessory, reproductive organs. The primary reproductive organs, or gonads, consist of the ovaries and testes. These organs are responsible for producing the egg and sperm cells and hormones. These hormones control the functions of the reproductive system, provide gender characteristics, and regulate the normal physiology of the reproductive system. All other organs, ducts, and glands in the reproductive system are considered secondary, or accessory, reproductive organs. These structures transport and sustain the developing offspring.

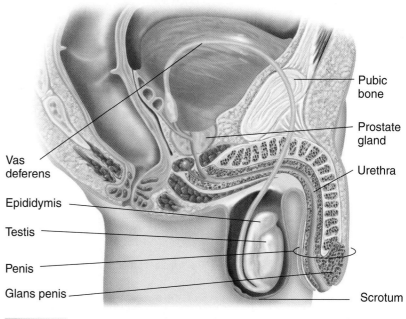

FIGURE 3.19 The male reproductive system.
© Jones & Bartlett Learning

Male Reproductive System

The male reproductive system operates interdependently with the urinary system. The primary structure of the male reproductive system is the testes. The urethra passes through the penis and is responsible for urine removal as well as the exit route for sperm. The testicles produce sperm and store sperm cells. After sperm are formed, they mature and are stored in the epididymis (tightly coiled tubes wrapped around the back of the testes) and then travel into the vas deferens, where peristaltic movements transport the sperm into the ejaculatory duct **FIGURE 3.19**.

The prostate encircles part of the urethra. The secretions of the prostate gland enhance the mobility of the sperm and provide an alkaline environment that protects it against the acidic environment of the vagina. The sperm and fluids pass through the urethra in the penis for ejaculation during sexual intercourse.

Male sex hormones are stimulated by the release of gonadotropin-releasing hormone (GnRH) from the hypothalamus. GnRH stimulates secretion of luteinizing hormone and follicle-stimulating hormone. Luteinizing hormones stimulate the cells to secrete testosterone. Testosterone and follicle-stimulating hormone stimulate the production of sperm in the testicles.

Practice defining a word associated with the reproductive system. Try breaking down the term spermatogenesis. Start with the suffix, -genesis, meaning "originating or beginning." Next, identify the prefix. In this case, there is no prefix. Finally, identify the word root or combining form, spermat/o, meaning "sperm." Putting it all together, the definition is "producing or originating sperm cells."

Female Reproductive System

The female reproductive system produces and transports ova from the ovary through the fallopian tube into the uterus. Most fertilization occurs in the fallopian tube. At the end of the fallopian tube is the uterus, where the fertilized ovum will implant. If implantation does not occur, the endometrium and ovum will be removed from the

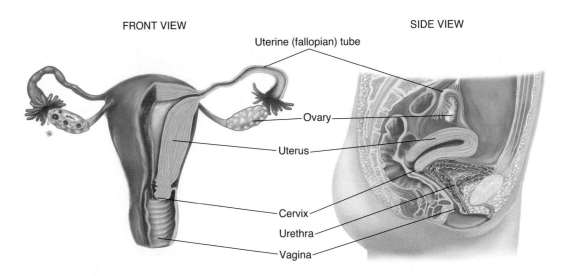

FRONT VIEW   SIDE VIEW

Uterine (fallopian) tube

Ovary

Uterus

Cervix

Urethra

Vagina

FIGURE 3.20 The female reproductive system.
© Jones & Bartlett Learning

body via menses. The average menstrual cycle occurs every 28 days. Ovulation takes place mid-cycle at or about the 14th day following the first day of the menstrual cycle. The primary structure of the female reproductive system is the ovaries. The accessory structures include the uterus, cervix, urethra, fallopian tubes, vagina, and breasts **FIGURE 3.20** .

Practice defining a word associated with the reproductive system. Try breaking down the term oophoroectomy. Start with the suffix, -ectomy, meaning "surgical removal of." Next, identify the prefix. In this case, there is no prefix. Finally, identify the word root or combining form, oophor/o, meaning "ovary." Putting it all together, the definition is "surgical removal of an ovary or ovaries."

The Immune System

The **immune system** is the body's defense mechanism. It protects the body by attacking and destroying invading pathogens. It adapts to its environment and evolves based on previous exposures. The immune system exhibits several characteristics:

- **Specificity**—The ability to distinguish between different pathogens
- **Memory**—The ability to mount a quick response to pathogens that are similar to previous pathogens
- **Mobility**—The ability of a local reaction to produce systemic effects
- **Replication**—The ability to reproduce cellular components of the immune system to amplify its response
- **Redundancy**—The ability to produce components with the same effect from multiple origins

The body's first line of defense against invading pathogens includes the skin, mucus, saliva, normal bacterial flora, the acidic environment of the stomach, and the flushing effect of tears, urination, diarrhea, vomiting, coughing, and sneezing. A disruption in normal body defenses can allow penetration by a pathogen.

The immune system is the body's defense mechanism. It helps protect the body against invading pathogens.
© auremar/ShutterStock, Inc.

An **antigen** is any substance or pathogen that elicits the immune system to produce an antibody. An **antibody** is a Y-shaped protein that identifies and neutralizes pathogens. The human body can respond to an antigen in many different ways.

If pathogens penetrate the body's first line of defense, the body will initiate an immune response. After an immune response is initiated, either from exposure to an invading pathogen or to a vaccine designed to stimulate the immune system, active immunity is developed. Active immunity means the immune system will be able to fight the same pathogen quickly on the next exposure. Passive immunity is the acquisition of antibodies without the immune system mounting a response. It does not confer lifelong protection, but provides defense until the host's own immune system can produce antibodies.

The lymphatic system is the part of the immune system that includes the lymph nodes, the lymphoid organs, and a network of vessels that carry lymph. The lymphatic system carries proteins and fluid that have leaked out of the circulatory system back to the blood. It also carries fat and fat-soluble vitamins absorbed from the gastrointestinal tract to the circulating blood.

Sensory Systems

There are five major senses: sight, hearing, touch, taste, and smell. Equilibrium is another sense; it is associated with the sense of hearing and plays a major role in our ability to maintain balance. The organs associated with these senses include the eyes, ears, skin, tongue, and nose.

The Eyes

As one of the five sensors of the body, the eyes perceive images and translate them into impulses. Each area of the eye has a specific function that works to protect it, maintain it, and enhance vision. Each eye is housed in a bony socket called the **orbit**. Covering the eyes are the eyelids. The eyelids are composed of four individual layers: the outer skin, the muscles, the connective tissue, and the conjunctiva. The **conjunctiva** is a thin mucous membrane that covers the inner surface of the eyelid and the **sclera**. The **cornea** is the clear, dome-shaped surface that covers the front of the eye and allows light into the eye for visual acuity. The **iris** filters light and is responsible for the color of the eye. The **retina** is the light-sensitive layer of tissue at the back of the eye that contains the nerve endings that transmit electrical impulses to the brain **FIGURE 3.21**.

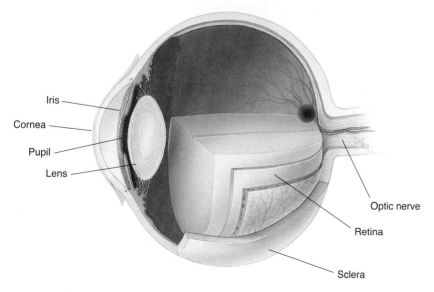

FIGURE 3.21 Anatomy of the eye.
© Jones & Bartlett Learning

Practice defining a word associated with the eyes. Try breaking down the term conjunctivitis. Start with the suffix, -itis, meaning "inflammation." Next, identify the prefix. In this case, there is no prefix. Finally, identify the word root or combining form, conjunctiv/o, meaning "conjuctiva." Putting it all together, the definition is "inflammation of the conjunctiva (mucous membrane around the eye)."

The Ears

The ears are responsible for hearing and maintaining balance. Each ear is composed of three sections: the external ear, middle ear, and inner ear. The external ear is composed of cartilage and skin. It transmits sound waves to the middle ear and protects the middle ear from foreign objects. The middle ear transmits sound waves that enter this cavity to the inner ear. As sound waves enter the inner ear, the inner ear transmits impulses to the brain. The inner ear also provides information to the brain about the orientation of the body at rest and when in motion, thus helping maintain balance and equilibrium **FIGURE 3.22**.

Practice defining a word associated with the ears. Try breaking down the term audiologist. Start with the suffix, -logist, meaning "one who studies." Next, identify the prefix. In this case, there is no prefix. Finally, identify the word root or combining form, audi/o, meaning "sound or hearing." Putting it all together, the definition is "one who studies sound or hearing."

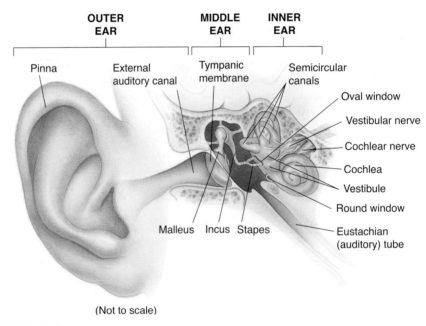

(Not to scale)

FIGURE 3.22 Anatomy of the ear.
© Jones & Bartlett Learning

WRAP UP

Chapter Summary

- Most medical terms are derived from Greek or Latin.

- A prefix is a word part found at the beginning of a word. It modifies the word root. It often indicates location, presence or absence, size, frequency, quantity, or position.

- A suffix is a word part found at the end of a word. It completes the word root. It often indicates a procedure, disease, condition, or disorder. Some suffixes are also words that stand alone, but when attached to a word root can provide more specificity.

- Combining forms are word roots that have a vowel added to the end of the word root to help in connecting suffixes or other word roots and combining forms.

- Dissecting a medical term is a good way to learn about its meaning. To break down or build a medical term, start with the suffix, then identify the prefix, and finally determine the word root or combining form.

- The study of the human body can be divided into two parts: anatomy and physiology. Anatomy is the study of the structures of the human body and its organs. Physiology is the study of the function and physical and chemical processes that take place in cells, tissues, and organs.

- Anatomic position describes the body when standing erect, with arms down at the sides, and with the palms of the hands facing forward. Anatomic directional terms describe the position of structures relative to other structures or locations in the body.

- A body can be divided into four planes (coronal or frontal, sagittal or lateral, axial or transverse, and median) by drawing an imaginary line through the side of the body from the top of the head to the feet and by drawing a horizontal line across the body.

- The body is divided into cavities or spaces that contain the internal organs or viscera. The two main cavities are the posterior or dorsal cavity and the anterior or ventral cavity. The ventral cavity is the larger cavity and is subdivided into two parts (thoracic and abdominopelvic) by the diaphragm. The lower part of the abdominopelvic cavity can be further subdivided into two parts: an upper abdominal portion and a lower pelvic portion.

- The cell is the basic building block of the human body. Cells organize to become tissues and tissues form organs. Organs work together and collectively form organ systems. Each organ system works to carry out specific and complex bodily functions. Systems are the most complex components of the human body.

- The integumentary system is composed of the skin, hair, nails, and glands. The skin is the largest organ of the human body. It is the body's first line of defense and acts as a barrier, protecting the body from chemical, physical, and microbial injury.

- This musculoskeletal system consists of bones and the tissues that connect them, such as tendons, ligaments, and cartilage. The skeletal system provides support for the human body.

- The cardiovascular system, sometimes called the circulatory system, includes the heart and blood vessels. The cardiovascular system plays a vital role in maintaining homeostasis.

- The respiratory system works with the circulatory system to provide oxygen and to remove the waste products of metabolism. It also helps to regulate the pH of the blood. It is composed of the nose and nasal cavities, pharynx, larynx, trachea, bronchial tree, and lungs.

- The gastrointestinal (GI) system breaks down food and fluids into small compounds that can be readily absorbed into the bloodstream and used by the body for energy production, for protein synthesis, and as enzymes for essential metabolic reactions. The four main functions of the GI system are digestion, absorption, metabolism, and excretion.

- The renal or urinary system maintains the body's balance of water, salts, and acids by removing excess fluids from the body or reabsorbing water as needed. It filters the blood to remove urea and other waste products from the bloodstream, converts these waste products and excess fluids into urine, and excretes them from the body via the bladder. The renal system is composed of two kidneys, two ureters, one bladder, and one urethra.

- The central nervous system (CNS) is the body's control center and includes the brain and spinal cord.

- The endocrine system is a system of glands that produce and secrete hormones. These hormones, or chemical messengers, are released directly into the bloodstream. They regulate mood, growth and development, tissue function, metabolism, sexual function, and reproduction.

- The reproductive system's function is to ensure survival of the species. The reproductive system has four main functions: to produce egg and sperm cells, to transport these cells, to develop offspring, and to produce hormones. There are separate reproductive systems for the male and female.

- There are five major senses: sight, hearing, touch, taste, and smell. Equilibrium is another sense; it is associated with the sense of hearing and plays a major role in our ability to maintain balance. The organs associated with these senses include the eyes, ears, skin, tongue, and nose.

Learning Assessment Questions

1. In the term bradycardia, what part of the word is the prefix?
   A. Cardia
   B. Brady
   C. Brad
   D. There is no prefix in this word.

2. In the term dysmenorrhea, what part of the word is the suffix?
   A. Rrhea
   B. Dys
   C. Meno
   D. There is no suffix in this word.

3. In the term endocarditis, what does the prefix endo mean?
   A. Outside
   B. Heart
   C. Inflammation
   D. Within

4. Which of the following is the correct medical term for "pertaining to above the stomach"?
   A. Hypogastric
   B. Epigastric
   C. Endogastric
   D. Gastric

5. Which of the following is the foundation of the word that identifies the structure or anatomy being described?
   A. Prefix
   B. Word root
   C. Suffix
   D. Combining form

6. Most often, the combining form ends with which of the following vowels: a, o, or i?
   A. A
   B. O
   C. I
   D. All of the above

7. Which of the following is the word root that has a vowel added to the end of the word root to help in connecting suffixes or other word roots and combining forms?
   A. Combining form
   B. Prefix
   C. Suffix
   D. Verb

8. Which of the following describes the body when standing erect, with arms down at the sides, and with the palms of hands facing forward?
   A. Frontal position
   B. Anatomic position
   C. Caudal position
   D. Coronal position

9. Which of the following is the study of the structures of the human body and its organs?
   A. Biology
   B. Chemistry
   C. Physiology
   D. Anatomy

10. Which of the following anatomic directional terms describes a position toward the midline of the body?
    A. Superior
    B. Anterior
    C. Medial
    D. Posterior

11. Which of the following anatomic directional terms describes a position toward the head of the body?
    A. Superior
    B. Anterior
    C. Posterior
    D. Lateral

12. Which of the following describes a vertical plane running from front to back?
    A. Coronal
    B. Sagittal
    C. Axial
    D. Medial

13. Which of the following describes a horizontal plane that divides the body or any of its parts into upper and lower parts?
    A. Coronal
    B. Sagittal
    C. Axial
    D. Medial

14. The integumentary system is composed of which of the following?
    A. Skin
    B. Hair
    C. Nails
    D. All of the above

15. The musculoskeletal system is composed of which of the following?
    A. Tendons
    B. Hair
    C. Stomach
    D. Lungs

16. The respiratory system is composed of which of the following?
    A. Trachea
    B. Larynx
    C. Pharynx
    D. All of the above

17. Which of the following body systems is the body's control center and includes the brain and spinal cord?
    A. Integumentary system
    B. Cardiovascular system
    C. Respiratory system
    D. Central nervous system

18. Which of the following body systems regulates mood, growth and development, tissue function, metabolism, sexual function, and reproduction?
    A. Integumentary system
    B. Endocrine system
    C. Respiratory system
    D. Reproductive system

19. Which of the following body systems is composed of two kidneys, two ureters, one bladder, and one urethra?
    A. Endocrine system
    B. Reproductive system
    C. Renal system
    D. Digestive system

20. Which of the following body systems is primarily responsible for digestion, absorption, metabolism, and excretion?

    A. Integumentary system

    B. Endocrine system

    C. Digestive system

    D. Reproductive system

21. Match the following medical terms:

    A. -stasis   1. stopping

    B. -pnea   2. vomiting

    C. -uria   3. paralysis

    D. -emesis   4. breath or breathing

    E. -plegia   5. abnormally fast

    F. iso-   6. between

    G. micro-   7. urine

    H. tachy-   8. small

    I. brady-   9. slow

    J. inter-   10. same

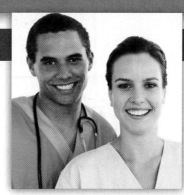

Communications: Medical Records and Documentation

OBJECTIVES

After reading this chapter, you will be able to:

- Identify the importance of communication.
- Understand the four basic elements of the communication cycle.
- Describe the four modes or channels of communication most pertinent in everyday exchanges.
- Discuss the importance of active listening in therapeutic communication.
- Identify the difference between verbal and nonverbal communication.
- Recognize the following body-language or nonverbal communication behaviors: facial expressions, personal space, position, posture, gestures/mannerisms, and touch.
- Discuss generalizations of cultural/religious effects on health care.
- Discuss the use of Maslow's hierarchy of needs in therapeutic communication.
- Compare and contrast cross-cultural concerns between patients and providers.
- Display cultural awareness.
- Identify the components of the medical health history and their documentation.
- Restate the function and meaning of SOAP/SOAPER and CHEDDAR documentation.
- Identify three areas of concern regarding HIPAA compliance and the patient's chart.
- Recall the rules for documentation and documenting in the patient's chart.
- List the advantages of electronic health records.
- Recall common documentation abbreviations.
- Describe the organization of a medical record.
- Mark on the schedule the arrival, registration, and admittance for patient appointments.
- Update registration information when a patient checks in.

- Record laboratory test orders in a patient record.
- Send laboratory test orders to the provider for approval.
- Upload the results of laboratory tests to a patient record.
- Schedule return appointments at the conclusion of the visit.

KEY TERMS

Acculturation	Electronic health record	Personal space
Active listening	(EHR)	Posture
Body language	Family history	Present illness
Certification Commission	Feedback	Receiver
for Healthcare	Five Cs of	Review of systems (ROS)
Information	communication	Scribe
Technology	Gestures and	Sender
(CCHIT)	mannerisms	SOAP method
CHEDDAR method	Hierarchy of needs	Social history
Chief complaint	Kinesics	Therapeutic
Chronological order	Medical history	communication
Communication	Medical transcriptionist	Touch
Culture	Message	Verbal communication
Dictate	Nonverbal	
Documentation	communication	

Chapter Overview

Communication and how people relate to each other during that process is one of the most important aspects of delivering competent, professional, and quality care to patients. Communication is defined as the act of transmitting information—an exchange of information between individuals using a common system of signs, symbols, or behavior.

Considering the communication problems that can arise from organizational and interpersonal contact, medical assistants should be aware that how they react and interact can have a direct relation to the patient's perception of the practice. Knowing the culture of your business will help you determine the type of communication and communication styles to use. What type of impression is your practice trying to make? Studies have shown that patients form an opinion of the practice in the first four minutes of contact. This is particularly important to keep in mind, as patients who are not happy with their treatment by the staff or physician will be more likely to share that information with others, making it difficult to attract new patients in the future. Physical appearance and dress are important, as are your attitude, degree of compassion, and a smile. Communication and attitude are everything. Your patients and employer will feel your genuine positive attitude.

The mastery of clinical and administrative skills will account for only 30 percent of what is necessary to be successful in your career. The other 70 percent of career success relates to your ability to provide service to patients and your applied communication skills.

Two major points of effective communication and service to patients can be defined as follows:

- The patient always comes first.
- The patient needs are satisfied.

The healthcare team must communicate effectively and efficiently to provide vital information during and after the decision-making processes for providers and patients alike. Working together using **verbal communication** (spoken words) and/or **nonverbal communication** (facial expressions, body movements, etc.) helps to provide the patient with the best possible quality health care and allows meaningful communication.

A medical assistant should be sensitive to and acknowledge cultural differences and religious beliefs when providing care to patients. For example, although touch may be accepted in some cultures, in others it is not. Keeping these issues in mind when working with patients from different cultures will improve the chances of effectively communicating and providing the patient with the best level of care.

Not all patients will be receptive to all types of communication and may have different needs depending on their psychological stability. Many patients have different ways of coping and dealing with stress when faced with a medical issue. Some patients may feel very ill when they visit the physician. Others may be upset and worried about impending test results. It is important for medical assistants to recognize psychological elements in their daily routine of working with patients.

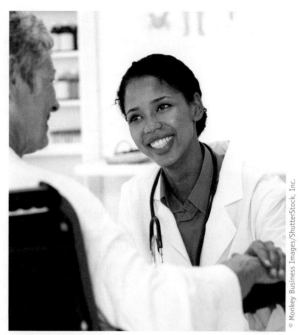

Communication and how people relate to each other during that process is one of the most important aspects of delivering competent, professional, and quality care to patients.

Another form of communication that the medical assistant must master is the art of documentation in the patient's record. In medicine, **documentation** is the act or an instance of supplying documents or supporting references of record. Medical records are legal documents, providing complete accounts of a patient's medical care and treatment. The patient's condition along with any changes that occur, medical history, evaluations, testing, and other pertinent information must be accurate when documented in the patient's chart. Healthcare providers make vital decisions based on the information contained in the patient's medical record. If an entry in the patient's record was omitted or an error occurred during documentation, the validity and accuracy of the patient's chart would not only be questioned, but may lead to positive judgment for the plaintiff if legal action were ever taken.

Over the years, the use of electronic health records (EHRs) has increased over paper documentation due to HIPAA compliance, patient continuity of care standards, and recent stimulus programs from the federal government. EHRs have proven to greatly improve the flow of information between providers, healthcare professionals, insurance carriers, and patients.

Preparing for the patient's office encounter is an important function that the medical assistant will most likely be responsible for managing throughout his or her workday. In medicine, not everything runs on time, even when the best plans are followed. But by using methods to control the flow of patients by proper scheduling, managing documents, and using effective time management, the healthcare team will have the essential tools to enhance patient care, increase compliance standards, and provide a strong anchor to a professional, competent practice.

The phrase "If it isn't documented, it wasn't done" in risk management reminds providers and healthcare professionals to document all interactions with patients regarding their medical care and treatment.

Communication and Its Role in the Healthcare Profession

Communication is key for any profession, but for medical professionals and their patients, it can mean the difference between life and death. This is just one of the many reasons effective communication is vital among the healthcare team and the patient. As a trained medical assistant, your ability to effectively communicate with other members of the healthcare team and with patients will set you apart from others in the field. In many accredited medical assisting programs, emphasis is placed not only on communication among patients and the healthcare team, but also on the extensive theories and principles behind law and ethics, verbal communication, nonverbal communication, clinical instruction, and the psychology behind each category. This enables the medical assistant to become a well-rounded health professional who is in tune with the care of the patient, which prepares him or her to deal with and communicate with all types of patients from different backgrounds and cultures.

One important style of communication is therapeutic communication. **Therapeutic communication** emphasizes empathy, enabling patients to feel a sense of comfort when faced with frightening news or feelings of apprehension with regard to healthcare information relayed to them. Patients will often look to the medical assistant for reassurance when faced with questions about the provider and the care that they will receive. Medical assistants can use specific therapeutic communication techniques throughout their careers. For a medical assistant, one of the most important skills in communicating with patients is the ability to develop a level of therapeutic communication after many years of experience.

In an optimal scenario, team members commit themselves to respectful and professional communication in a variety of forms and settings, allowing optimal care and compassion for their patients and coworkers alike.

Four Basic Elements in the Communication Cycle

For communication to occur, there must an exchange of information between at least two individuals, formally referred to as a sender and receiver. The actual cycle of communication includes four basic elements **FIGURE 4.1** :

- Sender
- Message and channel/mode of communication
- Receiver
- Feedback

The **sender** is the first part of the communication cycle and begins by creating or encoding whatever message will be sent. This is an important part of the cycle in which there should be some thought and care to form the message. Also, before actually forming the message, the person sending the message must determine whether the receiver will be able to understand and interpret the message and mode of communication to be used.

In the second part of communication, the **message** is formed, with the content varying in terms of complexity depending on the receiver's ability to understand the message. For instance, someone who has limited understanding of the English language may need for the message to be simplified in order to communicate with the sender. Another example may be a patient or a family member who is in shock or stressed due to health concerns; he or she may not be able to concentrate on the message at hand. Other ways of communicating messages may require a special skill, such as sign language or Braille.

Within the message part of the communication cycle are four subcategories that pertain to channels of communication:

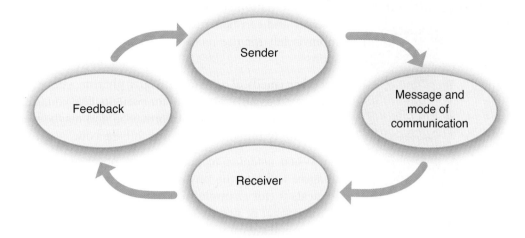

FIGURE 4.1 The four basic elements in the communication cycle.
© Jones & Bartlett Learning

- Speaking
- Listening
- Gestures or body language
- Writing

All of these will vary by the individual, his or her culture, his or her education, his or her life experiences, and how he or she feels about others and himself or herself as individuals. When considering the message and what channel of communication to use, the medical assistant must consider all these factors.

After the sender has formatted the message, the communication is sent to the receiver. The **receiver** is the person or persons who receive the message. In verbal communication, to interpret the message being sent, the receiver needs to listen to and concentrate on the message, aware not only of what is being spoken but also the tone, pitch, and rate of speech.

The last part of the communication cycle takes place when the receiver has interpreted the message and gives **feedback**, allowing the sender an opportunity to clarify any questions or misunderstandings about the original message sent by the sender.

In feedback, a vital part in that part of the cycle is listening. Being a good listener or being generally "in tune" regardless of whether the communication occurs verbally or nonverbally, is key in giving appropriate feedback. One method of listening is **active listening**, in which the receiver rewords the original message to verify the message from the sender. For a medical assistant, part of active listening is being aware of what a patient *isn't* saying by picking up on hints or observing body language that relays a different message from the one originally sent. Consider an example of a conversation between a patient and a medical assistant such as the following:

Sender (patient): Dr. Jones told me I have to take this medication every day without missing a dose, but I don't know if I can if my insurance doesn't cover it.

Receiver (medical assistant): Are you worried about not being able to afford the medication?

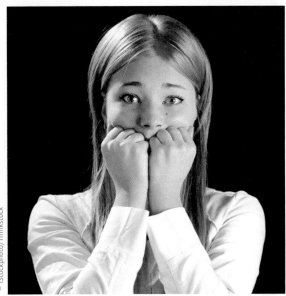

Tone of voice, gestures, and facial expressions are just some nonverbal ways that we communicate with others.

When a situation such as this one presents itself to the receiver and can be verified with the sender's message, room is left for the receiver to form a therapeutic response.

Receiver (medical assistant): Many pharmaceutical companies have programs for patients like you. Let me get some additional information and maybe we can apply for some assistance to help you.

When listening to patients, it is never appropriate to agree to lie to the physician, even when the patient requests it (for example, you notice a pack of cigarettes in the pocket of a patient who was just discharged from the hospital after undergoing open-heart surgery, and he asks you not to tell the physician that you've seen them). Even a small piece of information that is withheld from the provider can completely change the plan of treatment for the patient. If you are faced with this dilemma, you should remind the patient that you are bound to the rules of ethics within the office.

Verbal and Nonverbal Communication and the Differences Between Them

There are different types of communication that we engage in as individuals every day. Our tone of voice, body movements and gestures, facial expressions, and touch are just some ways that we communicate with others. Communication can be also categorized as positive or negative. Think about a form of negative nonverbal communication. What does it say to a person who is speaking when the other rolls his or her eyes?

Learning the different types of verbal and nonverbal communication is important for the medical assistant for working with patients and staff in the medical field. As a medical professional, you may need to pick up on certain clues during your interactions with patients and relay them to the provider in order for the provider to make an informed decision and plan of treatment for the patient.

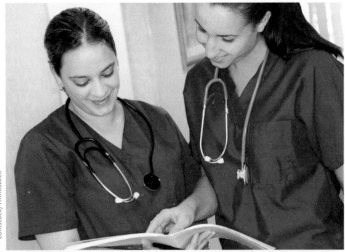

Learning different types of verbal and nonverbal communication is important for the medical assistant for working with patients and staff in the medical field.

Verbal communication takes place when a message is spoken. For verbal communication to be effective, both the sender and the receiver must use words that can be understood and both must perceive those words as having the same meaning; otherwise, the message will be misunderstood. You should be careful to enunciate your words. Also, the tone of your voice can completely change the message you are trying to send. Some factors that may positively influence verbal communication are being friendly, being warm and attentive, keeping eye contact with the person with whom you are communicating, listening carefully, and smiling. Examples of negative communication are mumbling, interrupting the patient, rushing through explanations, showing boredom, and forgetting common courtesies such as "please" and "thank you." Medical assistants should use the **five Cs of communication** to enable a positive exchange of information between parties:

What Would You Do?

A patient just finished a visit with a physician, who just prescribed a medication that needs to be taken at the same time every day without missing a dose. If the patient does not take the medication as prescribed, there is a potential for overdose and possible death. During the visit, the patient seemed fine and did not present any unusual issues. While leaving the office, you as the medical assistant noticed that the patient had a troubled look on her face on her way out to her car and appeared lost. The patient could not find her car in a parking lot with approximately 20 cars, where she parked less than one hour ago. What would you do?

© auremar/ShutterStock, Inc.

- **Complete**—The message must be complete, with all the information given.
- **Clear**—Clear information must be communicated to the patient to enable the patient to process and understand the meaning of the message. The patient should also be able to hear the message in order to understand it.
- **Concise**—When speaking to the patient, the message should be brief and to the point, with no unnecessary information. Avoid technical medical jargon when speaking to the patient to eliminate confusion.
- **Cohesive**—A logical and organized message should be delivered to the patient. The message should not be confusing, with information jumping from one subject to another.
- **Courteous**—Important in all aspects of communication, courtesy should always be shown to the patient. Greeting the patient with a smile, asking if the patient has any further questions during instructions/orders, and offering to assist the patient with any difficulties during ambulation will show the patient that you support and care for him or her, building a rapport between you, the office, and the patient.

Nonverbal communication is one of the most important forms of communication. Nonverbal communication accounts for 70 percent of a message's impact. The tone of the voice communicates about 23 percent, with the last 7 percent being just spoken word. Nonverbal communication can include body language, gestures, and mannerisms that may or may not be in agreement with the way the person is speaking. A person's facial expression can also change the message that is conveyed. **Body language** is defined as the unconscious body movements, gestures, and facial expressions that accompany speech. The study of body language is called kinesics. **Kinesics** catalogues these movements and attempts to define their meaning. Each culture is believed to possess a separate "language" of kinesics.

In nonverbal communication, a facial impression or expression is considered one of the most important observed factors. Consider something as simple as a frown or a smile. A smile conveys an approachable person, while a frown says "stay away." The eyes are considered the windows to a person's soul. Eye contact is another factor that may or may not give clues to the needs of patients, but may be considered impolite in certain cultures. As children, we were taught to never stare or point at others. In most Western cultures, a lack of eye contact when speaking to an individual is perceived as rude and disinterested. In other cultures, however, prolonged eye contact is considered rude and obtrusive. In addition to the patient's culture, the patient's eye contact may be influenced by his or her personality (shy versus outgoing),

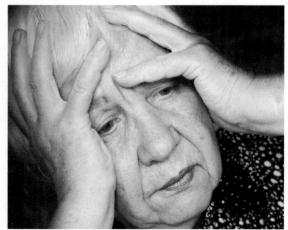

In nonverbal communication, a person's facial expression is one of the most important factors to observe.

© Oleg Golovnev/ShutterStock, Inc

nervousness, and emotional state as well as various medical conditions and health. As a medical assistant, you should never stare at a patient who may have different looks or needs when presenting to the office. The patient will be made uncomfortable, may feel dehumanized, and therefore is less likely to become a lifelong patient of the practice.

Another cultural and personal aspect of nonverbal communication is personal space. **Personal space** refers to the physical distance at which we feel comfortable from others while communicating. Personal space may sometimes be defined by individuals depending on the situation at hand. When attending a large concert in a small venue, you may be uncomfortable with the lack of personal space with strangers, but have no issues with friends in the same personal space. In the United States, personal space is defined normally by these space parameters:

- Intimate: touching to $1\frac{1}{2}$ feet
- Personal: $1\frac{1}{2}$ to 4 feet
- Social: 4 to 12 feet (this is most often observed)
- Public: 12 to 15 feet

Many times, you may hear "Keep out of my personal space" when working with another student or coworker on a project. This statement directly informs you that the other person feels uncomfortable and considers that space to be his own and does not want it violated. In other cultures, such as in China, crowding is viewed as a sign of warmth and intimacy, and it is not uncommon to define personal space at $1\frac{1}{2}$ to 2 feet. When meeting strangers, the distance is a little greater. It is also not uncommon for women to hold hands or link arms together while walking.

Also important is **posture**, which relates to the position of the body or parts of the body. A person who kicks back and puts his or her feet up on the desk may be very comfortable with his or her position of power or the person with whom he or she is engaged in conversation. Other examples are arm or leg crossings. Crossed arms during a conversation may indicate a closed opinion of the subject or an opinionated nature. Sometimes, a person who is angry or upset may cross his or her arms, showing displeasure in the conversation at hand.

When working with patients and others in the healthcare field, your position relative to the other person and can generate ease and a feeling of comfort. A grown adult standing over a small child can be very intimidating and threatening. As a medical assistant working with small children, it is best to get to their level, sometimes sitting beside them or bending down to speak to them in a nonthreatening manner.

A form of body language in which we "talk" with our hands can be defined as using **gestures and mannerisms**. This can be useful by emphasizing ideas, but can also be overused and irritating if not watched carefully. For instance, tapping your fingers and fidgeting may relay nervousness, clenching your fist may signify anger, and shrugging your shoulders may relay a feeling of indifference or lack of caring.

Touch communicates many different things. As a health professional, it is appropriate for you to use touch with patients as long as you use well-defined boundaries and good judgment. For example, a patient may need assistance with dressing before or after an exam, making it necessary to help with undergarments, etc. Another example is a patient who may be anxious or afraid during a procedure, in which case you may need to give reassurance by touching or holding his or her hand. Touch invades a person's personal space; as such, the medical assistant should always take into consideration the patient's culture and personality. Most patients understand that as a health professional, it is required that you touch them if doing so is related to their care. By explaining what type of touching is required verbally throughout a procedure, you allow the patient to understand what will happen and become more at ease. You must exercise sensitivity and special consideration with individuals who voice a concern over being touched or who have experienced violations in the past, such as child abuse, domestic abuse, or sexual assault.

Medical assistants should remember that many varied nonverbal cues can be used, but that a patient's culture may dictate how that patient should be approached. When it is necessary to touch the patient in order to perform a procedure, the medical assistant must be aware of his or her actions and communication, both verbal and nonverbal.

Cultural and Religious Factors That Affect Health Care

Healthcare providers in the United States have seen an increased need to understand the cultural and religious factors that could contribute to the effectiveness of a patient's care. Therapeutic effects can be compromised in certain religious cultures due to their members' beliefs. For example, followers of some religions do not believe in accepting blood for transfusions. This not only affects their health care should a transfusion be needed, but presents an ethical dilemma for the healthcare provider as well. It is important to recognize some of the factors that may influence a patient's decision on health care for himself or herself or for his or her family.

The medical assistant and other healthcare professionals should recognize and accept the diversity of others to improve health care and therapeutic communication with the patient. **Culture** is the customary beliefs, social norms, and material traits of a racial, religious, or social group **TABLE 4.1**. **Acculturation** is the process by which

Table 4.1 Ways in Which Cultural and Religious Factors Can Affect Health Care	
American/Western Culture	**Non-Western Culture**
Beliefs	
Being healthy means being free of disease.	Health is due to harmony, good luck, and reward.
Patients seek health care for treatment and prevention.	Patients seek medical attention for disease and illness.
Time is very important; to be late is impolite.	Time is flexible.
Being on a first-name basis builds rapport with a person.	Greeting a person by his or her first name is disrespectful.
Eye contact indicates respect and attentiveness.	Eye contact may be seen as disrespectful.
Many gestures have universal meanings.	Gestures may have a specific meaning (for example, a bow from a Japanese person).
The individual is the focus of healthcare decision making.	Family is the focus of healthcare decisions.
Direct communication prevents miscommunication.	Directness can indicate conflict.
Nuclear family bonds are important (wife/ husband/brother/sister).	Respect for authority and elders is important.
Values	
Independence over freedom.	Group acceptance.
Youth over elderly.	Family needs are more important than individual needs.
Individual interests.	Family networks and nuclear family are important.
Looking forward to the future, not just present.	Oriented to present, not future.

we learn the rules and values of our society. Self-esteem can sometimes play into the cultural factors affecting a patient's health care and status. An unemployed man who is seen as the head of the household in his culture could easily become depressed and withdrawn. The patient may not wish to proceed with any plans for future health care due to his economic stature and worries.

Being part of the healthcare team, it is important for the medical assistant to be aware of cultural diversity (which also includes race, gender, sexual orientation, age, disability, and social economic status) when performing duties. A general concept of cultures, how patients identify themselves, and a respect for others' individuality will enable the healthcare team to provide the best possible health care for its patients.

Therapeutic Communication Needs in Maslow's Hierarchy of Needs

Abraham Maslow is considered the founder of humanistic psychology and is best known for his **hierarchy of needs** **FIGURE 4.2**. The basic principle of the pyramid of needs is the theory that a person must satisfy one level of need before he or she can move on to the next. For example, on the bottom of the pyramid, the basic needs are air, water, sleep, and food. For a person to have his or her physiological needs met, he or she must have access to these. If these needs aren't being met, it would be very hard for the person to move on to the next level, which is security—finding a home, a job, and money.

There are five different levels in Maslow's hierarchy of needs:

- **Physiological**—These needs include air, water, sleep, and food.
- **Security**—Security needs include a home, a job, and money.
- **Social**—Social needs include acceptance, love, and friendship.
- **Esteem**—There are two types of esteem needs. The first is self-esteem, which results from competence/mastery of a task. The second is attention and recognition from others.
- **Self-actualization**—To be self-actualized is to become everything you are capable of becoming. Self-actualized people can maximize their potential. They can seek knowledge, peace, self-fulfillment, oneness in a religion, etc.

When a person finds a level of security and safety, he or she can feel a sense of belonging and love, and can give and receive affection. Helping us to manage this need

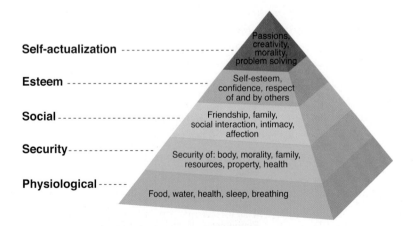

FIGURE 4.2 Maslow's hierarchy of needs is usually represented by this pyramid.
© Jones & Bartlett Learning

is connecting with others by being with family and friends, joining groups and organizations, and belonging to different groups in society.

The fourth level in this pyramid is esteem, which refers to a need for respect for ourselves and by others. When we satisfy these needs through recognition, status, or reputation, we have a feeling of self-confidence and self-worth.

The final level is self-actualization, in which we find our true calling—doing what fits us and makes us happy. This is the peak of the pyramid, when we've met all our needs. A person can rise and fall up and down in his or her needs depending on the circumstances.

Cross-Cultural Concerns for Patients and Healthcare Professionals

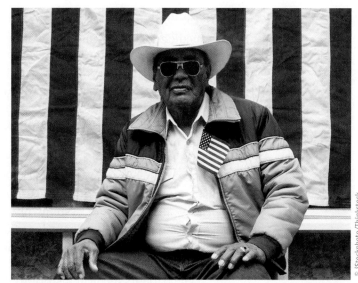

Healthcare professionals need to be aware of cultural concerns when interacting with their patients.

It is important for the medical assistant to understand that some patients may have different expectations with respect to their encounters with their provider. Some problems can occur with patients who feel they did not receive the care they expected, and interpret that as discrimination against foreigners or against their gender. Illness perspectives can also play a part, with some patients afraid to share information that may cause providers to diagnose them with a psychological illness or to share information that may cause others to ridicule them.

People in different cultures may also have different views on time. For example, some patients of different cultures may not understand the importance of arriving at their appointment on time. Knowing that patients communicate in different styles and have different perspectives on their health care will help heighten the awareness of potential communication pitfalls that the healthcare professional may encounter and help prevent them if possible.

Some cross-cultural considerations include the following:

- Having an awareness of potential sources of misunderstanding. Perspectives can lead to communication pitfalls. When possible, the healthcare provider should try to understand the patient's specific cultural beliefs.

- Having an awareness and knowledge of the patient's country of origin (politics, geography, religion). Showing interest and asking questions about the patient's country of origin will help to establish rapport.

- Recognizing difficulties in translating words and language. It is very difficult to translate medical concepts and terms. Less technical language is better when there is a language deficiency.

- Adapting to the patient's communication style. With many patients, closed questioning styles can be very difficult. A narrative approach is preferable—for example, encouraging the patient to offer any information that he or she feels is pertinent with the provider taking into consideration who is telling the story, who is hearing the story, and how the story or complaint is being relayed. This helps with therapeutic communication and improves the quality of information that is provided by patients.

Medical Health History and Purpose for Documentation

In medicine, the patient's medical history is the basis for all treatment by any and all of his or her medical providers. It is very important for the patient to answer questions truthfully when his or her medical history is being gathered so that the physician may make an informed decision regarding care.

Health history questionnaires normally ask for personal demographic data (such as date of birth, home address, phone numbers, Social Security information, marital status, employment information, and emergency contact information), the reason the patient has scheduled a visit with the provider (chief complaint), the patient's present illness, any medications or herbal supplements currently being used, allergies, medical history, family history, social history (smoking, alcohol, use of drugs), occupational history, and reviews of systems prepared by another physician or provider. Medical histories also contain a base for statistical data that is used for insurance analysis, research, and required information when necessary for state and local health departments or for criminal investigations.

The patient's medical history, in the patient's chart, is considered a legal document. It is essential that it reflect a concise and complete record of the patient's health. If information is missing or incorrect, medical and legal ramifications may arise that could easily have been avoided if proper documentation had been observed. The adage, "If it's not written, it didn't happen," holds true. The best policy is to write everything down concerning the patient and his or her care.

The medical assistant may be called upon to review and/or obtain the patient's information when the patient presents to the office or the provider for the first time. Many providers require patients to fill out in-depth questionnaires at home or in person prior to their office visit, procedure, or surgery. Questions asked in medical history questionnaires are very sensitive in nature, and patients' responses should be treated with respect. Be aware that some patients may not understand the questionnaires and may require assistance to answer the questions accurately.

Documentation in the Medical Record and Understanding Key Sections

Each physician and practice may have a preferred method of documentation in patients' records. As technology in medicine grows, different variations appear, with others losing favor over newer, more efficient, and less costly techniques to create an accurate, legal medical record.

Most of the time, the type of documentation used depends on whether your provider/practice uses paper or electronic health records to document in the patient record. In the more traditional paper method, information is gathered in the record by either handwritten or typed notes that the physician or other health professionals create when the patient contacts the office. All contact that is made with the patient via writing, verbal, telephone, online, or through another physician involved in the patient's care should be documented in the patient's chart. These notes are usually kept in **chronological order**, meaning that the most recent set of medical records and information is kept at the top of the chart (or, in an electronic chart, by the most recent date) for easy access, allowing an orderly progression.

In either an electronic or paper chart, errors should be corrected immediately, with dates and initials and the time of the correction being made.
© auremar/ShutterStock, Inc.

Documentation should always be done with care and thought. Make sure information is written legibly, using only standard abbreviations, and recorded accurately. A separate record should be made for each member of the family; it is strongly advised that you not use "family" charts (that is, a single chart for all

Cardiology Center Patient Procedure Chart

Date	Time	Patient	Appointment Type	Prior Balance	Last Visit Date
5/17/2011	3:00PM	Sarah Robinson	Office Visit	$0.00	5/8/2011

Ticket Number	Doctor	Facility	Date of Birth / Age	Prior Diagnosis
C6342	Dr. Longo	New York Medical Center	4/12/1974 37	Cardiac dysrhythmia

Patient ID Number	Responsible Party	Phone Number	
127635	Sarah Robinson	(555) 637-4548	

Sex: M F ✓

Address: 57 Orchard Street   City / State / ZIP: Rochester, NY 14601

Appointment Notes: *Pt. reports irregular heartbeat. EKG to R/O CAD. Schedule follow-up appointment for ~~one week~~. two weeks.*

Current ✓ Over 30 Over 60 Over 90 Over 120

Allocation Type   Financial Class   Social Security Number

Insurance Carrier 1   Insurance Carrier 2   Insurance Carrier 3

Height / Weight

CR 5/17/11 3:35 PM

Procedures

X	Service	Code	Charge	X	Service	Code	Charge
	H&P Low Complexity				Extrem Venous Eval, Low		
	H&P Mod. Complexity				Extrem Venous Eval, Comp		
	H&P High Complexity				Reveal Record Interp.		
	Consultation, Low				Defib Ck, Single, w/o Reprog.		
	Consultation, Med.				Defib Ck, Single, w/ Reprog.		
	Consultation, High				Defib Ck, Dual, w/o Reprog.		
	Office Visit, Minimal				Defib Ck, Dual Reprog.		
	Office Visit, Mod.				Single Pacer Check w/ Reprog.		
	Office Visit, High				Single Pacer Check		
X	EKG	0178T			Dual Pacer Check		
	Stress EKG (w/o Nuc Med)				Dual Pacer Check w. Reprog.		
	Rhythm Strip				Muga Scan		
	Holter Monitor				Cardiolite Stress Test Complete		
	Event Monitor				Adenosine Test, Complete		
	2D Echo w/ Color Doppler				Dobutamine Test, Complete		
	Codes Types:				Nuc Med Test, Incomplete (specify)		
	Stress Echo				CTA Heart Structure Only		
	Duplex Carotid Eval.				CTA Coronary Only		
	Ankle / Arm Indices (ABI)				CTA Heart & Coronary		
	Low Extrem, Art, Eval				CTA Other		
	Abdominal Ultrasound						

Diagnosis: 1. Cardiac dysrhythmia 2. _____ 3. _____

Next Appointment: 5/31/2011 11:30AM _____

Errors should be corrected immediately with dates, initials, and the time of correction being made.

the members of one family under a physician's care) for confidentiality purposes. Any allergies should be displayed prominently in the patient's chart and on every page of his or her record.

When omissions occur in a patient's records, the best way to handle any documentation after a recorded entry is to note it as an addendum, with the date and time that the addendum was added to the patient's record along with the author's initials. This will alleviate any questions later as to whether the record was altered or tampered with inappropriately.

Any patient's informed consent and/or refusal or unwillingness to act on advice or instructions from the provider should also be documented and signed with an acknowledgment from the ordering physician.

During an actual office exam or procedure, vital signs (temperature, pulse, respiration, and blood pressure) are normally obtained and documented by the medical assistant or other members of the healthcare team prior to the physician's contact with the patient. During the exam, the physician may want to document his or her findings by using a **scribe**, who remains in the exam room during the examination and writes down all information communicated verbatim for transcription later, or by dictating his or her findings into a small handheld digital or tape recording device either in front of the patient or after the visit. For our purposes, the definition of **dictate** is to say or read aloud so that the spoken words can be recorded or written down by someone else. If a recording device is used, the medial assistant or medical transcriptionist will type the information spoken from the physician into a document that becomes a permanent record in the chart. A **medical transcriptionist** is one who transcribes recorded dictation from providers to add patient-based information to medical records.

If an electronic format is used to chart patient information, a scribe may accompany the physician into the room and document his or her findings in an electronic format. Alternatively, in a twist of roles, the physician may chart his or her own findings on a computer using prefilled drop-down menus or templates, or may use digital dictation devices that automatically transcribe the dictation into the patient's chart using software that is compatible with the electronic health record company's format.

It is important for this information to be typed accurately and in a timely manner in the chart after each encounter to ensure quality care. Each and every contact with the patient in either form should be documented for legal as well as medical purposes.

Some of the key sections in a patient's chart are as follows:

- In the **chief complaint** (CC) section of a medical record, the reason the patient needs to be seen by the provider is recorded. This could be something very specific, such as a complaint that the patient makes when presenting to the office. For example, if the patient is asked why he made an appointment, and the patient responds that he has had a "sore throat for the past three days," then "sore throat" would likely be the patient's chief complaint. When working with patients and attempting to define their complaints, the medical assistant should try to record certain characteristics of the patient's complaint to allow the provider a clearer understanding of the patient's condition. These would include the location, severity, associated symptoms, radiation, quality, aggravating factors, alleviating factors, and how frequently the cause for complaint occurs.

- The **present illness** section addresses the chief complaint somewhat by identifying specific characteristics and details such as prior health problems or conditions, what other treatments or medications associated with the complaint have been taken, a list of current medications, and any allergies the patient may have. Using the preceding "sore throat" example, a history of present illness may include information such as "the patient has had a sore throat with fever of 102 degrees for the last three days on the right side, worse than the left. The patient has taken ibuprofen for the sore throat without any relief. The patient states that he has had an increase in a runny nose for the past week but denies any other contributing factors."

- The **medical history** section will include all of the patient's health problems, any major illnesses, childbirth information (if female), immunizations, surgeries, allergies, and any and all current and past medications and reasons if/when they were discontinued. Some physicians may document whether the illness is acute (such as in a sore throat) or chronic (such as a long-term illness like diabetes or heart disease) to monitor the frequency and the category of each episode of illness.

Patients may not be comfortable answering questions or have trouble remembering detailed information in front of the medical assistant or physician. Often, the sensitive and somewhat detailed questions are asked in writing in a questionnaire format at the beginning of the "new patient" intake process along with other paperwork required to establish the patient's care with the provider.

- The patient's **family history** section provides an insight and clues as to the patient's current and past conditions. Parents', grandparents', and siblings' medical history is very important for the provider to determine whether any familial or hereditary diseases exist, such as breast cancer, heart disease, or diabetes, or if there are other contributing aspects of the family history that may affect the patient. Important information such as causes of illness or death for grandparents, parents, and siblings can help the provider pinpoint whether the patient may be at risk for the condition(s) as well.

- The **social history** section includes information about the patient's status (married/single), sexual habits, occupations, hobbies, alcohol use, tobacco use, drug use (or use of any other chemical substances), and home environment. Note: In the case of a minor, the parent or caregiver may be asked to leave the room during this part of the history so that healthcare providers can obtain answers to any questions that the minor may feel uncomfortable answering in front of his or her parents.

- The **review of systems (ROS)** section is documented after the medical history has been taken and the patient is prepared for the medical examination. If there is any missing information or there are questions that you were unable to ask with the patient prior to the exam, a notation should be left for the physician to follow up during the exam. When the patient is with the physician for the physical examination, the ROS is performed. As the physician examines the patient, the physician asks questions and performs a systematic check of all relevant organs and body parts to make a diagnosis. The examination may start at the head and end at the feet. The physician would note any normal or abnormal findings during this exam. After completion, the physician will normally have a good idea of what the patient's condition and probable diagnosis is.

Each and every part of the patient's history and the review of systems are important for the provider to ascertain the most accurate and clinical diagnosis possible, based on the information provided.

In documentation, some common abbreviations can be used to save time and space as well as to document information **TABLE 4.2** . Recently, however, the use of medication abbreviations has been discouraged by many state medical boards and the Joint Commission and should not be used. Prescriptions should be written out in long hand or electronically to avoid any medication errors and enhance patient safety.

Organized Formats in the Medical Record

There are different organized formats for documentation in the patient's medical record. Depending on the provider and the practice, one of these methods may be preferred over another. This section reviews two formats: the SOAP method and the CHEDDAR method.

The SOAP Method

With the **SOAP method**, also referred to as the SOAPER method, you record the results of the patient's exam or his or her progress using a problem-oriented format. The acronyms SOAP and SOAPER stand for the following:

- S is for subjective data. This is obtained from the patient and others close to him.

What Would You Do?

You were working at the office and saw more than 35 patients in one day. In the middle of the night, you awaken and realize that an injection that you gave a patient didn't get recorded in that patient's chart. How would you correct the patient's chart—be it electronic or paper-based—to reflect this change?

© auremar/ShutterStock, Inc.

Table 4.2 Abbreviations Common in Documentation	
Abbreviation	**Meaning**
BP or B/P	Blood pressure
CBC	Complete blood count
CC	Chief complaint
CPE	Complete physical exam
D&C	Dilation and curettage
dx	Diagnosis
ECG, EKG	Electrocardiogram
EEG	Electroencephalogram
ER	Emergency room
GI	Gastrointestinal
GYN	Gynecology
HEENT	Head, eyes, ears, nose, and throat
I&D	Incision and drainage
MI	Myocardial infarction
N&V	Nausea and vomiting
NVD	Nausea, vomiting, and diarrhea
OPD	Outpatient department
OR	Operating room
P	Pulse
PERRLA	Pupils equal, round, reactive to light and accommodation
PT	Physical therapy
R	Respiration
ROM	Range of motion
ROS	Review of systems
SOAP	Subjective, objective, assessment, plan
SOB	Shortness of breath
T	Temperature
T&A	Tonsillectomy and adenoidectomy
URI	Upper respiratory infection
UTI	Urinary tract infection
WNL	Within normal limits
XR	X-ray

- O is for objective data. This is gleaned by observation, the physical exam, and studies performed.
- A is for assessment of the patient. This can be through an analysis of the patient's problem or of his or her status and any changes that have occurred.
- P is for plan. This is the designated plan for the patient.
- E is for education. This refers to measures to educate the patient.
- R is for response. This refers to the response given by the patient to education and the care given.

For example, a patient's physical exam may look as follows:

Jenny Jones, DOB 1/25/1975
Date of Visit: 6/12/2012

- S: Jenny returns today in follow-up from her right otitis media infection two weeks ago. She denies any problems today and states that her pain and earache have cleared up after being on amoxicillin for the past 10 days.
- O: Patient has no fever, blood, or drainage from the right ear.
- A: Right otitis media, resolved.
- P: Patient was advised to call office if she experiences recurring ear pain/ache.
- E: Patient was advised that if this is a continuing recurrent condition, we may order an ENT consult.
- R: Patient understands the above plan for her condition. She states that when she was a younger child, she was under consideration for tympanostomy tubes, but it was not pursued because her issues seemed to have resolved. She will contact the office if this condition returns and reoccurs.

The CHEDDAR Method

The **CHEDDAR method** is very similar to the SOAP method, but normally will be more detailed in nature. The documentation in the CHEDDAR method is more comprehensive, making it easier for the provider to form an opinion when evaluating the patient. The level of detail also improves the management of the levels of service, making it easier to document. The acronym CHEDDAR stands for the following:

- C is for chief complaint. This refers to the patient's chief complaint, subjective information, and presenting problems.
- H is for history. This refers to the social history and to the history of the problem at hand.
- E is for exam. This refers to the exam of the patient.
- D is for details. This refers to the details of the problem and of the patient's complaint.
- D is for drugs and dosages. This refers to the list of current medications and the frequency with which they are taken by the patient.
- A is for assessment. This refers to the patient's diagnosis after the exam and evaluation, plans for further testing, and medication changes.
- R is for return. This refers to the patient's return visit, when necessary.

Following is an example of the CHEDDAR method. Note that the CHEDDAR method is much more detailed in the description and disposition of the patient.

Patient: Jim Jones, DOB 6/1/1952 **Date of Visit:** 6/12/2012
Primary Physician: Dr. Rhonda Brown
CHIEF COMPLAINT (C)

Problems:

1) **Atheromatous coronary disease**
2) **Status post myocardial infarction**
3) **Status post coronary angioplasty**

This 60-year-old male patient first came to attention upon presentation 6/22/2004 at St. Mary's Medical Center with chest pain and acute inferior myocardial infarction. Prior to this the patient has no history of heart disease and no chronic illnesses.

HISTORY (H)

Past Medical History: Except as above, no chronic illnesses.

Family History: The patient has one brother with coronary disease. Father deceased at age 69 from lung cancer. Mother is 85 years old living with Alzheimer's in an extended care facility.

Social History: Nonsmoker and nondrinker. Married and lives with his wife. The patient is working currently as a Certified Public Accountant as a private practitioner.

EXAMINATION (E):

Review of Systems: 10 systems review was unremarkable as follows:

Neurosensory: No change in visual or auditory acuity. No tinnitus or vertigo. Patient denies change in gustatory or olfactory sensation.

Neurologic: No seizures, syncope, headaches, diplopia, or motor abnormality. No abnormalities of speech.

Skin/Integument: No rashes or nonhealing lesions.

Musculoskeletal: No joint deformities, erythema, or swelling.

Endocrine: No polydipsia or polyuria. No unusual intolerance to heat or cold. No major weight change in the recent past six months.

Pulmonary: No pleuritic chest pain, hemoptysis, cough, sputum, or wheezing.

Cardiac: No PND, orthopnea, or DOE. No palpitations or syncope. No chest pain. No peripheral edema.

GI: No nausea or vomiting. No melena or hematochezia. No abdominal pain.

Urologic: No dysuria or hematuria.

Psychiatric: No depression or suicidal ideation.

Physical Examination:

Vital Signs: Height 72 inches, weight 320 pounds, pulse 68, blood pressure 150/80.

HEENT: Anicteric, acyanotic.

Neck: No bruits or thyromegaly.

Lungs: Clear in all fields with bilateral equal chest expansion.

Heart: PMI displaced, quiet precordium, no abnormal lifts or thrills. S1 and S2 single. No murmur, gallop, rub, click, other adventitious sounds. CVP and carotids normal.

Abdomen: Peristaltic sounds normal. Nontender. No hepatosplenomegaly.

Extremities: Arterial pulses normal. No CCE.

DETAILS (D):

The patient was found to have a thrombotic occlusion of the mid LAD coronary artery, 90% stenosis in the diagonal branch, and 80% stenosis in the LCX. He underwent PTCA of the LAD coronary artery (not stented) so as to not occlude the diagonal branch, and had a successful course thereafter. He then underwent elective PTCA of the LCX coronary artery on 9/3/2004 with a drug-eluting stent placed in the LCX. The patient remained asymptomatic thereafter. The patient completed a course of cardiac rehabilitation.

Current Complaints: The patient denies chest pain, nitroglycerin usage, palpitations, syncope, PND, orthopnea, or other symptoms of coronary disease.

4) Hyperlipidemia.

The patient was started on an HMG Co-A reductase inhibitor at the time of his myocardial infarction. His initial lipid profile showed cholesterol 183 and LDL 119. Non-HDL cholesterol was 154, triglycerides 177, and HDL 29.

Current Complaints: The patient denies abdominal pain or nausea, headache, hematuria, or myalgias.

Laboratory:

1) Lipid profile with cholesterol 115 and LDL 44

2) Liver profile normal

3) Cardiolite stress test of 7/1/2009 was normal, with LVEF 60%

4) Echocardiogram with Doppler of 12/5/2007 showed normal LV size, systolic function, and intracardiac valves

5) ECG sinus rhythm, normal

DRUGS AND DOSAGES (D):

Current Medications:

Aspirin 81mg po qd

Crestor 20mg po qd

Toprol XL 50mg po qd

Nitroglycerin 0.4mg sublingual prn (none used).

Multivitamin one po qd

ASSESSMENT (A):

1) Atheromatous coronary disease

2) Status post myocardial infarction, anterior wall

3) Status post two vessel PTCAs, continued success

4) Hyperlipidemia, on treatment, within NCEP/ATP III primary guidelines but with secondary risk factors

5) Hypertension, adequate control, with hypertensive heart disease (LV diastolic dysfunction)

RETURN VISIT (R):

Disposition:

1) No change in medications.

2) EKG, basic metabolic profile, lipid profile, liver profile prior to next office visit.

3) ROV with me in six months.

The medical assistant should be aware of these basic formats and how they are used in medicine to understand the proper channels of documentation in the patient's record.

Electronic Health Records (EHRs)

Electronic health records (EHRs) are secured and stored confidentially and can be printed and viewed in part or in whole by the provider and the staff as necessary. This is a true advantage over a paper chart, which usually is only viewed by one person at a time and can easily become misplaced or lost. The EHR helps with planning and decisions with respect to patient care, as well as any ordered testing, medications, letters or communication between other health providers, and statistic information for local and state health departments and/or insurance analysis.

Many different versions of EHRs are available for providers based on specialty, size, and function. Some EHRs work seamlessly alongside billing and practice-management systems, while others do not. Implementing an EHR system is a very costly and time-consuming task, and should not be entered into quickly or without much investigation.

Certification Commission for Healthcare Information Technology (CCHIT) was developed to enact standards for vendors and their software in the EHR industry and to promote greater speed in adaptation of electronic healthcare information. In general, if the manufacturers meet these standards, the physician and/or facility can be somewhat confident that the software vendor they choose has met the standards required for HIPAA compliance (discussed in the next section) and other federal regulations regarding electronic health records.

HIPAA standards for privacy and security include security controls that dictate that a minimal necessity should be applied to the patient's confidential records, meaning that information should be available only for those who need access to it in the treatment of the patient. For example, a front desk receptionist may have less reason to view certain portions of the patient's medical records than the medical records clerk or physician who is treating the patient. Supersensitive medical records such as psychotherapy notes, HIV status, or mental health records should be segregated from the regular medical record and never sent with a regular release of records or consent.

HIPAA Compliance and the Patient's Chart

HIPAA paved the way for many changes in the way providers and staff communicate with patients, as well as changes required of health insurance carriers. Even though many privacy standards were observed and performed prior to HIPAA, it did establish certain standards for medical records, such as the following:

- Providing security of all electronic health information
- Establishing standards for all electronic health transmission claims
- Controlling and maintaining the privacy and security of private health information

Healthcare providers must develop and implement standard policies and procedures as defined by HIPAA, educate their staff of these standards, and appoint a compliance officer who is responsible for understanding the policies, keeping abreast of changes, and applying their knowledge to ensure conformity. Under the privacy rule section of HIPAA, a privacy officer is also appointed who designates and assigns or denies levels of access to staff to protected health information. This officer must also have an in-depth understanding of HIPAA and the privacy rules and policies to monitor the safety of these records. Employees who knowingly violate these standards can be penalized under federal regulations as follows:

- Fined not more than $50,000, imprisoned not more than one year, or both
- If the offense is committed under false pretenses, fined not more than $100,000, imprisoned not more than five years, or both
- If the offense is committed with intent to sell, transfer, or use individually identifiable health information for commercial advantage, personal gain, or malicious harm, fined not more than $250,000, imprisoned not more than 10 years, or both

As a medical assistant, you must always remember to handle this private healthcare information confidentially and follow any policies and procedures that fall under HIPAA compliance. Do not leave patient-related information unattended or within sight of other patients and staff. Depending on your role, you may have a limited access to patient records. Do not use anyone's password other than your own or access records to which either you or your physician do not have access. Do not release or send any patient records or information without proper HIPAA-complaint authorizations. Some states have stricter standards of confidentiality and medical-records compliance than those mandated by federally enacted HIPAA. If this is the case in your state, the state policies will be followed.

Remember, even after your initial HIPAA training at your employer, if you have any questions regarding HIPAA, its standards, patient confidentiality, release of information, or communication with patients and family members, the compliance and privacy officers are there to assist you in making the proper decision and taking the appropriate action.

Organizing Before and After Patient Encounters

Before the first patient is seen, some organization must occur to prepare for the day's appointments. In a paper-chart system, the physical chart needs to be pulled and reviewed and any loose papers should be filed in the chart (as long as the physician has signed off on all incoming information) prior to the patient's arrival.

Occasionally, obtaining these charts may take time, particularly if other staff or physicians in the practice need the chart to review testing, check messages, or for other various reasons between visits. Many offices pull patients' charts two or three days prior to the patient's appointments to prevent any last-minute issues that could arise when the chart is misplaced.

If possible, any updates or additional testing ordered between the patient's last visit and his or her present visit should be secured and available, as well as any hospitalization records or testing records created between visits. If electronic, all new records should be noted by the physician and scanned in the patient's electronic health record prior to the patient's arrival.

Greeting the Patient

One of the most important moments in a practice is when the patient arrives at the office. The receptionist, or the ambassador of the practice, should promptly greet the patient with a courteous smile while keeping eye contact with the patient.

Many medical assistants and receptionists in medical practices must perform more tasks than simply greeting the patient, but interacting with the patient takes priority. If a patient is in front of the receptionist and the telephone rings, the receptionist should make eye contact with the patient, letting the patient know that he or she will be attended to momentarily. Typically, the telephone should be answered within three rings. Then, the receptionist should take the call, but let the caller know that he or she is with a patient and ask if the caller is willing to hold. Finally, the receptionist should finish the conversation with the patient in front of him or her.

When others arrive at the same time as a scheduled patient—for example, a salesperson, pharmaceutical representative, or other vendor who may also require greeting—the patient should always be the focus at the front desk. Others should be asked to wait until after the patient's business is handled.

Sometimes, patients may arrive quite early or late for their scheduled appointment. Depending on your office policy, you may have to tactfully advise the patient of waiting until

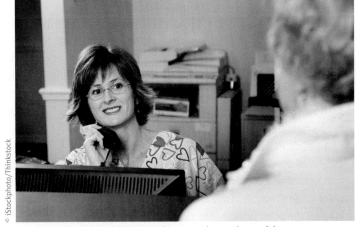

The receptionist should promptly greet the patient with a courteous smile while keeping eye contact with the patient.

his or her scheduled time, reminding the patient that others will be seen according to their appointment time, or, in the case of a patient arriving very late, you may have to ask the patient to reschedule if the appointment cannot be honored due to time constraints.

Other patients may walk in without an appointment and ask to be seen by the physician that day. These patients are normally treated no differently from someone who calls ahead for an appointment, other than the fact that obtaining information about the nature of their visit must be done carefully and confidentially if completed at the front desk. Subject to your office policy, however, walk-ins might not be seen depending on the severity (or lack thereof) and on time constraints of the schedule that day. It is always best to check with the practice manager or physician than to turn a patient away. Usually, walk-ins can be accommodated with a little imagination and some patience by the patient.

If a patient arrives at the front desk and is upset or confused for any reason, the medical assistant or receptionist should ascertain as quickly as possible how the patient should be assisted and act accordingly. Leaving a very ill or sick patient in the waiting area is not suggested, as his or her health condition may require immediate attention by a member of the clinical staff. Angry or confused patients also need special considerations and must be handled accordingly, as they may upset other patients in the waiting area. Practice managers should have policies in place to address these issues. If in doubt when faced with them, check with your supervisor for assistance.

It is important to mark immediately when the patient arrives to create a workflow and good practice repetition. In many electronic practice scheduling software programs, clicking on the patient's name will record the time and the name of the person who checked in the patient. This information can be tracked by others in the system, such as the clinical staff and physicians in other areas, to stay abreast of when patients arrive and how long they have been waiting. The medical assistant or receptionist must keep the patient flow moving at the front desk, as the clinical staff depends on a timely check-in to stay on schedule. If the physician is running behind due to an emergency with another patient at either the office or the hospital, patients scheduled for later visits should be forewarned that a delay is possible and given an estimate of how long the delay is likely to be. If the delay is more than 20 or 30 minutes, many practices attempt to reschedule later patients, offering an alternative day to those who are able and willing. The clinical staff should also notify patients in the clinical exam rooms if there is an unexpected delay due to a patient emergency. Most patients are very understanding once the reason for the delay is relayed to them and an offer of accommodation is made.

If you receive cancellations via telephone, voice mail, answering service, online, in writing, or through other means, the reason the patient canceled the appointment should be documented as well as any other attempts to reschedule with the patient in the patient's chart. Many patients will cancel at the last minute, creating a gap in the physician's schedule, which decreases practice income and efficiency. Many practices enact cancellation rules, such as three cancellations in one calendar year resulting in discharge by the physician from the practice, or possible cancellation fees if notice is not given at least 24 hours prior to the patient's appointment. Like many other policies discussed, this is practice-specific; not every office follows the same policy.

The medical assistant or receptionist is seen as the ambassador of the practice, as he or she is the first person patients will see when greeted upon arrival. Even though this position can be very busy and challenging, medical assistants should always remain calm and monitor their patients in the waiting area, noting any acutely ill, angry, or confused patients who may require immediate action.

Patient Registration and Intake Information

Depending on the registration process that occurs (online or via telephone) prior to the patient's arrival at the practice, some information may need to be obtained at the front desk prior to the patient being called back to see the physician. Most of this pertains to patient demographics, which include the patient's full name, date of birth, address, phone number, Social Security number, marital status, the name of the person responsible for the patient's health insurance, the patient's occupation and work phone number, the patient's spouse's occupation and phone number, health insurance information, a copy of patient's driver's license, signatures for release of information, and assignments of benefits for insurances purposes. Other forms, such as patient intake or history forms, HIPAA acknowledgments, and other office policies, may also need to be reviewed and acknowledged FIGURE 4.3 .

If the person is an established patient, it's important to update his or her records by asking whether any changes have occurred since the patient's last visit. Some practices update this information at each patient's appointment; others update it every three or six months, or sometimes yearly, although this approach is not particularly advisable. Information such as changes to phone numbers, addresses, insurance companies, or any other vital demographic information should be updated as quickly as possible in the billing system to ensure proper filing of claims as well as to ensure the patient's contact information is up to date.

Lab Results and the Patient Chart

Lab results ordered for patients by the physician can come in different forms. Many times, they may be faxed to a dedicated fax line, mailed from a resource laboratory, sent via a dedicated lab printer, or, in the case of urgent lab values, called to the office as an emergency report. Many medical-legal lawsuits come from lab testing ordered but never followed up on, with missing results or patients not being notified of the result by the ordering physician. Risk-management standards dictate that there should be a follow-up procedure for results to ensure all testing ordered is received and accounted for.

When taking results over the phone, it is always best to repeat results back as they are reported. For example, if the patient's BUN is reported over the phone as 21, the medical assistant should repeat directly after writing the result down as "BUN 21" to prevent discrepancies or errors. A notation should also be made as to the date, time, and caller's name, phone number, and department in case any future questions should arise. Upon receipt of urgent lab levels, the patient's chart should be accessed immediately and the physician should be notified of urgent lab levels for review.

The office must have policies in place for risk-management purposes to ensure that the ordering physician reviews all incoming results prior to the results being filed in the patient's record. Some physicians prefer to keep lab flow sheets that track regularly ordered testing to follow trends on their patients. Many times, they will ask that the medical assistant mark the results in the flow sheet to accurately chart any changes that may have occurred.

If lab results are handled through paper documentation, the results are normally placed with the patient's chart for the physician's review. If possible, any abnormal results should be shown to the physician as they are received. If in an electronic format, lab results are normally sent to the physician's inbox either by a lab interface that directly sends it to the ordering physician or as a document sent to the office as an e-result. The physician then reviews the results and makes any notations and recommendations. Depending on the result, it may then be sent to the medical assistant to follow through with any orders or to direct the results to the patient.

XYZ Family Practice

NOTICE OF PRIVACY PRACTICE / CONSENT

You have the right to request a restriction of your protected health information. This means you may ask us not to use or disclose any part of your protected health information for the purposes of treatment, payment, or healthcare operations. You may also request that any part of your protected health information not be disclosed to family members or friends who may be involved in your care or for notification purposes as described in this Notice of Privacy Practices. Your request must state the specific restriction requested and to whom you want the restriction to apply.

Your physician is not required to agree to a restriction that you may request. If a physician believes it is in your best interest to permit use and disclosure of your protected health information, your protected health information will not be restricted. If your physician does agree to the requested restriction, we may not use or disclose your protected health information in violation of that restriction unless it is needed to provide emergency treatment. With this in mind, please discuss any restriction you wish to request with your physician. You may request a restriction by submitting a written request to our Privacy Contact.

You have the right to request to receive confidential communications from us by alternative means or at an alternative location. We will accommodate reasonable requests. We may also condition this accommodation by asking you for information as to how payment will be handled or specification of an alternative address or other method of contact. We will not request an explanation from you as to the basis for the request. Please make this request in writing to our Privacy Contact.

You may have the right to have your physician amend your protected health information. This means you may request an amendment of protected health information about you in a designated record set for as long as we maintain this information. In certain cases, we may deny your request for an amendment. If we deny your request for amendment, you have the right to file a statement of disagreement with us and we may prepare a rebuttal to your statement and will provide you with a copy of any such rebuttal. Please contact our Privacy Contact if you have questions about amending your medical record.

You have the right to receive an accounting of certain disclosures we have made, if any, of your protected health information. This right applies to disclosures for purposes other than treatment, payment, or healthcare operations and valid authorizations or incidental disclosures as described in this Notice of Privacy Practices. It excludes disclosures we have made to you for a facility directory, to family members or friends involved in your care, or for notification purposes. You have the right to receive specific information regarding these disclosures that occurred after April 1, 2006. You may request a shorter time frame. The right to receive this information is subject to certain exceptions, restrictions, and limitations.

You have the right to obtain a paper copy of this notice from us, upon request, even if you have agreed to accept this notice electronically.

Complaints

You may complain to us or to the Secretary of Health and Human Services if you believe your privacy rights have been violated by us. You may file a complaint with us by notifying our Privacy Contact of your complaint. We will not retaliate against you for filing a complaint. You may contact our Privacy Contact, at (555) 555-1212 for further information about the complaint process.

This notice was published and becomes effective on April 1, 2006.

FIGURE 4.3 Sample notice of privacy consent.

Either way, after the physician has signed off on the results, the medical assistant should document the information relayed to the patient as requested by the physician, the date, the time at which the patient was contacted, as well as any other future orders or medications related to the documentation. For example in a paper document, if the physician read a patient's chemistry 12 lab results, which were normal, he may notate "Labs normal, repeat in 3 months, call patient, continue same meds" on the lab result. In turn, the medical assistant would attempt to contact the patient via telephone. If the patient was contacted, the exact message/order that the physician wrote would be communicated to the patient. The date, time, and phone number called as well as the disposition of the call ("patient understood instructions and was scheduled for a chemistry 12 lab test on xyz date") would be documented with the medical assistant's signature and credentials (CCMA). This way, whoever accesses that document later will be able to discern when the patient was contacted; that the patient was spoken to, instructed, and understood the physician's orders; and the person responsible for contacting the patient.

Many physicians prefer to contact patients themselves or follow through with abnormal or complicated results to help the patient understand the situation and to answer any questions the patient may have with regard to his or her plan of treatment.

Scheduling Return Appointments

After the patient's examination, the physician will review the plan of treatment with the patient, testing, recommended procedures or medications, and when the physician would like the patient to return to the office for a follow-up. Normally, this is communicated verbally to the patient and also written on an encounter form designating any testing, procedures, or additional scheduling along with a notation if any medications were introduced. Depending on the practice's workflow, the clinical medical assistant may review this in more detail with the patient prior to checkout or other staff may review this with the patient during the checkout process itself. Often, the physician correlates the patient's return visit with the start of a new medication or a test result. Having the patient come days earlier or later than the requested timeline may affect the outcome of the physician's plan. If the patient cannot return on the date that the physician requests and asks for a later or earlier date, it is best to check with the physician before scheduling.

When scheduling the return appointment, try to enter return information in the comment area or section of the appointment entry. For instance, if the patient is returning after a scheduled mammogram at Mercy Hospital on June 15th, a possible notation on the return appointment might be "One month patient recheck, discuss mammogram results from Mercy Hospital, done 6/15/xx." If you put this information in the return appointment entry, then whoever is reading the notes will be able to determine why the patient is returning, what testing was ordered, and where it was done. Also, if the testing isn't received prior to the return visit date, having this information handy helps prompt the staff to obtain the results from the hospital, thereby increasing efficiency and the quality of patient care.

If the patient does not wish to schedule his or her next appointment, the medical assistant or scheduler should tactfully ask why. If the patient does not wish to give you a reason, that information should be documented, as well as any other conversation pertaining to the refusal of a return appointment or of testing ordered by the physician. With fewer

What Would You Do?

As the front-desk medical assistant, you are having a busy day. Your coworkers are buzzing you on the intercom about a missing chart, there is a patient at your front window to check in, and the phone is ringing with an incoming call at the same time. How would you prioritize in this scenario? How could you manage this situation the most professionally?

© NorthGeorgiaMedia/ShutterStock, Inc.

and fewer patients being covered by employer-based insurance, the patient may not have the finances to return or to schedule the testing ordered by the physician. Or the patient might have felt embarrassed when presented with information by the physician after the exam. Showing sensitivity to these types of scenarios and treating the patient with dignity and respect will show the patient that you and your practice have a genuine concern for the patient and his or her health care.

The physician should be notified of any refusals, as he or she may wish to personally contact the patient by phone, send a letter advising the patient to continue the plan of treatment, make special arrangements, or, in severe situations, dismiss the patient from the practice for noncompliance with physician's orders.

Math Practice

Question: What is the copay amount if the patient's office visit was $75 and the patient is responsible for 20% of the charges?

Answer: $15

Question: If your schedule allows patients every 10 minutes, how many patients can your physician normally see within an hour?

Answer: 6

Question: What is the sum of 10.0 + 15.0 + 20.5 + 42.25 + 70.75?

Answer: 158.50

Question: What is the product of 514 × 5?

Answer: 2,570

Question: What is the product of $\frac{3}{4} \times \frac{2}{3}$?

Answer: $\frac{1}{2}$

Question: What is the difference of $\frac{2}{3} - \frac{7}{21}$?

Answer: $\frac{1}{3}$

Question: What is the difference of $\frac{3}{4} - \frac{4}{20}$?

Answer: $\frac{11}{20}$

Question: What is the product of $\frac{2}{4} \times \frac{5}{8}$?

Answer: $\frac{5}{16}$

Question: What is the quotient of $\frac{4}{5} \div \frac{1}{2}$?

Answer: $1\frac{3}{5}$

Question: **What is the quotient of $\frac{7}{8} \div \frac{3}{4}$?**

Answer: $1\frac{1}{6}$

Question: **What is the sum of 1.96 + 1.7 + 8.5?**

Answer: 12.16

Question: **What is the sum of 3.78 + 6.742 +3.2?**

Answer: 13.722

Question: **What is the difference of 7.96 − 5.4?**

Answer: 2.56

Question: **What is the difference of 12.9 − 5.67?**

Answer: 7.23

Question: **What is the product of 2.7 × 1.85?**

Answer: 4.995

Question: **What is the product of 4.6 × 2.3?**

Answer: 10.58

Question: **What is the quotient of 8.1 ÷ 0.9?**

Answer: 9

Question: **What is the quotient of 4.8 ÷ 0.8?**

Answer: 6

Question: **What is $\frac{4}{80}$ expressed as a percent?**

Answer: 5%

Question: **What is $\frac{3}{5}$ expressed as a percent?**

Answer: 60%

Question: **What is 50% expressed as a fraction?**

Answer: $\frac{1}{2}$

Question: **What is 80% expressed as a fraction?**

Answer: $\frac{4}{5}$

WRAP UP

Chapter Summary

- Communication is the act of transmitting information, or an exchange of information between individuals using a common system of signs, symbols, or behavior. Communication and how we relate to each other during that process is one of the most important aspects of delivering competent, professional, and quality care to patients.

- The ability of the healthcare team to communicate effectively and efficiently is directly related to providing vital information during and after the decision-making processes for providers and patients alike. Using either verbal or nonverbal communication helps by providing the patient with the best possible quality health care and allows for a meaningful exchange.

- Learning the different types of verbal and nonverbal communication is important for the medical assistant for working with patients and staff in the medical field.

- With therapeutic communication, the healthcare provider uses an element of empathy, allowing the patient to feel a sense of comfort when faced with frightening news or when feeling apprehensive about the information being relayed to him or her.

- Facial expressions are one of the most observed factors in nonverbal communication. A smile conveys an approachable person, while a frown says "stay away."

- Medical records are legal documents that provide complete accounts of the patient's medical care and treatment. The patient's condition and any changes that occur, medical history, evaluations, testing, and any other pertinent information must be accurate when documented in the patient's chart. Providers make vital decisions based on the information contained in a patient's medical record. If an entry in a patient's record was omitted or an error occurred during documentation, the validity and accuracy of the patient's chart would not only be questioned, but may lead to positive judgment for the plaintiff if legal action were ever taken.

- Personal space is the distance at which we feel comfortable with others while communicating. The most often observed space by individuals is social, which is usually between 4 and 12 feet.

- Touch communicates in many different ways. Being a healthcare professional, it is important for you to recognize the use of touch in the relationship with the patient as long as well-defined boundaries are used.

- Culture refers to the customary beliefs, social norms, and material traits of a racial, religious, or social group. It is important to recognize cultural factors that may influence patients' decisions on health care for themselves and their family.

- Abraham Maslow was the founder of humanistic psychology and is best known for his hierarchy of needs. The basic principle of the hierarchy of needs is that a person must satisfy one level of need before he or she can move onto the next.

- Some cross-cultural concerns may affect patients' expectations and encounters with healthcare professionals. The healthcare professional must be aware of potential sources of misunderstanding, the patient's origin, and difficulties in translation of word and language, and should adapt to the patient's communication style.

- The patient's medical history is the basis for treatment by any and all of the patient's providers. The medical assistant may play an important part in obtaining the patient's medical history and should understand the emphasis on collecting concise, complete, and accurate information when assisting patients with the completion of these documents.

- Documentation should always be done with care and thought. Make sure that the entries are legible, use standard abbreviations when applicable, and record information accurately. Any errors should be noted in a paper-based system with a line through the entry with initials and date, or electronically with an addendum noting the changes made. No entries should ever be discarded or removed.

- A medical transcriptionist types medical information spoken by the physician about the patient's examination or testing into a document that becomes a permanent part of the medical record. In the electronic format, templates or digital dictation devices may automatically transcribe the physician's dictation into the patient's chart using software that is compatible with the electronic health records format.

- Medical abbreviations can be used to save time and space as well as to document information. When using abbreviations, always remember to use common ones. Some medication documentation abbreviations have been discouraged by many state medical boards and the Joint Commission.

- The SOAP method of formatting in medical records uses a process of recording the patient's exam or progress notes based on a problem-oriented way. The CHEDDAR method is very similar to the SOAP method, but is normally more detailed in nature.

- Electronic health records store secure and confidential information about patients, but have the advantage of enabling the healthcare team to print and view the records in part or as a whole as necessary. Access to this information can be assigned by defined user groups, allowing minimal necessity to protected healthcare information and ensuring the patients' confidentiality.

- HIPAA requires providers to develop and implement standard policies and procedures for best practices. Staff education, compliance officers, and privacy officers promote understanding of the privacy policies necessary to work with patients' protected health information.

- A medical assistant who is responsible for front office reception duties must be organized and pleasant. Proper planning is required for the next day's patients as well as coordinating any paperwork or testing prior to the patients' arrival. Among other important duties, the receptionist is the ambassador of the practice and should always promptly greet patients with a smile. Patients can be difficult or have urgent issues develop while waiting for the physician, and the medical assistant needs to be attuned to patients in the reception area.

- When patients cancel or refuse appointments that are recommended by the physician, the medical assistant should always document this communication with the ordering physician for signature. Some offices adhere to a strict 24-hour cancellation policy with their patients, and may charge a fee for no-shows and last-minute cancellations.

- When patients present to the office at the reception desk, it is important for demographic information to be updated and made as accurate as possible. Denied claims, unprocessed statements, and inaccurate patient contact information may interfere with patient care or delay payments to the practice.

- Lab results that are reported to the practice can come in different formats. It is important to make sure that the physician reviews each and every report prior to filing the records in the paper or electronic health record. Urgent and abnormal results should be flagged for immediate viewing by the physician.

- Medical records are legal documents that follow patients throughout their entire encounter with the physician and staff. Any entries in the medical record must be accurate, legible, and detailed for the provider to make medical decisions and judgments.

Learning Assessment Questions

1. What is the personal space measurements for most citizens of the United States in normal conversation?

   A. Touching to 1.5 feet

   B. 1.5 feet to 4 feet

   C. 4 to 12 feet

   D. 5 to 7 feet

2. The term *culture* is defined how?

   A. Body language and the study of its different movements

   B. The customary beliefs, social norms, and material traits of a racial, religious, or social group

   C. The distance at which we are comfortable when communicating

   D. The manners used during dinner table service

3. In which of the following types of communication does the healthcare provider use empathy to give the patient a certain level of comfort when faced with frightening news or apprehension?

   A. Verbal communication

   B. Therapeutic communication

   C. Nonverbal communication

   D. Closed communication

4. Which of the following describes body language?

   A. Used to express feelings and emotions

   B. Makes up only 7 percent of message communicated

   C. Is less important than verbal communication

   D. Is used only in certain cultures

5. Which of the following is involved in the first part of the communication cycle, which begins by creating or encoding the message being sent?

   A. Receiver

   B. Sender

   C. Message

   D. Interpreter

6. Placing the most recent set of medical records and information at the top of the chart (or in an electronic chart, by most recent date) for easy access, allowing an orderly progression, is known as which of the following?

   A. Nonchronological order

   B. Chronological order

   C. Alphabetical order

   D. Numerical order

7. What are the five Cs of communication?

   A. Complete, clear, concise, cohesive, courteous

   B. Candid, complete, concise, cohesive, courteous

   C. Clear, candid, concise, cohesive, courteous

   D. Courteous, concise, caring, complete, curt

8. Which of the following is the process by which we learn the rules and values of our society?

   A. Acculturation

   B. Culture

   C. Maslow's theory of hierarchy

   D. Freud's theory

9. Which of the following is a very short and to-the-point statement that describes the reason a patient needs to be seen by the provider?

   A. Family history

   B. Chief complaint

   C. Social history

   D. History of present illness

10. HIPAA was designed to do which of the following?

   A. Provide security for all electronic health information

   B. Establish standards for all electronic health transmission claims

   C. Control and maintain the privacy and security of private health information

   D. All of the above

11. Which of the following is one of the most important things the medical assistant should do when greeting the patient upon his or her arrival?

   A. Smile and greet the patient promptly.

   B. Hand the patient paperwork and tell him or her to sit down and fill it out.

   C. Collect the patient's copay and review payment policies with the patient in detail.

   D. Offer the patient coffee and donuts to make him or her feel more comfortable.

12. How are walk-in appointments usually handled?

   A. By scheduling the patient immediately and working him or her in

   B. No differently than when someone calls for an appointment, and may not be honored depending on the lack of severity and time allowances

   C. By never scheduling on the same day

   D. By politely asking them to return tomorrow

13. How should patient cancellations that are left on office voice mails or with the answering service be handled?

   A. They should be noted and filed in the patient's chart.

   B. They should be noted and added to the patient's chart, and then forwarded to the physician for signature.

   C. They are not documented; they are merely relayed verbally to the physician.

   D. A call should be placed immediately to the patient to advise him or her of cancellation fees.

14. Why is it is important to update all patient demographic information upon registration?

   A. It can affect reimbursement to the practice as well as patient care.

   B. If not updated, it can cause the patient to be deactivated in the system.

   C. It doesn't matter. If the patient's address is wrong in the system, he or she will be forwarded information by the post office.

   D. You may need to be able to contact the patient at work in case of an appointment cancellation.

15. When taking critical lab values over the phone, it is recommend that you do which of the following?

   A. Repeat the words spoken by the person reporting the results so no errors are made, making a notation of the time, the date, the caller's name, and the caller's phone number.

   B. Inform the caller that you are too busy and tell him or her to fax you the information.

   C. Place the caller on hold until you can get the physician out of an exam room to take the call.

   D. None of the above

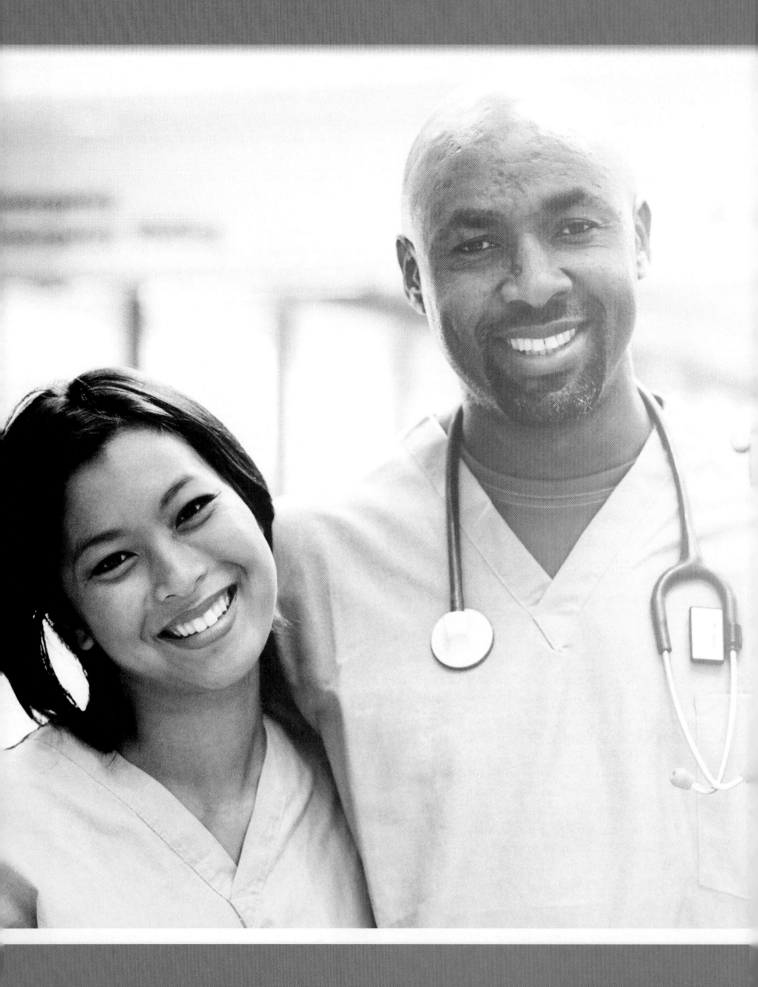

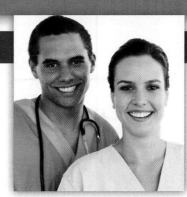

Infection Control and Medical Asepsis

OBJECTIVES

After reading this chapter, you will be able to:

- Define and state the critical importance of infection control in the ambulatory care setting.
- Describe the six links in the chain of infection.
- Define the five classifications of infectious microorganisms.
- Compare the routes of transmission of HIV and hepatitis B and C and discuss the risk of infection from needlestick.
- Describe the purpose of standard precautions and give six examples of ways healthcare providers should practice standard precautions.
- List eight types of body fluids and give an example of each.
- Describe personal protective equipment.
- Recognize five situations in which exposure to a patient's blood can occur, and discuss why standard precautions are important.
- Describe proper infectious waste disposal.
- List human fluids that may contain HIV, HBV, and HCV.
- Define medical asepsis.

KEY TERMS

Acquired
  immunodeficiency
  syndrome (AIDS)

Acute stage
Aerobes
Airborne precautions

Airborne transmission
Amniocentesis
Anaerobes

Aseptic technique	Gram-positive	Parasites
Bacteria	Hepatitis	Parenteral medications
Blood-borne transmission	Host	Pathogens
	Human immunodeficiency	Portal of entry
Chain of infection	virus (HIV)	Portal of exit
Contact precautions	Incubation stage	Prodromal stage
Convalescent stage	Indirect transmission	Reservoir
Declining stage	Infection control	Rhinorrhea
Direct transmission	Infectious agents	Rickettsiae
Droplet precautions	Infectious waste	Sharps
Epistaxis	Lochia	Standard precautions
Expanded precautions	Medical asepsis	Surgical asepsis
Facultative aerobes	Menses	Thoracentesis
Flora	Microorganisms	Universal precautions
Fomite	Mode of transmission	Vector transmission
Fungi	Morphology	Viruses
Gram-negative	Palliative	

Chapter Overview

This chapter covers the process of infection and describes the basics of infection control and standard precautions in the ambulatory care setting. Because medical assistants provide care to many patients and deal directly with other healthcare professionals, following proper procedures to minimize the spread of infection is essential. Following infection-control procedures, including standard precautions and medical asepsis, can limit the transmission of infection and provide barriers against transmission.

Infection Control

Many lives are lost because of the spread of infections. Healthcare workers can take steps to prevent the spread of infectious diseases in the ambulatory care setting. Procedures for **infection control** are precautions taken in the healthcare setting to prevent the spread of disease. Infection control is an essential component of healthcare delivery. There are two types of infection-control measures: medical asepsis and surgical asepsis. Infection-control measures can be as simple as following proper hand washing techniques or as complicated as disinfection of surgical instruments. Implementing these measures can break the chain of infection, prevent the transmission of disease, and create barriers against transmission in healthcare settings.

Infection-control procedures can help prevent the spread of disease.

Chain of Infection

For an infection to spread, several steps must occur. These steps are known as the **chain of infection**. Each step or link must be connected in sequential order for the spread of infection to occur. Healthcare providers use infection-control measures to break or interrupt the chain of infection and stop the spread of disease.

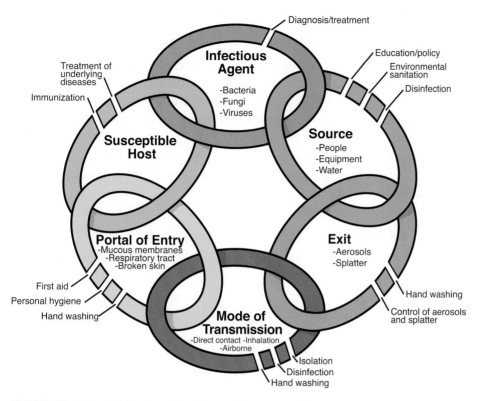

FIGURE 5.1 Chain of infection: Each link must be connected for infection to spread.
Adapted from http://www.healthcareessentials.co.nz/article/breaking-chain-infection

The steps or links in the chain of infection are as follows **FIGURE 5.1** :

- Infectious agent
- Reservoir
- Portal of exit
- Mode of transmission
- Portal of entry
- Susceptible host

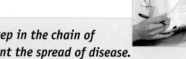

Interrupting one step in the chain of infection can prevent the spread of disease.
© auremar/ShutterStock, Inc.

What Would You Do?

What are the six steps in the chain of infection, and how can each one be interrupted?

© NorthGeorgiaMedia/ShutterStock, Inc.

Infectious Agents

Infectious agents are pathogens or microorganisms with the ability to cause disease. A **pathogen** is a bacterium, virus, or other microorganism that can cause disease. A **microorganism** is a microscopic organism such as a virus, bacterium, fungus, parasite, or rickettsiae. These microorganisms find a reservoir or host that provides the conditions necessary for its growth and multiplication. If steps are taken to interrupt and prevent the growth of these infectious agents, disease transmission can be reduced. Not all microorganisms are pathogenic. Some microorganisms are nonpathogenic and are part of the normal **flora**; they provide a balance in the body and destroy pathogens. Infection can occur when this normal balance is destroyed. Medical assistants must apply their knowledge of the process of infectious disease growth and transmission to reduce transmission and incidence of infectious diseases in patients and other healthcare professionals.

Microorganisms can be either pathogenic—or disease-causing—or nonpathogenic and part of the normal flora.

For microorganisms to grow and survive, the environment must be suitable for their growth. Following is a list of requirements that are necessary for their growth:

- **Oxygen**—Most pathogenic microorganisms need oxygen to grow and thrive. Microorganisms that need oxygen to thrive are called **aerobes**. Microorganisms that do not need oxygen or only a little oxygen to grow are called **anaerobes**.
- **Temperature**—The optimum temperature for microbial growth is body temperature (98.6 degrees Fahrenheit).
- **pH**—A slightly acidic pH can protect the body from infection. If the pH is higher, it indicates microbial growth. An environment that is too acidic will not support microbial growth.
- **Moisture**—Microorganisms grow best in a dark, moist environment.
- **Nutrients**—The body supplies nutrients necessary for microbial growth.

For an infection to occur, an infectious agent must be present. Infectious agents can be divided into five classifications:

- Viruses
- Bacteria
- Fungi
- Parasites
- Rickettsiae

Identification of the disease-causing organism can help determine the most appropriate type of treatment.

Identification of the causative infectious agent can help determine the most appropriate type of treatment.

Viruses

Viruses are pathogens that are classified by the type of DNA or RNA they have. (DNA, short for deoxyribonucleic acid, is a chemical substance in cells that carries the cell's genetic information. RNA, short for ribonucleic acid, acts as a messenger, carrying instructions from DNA for controlling the synthesis of proteins.) Viruses are the smallest of all the microorganisms and require a living host cell to replicate. Viruses invade a host cell and take over the cell's nucleus to multiply and produce other viruses. Viruses are not affected by chemical disinfectants and antibiotics. Viruses can also adapt to their environment so they remain resistant to treatment. Treatment of viral infections is usually **palliative**; that is, treatment merely relieves symptoms of the disease instead of curing the infection. Some viral infections can be prevented by vaccination. Commonly known viruses include HIV, herpes, hepatitis, influenza, and chicken pox, as shown in `TABLE 5.1`.

`FIGURE 5.2` outlines the CDC's recommended adult immunization schedule, while `FIGURE 5.3` shows the recommended immunization schedule for children aged 0 to 18 years.

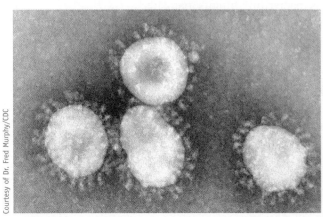

Viruses need a living host cell to replicate.

© auremar/ShutterStock, Inc.

Courtesy of Dr. Fred Murphy/CDC

A virus under an electron microscope.

Table 5.1 Common Viral Diseases

Disease	Mode of Transmission	Type of Infection	Symptoms	Vaccine Available
Herpes simplex virus 1	Direct contact with infected individual	Cold sores, fever blisters	Blisters or sores on or around the genitals or rectum	No
Herpes simplex virus 2	Direct contact with infected individual	Genital herpes	Painful blisters on lips and oral lesions, flulike symptoms, fever, swollen glands	No
Herpes zoster	Direct contact with infected individual	Shingles	Painful, blistering rash	Yes
HIV	Direct contact, anal or vaginal intercourse, sharing of IV drug needles, infected mother to child during pregnancy or childbirth, blood transfusions, direct contact with infected blood or body fluids	AIDS	Early: Fatigue, weight loss, loss of appetite, night sweats Late: Fever, cough, shortness of breath, infections	No
Rubella	Direct contact by respiratory droplets (coughing, sneezing)	German measles	Rash, fever	Yes
Rubeola	Direct contact by respiratory droplets (coughing, sneezing)	Measles	Fever, rash, cough, runny nose, conjunctivitis	Yes
Poliovirus	Fecal-oral transmission, fecal-contaminated food or water, direct contact with contaminated objects	Poliomyelitis	Fever, malaise, headache, sore throat, stiff neck and back	Yes
Influenza	Direct or indirect contact or droplet with infected individual	Flu, pneumonia	Fever, aches, loss of appetite, upper respiratory symptoms	Yes
Human papilloma-virus (HPV)	Vaginal, anal, or oral sex, rarely from infected mother to child during childbirth	Genital warts, cervical cancer	Genital warts, increased vaginal discharge, itching, genital warts on lips, mouth, tongue, and throat	Yes
Hepatitis (A, B, C)	HAV: Direct contact with stools or blood of infected person, fecal-contaminated food or water, oral-anal contact HBV: Contact with infected blood or body fluids, primarily through sharing of contaminated needles or syringes; less commonly through sexual contact	Liver	HAV: Dark urine, fatigue, itching, yellow skin, low-grade fever, loss of appetite HBV: Same as above HCV: Same as above	Only for HAV, HBV

(Continues)

Table 5.1   Common Viral Diseases *(Continued)*

Disease	Mode of Transmission	Type of Infection	Symptoms	Vaccine Available
	HCV: Contact with infected blood or body fluids, primarily through sharing of contaminated needles or syringes, infected mother to child during pregnancy or childbirth			
Epstein-Barr virus (EBV)	Direct contact with saliva of infected person	Infectious mononucleosis	Fever, sore throat, swollen lymph glands	No
Varicella zoster	Direct or indirect contact, droplet, or airborne secretion of infected person	Chicken pox (skin)	Vesicular eruptions on skin, low-grade fever, malaise	Yes
Conjunctivitis	Direct or indirect contact with discharge from eyes or upper respiratory tract secretions from infected person	Pink eye	Red and itchy eyes, crusted eyelashes	No

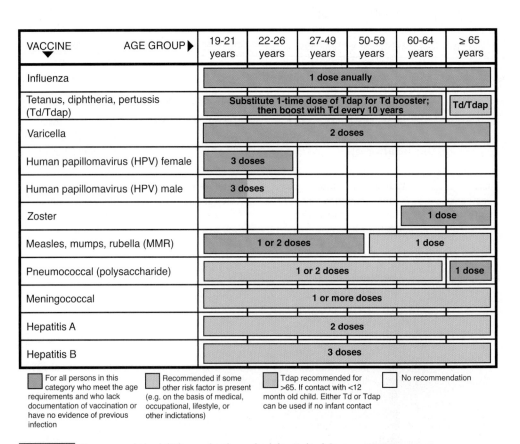

FIGURE 5.2 Recommended adult immunization schedule, United States, 2012.

Courtesy of the CDC

VACCINE AGE ▶	Birth	1 mth	2 mths	4 mths	6 mths	9 mths	12 mths	15 mths	18 mths	19-23 mths	2-3 years	4-6 years
Hepatitis B	HepB	HepB			HepB							
Rotavirus		RV	RV	RV								
Diphtheria, tetanus, pertussis		DTaP	DTaP	DTaP			DTaP					DTaP
Haemophilus influenzae type b		Hib	Hib	Hib		Hib						
Pneumococcal		PCV	PCV	PCV		PCV					PSSV	
Inactivated poliovirus		IPV	IPV		IPV							IPV
Influenza					Influenza (yearly)							
Measles, mumps, rubella							MMR					MMR
Varicella							VAR					VAR
Hepatitis A							Dose 1			HepA series		
Meningococcal							MCV4					

▉ Range of recommended ages for all children	▉ Range of recommended ages for certain high-risk groups	▉ Range of recommended ages for all children and certain high-risk groups

FIGURE 5.3 Recommended immunization schedule for persons 0–18 years, United States, 2012.
Courtesy of the CDC

Bacteria

Bacteria are microorganisms that have only one cell **FIGURE 5.4**. Under a microscope, bacteria have characteristic shapes, or **morphology**, and can look like balls (cocci), spirals (spirilla), or rods (bacilli). Bacteria can be classified according to their shape or by their ability to accept staining agents. Bacteria that stain red under a microscope are referred to as **Gram-negative** and bacteria that stain purple are referred to as **Gram-positive**. Many types of bacteria are beneficial (nonpathogenic), but some bacteria are infectious (pathogenic) and can make you sick. Bacteria that are nonpathogenic, such as those found on the skin or in the gastrointestinal tract, are part of the normal flora. When the balance of nonpathogenic bacteria is altered, the opportunity for

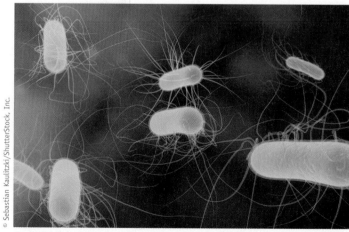

Escherichia coli.

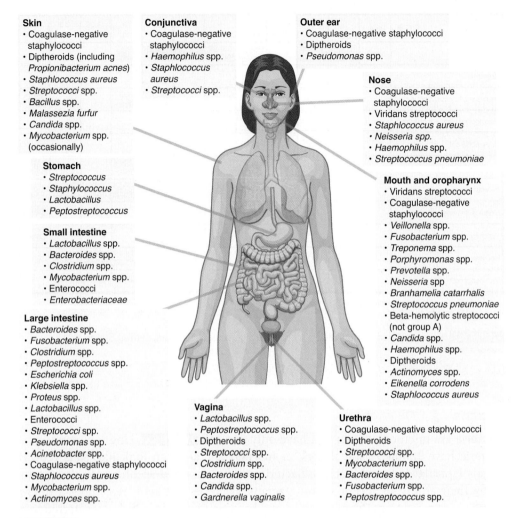

Skin
- Coagulase-negative staphylococci
- Diptheroids (including *Propionibacterium acnes*)
- *Staphlococcus aureus*
- *Streptococci* spp.
- *Bacillus* spp.
- *Malassezia furfur*
- *Candida* spp.
- *Mycobacterium* spp. (occasionally)

Stomach
- *Streptococcus*
- *Staphylococcus*
- *Lactobacillus*
- *Peptostreptococcus*

Small intestine
- *Lactobacillus* spp.
- *Bacteroides* spp.
- *Clostridium* spp.
- *Mycobacterium* spp.
- Enterococci
- *Enterobacteriaceae*

Large intestine
- *Bacteroides* spp.
- *Fusobacterium* spp.
- *Clostridium* spp.
- *Peptostreptococcus* spp.
- *Escherichia coli*
- *Klebsiella* spp.
- *Proteus* spp.
- *Lactobacillus* spp.
- Enterococci
- *Streptococci* spp.
- *Pseudomonas* spp.
- *Acinetobacter* spp.
- Coagulase-negative staphylococci
- *Staphlococcus aureus*
- *Mycobacterium* spp.
- *Actinomyces* spp.

Conjunctiva
- Coagulase-negative staphylococci
- *Haemophilus* spp.
- *Staphlococcus aureus*
- *Streptococci* spp.

Vagina
- *Lactobacillus* spp.
- *Peptostreptococcus* spp.
- Diptheroids
- *Streptococci* spp.
- *Clostridium* spp.
- *Bacteroides* spp.
- *Candida* spp.
- *Gardnerella vaginalis*

Outer ear
- Coagulase-negative staphylococci
- Diptheroids
- *Pseudomonas* spp.

Nose
- Coagulase-negative staphylococci
- Viridans streptococci
- *Staphylococcus aureus*
- *Neisseria* spp.
- *Haemophilus* spp.
- *Streptococcus pneumoniae*

Mouth and oropharynx
- Viridans streptococci
- Coagulase-negative staphylococci
- *Veillonella* spp.
- *Fusobacterium* spp.
- *Treponema* spp.
- *Porphyromonas* spp.
- *Prevotella* spp.
- *Neisseria* spp
- *Branhamelia catarrhalis*
- *Streptococcus pneumoniae*
- Beta-hemolytic streptococci (not group A)
- *Candida* spp.
- *Haemophilus* spp.
- Diptheroids
- *Actinomyces* spp.
- *Eikenella corrodens*
- *Staphylococcus aureus*

Urethra
- Coagulase-negative staphylococci
- Diptheroids
- *Streptococci* spp.
- *Mycobacterium* spp.
- *Bacteroides* spp.
- *Fusobacterium* spp.
- *Peptostreptococcus* spp.

FIGURE 5.4 Normal microbial flora: Many such nonharmful bacteria are found on the skin or in the intestinal tract.

© Jones & Bartlett Learning

pathogenic bacteria to grow and cause infectious disease increases. Bacteria reproduce quickly and release toxins, which can damage tissues. Examples of infectious bacteria include *Escherichia coli*, *Streptococcus*, and *Staphylococcus* **TABLE 5.2**.

Fungi

Fungi are plantlike organisms that can grow on cloth, food, showers, or people, or in any warm, moist environment. Fungi are different from bacteria. The DNA of a fungus is contained within a nuclear membrane. Fungi are single-celled or multicellular parasites. That means they absorb nutrients from the environment or from hosts such as animals and human beings. Fungi are aerobes (that is, they need oxygen to survive) or **facultative aerobes** (that is, they can survive with or without oxygen). Fungi are opportunistic pathogens that can cause infections in immunocompromised patients. Immunocompromised patients are those whose immune system is weakened or absent and who are incapable of producing a normal immune response. Molds are multicelled fungi that grow best in warm and damp places. They can infect and ultimately destroy

Table 5.2 Common Bacterial Diseases

Disease	Infectious Agent	Mode of Transmission
Anthrax	*Bacillus anthracis*	Direct contact with spores through a cut or scrape on skin, inhalation, or ingestion of tainted meat
Chlamydia	*Chlamydia trachomatis*	Sexual contact
Escherichia coli	Gram-negative bacilli	Fecal-contaminated food, water, meat, direct contact through an injury or open wound
Gonorrhea	*Neisseria gonorrhoeae*	Sexual contact
Nosocomial infection (hospital-acquired infection)	Gram-negative bacteria	In the hospital
Pneumococcal	*Streptococcus pneumoniae*	Respiratory
Staphylococcal infection (strep throat, otitis media, pneumonia)	Usually group A beta-hemolytic *Streptococcus*	Respiratory
Syphilis	*Treponema pallidum*	Sexual contact
Tetanus	*Clostridium tetani*	Direct contact with spores through an injury or open wound
Tuberculosis	*Mycobacterium tuberculosis*	Inhalation
Typhoid fever	*Salmonella typhi*	Contaminated food or beverages

plants and food. Yeasts are the only fungi that are not multicellular, but they, too, absorb nutrients from plants. Fungi play an important role in the environment. Compared with humans, plants are more susceptible to fungal infections. Many fungi do not cause illness; however, infection from specific species can occur. Examples of fungal infections include *Candida albicans* (yeast infection) and *Tinea pedis* (athlete's foot).

> Fungi absorb nutrients from the environment or from their host.

Tinea pedis, commonly known as athlete's foot.

Ccourtesy of Dr. Lucille K. Georg/CDC

Parasites

Parasites are organisms that benefit at the expense of another living organism. The host is the organism that is being used by the parasite for nourishment. Parasites can be single-celled or multicellular. Parasites are classified as follows:

- **Protozoa**—These are single-celled parasites that have a nucleus and can only divide in a host organism. These organisms can cause malaria and trichomoniasis.
- **Metazoa**—These are multicellular parasites that can cause hookworms, ringworms, and tapeworms.
- **Ectoparasite**—These are multicellular parasites that live on the surface of the host. These organisms can cause scabies and lice.

> *Parasites can be classified as protozoa, metazoa, or ectoparasite.*

© auremar/ShutterStock, Inc.

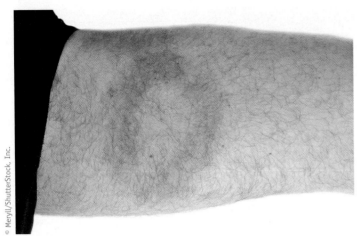

Lyme disease is transmitted by deer ticks and often first appears as a rash near the bite.

What Would You Do?

What are the five classifications of infectious agents? Give examples in each category.

© NorthGeorgiaMedia/ShutterStock, Inc.

Rickettsiae

Rickettsiae are intracellular parasites that depend completely on their host for survival. Rickettsiae are larger than viruses and can be seen under conventional microscopes after staining procedures. Most rickettsial pathogens are transmitted by fleas, ticks, mites, or lice. Examples of this type of infection include Rocky Mountain spotted fever and Lyme disease.

Reservoir

A **reservoir** is where a microorganism can thrive and reproduce. For example, microorganisms thrive in people, animals, insects, and inanimate objects such as food, water, tabletops, and doorknobs. Proper hygiene and cleaning of supplies, linen, and equipment can break this link in the chain of infection.

The reservoir is the second link in the chain of infection. Proper hygiene and cleaning of supplies, linen, and equipment can break this link in the chain of infection.

Portal of Exit

In order for a microorganism to cause an infection, it must leave the reservoir. In people, this **portal of exit** can be through the discharge of body secretions or excretions or respiratory droplets. It can also be through open wounds, the vagina, or rectum. Respiratory hygiene and cough etiquette, isolation techniques, and application of sterile dressings to wounds can break this link in the chain of infection.

The portal of exit is the third link in the chain of infection. Respiratory hygiene and cough etiquette, isolation techniques, and application of sterile dressings to wounds can break this link in the chain of infection.

Mode of Transmission

The next link in the chain of infection is the **mode of transmission**. This is the means by which the microorganism travels from the portal of exit to another host. Diseases can be transmitted directly or indirectly. **Direct transmission** involves direct contact between the infectious person or infected body fluids and the susceptible host. Direct contact includes eating, drinking, sexual intimacy, and **blood-borne transmission** (in which infected blood enters a susceptible host through blood or body fluids). **Indirect transmission** involves an intermediate means that carries the infectious agent to the host. Indirect transmission can occur from inhaling contaminated air or handling or touching an infectious object (**fomite**). Infections can also be transmitted indirectly via tiny droplets of vapor in the air (**airborne transmission**) or from disease-carrying insects (**vector transmission**). Proper hand hygiene, use of personal protective equipment, medical and surgical asepsis, and disposal of contaminated objects can break this link in the chain of infection.

The mode of transmission is the fourth link in the chain of infection. Proper hand hygiene, use of personal protective equipment, medical and surgical asepsis, and disposal of contaminated objects can break this link in the chain of infection.

Portal of Entry

The **portal of entry** is where the infectious microorganism enters the host's body. It allows the agent access to another person. Portals of entry include the mouth, nose, eyes, ears, throat, intestinal tract, urinary tract, reproductive tract, and open skin. Portals can also result from tubes placed in body cavities or from punctures from invasive procedures. Proper hand hygiene, use of personal protective equipment, application of sterile dressings to wounds, and disposal of contaminated objects can break this link in the chain of infection.

The portal of entry is the fifth link in the chain of infection. Proper hand hygiene, use of personal protective equipment, application of sterile dressings to wounds, and disposal of contaminated objects can break this link in the chain of infection.

Susceptible Host

The last link in the chain of infection is the **host**. This is a person who is susceptible to infection by a pathogen. For the infectious process to continue, microorganisms must enter another host who is susceptible to infection. The host is susceptible to disease because it lacks the immunity or physical resistance to overcome invasion by the pathogen. The elderly, immunosuppressed, or those with chronic disease can be at increased risk. Susceptibility can also depend on the type of pathogen, the duration of exposure to the pathogen, the psychological and physical health of the host, and age of the host. Maintaining a healthy lifestyle and getting immunized can break this link in the chain of infection.

A susceptible host is the sixth link in the chain of infection. Maintaining a healthy lifestyle and getting vaccinated can break this link in the chain of infection.

Defense Mechanisms

The body has many specialized defense mechanisms and barriers in place to help prevent exposure to pathogens and infection. These barriers can be mechanical/physical, chemical, or cellular. Mechanical/physical barriers include the hairlike cilia that filter out pathogens in the respiratory tract, intact skin, and mucous membranes **FIGURE 5.5**. Chemical barriers include a highly specific and complex immune system and secretions such as tears, sweat, urine, mucus, and saliva. Cellular mechanisms, such as white blood cells, are the body's defense mechanisms that fight against infection in tissues, blood, and lymph.

The immune system protects against pathogens and abnormal cell growth. Inflammation is the body's normal response to invasion by a pathogen or foreign body or physical trauma. Inflammation does not always indicate an infection, but an infection does not occur without inflammation. The body's inflammatory response is designed to help fight infection and destroy invading pathogens. If the inflammatory response is not effective, accumulation of pus, lymph-node enlargement, or septicemia can occur.

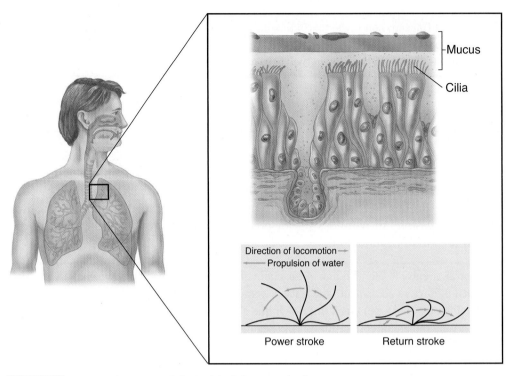

FIGURE 5.5 Hairlike cilia is one of the body's defense mechanisms.
© Jones & Bartlett Learning

Stages of Infectious Diseases

After exposure to a disease-causing pathogen, several stages occur from the time of exposure to full recovery from the disease. These stages generally occur in order and can be useful in providing patient education and opportunities for treatment:

What Would You Do?

What are the stages of infectious diseases?

© NorthGeorgiaMedia/ShutterStock, Inc.

- Incubation stage—The **incubation stage** is the time between the exposure to a pathogen and when the first signs and symptoms of the disease appear. The length of the incubation period can vary depending on the disease.
- Prodromal stage—The **prodromal stage** occurs between the onset of initial symptoms and the onset of symptoms that show a disease process is occurring. It is often characterized by fever and malaise.
- Acute stage—The disease process reaches its peak during the **acute stage**. Symptoms during this stage can help identify the disease process.
- Declining stage—During the **declining stage**, symptoms begin to subside. The infection is still present, but the patient will begin to feel better.
- Convalescent stage—During the **convalescent stage**, the patient begins to recover and regain strength.

Transmission of Disease

Medical assistants run the risk of acquiring an infection because they are in constant contact with patients who may have such pathogens as viruses, bacteria, or fungi. These pathogens can be found in the patient's blood or body fluids. Pathogens can be transmitted from one person to another, especially if measures are not taken to prevent the spread of infection. Consistent adherence to infection-control measures can reduce the risk of disease transmission. The CDC recommends that all healthcare providers consider each person to be potentially infectious with blood-borne pathogens such as HIV/AIDS, hepatitis B, and hepatitis C.

The CDC recommends that all healthcare providers consider each person to be potentially infectious with blood-borne pathogens such as HIV/AIDS, hepatitis B, and hepatitis C.
© auremar/ShutterStock, Inc.

Human Immunodeficiency Virus and AIDS

Human immunodeficiency virus (HIV) is a blood-borne virus similar to other viruses that cause the flu or common cold except that with HIV, over time, your immune system cannot clear most of the virus out of the body. There are two types of HIV: HIV-1 and HIV-2. The term HIV generally refers to HIV-1. HIV is carried in blood, blood products, semen, and other body fluids such as vaginal secretions, and possibly breast milk. It can also penetrate mucous membranes. HIV gradually attacks CD4+ T-cells, a key component of the immune system responsible for providing immunity. The body must have these white blood cells to fight infections and disease, but over time, HIV invades them and uses them to make more copies of itself. As HIV progressively damages these cells, the body becomes more vulnerable to infections and has difficulty fighting off infections. When a patient has advanced HIV or when the patient's T-cell count falls below 200, that person is said to have **acquired immunodeficiency syndrome (AIDS)**. There is no curative treatment for HIV or AIDS and no vaccine available to prevent contracting HIV. Antiviral drugs are used to weaken cell protein, which is important for viral replication and for preventing opportunistic infections.

HIV is spread primarily by the following:

- Not using a condom when having sex with a person who has HIV, with unprotected anal sex carrying a greater risk than unprotected vaginal sex
- Having multiple sex partners or partners with other sexually transmitted diseases
- Sharing needles, syringes, rinse water, or other items used to make illicit drugs for injection
- Transmission from an infected mother to child during pregnancy, delivery, or while breastfeeding

Less common modes of transmission include the following:

- Needlesticks from an HIV-contaminated needle or sharps
- HIV-contaminated blood transfusions, blood products, or organ/tissue transplants
- Contact of HIV-infected blood or blood contaminated body fluids and broken skin, wounds, or mucous membranes
- Open-mouth kissing
- Tattooing or body piercing

HIV is not spread by the following:

- Water
- Air
- Insects

- Animals
- Closed-mouth kissing
- Coughing
- Casual contact such as hugging
- Saliva, tears, or sweat

Healthcare workers should assume that the blood and body fluids from all patients are potentially infectious. They should follow standard precautions at all times. These precautions include the following:

- Routinely using personal protective equipment when anticipating contact with blood or body fluids
- Washing hands and other skin surfaces immediately after contact with blood or body fluids
- Carefully handling and disposing of sharps during and after use

Viral Hepatitis

Hepatitis means inflammation of the liver. There are several types of viral hepatitis: hepatitis A (HAV), hepatitis B (HBV), hepatitis C (HCV), hepatitis D (HDV), and hepatitis E (HEV). HAV, HBV, and HCV are the three most common types of viral hepatitis. In all cases of viral hepatitis, the liver becomes inflamed or swollen.

HAV infection occurs frequently in the United States and is endemic in certain western and southwestern states and in Alaska. Since 1996, hepatitis A vaccination (Havrix, Vaqta) is part of routine pediatric immunization in the United States. Hepatitis A vaccine is recommended for adults with a medical, occupational, or behavioral risk of infection. Medical indications include clotting factor disorders or chronic liver disease, such as chronic active hepatitis C and/or B virus infection. Occupational indications include working with HAV in a laboratory setting. Behavioral indications include illicit (injection and noninjection) drug users and men having unprotected sex with men.

Universal vaccination (Engerix-B, Recombivax-HB) of infants against HBV has been standard in the United States since 1991. Hepatitis B immunization is recommended for adults with a medical, occupational, or behavioral risk of infection. Medical indications include hemodialysis, treatment with clotting-factor concentrates, or HIV infection. Occupational indications include healthcare or public safety work with potential exposure to blood or body fluids such as vaginal secretions, semen, and saliva. Behavioral indications include injection drug use, sex with more than one partner in the previous six months, kissing or close family contact with an infected individual, recently acquired sexually transmitted infection, and men having unprotected sex with men. Unvaccinated adults with diabetes; clients of facilities that treat sexually transmitted infections, HIV, or drug abuse; residents and staff members of institutions for the developmentally disabled; and household contacts and sex partners of those with chronic hepatitis B infection should also be vaccinated for HBV.

There is no vaccine to prevent HCV and no treatment after exposure to prevent infection. The virus is spread through blood, body fluids, needle sharing, or needlesticks, or from mother to baby during labor and delivery. Patients with HCV may also be at risk

What Would You Do?

What are the modes of transmission for HIV and viral hepatitis?

for infection with HBV, HAV, and HIV. These patients should be vaccinated for HAV and HBV.

The Occupational Safety and Health Administration (OSHA) established the blood-borne pathogen standard to reduce the risk of occupational exposure to infectious microorganisms such as hepatitis B virus, hepatitis C virus, and HIV virus present in blood that can cause disease **FIGURE 5.6** .

Mandatory Reporting of Infectious Diseases

Certain infectious diseases must be reported to the state or local authority. The Centers for Disease Control and Prevention (CDC) also require that this information be reported to them. Each year, the CDC publishes a summary of the cases of notifiable disease reported for the most recent year data is available. This data helps the CDC prevent and control the spread of infection. Forms for reporting infectious diseases are available at each state health department. The state health department then forwards the information to the CDC. Orders for tests and procedures and follow-up orders may be requested when the appropriate agency has received the information. **TABLE 5.3** lists diseases that must be reported to the CDC.

OSHAFactSheet

OSHA's Bloodborne Pathogens Standard

Bloodborne pathogens are infectious microorganisms present in blood that can cause disease in humans. These pathogens include, but are not limited to, hepatitis B virus (HBV), hepatitis C virus (HCV), and human immunodeficiency virus (HIV), the virus that causes AIDS. Workers exposed to bloodborne pathogens are at risk for serious or life-threatening illnesses.

Protections Provided by OSHA's Bloodborne Pathogens Standard

All of the requirements of OSHA's Bloodborne Pathogens standard can be found in Title 29 of the Code of Federal Regulations at 29 CFR 1910.1030. The standard's requirements state what employers must do to protect workers who are occupationally exposed to blood or other potentially infectious materials (OPIM), as defined in the standard. That is, the standard protects workers who can reasonably be anticipated to come into contact with blood or OPIM as a result of doing their job duties.

In general, the standard requires employers to:

- **Establish an exposure control plan.** This is a written plan to eliminate or minimize occupational exposures. The employer must prepare an exposure determination that contains a list of job classifications in which all workers have occupational exposure and a list of job classifications in which some workers have occupational exposure, along with a list of the tasks and procedures performed by those workers that result in their exposure.

- **Employers must update the plan annually** to reflect changes in tasks, procedures, and positions that affect occupational exposure, and also technological changes that eliminate or reduce occupational exposure. In addition, employers must annually document in the plan that they have considered and begun using appropriate, commercially-available effective safer medical devices designed to eliminate or minimize occupational exposure. Employers must also document that they have solicited input from frontline workers in identifying, evaluating, and selecting effective engineering and work practice controls.

- **Implement the use of universal precautions** (treating all human blood and OPIM as if known to be infectious for bloodborne pathogens).

- **Identify and use engineering controls.** These are devices that isolate or remove the bloodborne pathogens hazard from the workplace. They include sharps disposal containers, self-sheathing needles, and safer medical devices, such as sharps with engineered sharps-injury protection and needleless systems.

- **Identify and ensure the use of work practice controls.** These are practices that reduce the possibility of exposure by changing the way a task is performed, such as appropriate practices for handling and disposing of contaminated sharps, handling specimens, handling laundry, and cleaning contaminated surfaces and items.

- **Provide personal protective equipment (PPE), such as gloves, gowns, eye protection, and masks.** Employers must clean, repair, and replace this equipment as needed. Provision, maintenance, repair and replacement are at no cost to the worker.

- **Make available hepatitis B vaccinations to all workers with occupational exposure.** This vaccination must be offered after the worker has received the required bloodborne pathogens training and within 10 days of initial assignment to a job with occupational exposure.

- **Make available post-exposure evaluation and follow-up to any occupationally exposed worker who experiences an exposure incident.** An exposure incident is a specific eye, mouth, other mucous membrane, non-intact skin, or parenteral contact with blood or OPIM. This evaluation and follow-up must be at no cost to the worker and includes documenting the route(s) of exposure and the circumstances

FIGURE 5.6 OSHA's blood-borne pathogen standards.
Courtesy of OSHA

Table 5.3 Some Diseases That Must Be Reported to the CDC		
Anthrax	Botulism	Chancroid
Chlamydia trachomatis infections	Cholera	Diphtheria
Giardiasis	Gonorrhea	Hepatitis A, B, and C
Legionellosis	Lyme disease	Malaria
Measles	Meningococcal disease	Mumps
Pertussis	Poliomyelitis	Rabies (animal and human)
Rocky Mountain spotted fever	Rubella	Salmonellosis
Syphilis	Tetanus	Toxic-shock syndrome
Tuberculosis	Tularemia	Typhoid fever
Varicella	West Nile virus	Yellow fever

Universal Precautions

Universal precautions were a set of precautions recommended in 1987 by the CDC to prevent transmission of blood-borne infections such as HIV/AIDS, hepatitis B, and hepatitis C to healthcare personnel. Under universal precautions, all blood and body fluids should be considered potentially infectious. In 1996, these precautions were expanded and called standard precautions.

Standard Precautions

Standard precautions are the minimum level of infection-control practices recommended by the CDC that should be used by all healthcare professionals all of the time when caring for people. Standard precautions are designed for all patients, regardless of their diagnosis or presumed infection status. Using standard precautions in the care of all patients can help reduce the risk of transmission of microorganisms from recognized and unrecognized sources of infection. These practices not only protect the patient from the spread of infection, but also protect you from becoming infected. Standard precautions apply to blood, all body fluids, and secretions and excretions (except sweat) whether or not they contain visible blood, nonintact skin, and mucous membranes. Appropriate protection against exposure to blood and body fluids should be routine practice for all healthcare providers.

Standard precautions include the following **FIGURE 5.7**:

- Hand hygiene
- Personal protective equipment
- Injection safety
- Environmental cleaning
- Medical equipment
- Respiratory hygiene/cough etiquette

> Standard precautions in the care of all patients can help reduce the risk of transmission of infection.

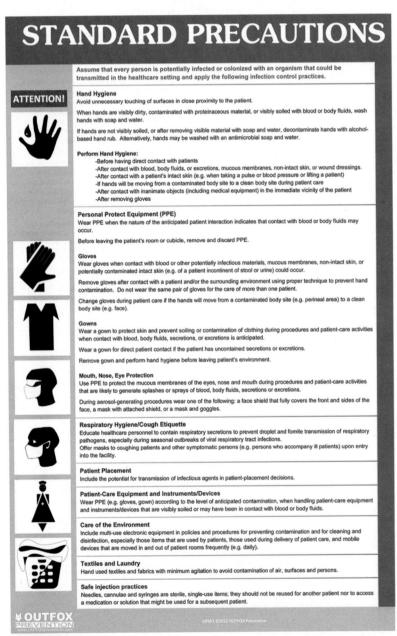

FIGURE 5.7 Centers for Disease Control and Prevention's standard precautions for infection control.
Courtesy of OUTFOX Prevention

Hand Hygiene

Washing your hands is one of the most effective ways to prevent transmission of pathogens. Good hand hygiene can reduce the risk of spreading infections in ambulatory care settings. Use of an alcohol-based hand rub is the primary method of hand hygiene recommended by the CDC and the World Health Organization (WHO) in ambulatory care settings because of its activity against a broad spectrum of pathogens. Use of an alcohol-based hand rub is the preferred method for hand hygiene when the hands are not visibly soiled

Standard precautions apply to blood, all body fluids, and secretions and excretions (except sweat) whether or not they contain visible blood, nonintact skin, and mucous membranes.
© auremar/ShutterStock, Inc.

by body fluids or dirt. Using an alcohol-based hand rub also requires less time, is less irritating to the hands, and is more convenient because it can be applied at the patient's bedside, unlike soap and water. Use of soap and water is the preferred method of hand hygiene when the hands are visibly soiled or when one is caring for patients with known or suspected infectious diarrhea.

Hand hygiene should be performed in the following ambulatory care situations:

- Before touching a patient, after direct contact with a patient, and in between patients, even if gloves are worn
- Immediately after glove removal or after removal of personal protective equipment
- Before performing an aseptic task, such as placing an IV or handling an invasive device

Good hand hygiene is one of the most effective methods to prevent transmission of infection in ambulatory care settings.
© auremar/ShutterStock, Inc.

- After touching blood, body fluids, secretions, excretions (except sweat), wound dressings, intact skin, nonintact skin, and contaminated items, even if gloves are worn
- During patient care when moving hands from a contaminated body site to a clean body site
- After contact with inanimate objects in the vicinity of the patient

When the hands are visibly soiled or when caring for patients with known or suspected infectious diarrhea, the technique for hand hygiene in ambulatory care settings is as follows:

1. Wet your hands.
2. Apply soap and rub all surfaces for 40–60 seconds.

The Centers for Disease Control and Prevention recommend washing your hands for as long as it takes to sing the "happy birthday" song twice (60 seconds).

3. Rinse with warm water and dry hands thoroughly with a single-use towel.
4. Use the towel to turn off the faucet.
5. Dispose of the used towel without touching the garbage can.

When the hands are not visibly soiled by body fluids or dirt, the technique for hand hygiene in ambulatory care settings is as follows:

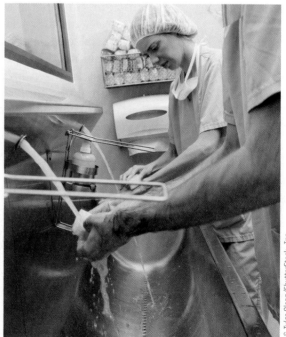

Hand hygiene can prevent the transmission of pathogens.
© Tyler Olson/ShutterStock, Inc.

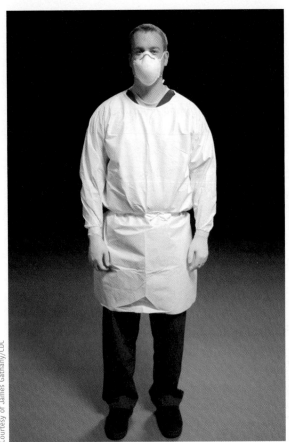

Medical assistants should wear personal protective equipment to protect against exposure to infectious agents.

1. Apply enough alcohol-based hand rub to cover all areas of the hands.
2. Rub all surfaces for 20–30 seconds.
3. Rub hands until dry.

Personal Protective Equipment

Personal protective equipment (PPE) protects healthcare providers from exposure to or contact with infectious agents. Examples of PPE include gloves, gowns, goggles, masks, and face shields. The selection of PPE is determined by the potential for exposure to blood, body fluids, or infectious agents and the type of exposure anticipated.

When you are selecting PPE, consider three key things:

■ The type of anticipated exposure, such as touch, splashes, or sprays, or large volumes of body fluids that might penetrate the clothing.
■ The appropriateness of the PPE for the task.
■ The fit. PPE must fit the individual user. The employer must ensure that all PPE are available in sizes appropriate for all personnel.

> Personal protective equipment includes gloves, gowns, masks, goggles, glasses, and face shields.

Gloves protect hands and are the most common type of PPE used in the healthcare setting. Most patient-care activities require the use of a single pair of nonsterile gloves made of latex, nitrile, or vinyl. Some facilities have eliminated or limited latex products, including gloves, and now use gloves made of nitrile or other material because of allergy concerns. Gloves should fit the user's hands, should not be too loose or too tight, and should not tear or damage easily. Be aware that gloves protect the hands from contamination, but do not prevent needlesticks or other sharp instruments from penetrating the skin.

Gloves should be worn in the following situations:

■ In situations involving direct or indirect contact with blood, body fluids, secretions, excretions, mucous membranes, nonintact skin, or potentially infectious material
■ When changing between tasks and procedures on the same patient after contact with infectious material
■ Before going to another patient
■ During surgical or invasive procedures

Facial protection (face, eyes, nose, and mouth) should be worn in the following situation:

■ During activities that are likely to generate splashes of blood, body fluids, secretions, or excretions

A gown should be worn to protect skin and clothing during the following situation:

■ During activities or procedures where contact with blood, body fluids, secretions, or excretions is anticipated

Following are recommendations for personal protective equipment in ambulatory care settings:

■ Remove and discard all PPE before leaving the patient's room.
■ Do not reuse the same pair of gloves or other PPE on more than one patient.
■ Wash hands with an alcohol-based rub or soap and water immediately after removing gloves.

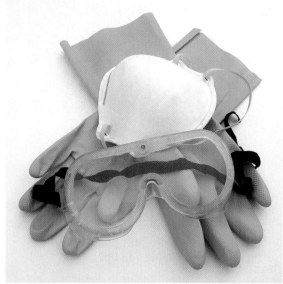
Personal protective equipment.

Injection Safety

Injection safety includes methods designed to prevent transmission of infectious disease from one patient to another, or from a patient to a healthcare provider during administration of **parenteral medications** or handling of needles, scalpels, and other sharp instruments or devices.

Unsafe injection practices include the use of one syringe or needle to administer medication to more than one patient, reinsertion of a used syringe into a vial of medication or solution container and then using that same vial or solution for another patient, and preparation and administration of medications near contaminated supplies or equipment.

Recommendations for safe injection practices in ambulatory care settings include the following:

■ Use aseptic technique when preparing and administering parenteral medications. **Aseptic technique** is a set of practices or procedures performed under controlled conditions with the goal of minimizing contamination by pathogens.
■ Use alcohol wipes to clean the top of a vial before inserting a needle into the vial.
■ Use a new needle and syringe for each patient and for each entry into a vial or bag of solution.
■ Do not administer medications from one syringe to multiple patients.
■ Single-dose or single-use vials should only be used for one patient.
■ Multidose vials, when used on multiple patients, should not enter patient care areas.
■ Do not use the same IV tubing or administration set for multiple patients.

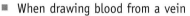

What Would You Do?

What type of PPE would you wear in the following situations?

■ When drawing blood from a vein
■ When taking blood pressure measurements
■ When irrigating a wound

© NorthGeorgiaMedia/ShutterStock, Inc.

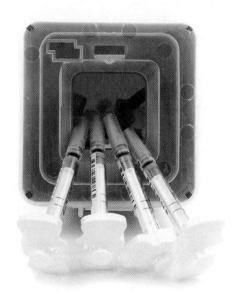
Dispose of used syringes and needles in a sharps container.

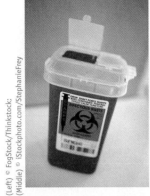
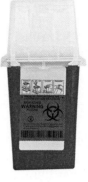
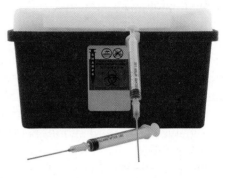

(Left) © FogStock/Thinkstock;
(Middle) © iStockphoto.com/StephanieFrey

(Right) © Bhathaway/ShutterStock, Inc.

Puncture-proof sharps containers should be sent to a biohazard agency for safe disposal.

What Would You Do?

You are in charge of developing a plan to eliminate an employee's risk for exposure to infectious blood or bodily fluids. What measures would you take to eliminate or lessen the risk for exposure to these infectious agents?

© NorthGeorgiaMedia/ShutterStock, Inc.

- Dispose of used sharp instruments, syringes, and needles in a sharps container. Never break needles off or handle needles after they are used.

When exposure to a blood-borne pathogen occurs, OSHA blood-borne pathogens standards require employers to make medical evaluation and follow-up available to all workers at no cost to the patient. Exposure should be reported immediately to the employer. This will facilitate immediate evaluation and, if necessary, treatment. It can also prevent the worker from spreading the blood-borne pathogen to others. Post-exposure prophylaxis for HIV, HBV, and HCV must also be offered to employees when medically indicated.

Environmental Cleaning

Removing visible soil and contamination from a device or surface by scrubbing with a surfactant (a substance that reduces the surface tension of a liquid in which it is dissolved) or detergent and water or with chemical agents can remove large numbers of microorganisms. Surfaces that are most likely to become contaminated with pathogens include those in close proximity to the patient and those that are frequently touched in patient-care areas.

Recommendations for environmental cleaning in ambulatory care settings include the following:

- Clean or disinfect frequently touched surfaces in close proximity to the patient.
- Clean up spills immediately. Spilled blood or body fluids should be cleaned using a liquid germicide or a 1:10 bleach solution.
- Use EPA-registered cleaners or disinfectants specific for healthcare use.
- Follow the manufacturer's guidelines on proper use of the product.
- Place materials used to clean up a spill in a biohazard waste bag.

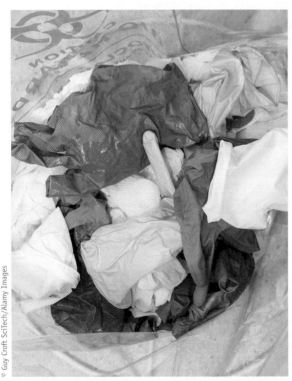

© Guy Croft SciTech/Alamy Images

Materials used to clean up a spill should be placed in a biohazard waste bag.

Medical Equipment

Medical equipment can either be reusable or for single use. Reusable medical equipment should be accompanied by instructions from the manufacturer for cleaning and disinfection or sterilization. Single-use devices should not be reprocessed. All reusable medical equipment must be cleaned and disinfected or sterilized and maintained to prevent transmission of infectious agents.

Recommendations for cleaning, disinfection, and sterilization of medical equipment in ambulatory care settings include the following:

■ All reusable medical equipment should be cleaned and disinfected or sterilized according to the manufacturer's specifications before it is used on another patient.

■ All healthcare professionals should wear appropriate personal protective equipment when handling contaminated medical equipment.

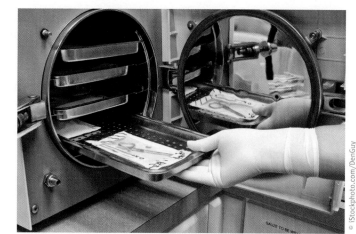

All reusable medical equipment should be cleaned, disinfected, or sterilized.

Respiratory Hygiene/Cough Etiquette

Respiratory hygiene/cough etiquette is a standard precaution of infection control that targets patients and their family members with undiagnosed transmissible respiratory infections, including cough, **rhinorrhea** (runny nose), and increased respiratory secretions at the point of entry into the healthcare facility, such as reception and triage areas.

Recommendations for respiratory hygiene/cough etiquette practices in ambulatory care settings include the following:

■ Contain respiratory secretions in those who have signs and symptoms of a respiratory infection.

■ Post signs at the entrance of healthcare facilities with instructions to cover their mouths/noses when coughing or sneezing, use and dispose of tissues, use masks when available, and use proper hand washing techniques.

■ If possible, place febrile respiratory symptomatic patients at least 3 feet away from others in common waiting areas.

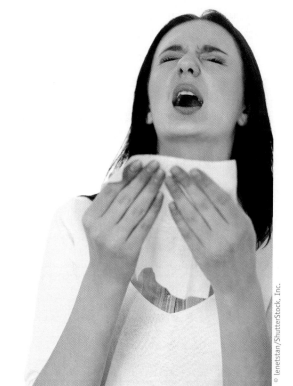

All patients should cover their mouth/nose when coughing or sneezing.

Explain standard precautions and how they can prevent transmission of infection.

Expanded Precautions

In addition to standard precautions, the CDC developed guidelines intended for patients diagnosed with or suspected of having specific highly transmissible diseases.

These are known as **expanded precautions** (formerly known as transmission-based precautions).

> *Expanded precautions should be followed in addition to standard precautions for all patients diagnosed with or suspected of having highly transmissible diseases.*
>
> © auremar/ShutterStock, Inc.

These precautions are designed to reduce the risk for contact, droplet, or airborne transmission of pathogens. These precautions should be used in addition to standard precautions.

Contact Precautions

Contact precautions apply to patients with the presence of stool incontinence, draining wounds, uncontrolled secretions, pressure ulcers, presence of tubes or bags of draining body fluids, or generalized rash. These patients should be placed in an exam room as soon as possible. Standard precautions should be performed, including hand hygiene; respiratory hygiene and cough etiquette; use of personal protective equipment such as a face mask, gown, and goggles; and disinfecting the exam room **FIGURE 5.8**.

What Would You Do?

A patient known or suspected to be infected with *Mycobacterium tuberculosis* comes into your healthcare facility. What measures would you take to eliminate or lessen the risk for exposure to or transmission of these infectious agents?

© NorthGeorgiaMedia/ShutterStock, Inc.

Droplet Precautions

Droplet precautions apply to patients known or suspected to be infected with a pathogen that can be transmitted via a droplet such as respiratory viruses and bordetella pertussis. These patients should be placed in an exam room with a closed door as soon as possible. If an exam room is unavailable, the patient should use a face mask and wait in a separate area as far away as possible from other patients. Standard precautions should be performed, including hand hygiene; respiratory hygiene and cough etiquette; use of personal protective equipment such as a face mask, gown, and goggles; and disinfecting the exam room **FIGURE 5.9**.

Airborne Precautions

Airborne precautions apply to patients known or suspected to be infected with a pathogen that can be transmitted via the air such as tuberculosis, measles, and chicken pox. These patients should enter the healthcare facility through a dedicated isolation entrance and be placed immediately in an airborne infection isolation room with a closed door. If this type of room is unavailable, the patient should be instructed to wear a face mask until

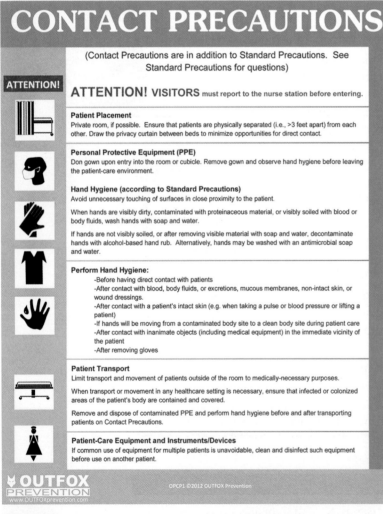

FIGURE 5.8 Contact precautions are one component of expanded precautions.
Courtesy of OUTFOX Prevention

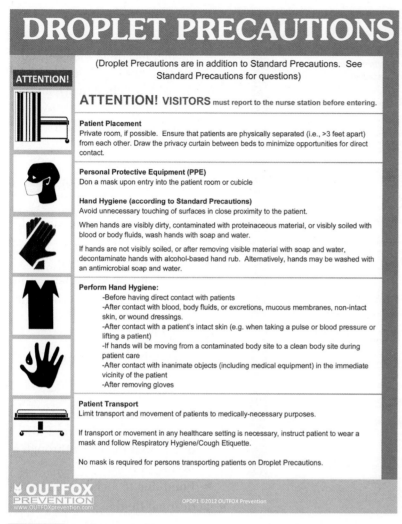

FIGURE 5.9 Droplet precautions are one component of expanded precautions.
Courtesy of OUTFOX Prevention

transfer to a healthcare facility capable of managing this patient can occur. Standard precautions should be performed, including hand hygiene; respiratory hygiene and cough etiquette; use of personal protective equipment such as a face mask, gown, and goggles; and disinfecting the exam room **FIGURE 5.10**.

Blood and Body Fluids

Blood and body fluids refer to blood, secretions, and excretions of a patient. Pathogens found in the patient's blood or body fluids can be transmitted from the infectious person or infected body fluids to a susceptible host, especially if measures are not taken to prevent the spread of infection. The potential for exposure to these pathogens increases whenever invasive procedures are being performed. Examples of blood and body fluids and areas where the medical assistant may be exposed to them are listed here:

- Blood:
  - Drawn during venipuncture
  - Administering an injection

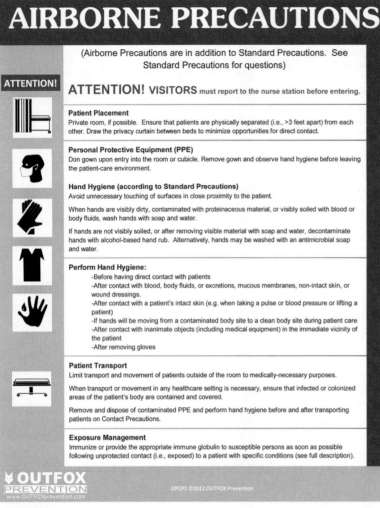

FIGURE 5.10 Airborne precautions are one component of expanded precautions.
Courtesy of OUTFOX Prevention

- **Epistaxis** (nosebleeds)
- Open wounds or lesions
- Vaginal bleeding, **menses** (during menstruation), **lochia** (discharge after childbirth), and hemorrhage
- Feces, vomit, or other body fluids
- Vaginal secretions:
  - Vaginal discharge (with or without infection)
  - During pap smears or vaginal exams
- Cerebrospinal fluid:
  - Drawn during spinal tap
  - Fluid from trauma to the brain or spinal cord
- Synovial fluid:
  - Drawn during arthroscopic procedures
- Pleural fluid:
  - Drawn during **thoracentesis** (a procedure that removes fluid or air from the chest through a needle or tube)
  - Fluid due to a chest trauma
- Pericardial fluid:
  - Exposure to fluid during cardiac surgery or cardiac trauma
- Peritoneal fluid:
  - Exposure to fluid during abdominal surgery
- Semen:
  - Exposure to seminal fluid during fertility testing
- Amniotic fluid:
  - Drawn during **amniocentesis** (a procedure used to diagnose fetal defects in the early second trimester of pregnancy)
- Breast milk:
  - Not likely to occur
- Saliva:
  - Expectorated sputum
  - Exposure during dental procedures

Needlesticks

Healthcare workers use many types of needles and other sharp devices to provide patient care. Medical assistants are at risk of exposure to blood-borne pathogens such as

HIV, hepatitis B (HBV), and hepatitis C (HCV) from needlesticks and other sharps-related injuries in the workplace. **Sharps** are objects that can penetrate the skin, such as needles, scalpels, glass, and capillary tubes. The risk of HBV or HCV infection caused by a needlestick is significantly greater than the risk of HIV infection from a needlestick.

To prevent needlestick injury and reduce the risk of infection, healthcare workers should do the following:

- Avoid the use of needles if safe and effective alternatives are available.
- Never recap used needles.
- Avoid removing needles from syringes.
- Dispose of used needles in sharps disposal containers immediately.

Use the one-handed scoop method when recapping, bending, or removing needles.

To address the problem of exposure to blood-borne pathogens from accidental sharps injuries, the Needlestick Safety and Prevention Act was created by OSHA. It mandates the following:

- Employers must use safer medical devices such as those that are needleless or that have built-in protection to guard against contact with contaminated sharps.
- Employers must involve employees in identifying, evaluating, and selecting safer medical devices.
- Employers must maintain a sharps injury log for contaminated sharps.
- Sharp containers must be readily accessible.
- Recapping, bending, or removing needles is allowed only if it is required for a medical or dental procedure.
- When recapping, bending, or removing needles, a one-handed scoop technique may be used. This technique uses the needle itself to scoop up the cap; after that, the capped needle is carried to the sharps container.
- If a sharps disposal container is not in close proximity, the scoop technique of recapping may be used.

Infectious Waste

Infectious waste is any item that has come in contact with blood or body fluids. These items should be handled with PPE such as gloves and placed in appropriate biohazard containers. Infectious waste is either burned or autoclaved before it is disposed of. Contact your local department of health for specific procedures you must follow to dispose of sharps and infectious waste. They can also refer you to a company that specializes in disposal of sharps and infectious waste. Most companies will set up a pickup schedule; charges may be based on the frequency of pickup or the amount of infectious waste that needs to be disposed of.

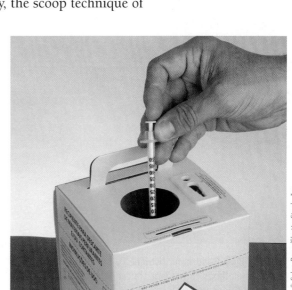

Dispose of all infectious waste in a biohazard container.

Infectious waste and all items used to handle it should be placed in a biohazard container.

Medical Asepsis

One measure of infection control is medical asepsis. The other measure of infection control is surgical asepsis. **Surgical asepsis** is the use of practices to prevent transmission of infectious organisms and eliminate microorganisms during surgery. **Medical asepsis** is the use of practices to help contain and prevent the transmission of infectious organisms and to maintain an environment free from contamination. Following these practices greatly reduces the presence of pathogens that could cause disease in others. Techniques used to maintain medical asepsis include hand washing, gowning, wearing face masks, cleaning and disinfecting contaminated surfaces and equipment, and adherence to standard and expanded precautions. Standard and expanded precautions are considered methods of medical asepsis.

Equipment should be medically aseptic if it is to be used in procedures that enter into the body or into sterile areas of the body. Not all objects need to be sterile. Stethoscopes and sphygmomanometers are used on many patients daily, but do not enter into sterile areas of the body. These objects should be cleaned and disinfected routinely with alcohol-based wipes.

Examples of medical asepsis include the following:

- Following hand washing guidelines outlined in standard precautions
- Use of PPE as outlined in standard precautions
- Disposal of biohazardous waste in appropriate sharps containers
- Cleaning or sterilizing equipment or supplies before use
- Covering open wounds with a sterile dressing

Skills for the Medical Assistant

A medical assistant must be proficient in the skills necessary to minimize the spread of infection. The procedures outlined in this section cover the basics of infection control and standard precautions in the ambulatory care setting. Following these infection-control procedures, including standard precautions and medical asepsis, can limit the transmission of infection and provide barriers against transmission.

Performing Hand Hygiene When Hands Are Visibly Soiled

Good hand hygiene is one of the most effective methods to prevent direct and indirect transmission of pathogens in ambulatory care settings. Hand washing must be performed on a regular basis before and after each patient contact and procedure.

In this exercise, you will learn the procedure for washing hands that are visibly soiled or when caring for patients with known or suspected infectious diarrhea. The duration of the entire procedure is 40–60 seconds.

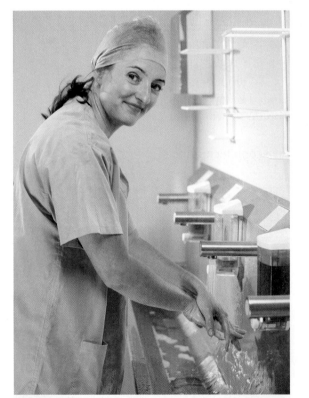

FIGURE 5.11 Good hand hygiene is one of the most effective methods to prevent transmission of pathogens in an ambulatory care setting.
© iStockphoto.com/sturti

Equipment Needed

- Sink, preferably with foot-operated controls
- Liquid soap (preferably) with foot-operated dispenser
- Disposable paper towels
- Nail brush or stick

Steps

1. Remove all jewelry. (A plain wedding band is acceptable.)
2. Turn on the faucet using the foot-operated controls or with a dry paper towel **FIGURE 5.11**. Discard the paper towel after turning on the faucet.
3. Wet hands with water **FIGURE 5.12**.
4. Apply enough soap to cover all hand surfaces **FIGURE 5.13**.
5. Rub together the palms of both hands in a circular motion **FIGURE 5.14**.
6. Rub with the right palm over the back of the left hand with interlaced fingers, and vice versa **FIGURE 5.15**.
7. Rub palm to palm with fingers interlaced **FIGURE 5.16**.
8. Rub the backs of the fingers to the opposing palms with fingers interlocked **FIGURE 5.17**.

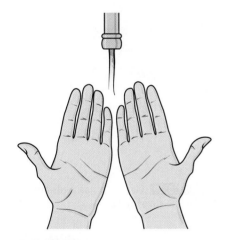

FIGURE 5.12 Wet hands with water.
© Jones & Bartlett Learning

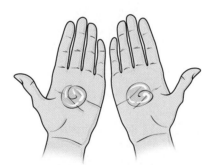
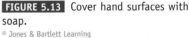

FIGURE 5.13 Cover hand surfaces with soap.
© Jones & Bartlett Learning

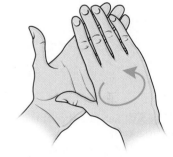

FIGURE 5.14 Rub together in a circular motion the palms of both hands.
© Jones & Bartlett Learning

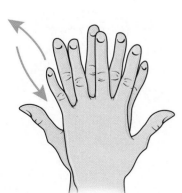
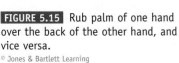

FIGURE 5.15 Rub palm of one hand over the back of the other hand, and vice versa.
© Jones & Bartlett Learning

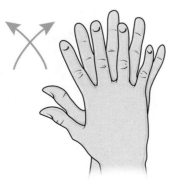

FIGURE 5.16 Rub palm to palm with fingers interlaced.
© Jones & Bartlett Learning

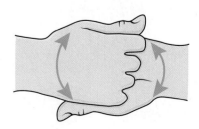

FIGURE 5.17 Rub the backs of the fingers to the opposing palms.
© Jones & Bartlett Learning

9. Rub in a circular motion counterclockwise with the left thumb clasped in the right palm and vice versa **FIGURE 5.18**.
10. Rub in a circular motion backward and forward with clasped fingers of the right hand in the left palm and vice versa **FIGURE 5.19**.
11. Use a nail brush or stick to clean the nail beds for the first hand washing of each day **FIGURE 5.20**.
12. Rinse hands with water **FIGURE 5.21**.
13. Dry hands thoroughly with a single-use disposable paper towel. Do not touch the towel dispenser after hand washing. Prepare a towel in advance if you will have to touch the paper towel dispenser **FIGURE 5.22**.
14. Use the foot pedal or a clean disposable towel to turn off the faucet **FIGURE 5.23**.
15. Discard the used paper towel **FIGURE 5.24**.

After hand washing, do not touch any contaminated surface and never allow your clothing to touch the sink.

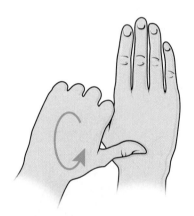

FIGURE 5.18 Rub in a circular motion counterclockwise.
© Jones & Bartlett Learning

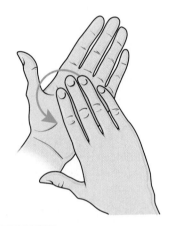

FIGURE 5.19 Rub in a circular motion backward and forward with clasped fingers.
© Jones & Bartlett Learning

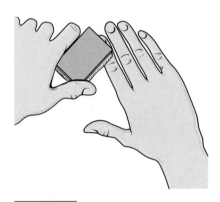

FIGURE 5.20 Clean the nail beds and under the fingernails.
© Jones & Bartlett Learning

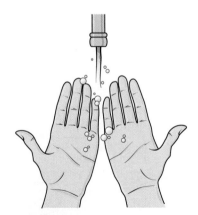

FIGURE 5.21 Rinse hands with water.
© Jones & Bartlett Learning

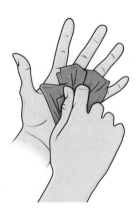

FIGURE 5.22 Dry hands thoroughly with a single-use paper towel.
© Jones & Bartlett Learning

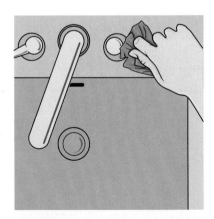

FIGURE 5.23 Use a clean disposable towel to turn off the faucet (if not lever operated).
© Jones & Bartlett Learning

Performing Hand Hygiene When Hands Are Not Visibly Soiled

Good hand hygiene is one of the most effective methods to prevent direct and indirect transmission of pathogens in ambulatory care settings. Hand rubbing, when hands are not visibly soiled, must be performed on a regular basis before and after each patient contact and procedure.

In this exercise, you will learn the procedure for hand hygiene when hands are not visibly soiled by blood, body fluids, or dirt. The duration of the entire procedure is 20–30 seconds.

Equipment Needed

- Alcohol-based hand rub

Steps

1. Remove all jewelry. (A plain wedding band is acceptable.)
2. Apply a palmful of alcohol-based hand rub in a cupped hand, covering all surfaces.
3. Rub together the palms of both hands in a circular motion.
4. Rub with the right palm over the back of the left hand with interlaced fingers, and vice versa.
5. Rub palm to palm with fingers interlaced.
6. Rub the backs of the fingers to the opposing palms with fingers interlocked.
7. Rub in a circular motion counterclockwise with the left thumb clasped in the right palm and vice versa.
8. Rub in a circular motion backward and forward with clasped fingers of the right hand in the left palm and vice versa.
9. Allow hands to air dry.

After performing the hand rub procedure, do not touch any contaminated surface.

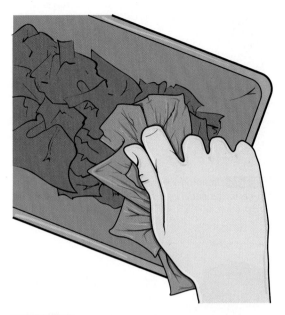

FIGURE 5.24 Discard the used paper towel.
© Jones & Bartlett Learning

Donning Personal Protective Equipment

Donning personal protective equipment protects the medical assistant from exposure to or contact with infectious agents.

Equipment Needed

- Disposable gloves
- Disposable gown
- Disposable mask
- Face shield
- Respirator

Sequence for Donning PPE

1. Gown
2. Mask or respirator

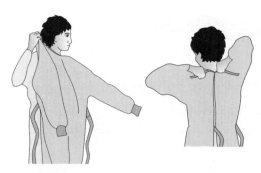

FIGURE 5.25 Donning a gown: The opening should be in the back.
Courtesy of CDC

3. Goggles or face shield
4. Gloves

The PPE needed and the sequence for donning will be determined by the precautions that need to be taken.

Steps for Donning a Gown

1. Select the appropriate size and type of gown.
2. The opening of the gown should be in the back. Secure the gown at the neck and waist. If the gown is too small to cover you, use a second gown. Put the first gown on with the ties in the front and the second gown on over the first with the ties in the back **FIGURE 5.25**.

Steps for Donning a Mask

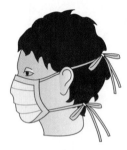

FIGURE 5.26 Place the mask over your nose, mouth, and chin, and secure it with ties or elastic.
Courtesy of CDC

1. Place the mask over the nose, mouth, and chin.
2. Fit the flexible nosepiece over the nose bridge.
3. Secure the mask on with ties or elastic and adjust to fit. If the mask has ties, tie the top set of ties at the back of your head above the ears and the lower set of ties at the base of your neck. If the mask has elastic bands, separate the elastic bands with one hand and the mask with the other hand. Next, place and hold the mask over your mouth, nose, and chin with one hand and using the other hand stretch the bands over your head. Place the top elastic band at the upper back of your head above the ears and the lower elastic band below the ears at the base of the neck **FIGURE 5.26**.

Steps for Donning a Particulate Respirator

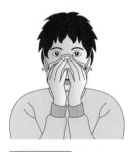

FIGURE 5.27 Donning a respirator: Select one that fits you well.
Courtesy of CDC

1. Select a fit-tested respirator (a respirator that provides the most acceptable fit).
2. Place the respirator over the nose, mouth, and chin.
3. Fit the nosepiece of the respirator over the nose bridge.
4. Secure on the head with elastic and adjust to fit.
5. Perform a fit check **FIGURE 5.27**.

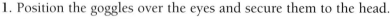

Always follow the manufacturer's instructions for the specific respirator, as they may vary from one device to another.

Steps for Donning Goggles or a Face Shield

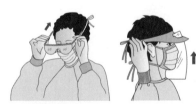

FIGURE 5.28 Donning goggles or a face shield: Secure a face shield on the forehead with a headband.
Courtesy of CDC

1. Position the goggles over the eyes and secure them to the head.
2. If using a face shield, position the face shield over the face and secure it on the forehead with a headband.
3. Adjust to fit **FIGURE 5.28**.

Steps for Donning Gloves

1. Select the proper type and size of gloves.
2. Insert hands into gloves.

3. If you are wearing an isolation gown, extend the gloves over the isolation gown cuffs FIGURE 5.29 .

Removing Personal Protective Equipment

Correctly removing personal protective equipment protects the medical assistant from exposure to contaminated materials and limits opportunities for self-contamination. The location for removal of PPE will depend on the category of isolation precautions a patient is on and the amount and type of PPE worn by the medical assistant. If gloves are the only PPE that is worn, they may be discarded in the patient's room. Gowns, goggles, and face shields should be removed at the doorway or in the anteroom. Respirators should always be removed after leaving the patient's room and only when the door of the room has been closed. Proper hand hygiene, either hand washing or hand rubbing, should be performed after removal of PPE.

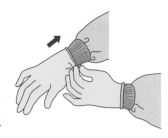

FIGURE 5.29 Don gloves last, making sure to use the proper size.
Courtesy of CDC

Equipment Needed

- Sink, preferably with foot-operated controls
- Liquid soap (preferably) with foot-operated dispenser or alcohol-based hand rub
- Disposable paper towels

Sequence for Removing PPE

1. Gloves
2. Goggles or face shield
3. Gown
4. Mask or respirator

Steps for Removing Gloves

1. Gloves should be removed first because they are considered to be the most contaminated. Using one gloved hand, pull the outside edge of the opposite glove near your wrist toward your fingertips and pull and peel the glove away from the hand, turning the glove inside out. Pull the fold until the glove is almost off. Continue to hold the removed glove and completely remove the glove. The contaminated side should now be in the inside.
2. Hold the glove that was just removed with the gloved hand.
3. Using the pointer finger of the ungloved hand, slide your finger under the remaining glove.
4. Pull the glove off from the inside and create a bag for both gloves.
5. Discard FIGURE 5.30 .

Steps for Removing Goggles or a Face Shield

1. Using both ungloved hands, lift the goggles or face shield away from the face.
2. If the goggles and face shield are disposable, discard them in the appropriate biohazard waste container. If

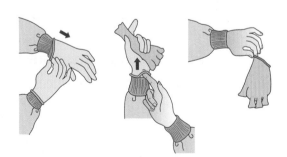

FIGURE 5.30 Remove gloves first because they are likely the most contaminated.
Courtesy of CDC

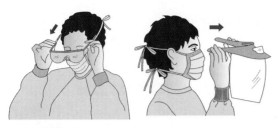

FIGURE 5.31 Removing goggles or a face shield.
Courtesy of CDC

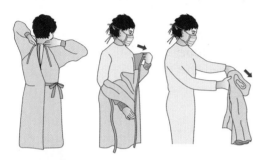

FIGURE 5.32 When removing a gown, turn the contaminated outside toward the inside.
Courtesy of CDC

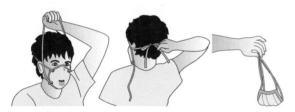

FIGURE 5.33 Removing a mask or respirator: Be careful not to touch the front of the mask as it is considered contaminated.
Courtesy of CDC

they aren't disposable, place them in the appropriate container for disinfection **FIGURE 5.31**.

Steps for Removing a Gown

1. Unfasten ties.
2. Using your hands, take the gown off from the neck and shoulders while touching the inside of the gown.
3. Turn the contaminated outside of the gown toward the inside.
4. Roll the gown into a bundle.
5. Discard the gown **FIGURE 5.32**.

Steps for Removing a Mask

1. Untie the bottom tie of the mask.
2. Untie the top tie. Be careful not to touch the front of the mask as it is considered contaminated.
3. Lift the mask away from the face.
4. Discard **FIGURE 5.33**.

Steps for Removing a Particulate Respirator

1. Lift the bottom elastic over your head.
2. Lift off the top elastic.
3. Discard.

After removal of all PPE, perform hand hygiene immediately. If hands are contaminated during removal of PPE, wash hands thoroughly if visibly soiled or with an alcohol-based hand rub if not visibly soiled before continuing to remove remaining PPE.

Sanitizing Instruments

Instruments must be cleaned to remove all tissue and debris prior to use. Sanitization is the process of washing and scrubbing to remove all blood, body fluids, and tissue.

Equipment Needed

- Sink, preferably with foot-operated controls
- Sanitizing agent with enzymatic action
- Soft brush
- Liquid soap (preferably) with foot-operated dispenser or alcohol-based hand rub
- Disposable paper towels
- Protective apron
- Gloves
- Goggles

Steps

1. Don PPE: goggles, apron, and gloves.
2. Follow standard precautions. If the instruments need to be transported, place the instruments in a biohazard container before transporting.
3. Rinse the instruments in cold water.
4. Place the instruments in the sanitizing agent.
5. Clean and scrub each instrument with detergent and water using a soft brush to remove all debris.
6. Rinse the instruments with hot water to remove any residue.
7. Dry each instrument with a disposable paper towel.
8. Remove PPE.
9. Wash hands thoroughly.

What Would You Do?

Your personal protective equipment came in contact with a patient's blood and body fluids. What would you do to handle and dispose of these items?

© NorthGeorgiaMedia/ShutterStock, Inc.

Performing Chemical Disinfection of Instruments

Heat-sensitive items must be sterilized using chemical disinfectants before use.

Equipment Needed

- Sink, preferably with foot-operated controls
- Liquid soap (preferably) with foot-operated dispenser or alcohol-based hand rub
- Chemical disinfectant
- Timer
- Sterile water
- Airtight container
- Disposable paper towels
- Poly-lined towels
- Sterile towels
- Protective apron
- Sterile gloves

Steps

1. Make sure the instrument has been sanitized and dried prior to chemical disinfection.
2. Don PPE.
3. Prepare the solution according to the manufacturer's instructions.
4. Pour the solution into an airtight container. Be careful to avoid splashing the solution.
5. Submerge the instrument in the solution and close the lid of the container.
6. Label the container with the name of the solution, date, and time required (according to the manufacturer) for sterilization.
7. When the required time has passed, remove the instrument using sterile gloves.
8. Rinse the instrument in sterile water.
9. Place the instrument on sterile poly-lined towels.

10. Dry the instrument completely using a sterile towel.

11. Store the instrument in a sterile area.

12. Remove PPE.

13. Wash hands thoroughly.

Wrapping Items for Autoclaving

Once an instrument has been sanitized, it can be wrapped for autoclaving. Articles must be wrapped in a special porous autoclave paper or cloth wrap. The manufacturer's instructions should be followed to ensure that sterility is achieved.

Equipment Needed

- Sink, preferably with foot-operated controls
- Liquid soap (preferably) with foot-operated dispenser or alcohol-based hand rub
- Autoclave paper or cloth
- Disposable plastic sealed pouches
- Autoclave tape
- Cotton balls
- Gauze
- Tip protectors
- Sterile gloves
- Sterilization indicator
- Sanitized instrument

Steps

1. Wash your hands.
2. Assemble all necessary items.
3. Make sure the instrument has been sanitized prior to wrapping for autoclaving **FIGURE 5.34**.
4. Place two squares of autoclave paper on a clean, flat surface with one corner of the paper facing you **FIGURE 5.35**.
5. Use a cotton ball for hinged instruments.
6. Wrap the item using the first square of the autoclave paper by folding the corner of the paper toward the center and turning a small corner back toward you **FIGURE 5.36**.
7. Next, fold two other sides toward the center in the same way as in step 6 **FIGURE 5.37**.
8. Fold the last corner of the autoclave paper up from the bottom in the same manner as the other three corners **FIGURE 5.38**.
9. Wrap the package in the second piece of autoclave paper using the same technique **FIGURE 5.39**.
10. Using autoclave tape, tape the package. Write the contents, date, and your initials on the tape **FIGURE 5.40**.

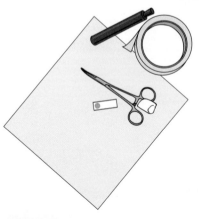

FIGURE 5.34 After washing your hands, assemble all of the necessary items and make sure that the instrument has been sanitized.

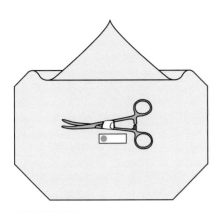

FIGURE 5.35 Place the instrument and the sterilization indicator on a square of clean autoclave paper.
© Jones & Bartlett Learning

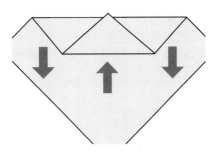

FIGURE 5.36 Wrap the item by folding the corner of the paper toward the center and back toward you.
© Jones & Bartlett Learning

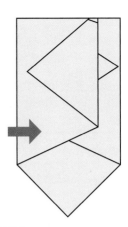

FIGURE 5.37 Wrap the item by folding the other two corners of the paper toward the center and back toward you.
© Jones & Bartlett Learning

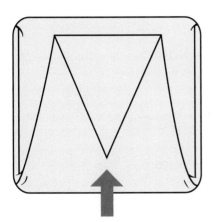

FIGURE 5.38 Fold the last corner of the autoclave paper.
© Jones & Bartlett Learning

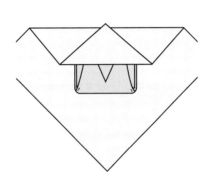

FIGURE 5.39 Wrap the package in the second piece of autoclave paper using the same technique.
© Jones & Bartlett Learning

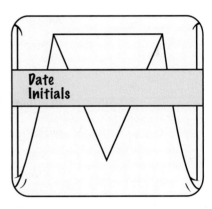

FIGURE 5.40 Label the contents of the autoclave package.
© Jones & Bartlett Learning

Math Practice

Question: **What is the sum of $\frac{1}{5} + \frac{5}{7}$?**

Answer:

Step 1: To obtain the sum, first determine the lowest common denominator: $\frac{1}{5} \times \frac{7}{7} = \frac{7}{35}$ and $\frac{5}{7} \times \frac{5}{5} = \frac{25}{35}$

Step 2: Complete the addition operation: $\frac{7}{35} + \frac{25}{35} = \frac{7+25}{35} = \frac{32}{35}$

Question: **What is the difference of $\frac{8}{11} - \frac{2}{11}$?**

Answer: $\frac{6}{11}$

Question: **What is the product of $^4/_8 \times {}^3/_5$?**

Answer: $^{12}/_{40}$, then simplify to $^3/_{10}$

Question: **What is the sum of 4.2 + 2.35 + 7.309?**

Answer: 13.859

Question: **What is the sum of 2.95 + 5.18 + 74.678?**

Answer: 82.808

Question: **What is the difference of 11.38 − 2.69?**

Answer: 8.69

Question: **How do you write $^8/_{50}$ as a percent?**

Answer:

Step 1: Find the equivalent fraction with a denominator of 100: $^8/_{50} \times {}^2/_2 = {}^{16}/_{100}$
Step 2: Convert the fraction to a percent: $^{16}/_{100} = 16\%$

Question: **How do you write $^7/_{10}$ as a percent?**

Answer:

Step 1: Find the equivalent fraction with a denominator of 100: $^7/_{10} \times {}^{10}/_{10} = {}^{70}/_{100}$
Step 2: Convert the fraction to a percent: $^{70}/_{100} = 70\%$

Question: **What is the quotient of $^3/_8 \div {}^2/_3$?**

Answer: $^9/_{16}$

Question: **What is the difference of $^9/_{15} − {}^2/_5$?**

Answer:

Step 1: Determine the lowest common denominator: $^9/_{15} \times {}^1/_1 = {}^9/_{15}$ and $^2/_5 \times {}^3/_3 = {}^6/_{15}$
Step 2: Complete the subtraction operation: $^9/_{15} − {}^6/_{15} = {}^3/_{15}$
Step 3: Simplify the fraction: $^1/_5$

Question: **What is the product of $^4/_7 \times {}^3/_5$?**

Answer: $^{12}/_{35}$

Question: **What is the product of $^3/_5 \times {}^5/_6$?**

Answer: $^{15}/_{30}$, which simplifies to $^1/_2$

Question: **What is the quotient of $^4/_7 \div {}^5/_8$?**

Answer: $^{32}/_{35}$

WRAP UP

Chapter Summary

- Infection-control procedures such as medical asepsis and surgical asepsis are precautions taken in the healthcare setting to prevent the spread of disease. These measures can break the chain of infection and prevent the transmission of disease.

- The chain of infection is the steps or links that must be connected in sequential order for the spread of infection to occur.

- An infectious agent is a microorganism that has the ability to cause a disease. It is the first step in the chain of infection. Infectious agents can be divided into five classifications: viruses, bacteria, fungi, parasites, and rickettsiae.

- Viruses are the smallest of all microorganisms and require a living host cell to replicate. Viruses are not affected by chemical disinfectants and antibiotics and can adapt to their environment so they remain resistant to treatment. Some viral infections can be prevented by vaccination.

- Bacteria are microorganisms that have only one cell. Many types of bacteria are beneficial, but some bacteria are pathogenic and can make you sick.

- Fungi are plantlike organisms that can grow on cloth, food, showers, or people, or in any warm, moist environment. Many fungi do not cause illness; however, infection from specific species can occur.

- Parasites are organisms that benefit at the expense of another living organism. Parasites are classified as protozoan, metazoan, and ectoparasitic.

- Rickettsiae are intracellular parasites that depend completely on their host for survival. Most rickettsial pathogens are transmitted by fleas, ticks, mites, or lice.

- A reservoir is a place where the microorganism can thrive and reproduce. It is the second link in the chain of infection.

- For a microorganism to cause an infection, it must leave the reservoir through a portal of exit. A portal of exit can be through the discharge of body secretions or excretions or respiratory droplets. It can also be through open wounds, the vagina, or the rectum. A portal of exit is the third link in the chain of infection.

- The means by which the microorganism travels from the portal of exit to another host is the mode of transmission. Diseases can be transmitted via direct contact between the infectious person or infected body fluids and the susceptible host or indirectly via an intermediate means that carries the infectious agent to the host. The mode of transmission is the fourth link in the chain of infection.

- The portal of entry is the place where the infectious microorganism enters the host's body. It allows the agent access to another person. It is the fifth link in the chain of infection.

- The last link in the chain of infection is the host. The host is the person who is susceptible to infection by a pathogen. For the infectious process to continue, microorganisms must enter another host who is susceptible to infection. The elderly, the immunosuppressed, and those with chronic conditions are at increased risk.

- The body has mechanical/physical, chemical, and cellular defense mechanisms that help prevent exposure to pathogens and infection.

- There are five stages of infectious diseases. The incubation stage is the time between exposure to a pathogen and the time the first signs and symptoms of the disease appear. The prodromal stage is the time between the initial symptoms and the symptoms that show a disease process is occurring. The acute stage is when the disease process reaches its peak. The declining stage is when symptoms begin to subside, but the infection is still present. The convalescent stage is when the patient begins to recover and regain strength.

- Human immunodeficiency virus (HIV) is a retrovirus carried in blood, blood products, semen, and other body fluids that gradually attacks T-cells. AIDS is advanced HIV infection. There is no curative treatment for HIV or AIDS.

- Hepatitis is an inflammation of the liver. The three most common types of hepatitis are hepatitis A, hepatitis B, and hepatitis C. Vaccinations are available to prevent hepatitis A and B, but not C.

- The Centers for Disease Control and Prevention (CDC) publish a list of notifiable diseases. These diseases must be reported to the state health department and the CDC.

- Universal precautions are a set of measures from the Centers for Disease Control and Prevention (CDC) designed to prevent the transmission of blood-borne infections. Under universal precautions, all blood and bodily fluids should be considered potentially infectious.

- Standard precautions are a set of measures from the Centers for Disease Control and Prevention (CDC) that should be used by all healthcare professionals, regardless of the patient's diagnosis or presumed infection status. Standard precautions include hand hygiene, personal protective equipment, injection safety, environmental cleaning, medical equipment, and respiratory hygiene/cough etiquette.

- Expanded precautions (formerly known as transmission-based precautions) are second-tier guidelines from the Centers for Disease Control and Prevention (CDC) intended for patients diagnosed with or suspected of having specific highly transmissible diseases. They should be used in addition to standard precautions. Contact precautions, droplet precautions, and airborne precautions are all expanded precautions.

- Blood and body fluids refer to blood, secretions, and excretions of a patient. Examples of body fluid include vaginal secretions, cerebrospinal fluid, synovial fluid, pleural fluid, pericardial fluid, peritoneal fluid, semen, amniotic fluid, breast milk, and saliva.

- The Needlestick Safety and Prevention Act was created by OSHA to prevent needlestick injury and reduce the risk of infection in the workplace.

- Infectious waste is any item that has come in contact with blood or body fluids. Infectious waste should be burned or autoclaved before it is disposed of.

Learning Assessment Questions

1. Which of the following is *not* a link in the chain of infection?

    A. Infectious agent

    B. Medical asepsis

    C. Mode of transmission

    D. Susceptible host

2. Which of the following microorganisms is classified by its type of DNA or RNA and requires a living host cell to replicate?

    A. Virus

    B. Bacteria

    C. Parasite

    D. Rickettsiae

3. Which of the following microorganisms have only one cell?

    A. Virus

    B. Parasite

    C. Bacteria

    D. Rickettsiae

4. Which of the following is an intracellular parasite that depends completely on its host for survival?

    A. Virus

    B. Parasite

    C. Bacteria

    D. Rickettsiae

5. Which of the following is a place where a microorganism can thrive and reproduce?

   A. Portal

   B. Reservoir

   C. Pathogen

   D. None of the above

6. Fungi that need oxygen to survive are called which of the following?

   A. Anaerobes

   B. Aerobes

   C. Facultative anaerobes

   D. Rickettsial pathogens

7. Which of the following describes the means by which the microorganism travels from the portal of exit to another host?

   A. Mode of transmission

   B. Portal of exit

   C. Susceptible host

   D. Portal of entry

8. Which of the following is the last link in the chain of infection?

   A. Portal of entry

   B. Susceptible host

   C. Portal of exit

   D. Reservoir

9. Which of the following is the stage of infectious disease in which the disease processes reach their peak?

   A. Incubation stage

   B. Prodromal stage

   C. Convalescent stage

   D. Acute stage

10. Which of the following describes the human immunodeficiency virus?

    A. Is an airborne virus

    B. Is transmitted by a vector

    C. Is a blood-borne virus

    D. Is transmitted by shaking hands

11. Hepatitis refers to inflammation of which organ?

    A. Liver

    B. Pancreas

    C. Stomach

    D. Gall bladder

12. Which of the following is the minimum level of infection-control practices recommended by the Centers for Disease Control and Prevention?

    A. Contact precautions

    B. Universal precautions

    C. Droplet precautions

    D. Airborne precautions

13. Which of the following is *not* a standard precaution?

    A. Hand hygiene

    B. Personal protective equipment

    C. Injection safety

    D. None of the above

14. Standard precautions are issued by which of the following?

    A. Centers for Disease Control and Prevention

    B. Department of Health and Human Services

    C. Food and Drug Administration

    D. Occupational Safety Commission

15. Which of the following refers to the use of practices such as hand washing, general cleaning, and disinfecting of contaminated surfaces?

    A. Medical asepsis

    B. Surgical asepsis

    C. Medical decontamination

    D. Sanitization

16. Which of the following measures apply to patients with the presence of stool incontinence, draining wounds, uncontrolled secretions, or generalized rash?

    A. Respiratory hygiene

    B. Droplet precautions

    C. Airborne precautions

    D. Contact precautions

17. Which of the following are second-tier guidelines of the CDC that apply to specific categories of patients and that include air, contact, and droplet precautions?

    A. Standard precautions

    B. Universal precautions

    C. Expanded precautions

    D. None of the above

18. Which of the following describes latex gloves, face masks, and goggles?

    A. Personal protective equipment

    B. Standard precautions

    C. Universal precautions

    D. Expanded precautions

19. Which of the following is a body fluid?

    A. Semen

    B. Breast milk

    C. Saliva

    D. All of the above

20. Which of the following pathogens *cannot* be transmitted via air?

    A. HIV

    B. Tuberculosis

    C. Measles

    D. Chicken pox

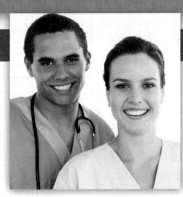

Medical History, Patient Screening, and Exams

KEY TERMS

Afebrile	Inspection	Problem-oriented
Aneroid	Knee-chest position	interview
sphygmomanometer	Korotkoff sounds	Prone position
Auscultation	Lateral position	Pulse
Auscultory gap	Lithotomy position	Pulse rate
Blood pressure	Manipulation	Pyrexia
Complete physical	Mensuration	Respiratory rate
examination	Nasal speculum	Sign
Diastolic blood pressure	Objective information	Sims' position
Digital	Observation	Subjective information
sphygmomanometer	Ophthalmoscope	Supine position
Dorsal recumbent	Otoscope	Symptom
position	Palpation	Systolic blood pressure
Febrile	Past medical history	Temporal artery
Fowler's positions	(PMH)	thermometer
General survey	Peak inflation level	Trendelenburg position
Health history	Percussion	Tuning fork
Horizontal recumbent	Personal and social	Tympanic thermometer
position	history	White-coat syndrome

Chapter Overview

A thorough medical history and physical examination are essential for gathering sensitive information and providing appropriate patient care. By completing accurate assessments, you will build strong patient relationships and direct clinical thinking. A poor or incomplete history and physical examination will lead to poor or incomplete care. Likewise, a comprehensive history and physical examination will lead to comprehensive and complete patient care.

Several skills are necessary for appropriate history taking and examination, including empathetic listening, the ability to interview patients of various ages and cultural backgrounds, and the competence to discern important items and present them to a clinician for further review. By perfecting the skills of history taking and physical examination, you will be able to assist in the provision of quality, patient-centered health care.

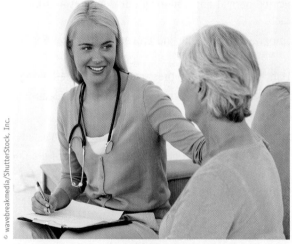

Use empathetic listening skills and nonverbal communication to establish rapport and elicit a thorough medical history.

Terminology

TABLE 6.1 lists terms used in the medical history and physical examination.

Table 6.1 Terms Used in the Medical History and Physical Examination	
Term	**Meaning**
Chief complaint	The reason a patient is seeking care
Family history	The health status of a patient's family members; used to assess the risk of certain illnesses and conditions
Health history	A patient's clinically relevant history of medical issues and conditions
Korotkoff sounds	The sounds heard during a blood-pressure measurement, made by blood flowing through the brachial artery
Past medical history	A summary of a patient's health status prior to the present illness
Personal and social history	The aspects of a patient's personal life that contribute to health status
Physical	A complete physical examination, usually completed on an annual basis
Present illness	A summary of the symptoms associated with the chief complaint

Abbreviations Related to the Medical History and Physical Examination

The following are abbreviations related to the medical history and physical examination:

- Ax—Axillary temperature
- BP—Blood pressure
- CBC—Complete blood count
- CC—Chief complaint
- C/O—Complaint of
- CPE—Complete physical examination
- DTR—Deep tendon reflexes
- Dx—Diagnosis
- ER—Emergency room
- EtOH—Alcohol
- FH—Family history
- Ft—Feet
- HEENT—Head, eyes, ears, nose, and throat
- H/O—History of
- H&P—History and physical
- HPI—History of present illness
- Ht—Height
- Imp—Impression
- In—Inches
- Lbs—Pounds
- NKDA—No known drug allergies
- N/V or N&V—Nausea and vomiting
- OTC—Over-the-counter
- P—Pulse
- PERRLA—Pupils equal, round, and reactive to light and accommodation
- PI—Present illness
- PMH—Past medical history
- R—Rectal temperature
- R—Respiration
- R/O—Rule out
- ROS—Review of systems
- SOB—Shortness of breath
- s/p—Status post (after a significant event has occurred)
- T—Temperature
- TA—Temporal artery temperature
- Tym—Tympanic membrane temperature
- UCHD—Usual childhood diseases
- VSS—Vital signs stable
- WNL—Within normal limits
- Wt—Weight

Medical History

A medical history or **health history** is the clinically relevant information obtained from the patient during a structured interview, usually prior to a physical examination. Several elements are required for a comprehensive health history for an adult. You must be able to talk to a patient and obtain and organize each element of the patient's health. As you hone your skills as a medical assistant, you will learn to elicit information from a patient and identify the most important parts of a patient's story.

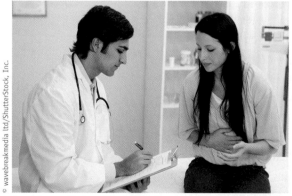

Signs are what you see; symptoms are what a patient feels. Signs are objective; symptoms are subjective.

© auremar/ShutterStock, Inc.

Some situations or patients do not require a comprehensive history. Instead, a focused or **problem-oriented interview** is appropriate. In these cases, you will tailor your history taking to the patient's specific concern, the goals for assessment, the setting of the interview or examination, and the amount of time available for evaluation. Again, as you grow as a medical assistant, you will learn to adapt your questions and assessment techniques to obtain relevant information.

The primary components of a medical history provide structure to a patient's story, as well as your written record of the interview. However, the sequence of the interview should be dictated by the patient's cues. In general, a medical history will be more fluid than the structure provided here. However, you will learn to listen and arrange information into the correct category.

An important distinction to remember while compiling the patient medical history is the difference between subjective information and objective information. **Subjective information** is something that the patient tells you. This information cannot be easily measured or quantified. Subjective information is provided by the patient in the interview. **Objective information** is something that you collect by using your senses and can easily quantify. Objective information is obtained from the physical examination. A similar distinction exists between signs and symptoms of a disease or condition. A **symptom** is a subjective experience that a patient feels. Symptoms cannot be verified. A **sign** is an objective identifier of a disease or condition. Signs can be felt, heard, seen, and measured. Chills, shivering, and nausea are symptoms. Bleeding, swelling, and elevated blood pressure are signs.

Identifying Data

The first item to note when obtaining a medical history is the date and time of the history. You should routinely document the date and time of patient evaluation in all clinical settings.

Next, identify the patient's age, gender, marital status, and occupation. The source for this information may be the patient, a caregiver, or the record from a previous visit. Also, document the reliability of the medical history. Provide a judgment as to the patient's mental status or mood. This opinion, though recorded at the end of the interview, should be continuously assessed throughout the interview. For example, you may report that the patient was vague and unable to remember details or that the patient was able to provide many details and specific information. The reliability of the medical history will vary, depending on the patient's memory, trust, and mood.

A patient will describe subjective symptoms during a medical history.

© wavebreakmedia ltd/ShutterStock, Inc.

Chief Complaint

The chief complaint (CC) is the issue or issues for which the patient is currently seeking care. Try to quote the patient's own words when describing the symptoms associated with the CC. If patients have no specific complaints, such as when they present for an annual or routine examination, you may report their goals for the visit instead.

During a medical history, the patient will provide information spontaneously, but you must organize it.
© auremar/ShutterStock, Inc.

Present Illness

The description of the present illness (PI) expands the CC and explains how and when each symptom developed. Include the patient's thoughts and feelings about the illness. Provide a clear, chronological account of the current issues the patient is experiencing, including any treatments or medications that the patient has used in an attempt to alleviate the symptoms. Provide descriptions of the location, quality, severity, timing, setting, aggravating or relieving factors, and associated manifestations of the symptoms.

When discussing the PI, also note the patient's current medications, including prescription and nonprescription drugs and remedies. Ask about allergies to medications or environmental exposures and state the reaction to each. Also note tobacco, alcohol, and drug use. These items may be noted in the personal and social history section of the medical history, but because these items are often relevant to the present illness, you may choose to record them here as well.

Past Medical History

Identify the patient's **past medical history (PMH)**, which summarizes the patient's health status prior to the PI. Record any previous childhood and adult illnesses and include any chronic conditions. Categorize adult illnesses into medical issues, surgical history, obstetric and gynecological history, and psychiatric history. Provide dates, diagnoses, and treatments associated with each category. Document health-maintenance information such as immunizations, screenings, lifestyle issues, and home safety. Record dates and results of pertinent screening tests.

Family History

A family history outlines the age and health, or age and cause of death, of siblings, parents, grandparents, children, and grandchildren. Document the presence or absence of specific family illnesses. Specifically, note if any of the following common illnesses are present in immediate family members: hypertension, coronary artery disease, elevated cholesterol levels, stroke, diabetes, thyroid disease, kidney disease, cancer, arthritis, tuberculosis, asthma or lung disease, headache disorders, seizure disorders, mental illness, suicide, substance abuse, and allergies. Also note any other conditions or illnesses provided by the patient.

Personal and Social History

The **personal and social history** identifies the aspects of a patient's personal life that can contribute to his or her health status. Describe the patient's educational level, household, interests, and lifestyle. This section illustrates the patient's personality and identifies sources of support, coping style, and fears or anxieties. Include significant life experiences, financial situation, job history, major sources of stress, religious affiliation, and leisure activities or hobbies. Provide detail about the patient's exercise and dietary habits, as well as complementary and alternative healthcare practices.

Review of Systems

As part of the medical history, the review of systems (ROS) documents the presence or absence of common symptoms associated with each major body system. Ask the patient questions about his or her entire body, moving from head to toe. The ROS allows an opportunity for the patient to provide subjective data about his or her body. The ROS will help guide the physical examination.

The Attributes of a Symptom

Location—Where is it?

Quality—What is it like?

Severity—How bad is it?

Timing—When did it start? How long does it last? How frequently does it occur?

Setting—What circumstances or situations may have contributed to the symptom?

Relieving or exacerbating factors—What makes it better or worse?

Associated manifestations—What else accompanies the symptom?

General

Note any recent changes in weight, or even if the patient notes that his or her clothes fit differently than before. Include the presence or absence of weakness, fatigue, and fever. Report the patient's overall perception of his or her general state of health, and if the current state is different from his or her usual state.

Skin

Note if the patient complains of rashes, lumps, sores, dryness, itching, color changes, or hair or nail changes. Note any changes to the size, shape, or color of moles. Also note the amount of time spent in the sun and the use of sunscreen.

Head, Eyes, Ears, Nose, Throat (HEENT)

Note the presence or absence of headache, dizziness, or lightheadedness. Note vision changes, eyeglasses or contact-lens use, blurred or double vision, pain, redness, or other visual disturbances. Record the date of the patient's last eye examination. Note changes in hearing, tinnitus, earaches, ear drainage, and hearing-aid use. Note the presence of frequent colds or respiratory infections, nasal congestion, nosebleeds, or sinus pain. Note the condition of the teeth and gums, the use of dentures, sore tongue or mouth, or hoarseness. Record the date of the patient's last dental examination. Also note difficulties chewing or swallowing, bad breath, or changes in salivation.

Neck

Note lumps, pain, or stiffness in the neck.

Breasts

Note lumps or pain in the breasts and any nipple discharge. Also note changes in breast size, shape, or appearance. Note self-examination practices. If the patient is a female, record the date of her last mammogram.

Respiratory

Note cough, sputum, shortness of breath, and wheezing. Record the date of the patient's last chest X-ray.

Cardiovascular

Note chest pain or discomfort, palpitations, and edema. Record the dates of previous cardiovascular test results. Note leg cramps and varicose veins.

Gastrointestinal

Note trouble swallowing, indigestion, changes in appetite, nausea, vomiting, bowel movements, hemorrhoids, constipation, diarrhea, abdominal pain, and belching or passing gas.

Urinary

Note the frequency of urination, changes in urination, pain on urination, blood in the urine, and incontinence.

Genital

For males, note discharge from the penis and testicular lumps. For females, note the age at the onset of menstrual cycles, the regularity of menstrual periods, the date of the last menstrual period, or age at menopause. Also note the number of pregnancies, the number and type of deliveries, pregnancy- or birth-related complications, and birth-control method. Also note vaginal discharge or changes to the genitalia. For all patients, note sexual orientation or preference, interest in sexual activity, and pain associated with sexual intercourse.

Musculoskeletal

Note muscle or joint pain or stiffness, arthritis, and back pain. For pain, note the quality of the pain, the timing of the pain, factors that worsen or relieve the pain, and the duration and frequency of the pain.

Neurologic

Note fainting, seizures, blackouts, paralysis, numbness, tingling in the extremities, and tremors. Also note changes in balance or coordination, changes in sensory perception, changes in speech, and involuntary movements.

Hematologic

Note bruising, excessive bleeding, and transfusions. Also note blood type.

Endocrine

Note intolerance to heat or cold, excessive sweating, excessive thirst, excessive hunger, excessive urination, and changes in shoe size. Also note changes in hair growth, loss of hair, and changes in fingernail and toenail growth.

Psychiatric

Note nervousness, anxiety, mood, memory changes, irritability, changes in concentration, sources of stress, and suicide attempts.

Patient Interview

When interacting with patients, the medical assistant must put the patient at ease to facilitate information gathering. You must guide the conversation and obtain the information required for the physician to determine the best care possible. Although you want to be pleasant and friendly, do not let the patient guide the conversation and stray from the focus of the medical visit. Also, maintain your composure and professionalism when listening to the patient's answers. Some of the information provided may be private and embarrassing for the patient to share.

Before the Interview

Prior to seeing the patient, ensure that the examination room is clean and ready for the patient and gather all necessary supplies that will be needed for the interview and the physical examination. Review the patient's chart and identify the reason for the patient's visit. Take this opportunity to set goals for the patient interview. The goal may be as simple as obtaining a complete health history or follow-up on an issue from a previous visit. Or, you may have a goal that is directed by your place of employment, such as completing specific forms or obtaining specific information, or the patient may require a specific type of examination, such as for school or work requirements or a physical prior to participating in sports.

When meeting the patient, accompany him or her to the examination room and assist as necessary if mobility issues are a concern. Greet the patient in a friendly and professional manner. Remember to introduce yourself and explain your role in the examination process. Do not begin the interview process until the patient is seated comfortably in a private examination room. To avoid the patient providing too much detail about the CC or PI before you are prepared for the interview, ask general questions while he or she gets settled. For example, ask "Have you had a good day today?" or "Did you have any trouble finding the office?" Similarly, you may choose to ask about the weather or another impersonal subject. Asking "How are you today?" might prompt the patient to begin sharing details of the CC or PI.

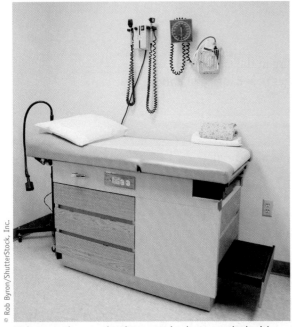

Make sure the examination room is clean, stocked with supplies, and ready for the patient before the interview.

© Rob Byron/ShutterStock, Inc.

During the Interview

The interview should be conducted in the privacy of an examination room with the door closed and the patient comfortable. Build rapport with the patient and maintain a professional demeanor. Maintain eye contact and speak slowly and clearly when communicating with the patient. Be aware of any communication barriers the patient may have. Also be aware of any cultural boundaries or customs that may affect your ability to effectively communicate with the patient. Every patient's beliefs about medical care and his or her own medical condition are influenced by his or her background, family, belief system, and cultural heritage. For a more complete discussion of communicating with patients with visual or hearing impairments, see Chapter 19.

Be sensitive to patient fears and concerns. Patients may require nurturing and validation, but maintain professional separation and patient privacy. If a patient is defensive when answering questions or refuses to provide information, do not press for more information. When discussing sensitive topics, pose questions matter-of-factly and adopt a nonjudgmental tone and demeanor. Try to ask questions regarding drug or alcohol use, sexual behaviors, or other potentially sensitive subjects late in the interview, once rapport has been established and you have assessed the patient's comfort level and willingness to share information.

Many medical offices and clinical settings use computerized medical records. In this case, you may be entering patient information gathered from the interview and medical history directly into a computer. Remember to continue to make eye contact with the patient throughout the interview. Computerized systems are efficient tools for gathering and sharing medical information, but not looking at the patient damages rapport and can make the patient feel disengaged from the interview process. Give the patient as much undivided attention as possible.

Ask the patient open-ended questions that allow freedom of response. Do not ask questions that can be answered with a "yes" or "no." Use verbal and nonverbal communication to encourage the patient to share his or her story and provide as much detail as possible.

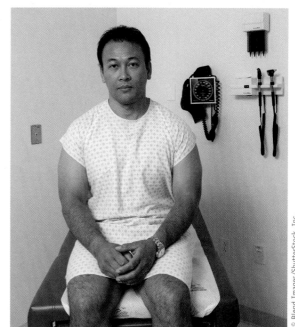

After the patient interview has been completed, help the patient get ready for the physical examination.

Remember that you are not the patient's healthcare provider. Refrain from making judgments or assessments about the patient's health. Refer all patient questions to the provider. Your role is to gather information and record it accurately.

After the Interview

After the patient interview is complete and the medical history has been obtained, the patient should be prepared for the physical examination. First, obtain the patient's vital signs and record them in the medical chart. If instructed by the physician, ask the patient to empty his or her bladder before the examination, and provide a specimen cup if a urine sample is needed. Provide the patient with a gown and instruct him or her to undress and put the gown on with the opening to the back. Also provide a drape to cover the patient. A drape provides modesty and warmth for the patient.

Instruct the patient to sit at the end of the examination table when he or she is dressed. You may need to offer assistance with undressing and donning the gown if patients are weak, frail, or disoriented. Never leave disoriented, dizzy, or ill patients alone; ask for help from another healthcare provider or the patient's family or caregiver. When the patient is ready, notify the physician and be prepared to assist with the examination as requested.

The written record of your encounter with the patient should organize the information and communicate all of the patient's clinical issues and pertinent data to the rest of the healthcare team.

Physical Examination

A **complete physical examination**, often simply called a "physical," is performed to assess the general health status of a patient. The examination evaluates all major body systems and organs. From the results and observations made during the examination, a healthcare provider can formulate an assessment of the patient's health and establish a plan for future care, diagnoses, treatments, and follow-up.

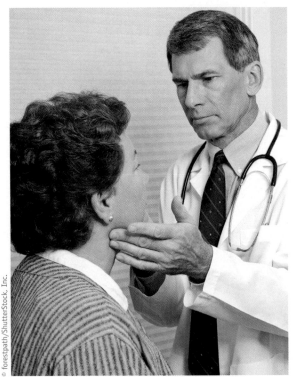

A physician uses palpation to assess a patient's neck.

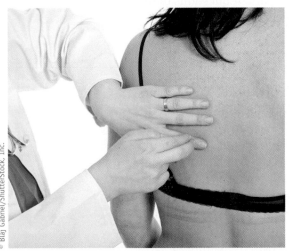

A physician uses indirect percussion on a patient's back to evaluate the lungs.

As a medical assistant, you will not complete a physical examination by yourself, but you will assist the provider and patient. You may need to gather instruments and supplies or take notes or record findings for the provider. You may also need to help position the patient or provide comfort or emotional support during the examination.

Examination Techniques

Providers use several methods of evaluation during a physical examination. Each of the six basic techniques provides objective information about the condition of a body system or organ. A provider will use different techniques, depending on the body part being examined.

Inspection

Inspection, also called **observation**, is evaluation using sight. This technique is used to evaluate a patient's general appearance, the color and condition of the skin, the patient's ability to move freely and independently, and the presence of any deformities or injuries. Body posture, grooming, and mannerisms can be noted with observation. Speech patterns or breathing difficulties may also be noted simply by observing the patient.

Palpation

Palpation is evaluation using touch. Palpation can confirm findings made by observation. A provider may use fingertips, one or both hands, or the palms of the hands to evaluate different body parts. Palpation is used to assess body temperature; size, shape, and location of organs; size, shape, and location of abnormal structures; abdominal rigidity; and the quality of pulsations. Skin moisture and texture can be felt, as well as the position of limbs, bones, and joints.

Percussion

Percussion is the process of producing sounds by tapping on body parts. The quality, pitch, duration, and resonance of each sound helps the provider to identify the size, density, and location of internal organs, structures, and cavities. Direct percussion is the process of tapping the patient's body directly. Indirect percussion is the process of placing a hand or finger on the patient's body, then striking that finger or hand with the opposite hand.

Solid, dense structures produce a dull sound on palpation. Air-filled structures produce a hollow, drumlike sound.

Auscultation

Auscultation is evaluation by listening. Indirect auscultation uses an instrument such as a stethoscope to listen to body sounds. Direct auscultation involves placing the

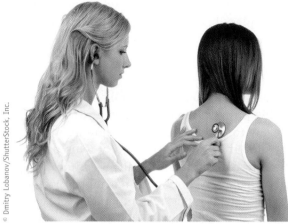

A physician uses indirect auscultation on a patient's back to evaluate the lungs.

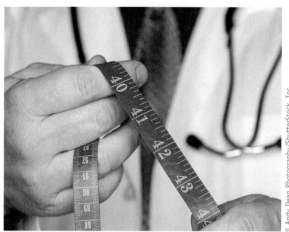

A physician uses mensuration to evaluate the size and length of body areas.

ear directly on a bare surface of the body. Commonly, providers auscultate the heart, lungs, and bowels during a physical examination.

Auscultation is a difficult skill. Many sounds are faint and quick; a provider must be able to discriminate normal from abnormal sounds. These skills are acquired with practice and experience.

Mensuration

Mensuration is the process of taking measurements. Measurements obtained during a physical examination may include height, weight, head circumference, chest circumference, temperature, respiration rate, pulse, and blood pressure. Degree of joint flexion or extension and limb length can also be measured. Record measurements in the units preferred by the provider and be consistent with the units throughout exams.

Manipulation

Manipulation is the passive movement of a joint. Manipulation is useful for patients with joint injuries or deformities, and for evaluating recovery and rehabilitation after joint-related surgeries.

Examination Positions

Various patient positions are required for the physical examination. Each position enables the provider to more easily examine the appropriate body area. As a medical assistant, you may be asked to help patients move into each position and provide a drape or covering for his or her privacy and comfort. Always ensure patient safety when assisting patients into positions. Seven positions are available for physical examination. Trendelenburg position is not used during the physical examination, but may be required for treatment and surgery.

Supine

The **supine position** or **horizontal recumbent position** requires the patient to lie flat on his or her back. This

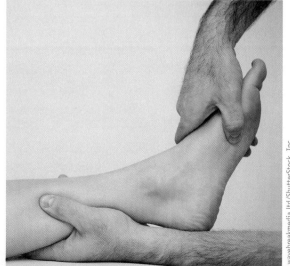

A physician uses manipulation to evaluate joints.

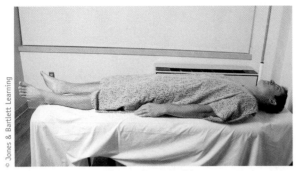

Supine or horizontal recumbent position.

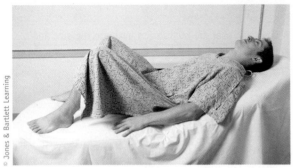

Dorsal recumbent position.

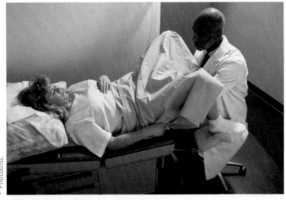

Lithotomy position.

position is used to examine the front of the body. A drape may be placed over the patient's lower body in a horizontal position.

Dorsal Recumbent

The **dorsal recumbent position** is similar to the supine position. This position requires a patient to lie on his or her back with feet flat on the examination table. The knees should be separated slightly. This position is usually more comfortable for patients with back or abdominal pain than the horizontal recumbent position. Examinations of the genitals, rectum, head, neck, chest, and abdomen can be performed in the dorsal recumbent position. A drape should be placed over the patient's lower body in a diamond shape. In this position, one corner of the drape may be lifted to examine the genitals without exposing the rest of the body.

Lithotomy

The **lithotomy position** is similar to the dorsal recumbent position, except that the feet are placed in stirrups attached to the end of the examination table. The patient is lying on his or her back and the buttocks are as close to the end of the table as possible. The lithotomy position is used for examinations of the pelvis and genitals.

Fowler's

Fowler's positions are modified seated positions. The patient sits with his or her back against the examination table, which is raised to 45 or 90 degrees, and the legs rest flat on the table. At a 45-degree angle, the position is called semi-Fowler's position; at a 90-degree angle, the position is called high Fowler's position. Fowler's positions are used for examinations of the head and upper body.

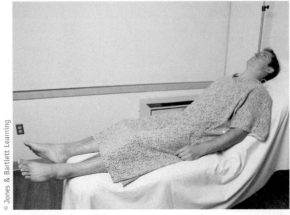

Semi-Fowler's position.

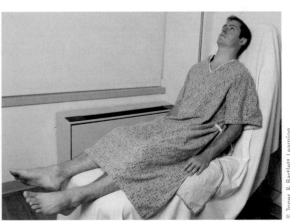

High Fowler's position.

Knee-chest

The **knee-chest position** requires a patient to kneel on the examination table with his or her buttocks elevated and chest resting on the table. It is an uncomfortable position for most patients to maintain, as well as embarrassing. As such, it is rarely used. The knee-chest position was used for examinations of the rectum, but the use of the proctologic table has made the position unnecessary. The table is situated to assist patients into a position that makes examinations of the lower body more comfortable. The proctologic table supports the head and chest and the table is elevated to expose the buttocks.

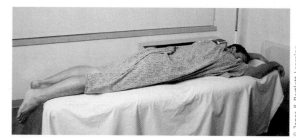

Prone position.

Prone

The **prone position** requires a patient to lie face down on the examination table. His or her head should be turned to the side and the arms placed next to the body or above the head. This position is used to examine the back of the body, including the spine. A drape may be placed over the patient in a horizontal position to cover the patient's mid-back to the legs.

Sims'

Sims' position or **lateral position** requires a patient to lie on his or her left side. The left knee is flexed to provide support for the body and the left arm and shoulder should be behind the patient. The right knee is also flexed. A pillow may be placed between the knees for patient comfort as long as it will not interfere with the examination. A pillow may also be placed under the patient's head. Sims' position is used for examinations of the vagina and rectum. A drape may be placed in a diamond shape to cover the patient from the shoulders to the knees. In this orientation, one corner of the drape may be lifted to expose the rectum without exposing the rest of the body.

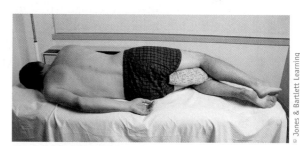

Sims' or lateral position.

Trendelenburg

Trendelenburg position is not routinely used for physical examinations. This position requires a patient to lie in a supine position with the head of the table or bed lowered and the legs elevated. This position aids a person in shock by assisting blood to move from the lower body to the upper body and brain, which can elevate blood pressure until emergency treatment is initiated. Trendelenburg position is also used for abdominal and pelvic surgery. This position improves visualization and maneuverability of the abdominal and pelvic organs.

Examination Format

Every provider may approach the physical examination with a slightly different format or technique, as long as a thorough and complete examination is performed. You will learn to work with all styles of providers and accommodate each provider's preferences. The following descriptions are only a guide to conducting a physical examination. The format or order of examination may be altered, depending on the needs of the patient or provider.

Vital Signs

As a medical assistant, you will likely obtain the patient's vital signs before the physician begins the physical examination. You will assess the blood pressure, pulse, respiratory rate, and body temperature. The following section describes general principles behind obtaining and recording vital signs. You will learn the techniques for obtaining vital signs in the "Skills for the Medical Assistant" section later in this chapter. Normal values for vital signs are provided for various age groups in TABLE 6.2.

Blood pressure or pulse should be assessed first. **Blood pressure** is an assessment of the function of the heart and measures the force exerted on the arteries during one heartbeat. The blood-pressure measurement consists of two parameters: systolic blood pressure and diastolic blood pressure. The **systolic blood pressure** is the pressure in the arteries during systole, or the contraction phase of the heartbeat. The **diastolic blood pressure** is the pressure in the arteries during diastole, or the relaxation phase of the heartbeat. The blood-pressure measurement is recorded as a fraction, with the systolic blood pressure as the numerator and the diastolic blood pressure as the denominator. The ideal adult blood pressure is 120/80mmHg.

Blood pressure is affected by age, gender, medications, disease or illness, emotions, and diet. If the blood pressure is elevated, you may want to measure it again later in the examination.

It is essential to choose the correct cuff size when assessing blood pressure. A cuff that is too small will lead to falsely high blood-pressure measurements and a cuff that is too large will lead to falsely low measurements.

Before obtaining a blood-pressure reading, ensure that the patient has abstained from smoking or ingesting caffeine for at least 30 minutes. Also, the patient should be seated, with both feet supported, and resting comfortably for at least five minutes before measuring blood pressure. The examination room should be quiet and free of distractions and the arm that you use to measure blood pressure should be free of

Table 6.2 Normal Vital Signs

Age Group	Vital Sign Blood Pressure	Heart Rate	Respiratory Rate	Core Body Temperature
Birth	65–85/45–55 mmHg	90–190 beats per minute	30–60 breaths per minute	97.5–100.0°F
0–6 months	70–90/50–65 mmHg	80–180 beats per minute	24–38 breaths per minute	97.5–100.0°F
6–12 months	80–100/55–65 mmHg	75–155 beats per minute	22–30 breaths per minute	97.5–100.0°F
1–2 years	90–105/55–70 mmHg	70–150 beats per minute	22–30 breaths per minute	97.5–100.0°F
2–6 years	95–110/60–75 mmHg	68–138 beats per minute	20–24 breaths per minute	97.5–100.0°F
6–10 years	100–120/60–75 mmHg	65–125 beats per minute	16–22 breaths per minute	97.5–100.0°F
10–14 years	110–135/65–85 mmHg	55–155 beats per minute	16–22 breaths per minute	98.2–100.2°F
14 years–adult	Less than 130/85 mmHg	60–100 beats per minute	14–20 breaths per minute	98.2–100.2°F
65 years and older	Less than 130/85 mmHg	50–65 beats per minute	12–20 breaths per minute	96.6–98.8°F

clothing, injuries, or scars. Support the patient's arm slightly above waist level. Provide a table or other support for the patient, as the patient's own effort to elevate his or her own arm can lead to increased blood pressure.

Patients frequently experience anxiety and apprehension when visiting a physician's office, which can lead to elevated blood pressure. This phenomenon, known as **white-coat syndrome**, can lead to inaccurate blood-pressure readings. Patients may require blood-pressure assessment at home or in a community setting to relieve the anxiety.

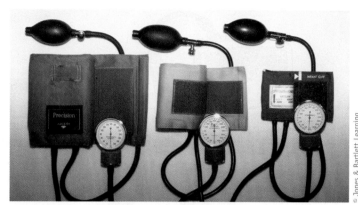

Blood-pressure cuffs are available in many sizes.

The **pulse** is felt by compressing an artery at various points on the body. The pressure in the artery is created by the contraction and relaxation of the heart. The radial pulse, felt at the radial artery on the thumb side of the wrist, is the most common site for measuring pulse. The apical pulse is located at the apex of the heart, on the left side of the chest, between the fifth and sixth ribs. A stethoscope is required to auscultate the apical pulse. Apical pulse is appropriate for patients with heart abnormalities or arrhythmias. A pulse can also be felt at the temporal artery, the carotid artery, the brachial artery, the femoral artery, the popliteal artery, and the dorsalis pedis artery **FIGURE 6.1**.

The **pulse rate** is the number of beats felt or heard in one minute. Pulse rates vary according to gender, age, fitness level, medications, pain, and emotions. To measure the pulse rate, count the number of beats for 15 seconds and multiply the result by four to obtain the number of heartbeats per minute. A normal adult heart rate is 60 to 100 beats per minute. If the heart rate is unusually fast or slow or is irregular in rhythm, count the beats for one full minute to measure an accurate pulse rate.

The **respiratory rate** is the number of breaths completed by the patient in one minute. Like the pulse, respiration varies with age, emotions, illness, medications, and activity level. Normally, adults have a respiratory rate of 12 to 20 breaths per minute.

Measure the patient's temperature using a thermometer or digital electronic probe. Ensure that the patient has abstained from drinking or eating hot or cold substances for at least 30 minutes. Unless otherwise indicated, such as in unconscious or restless patients or patients who are unable to close their mouths, the body temperature of an adult can be assessed orally. The oft-reported normal body temperature of 98.6°F (37°C) fluctuates dramatically among patients and at different times of the day. Also, the type of measurement influences the temperature reading. A rectal temperature is generally 0.7 to 0.9°F (0.4 to 0.5°C) higher than an oral temperature. An axillary temperature, taken under the arm, is generally 1°F (0.6°C) lower than an oral temperature and is considered less accurate. A tympanic

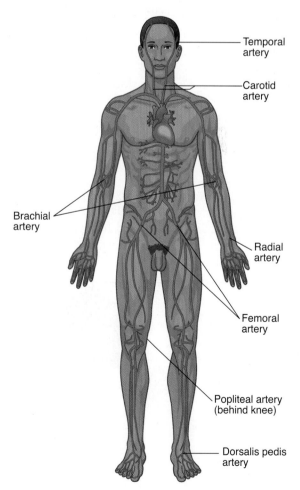

Temporal artery

Carotid artery

Brachial artery

Radial artery

Femoral artery

Popliteal artery (behind knee)

Dorsalis pedis artery

FIGURE 6.1 Pulse sites.
© Jones & Bartlett Learning

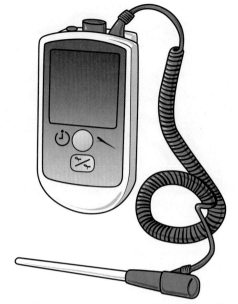

Electronic thermometers have interchangeable probes for measuring body temperature by oral and rectal routes.

membrane temperature, which is measured in the ear canal, is generally 1.4°F (0.8°C) higher than an oral temperature.

Different Location, Different Temperature

Body temperature measurements vary, depending on the location of the measurement. Rectal measurements are 0.7–0.9°F higher than oral measurements. Axillary measurements are 1°F lower than oral measurements. Tympanic membrane measurements are 1.4°F higher than an oral temperature.

General Survey

The examination begins with a **general survey**, which includes initial assessments of the patient's stature, height, weight, and overall appearance. The patient's level of consciousness, alertness, and responsiveness will be assessed, as well as apparent signs of distress. The physician will use inspection techniques to assess the skin color and lesions, as well as body odors or bad breath that may indicate an underlying condition. After the general survey, the physician will examine each body system in turn, usually following the same pattern as the ROS obtained in the initial interview.

Skin

The skin is evaluated by inspection and palpation. The patient will be standing or seated and the physician will note the color, condition, lesions, and deformities of the skin, as well as the condition of the fingernails and toenails.

Head, Eyes, Ears, Nose, Throat (HEENT)

The HEENT are evaluated by inspection and palpation. The patient will be seated. The physician will observe each body part and use an **opthalmoscope** and **otoscope** to evaluate the internal structures of the eyes and ears, respectively. Pupils will be assessed for symmetry and reactivity to light by shining a pen light into the eye. A **tuning fork** can be used to assess hearing and a **nasal speculum** can allow visualization of nasal passages. Oral hygiene is evaluated and the mouth, throat, and tongue are inspected for lesions or deformities.

Neck

The neck is evaluated by inspection, palpation, auscultation, and manipulation. The patient will be seated. The physician will note range of motion, the size of the thyroid, and the size of the lymph nodes. The physician may also observe swallowing and auscultate the carotid artery to listen for sounds that indicate a blockage.

Breasts

The breasts are examined by inspection and palpation. The patient is in a seated or recumbent position. The

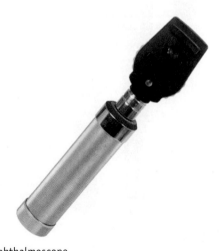

An ophthalmoscope.

physician observes the size, shape, and symmetry of the breasts, as well as any deformities or injuries.

Chest and Respiration

The chest is evaluated by inspection and palpation. The patient is seated and the provider observes the chest for deformities or masses. The structure of the chest is noted, as well as the chest's movement during respiration.

The lungs are evaluated with auscultation and percussion. The physician uses a stethoscope to auscultate the lungs on the anterior and posterior chest. Percussion can be used to detect fluid, excess air, or abnormal masses in the lungs.

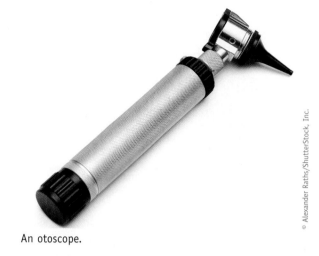

An otoscope.

Heart

The heart is evaluated by auscultation. The patient is seated and the physician uses a stethoscope to auscultate the heart from the anterior and posterior chest wall.

Abdomen

The abdomen is evaluated by inspection, auscultation, palpation, and percussion. The patient will be in a horizontal or dorsal recumbent position. The physician will observe the symmetry of the abdomen and use a stethoscope to listen to bowel sounds. The physician will also palpate the abdomen to assess pulse, the presence of masses, hernias, and muscle and organ tenderness. The physician will use percussion to evaluate the size of the liver, spleen, and stomach, and the presence of air.

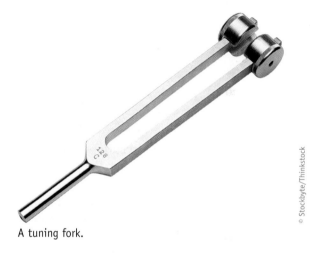

A tuning fork.

Genitals, Urinary System, and Rectum

A male's genitals, urinary system, and rectum are examined by inspection and palpation. The patient is standing and a physician inspects the external genitalia first. The physician will also evaluate the presence of hernias. The patient is then asked to bend over the table and the physician inserts a gloved finger into the anus and rectum to determine the presence of hemorrhoids or other abnormalities and evaluate the size and tenderness of the prostate gland, as well as the presence of nodules on the prostate.

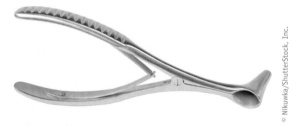

A nasal speculum.

A female's genitals, urinary system, and rectum are also examined by inspection and palpation. The patient is in the lithotomy position and the physician inspects the external genitalia first. A vaginal speculum is used to view internal pelvic structures. Next, the physician will insert two gloved fingers into the vagina to evaluate the size, position, tenderness, and symmetry of internal female organs. A single gloved finger may also be inserted into the anus for evaluation of the rectum.

Musculoskeletal

The back is evaluated by inspection, palpation, and manipulation. The patient is standing and the physician observes the spine and the symmetry of the back. The

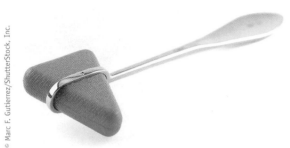

Reflexes can be assessed with a percussion hammer.

physician may stand to the side of the patient to obtain a lateral view, which would reveal abnormal curvatures of the spine.

The legs and feet are evaluated by inspection, palpation, manipulation, and mensuration. The patient is in a recumbent position and the physician evaluates the lower extremities for length, range of motion, the presence of edema, and deformities or injuries.

Muscle strength may be examined by asking the patient to perform a set of movements while the physician provides resistance to the movements. Strength of small and large muscle groups may be assessed.

Reflexes are assessed by percussion. The patient is seated and the physician taps tendons, either with his fingers or a percussion hammer, at various places on the body to stimulate the sensory nerves and cause an involuntary reaction. Tests for balance and coordination may also be completed during a physical examination if the physician desires or if guided by the patient history.

Examination Follow-Up

After a complete physical examination, the physician will develop an assessment of the patient's medical condition and determine a plan for treatment or follow-up care. As the medical assistant, you may be asked to complete additional tests, obtain blood or urine samples for further testing, provide patient-education information, or assist in screening tests. Record all your findings accurately in the patient's medical chart.

When the patient is ready and able to leave the examination room, ensure that the patient is safe and oriented. Assist with moving or dressing, as required. If a patient has been lying down on the examination table for a prolonged period, he or she may feel dizzy or lightheaded upon sitting or standing. Do not rush the patient. Allow him or her plenty of time to become comfortable.

Answer any of the patient's questions to the best of your ability, and advise him or her of follow-up appointments and how he or she will be informed of laboratory results, if applicable. Direct the patient out of the examination room and then prepare the room for the next patient.

Skills for the Medical Assistant

As a medical assistant, it will likely be one of your primary responsibilities to obtain patient histories and assist with physical examinations. Always be professional and courteous when discussing sensitive or embarrassing health-related topics with patients and caregivers. Your professionalism will establish a positive rapport with patients and improve health care.

Accuracy when obtaining and recording vital signs is essential. Changes in vital signs are used to guide a physician's assessment and plan for a patient's health, so precise and accurate measurements are important. Several pieces of equipment are available for obtaining body-system measurements and vital signs, so be familiar with each piece of equipment used in your practice setting and understand its proper use, function, and calibration.

Measure Height and Weight

Height and weight are not considered vital signs, but are important and routinely obtained during physical examinations. Height and weight are normally measured simultaneously. Accuracy in measuring and recording a patient's height and weight is necessary because changes in either of these parameters might indicate an underlying condition or abnormality in overall health or well-being. In this exercise, you will learn how to obtain and record a patient's height and weight.

Equipment Needed

- Balance beam scale with measuring bar
- Paper towels

Steps

1. Wash your hands.
2. Identify the patient and explain the procedure. Ensure that the patient understands and is willing and able to cooperate with your instructions. Ask the patient to remove his or her shoes and heavy clothing or outerwear. Also ask the patient to remove any heavy objects from his or her pockets.
3. Place a paper towel on the scale. Instruct the patient to stand on the paper towel with his or her back against the measuring bar, looking straight ahead. Because the platform is movable, assist an unsteady patient to step on to the scale. Always ensure patient safety.

A patient should face backward when measuring height, since the measuring bar may cause injury to the eyes or face when it is lifted.

---

4. Instruct the patient to stand up tall, with back straight and head level, and lower the measuring bar to rest firmly on top of the patient's head **FIGURE 6.2**.
5. Read the line where the measuring bar rests. This is the patient's height **FIGURE 6.3**.
6. Lift the measuring bar and allow the patient to step off the scale. Assist the patient as needed. Return the measuring bar to its original position.
7. Record the patient's height in the medical record. For example, write "1400: Ht. 5 ft 4 in. J. Jones, CMA."

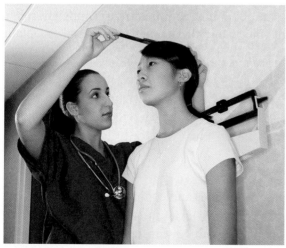

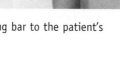

FIGURE 6.2 Lower the measuring bar to the patient's head.
© Comstock/Thinkstock

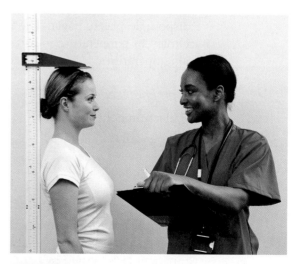

FIGURE 6.3 The patient's height is read at the line where the measuring bar rests.
© Jupiterimages/Polka Dot/Thinkstock

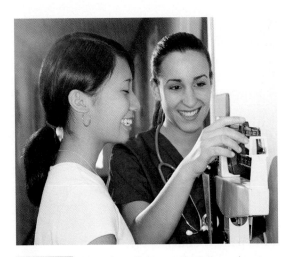

FIGURE 6.4 Move the weights on the balance beam until it is centered.
© Comstock/Thinkstock

8. Instruct the patient to step back on to the center of the scale, providing assistance as necessary. This time, the patient can be facing the scale.

9. Move the lower weight bar to the nearest 50-pound increment below the patient's approximate weight.

10. Move the upper weight bar until the balance beam is centered **FIGURE 6.4**.

11. Obtain the patient's weight by adding the reading from the lower bar to the reading from the upper bar.

12. Record the patient's weight in the medical chart. For example, write "1405: Wt. 118 lb. J. Jones, CMA."

13. Assist the patient to step off the scale. Provide a chair for the patient to replace his or her shoes. Allow the patient time to gather personal items that were removed. Assist the patient as needed.

14. Return the weights on the balance beam to zero.

15. Wash your hands.

Measure Oral Temperature

Many factors influence body temperature. The average adult temperature is 98.6°F (37.0°C), but every individual will have a unique body temperature. The terms **febrile** and **pyrexia** indicate that a patient has a fever or elevated body temperature. **Afebrile** means the absence of a fever.

There are several types of thermometers available today, but the most common type of thermometer for assessing body temperature is an oral electronic or digital thermometer. Due to safety hazards, glass thermometers containing mercury have been phased out of use in the last 20 years. There are no safety concerns with any thermometers currently in use. In the following exercises, you will learn how to obtain and record a patient's body temperature using several common methods and types of thermometers. Familiarize yourself with each manufacturer's device that is used in your practice setting. Understand how to calibrate the thermometer as well as its proper use, cleaning, and storage.

Electronic and digital thermometers are easy to use and have display screens that indicate the results. Probes are attached to the thermometer and covered with a disposable plastic cover. The results are obtained within a few seconds and offer accuracy in temperature measurement. Electronic thermometers are used to obtain oral temperatures.

Equipment Needed

■ Electronic thermometer
■ Probe cover

Steps

1. Wash your hands. Gather all necessary supplies and equipment.

2. Identify the patient and explain the procedure. Ensure that the patient understands and is willing and able to cooperate with your instructions. Allow the patient to be seated in a comfortable position.

3. Select a blue (oral) probe and attach it to the thermometer. Cover the probe with a disposable cover.

4. Insert the probe under the tongue, on either side of the mouth **FIGURE 6.5**. Instruct the patient to close his or her mouth around the probe but not to place his or her teeth on the probe.

5. Leave the probe in place until the thermometer indicates that a result has been obtained.

6. Remove the thermometer's probe from the patient's mouth and read the temperature result on the display screen.

7. Discard the probe cover in the biohazard waste container.

8. Replace the probe in the base of the thermometer.

9. Wash your hands.

10. Record the temperature in the patient's chart. For example, write "1410: T 98.4°. J. Jones, CMA."

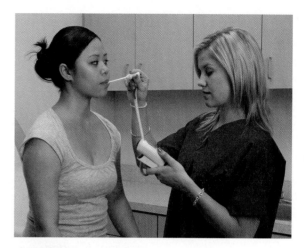

FIGURE 6.5 Insert the probe of the electronic thermometer under the patient's tongue.
© J.R. Bale/Alamy Images

Measure Rectal Temperature

Rectal temperatures are commonly obtained in young children or patients who are unable or unwilling to cooperate with an oral measurement. However, due to the increased use of other types of thermometers, rectal temperatures are no longer obtained as frequently in ambulatory settings.

Equipment Needed

- Electronic thermometer
- Probe cover
- Lubricating jelly
- Disposable gloves

Steps

1. Wash your hands. Gather all necessary supplies and equipment. Don a pair of gloves.

2. Identify the patient and explain the procedure. Ensure that the patient understands and is willing and able to cooperate with your instructions. The patient should be placed into Sims' position and draped.

3. Select a red (rectal) probe and attach it to the thermometer. Cover the probe with a disposable cover. Apply lubricating jelly to the probe.

4. Gently spread the buttocks and insert the probe into the rectum approximately 1.5 inches.

5. Hold the buttocks together with one hand and hold the thermometer in place with the other. Leave the probe in place until the thermometer indicates that a result has been obtained.

6. Remove the thermometer's probe and read the temperature result on the display screen.

7. Discard the probe cover in the biohazard waste container.

8. Replace the probe in the base of the thermometer.

9. Remove the gloves and wash your hands. Offer a tissue to the patient to wipe his or her buttocks clean. Assist the patient with dressing or changing positions as required.

10. Record the temperature in the patient's chart. For all routes other than oral, record the route by which the temperature was obtained. For example, write "1410: T 99.4° (R). J. Jones, CMA."

When using an electronic thermometer, blue probes are used for oral temperatures and red probes are used for rectal temperatures.

Measure Axillary Temperature

Axillary temperature is measured underneath the arm. Similar to the rectal route, axillary temperature measurement is falling out of favor and being replaced by simpler, more comfortable, and more accurate techniques.

Equipment Needed

- Digital thermometer
- Probe cover
- Paper towel

Steps

1. Wash your hands. Gather all necessary supplies and equipment.
2. Identify the patient and explain the procedure. Ensure that the patient understands and is willing and able to cooperate with your instructions.
3. Instruct the patient to remove clothes to provide access to the axilla or underarm area. Wipe the underarm clean and dry with a paper towel. Provide a drape or gown if necessary to allow for patient comfort and modesty. Allow the patient to be seated in a comfortable position.
4. Select a blue (oral) probe and attach it to the thermometer. Cover the probe with a disposable cover.
5. Place the thermometer under the arm, in the axilla. Instruct the patient to hold his or her arm against his chest to keep the thermometer in place **FIGURE 6.6**.
6. Leave the probe in place until the thermometer indicates that a result has been obtained. This may take up to 10 minutes, depending on the manufacturer's instructions.
7. Remove the thermometer from the patient's axilla and read the temperature result on the display screen.
8. Discard the probe cover in the biohazard waste container.
9. Clean or sanitize the thermometer according to the manufacturer's instructions.
10. Wash your hands.
11. Record the temperature in the patient's chart. For all routes other than oral, record the route by which the temperature was obtained. For example, write "1410: T 97.4° (Ax). J. Jones, CMA."

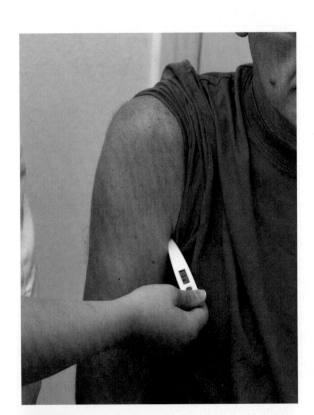

FIGURE 6.6 Insert the probe of the electronic thermometer under the patient's arm.
© Art Directors & TRIP/Alamy Images

Measure Aural Temperature

An aural temperature is assessed in the ear canal with the use of a **tympanic thermometer** FIGURE 6.7. Tympanic thermometers are increasingly popular due to their simplicity, ease of use, comfort, and accuracy in measuring core body temperature. Tympanic thermometers can be used on adults as well as children older than two years. Excess cerumen (earwax) in the ear canal can cause inaccurate readings, however. Also, an ear infection can cause an elevated temperature reading.

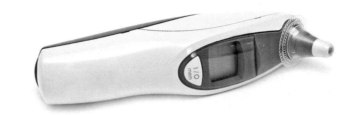

FIGURE 6.7 A tympanic thermometer.
© Anna Stasevska/ShutterStock, Inc.

Equipment Needed

- Digital tympanic thermometer
- Probe cover

Steps

1. Wash your hands. Gather all necessary supplies and equipment.
2. Identify the patient and explain the procedure. Ensure that the patient understands and is willing and able to cooperate with your instructions. Allow the patient to be seated in a comfortable position.
3. Cover the thermometer with a disposable probe cover.
4. Straighten the ear canal by gently pulling up and back slightly on the ear for adults and older children and by pulling the ear down and back for infants and small children. Place the thermometer into the ear canal and activate the thermometer, according to the manufacturer's instructions FIGURE 6.8.

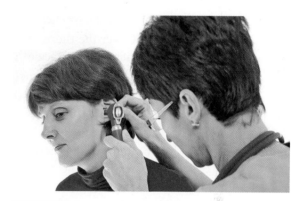

FIGURE 6.8 Insert the thermometer into the patient's ear canal.
© jordache/ShutterStock, Inc.

5. Leave the probe in place until the thermometer indicates that a result has been obtained.
6. Remove the thermometer from the patient's ear and read the temperature result on the display screen.
7. Discard the probe cover in the waste container.
8. Clean and store the thermometer according to the manufacturer's instructions.
9. Wash your hands.
10. Record the temperature in the patient's chart. For all routes other than oral, record the route by which the temperature was obtained. For example, write "1410: T 98.4° (Tym). J. Jones, CMA."

Measure Body Temperature With a Temporal Artery Thermometer

A **temporal artery thermometer** FIGURE 6.9 offers a noninvasive means of assessing body temperature. These thermometers, which measure the temperature of the skin sur-

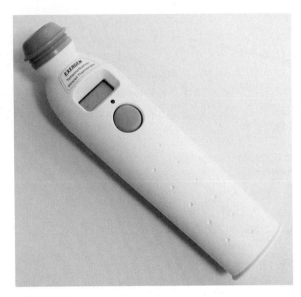

FIGURE 6.9 A temporal artery thermometer.
© Jones & Bartlett Learning

face over the forehead, offer better accuracy than aural and rectal thermometers, according to several studies. Temporal artery thermometers can be used in patients of all ages and the procedure is quick, painless, and safe. Perspiration on the forehead, as well as scanning too rapidly, can cause inaccurate readings.

Equipment Needed

- Temporal artery thermometer
- Probe cover or alcohol wipe

Steps

1. Wash your hands. Gather all necessary supplies and equipment.
2. Identify the patient and explain the procedure. Ensure that the patient understands and is willing and able to cooperate with your instructions. Allow the patient to be seated in a comfortable position. Remove perspiration from the forehead, if necessary.
3. Cover the thermometer with a disposable probe cover or use an alcohol wipe to clean the surface of the thermometer that will touch the patient.
4. Place the thermometer against the center of the patient's forehead. Press the Scan button as you slide the thermometer across the forehead toward the temple **FIGURE 6.10**.
5. Slide the probe until the thermometer indicates that a result has been obtained.
6. Remove the thermometer from the patient's forehead and read the temperature result on the display screen.
7. Discard the probe cover, if applicable, in the waste container.
8. Clean and store the thermometer according to the manufacturer's instructions.
9. Wash your hands.
10. Record the temperature in the patient's chart. For all routes other than oral, record the route by which the temperature was obtained. For example, write "1410: T 99.6° (TA). J. Jones, CMA."

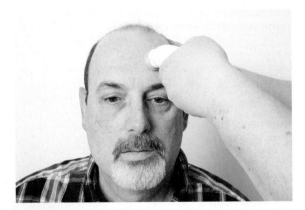

FIGURE 6.10 Slide the thermometer across the patient's forehead.
© Jones & Bartlett Learning

Measure Radial Pulse and Respirations

The pulse is easily felt at points on the body where an artery is close to the surface of the skin and a solid structure, such as a bone. The radial pulse is measured at the patient's wrist. Use the tips of your index and middle fingers to measure the pulse; do not use your thumb, which has its own pulse and can interfere with accurate measurement of the patient's pulse.

The respiratory rate and the radial pulse are often obtained simultaneously. Try to count the respiratory rate without alerting the patient. Often, breathing patterns change if a patient knows he or she is being watched. Count the number of cycles of inhalation and exhalation in one minute. Note any abnormalities in the quality, pattern, or sounds of breathing. In the following exercise, you will learn how to measure and record a radial pulse and respiratory rate.

Equipment Needed

- Watch with a second hand

Steps

1. Wash your hands. Gather all necessary supplies and equipment.
2. Identify the patient and explain the procedure. Ensure that the patient understands and is willing and able to cooperate with your instructions. Allow the patient to be seated in a comfortable position.
3. Position the patient with one of his or her wrists resting on a table or the lap.
4. Locate the radial pulse with your fingertips. Gently press on the radial artery so that you feel strong pulsations **FIGURE 6.11**.
5. Count the pulsations for the appropriate length of time. In patients with heart disease or dysfunction, count pulsations for one full minute. In healthy patients with no diagnosed heart abnormalities, you may count for only 15 or 30 seconds; multiply the number of pulsations by four or two, respectively, to obtain the pulsations in one minute.
6. While still holding the patient's wrist, and without alerting the patient, observe the respirations completed by the patient in one minute.
7. Wash your hands.
8. Record the pulse and respiratory rate in the patient's chart. Also record any abnormalities or irregularities in the pulse or breathing if any were noted. For example, write "1420: P 64, R 16. J. Jones, CMA."

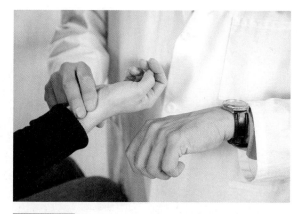

FIGURE 6.11 Gently press on the radial artery to feel a pulse.
© iofoto/ShutterStock, Inc.

Measure Apical Pulse

Apical pulse is measured in patients with known heart-rate dysfunction or irregularity, as it allows a more accurate assessment of heart rate. In the following exercise, you will learn how to measure and record an apical pulse.

Equipment Needed

- Stethoscope
- Watch with a second hand
- Alcohol wipes

Steps

1. Wash your hands. Gather all necessary supplies and equipment.
2. Identify the patient and explain the procedure. Ensure that the patient understands and is willing and able to cooperate with your instructions. Assist the patient to disrobe from the waist up and assume a supine position.
3. Wipe the earpieces of the stethoscope with an alcohol wipe. Locate the apex of the heart, between the fifth and sixth ribs at the mid-clavicular line, just left of

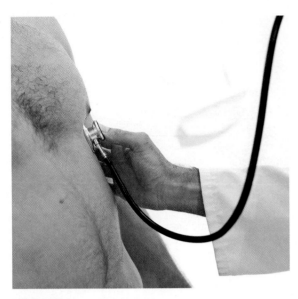

FIGURE 6.12 Measure the apical pulse by placing a stethoscope over the apex of the heart.
© iStockphoto/Thinkstock

the sternum. Place the stethoscope over the apex of the heart and listen for each "lub-dub" sound, indicating a heartbeat **FIGURE 6.12** .

4. Count the pulses or heartbeats for one full minute.

5. Assist the patient to sit up and dress.

6. Wash your hands. Clean the earpieces, diaphragm, and tubing of the stethoscope with an alcohol wipe.

7. Record the pulse in the patient's chart, noting that the pulse was an apical pulse. For example, write "1425: P 88 (AP), slightly irregular. J. Jones, CMA."

Measure Blood Pressure

Blood pressure is measured by auscultation using a stethoscope and a sphygmomanometer. Though once the standard, mercury-containing sphygmomanometers are rarely used today, due to the health risks associated with mercury exposure. Most sphygmomanometers are aneroid or digital. An **aneroid sphygmomanometer** **FIGURE 6.13** is a manual device that consists of a cuff attached to rubber tubing and a dial that indicates pressure in millimeters of mercury (mmHg). A **digital sphygmomanometer** **FIGURE 6.14** is automatic and produces a digital display of the blood pressure.

The sounds heard through the stethoscope during a blood-pressure measurement are called **Korotkoff sounds**. There are five distinct sounds that are heard, though hearing all of them and discriminating among the sounds is difficult. As you gain experience, you will become more proficient at perceiving each sound. The first and last Korotkoff sounds are most important for measuring blood pressure. In the following exercise, you will learn how to measure blood pressure with an aneroid sphygmomanometer.

Equipment Needed

- Aneroid sphygmomanometer
- Stethoscope
- Alcohol wipes

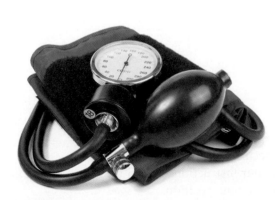

FIGURE 6.13 An aneroid sphygmomanometer.
© Vladislav_studio/ShutterStock, Inc.

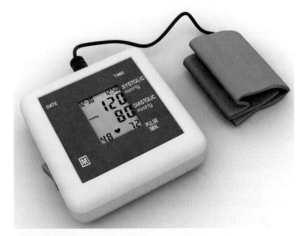

FIGURE 6.14 A digital sphygmomanometer.
© rose designs/ShutterStock, Inc.

Steps

1. Wash your hands. Gather all necessary supplies and equipment. Select the correctly sized cuff for the patient. Blood-pressure cuffs are available to fit small pediatric patients up to obese adults.

Selecting the Correct Blood-Pressure Cuff

The width of the inflatable bladder should cover approximately 40 percent of the circumference of the patient's limb being used for measurement. The length of the inflatable bladder should cover approximately 80 percent of the limb circumference. Remember, the width and length of the blood-pressure cuff refer only to the inflatable portion of the cuff, not the entire cuff.

---

2. Identify the patient and explain the procedure. Ensure that the patient understands and is willing and able to cooperate with your instructions. Allow the patient to be seated in a comfortable position. Feet should be placed flat on the floor with legs uncrossed. The arm should be resting at heart level, supported on the lap or a table. Remove clothing from the arm that will be used for the measurement.

3. Wipe the earpieces of the stethoscope with an alcohol wipe.

4. Locate the brachial artery. Center the blood-pressure cuff over the brachial artery and slightly above the elbow. Secure the cuff and ensure it is completely deflated.

If you inflate the blood-pressure cuff too slowly, the diastolic blood pressure will be falsely high and the patient will experience discomfort. If you deflate the blood-pressure cuff too quickly, the systolic blood pressure will be low and the diastolic blood pressure will be high. If you deflate the blood-pressure cuff too slowly, the diastolic blood pressure will be falsely high.
© auremar/ShutterStock, Inc.

5. Locate the radial pulse. Inflate the cuff by turning the knob on the bulb to the right and pumping the bulb until the pulse is no longer felt. Watch the dial on the sphygmomanometer and note the pressure when the radial pulse disappears. This is the **peak inflation level**.

6. Deflate the cuff by turning the knob on the bulb to the left and allow the arm to rest for approximately one minute.

7. Place the diaphragm of the stethoscope over the brachial artery **FIGURE 6.15**. The stethoscope should not be touching the blood-pressure cuff. If it does, move the cuff up the arm until it no longer touches the stethoscope. Hold the stethoscope in place gently with your fingers.

8. Inflate the cuff smoothly and quickly to the peak inflation level plus 30mmHg.

9. Deflate the cuff at a rate of 2–4mmHg per heartbeat, roughly equivalent to 2mmHg per second in most adults. Listen for the first Korotkoff sound. This will be the first sound heard when deflating the cuff. It is a sharp, tapping sound. The pressure at which this first sound occurs is the systolic blood pressure or the top number of the blood pressure.

10. Continue deflating the blood-pressure cuff. When the last Korotkoff sound disappears, note the pres-

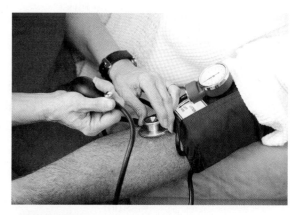

FIGURE 6.15 Place the stethoscope over the brachial artery.
© Lisa F. Young/ShutterStock, Inc.

sure. When blood is flowing freely through the artery, no more sounds will be heard. The pressure at which all sounds disappear is the diastolic blood pressure or the bottom number on the blood pressure.

11. Continue deflating the blood-pressure cuff another 10mmHg to ensure that all sounds have disappeared.

An **auscultory gap** is heard in some patients. Korotkoff sounds will disappear and reappear at a lower pressure. Always inflate the blood-pressure cuff above the peak inflation level and deflate the cuff below the last Korotkoff sound to rule out an auscultory gap.

---

12. Deflate the cuff quickly and remove it.

13. Wash your hands. Clean the earpieces, diaphragm, and tubing of the stethoscope with an alcohol wipe.

14. Record the blood-pressure measurement in the patient's chart. Always record which arm was used for the measurement. For example, write "1425: BP 134/86 in right arm. J Jones, CMA."

Prepare a Patient for and Assist With a Physical Examination

As a medical assistant, one of your primary responsibilities on a daily basis will likely be preparing for and assisting with physical examinations. You will prepare the examination room and equipment for the physical examination. You will also be responsible for interviewing the patient, recording the chief complaint and patient history, and obtaining vital signs prior to the physician or other healthcare provider examining the patient. In this exercise, you will learn the basic principles behind preparing for and assisting with a physical examination.

Equipment Needed

- Gown
- Drape
- Stethoscope
- Ophthalmoscope
- Otoscope
- Tongue depressors
- Sterile gauze pads
- Tuning fork
- Nasal speculum
- Tape measure
- Percussion hammer
- Vaginal speculum, if the patient is female
- Test kit for fecal occult blood test
- Disposable examination gloves
- Lubricant
- Tissues
- Towel
- Stool
- Lamp
- Waste container

Steps

1. Prepare the examination room by cleaning equipment, stocking supplies, disinfecting the examination table, and placing clean paper on the table.
2. Review the patient's chart and ensure that a form is ready to record the findings from the history and physical.
3. Wash your hands and assemble the equipment that will be used during the examination.
4. Pull the step out from the bottom of the examination table. Place a clean drape and gown on the table.

5. Identify the patient and introduce yourself. Ask the patient to follow you to the examination room. Assist the patient if necessary. Explain the forthcoming procedures and examination to the patient. Ensure that the patient understands and is willing and able to cooperate with your instructions.
6. Instruct the patient to empty his or her bladder prior to the examination. If a urine sample is requested by the physician, provide a specimen cup to the patient.
7. Interview the patient. Inquire as to the reason for his or her visit and record the chief complaint in the patient's own words. Solicit information on the patient's present illness, past medical history, family history, and social history. Conduct a review of systems and record any abnormalities or concerns offered by the patient.
8. Measure and record the patient's height, weight, and vital signs.
9. Instruct the patient to undress, don the gown, sit at the end of the table, and cover his or her legs with the drape. Assist the patient with this step if required.
10. When the patient is prepared, notify the physician.
11. Assist the provider throughout the examination by taking notes, providing supplies and equipment, adjusting the lights, or supporting the patient.
12. After the examination, assist the patient to a comfortable, seated position. Provide tissues or towels for the patient to clean himself or herself if needed.
13. Instruct the patient to dress. Assist as needed.
14. Take any specimens or samples obtained during the examination to the laboratory, along with proper requisition forms or identifying paperwork.
15. Return to the room and provide patient instruction or education as directed by the physician. Help the patient schedule any follow-up appointments or procedures. Walk the patient out of the office.
16. Clean the examination room and prepare it for the next patient.

Math Practice

Question: **What is the simplest form of the fraction $^{45}/_{90}$?**

Answer: $^1/_2$

Question: **Which of the following quantities is the smallest: $^1/_8$mL, $^2/_3$mL, $^5/_6$mL, or $^4/_7$mL?**

Answer: $^1/_8$mL

Question: **Which of the following quantities is the largest: $^3/_{10}$mg, $^4/_8$mg, $^7/_{100}$mg, or $^2/_5$mg?**

Answer: $^4/_8$mg

Question: **What is the sum of $^7/_8 + ^3/_{10}$?**

Answer: $1^7/_{40}$

Question: **What is the sum of $^5/_8 + ^2/_3$?**

Answer: $1^7/_{24}$

Question: **What is the difference of $^2/_7 - ^5/_{21}$?**

Answer: $^1/_{21}$

Question: **What is the difference of $^4/_5 - ^6/_{11}$?**

Answer: $^{14}/_{55}$

Question: **What is the product of $^2/_7 \times ^1/_3$?**

Answer: $^2/_{21}$

Question: **What is the product of $^3/_5 \times ^2/_8$?**

Answer: $^3/_{20}$

Question: **What is the quotient of $^4/_7 \div ^1/_3$?**

Answer: $1^5/_7$

Question: **What is the quotient of $^5/_8 \div ^4/_5$?**

Answer: $^{25}/_{32}$

Question: What is the sum of 5.18 + 3.2 + 13.5?

Answer: 21.88

Question: What is the sum of 8.24 + 12.3 + 3.19?

Answer: 23.73

Question: What is the difference of 10.29 − 8.13?

Answer: 2.16

Question: What is the difference of 9.17 − 3.5?

Answer: 5.67

Question: What is the product of 6.4 × 2.83?

Answer: 18.112

Question: What is the product of 2.7 × 9.4?

Answer: 25.38

Question: What is the quotient of 5.525 ÷ 0.85?

Answer: 6.5

Question: What is the quotient of 9.6 ÷ 1.6?

Answer: 6

Question: What is $^{2}/_{80}$ expressed as a percent?

Answer: 2.5%

Question: What is $^{7}/_{10}$ expressed as a percent?

Answer: 70%

Question: What is 30% expressed as a fraction?

Answer: $^{3}/_{10}$

Question: What is 65% expressed as a fraction?

Answer: $^{13}/_{20}$

WRAP UP

Chapter Summary

- A medical history and physical examination gather health information and guide the physician's assessment and plan for patient care. You will learn to communicate effectively with patients of all ages and cultures to obtain sensitive and clinically relevant information that you will present to the healthcare provider.

- A complete medical history consists of the patient's chief complaint, a description of the present illness, the past medical history, the family history, a personal and social history, and a review of systems. The patient will provide you with subjective information, which you will organize and categorize to present to the physician.

- When interviewing the patient, maintain a professional demeanor, establish rapport with the patient, and ensure patient comfort and safety at all times. Communicate clearly, using verbal and nonverbal communication skills, and ask the patient open-ended questions to facilitate information gathering.

- A complete physical examination is performed to assess the general health status of a patient. The information provided in the medical history will guide the physical examination. A physician will obtain objective information about each body system during the examina-

tion using techniques including inspection, palpation, percussion, auscultation, mensuration, and manipulation. Patients will be placed in a variety of different positions to allow for visualization of the body area of interest. You will be called upon to assist and aid the patient and the physician during the physical examination.

- You will likely obtain the patient's height, weight, blood pressure, pulse, respiratory rate, and body temperature before the examination begins. Many factors influence accurate measurements. You must be familiar with various techniques and equipment used to assess vital signs to maintain accuracy and precision. Vital sign changes may indicate an underlying health condition, so inaccurate measurements may lead to incorrect diagnoses.

- As a medical assistant, you will have the opportunity to obtain patient histories and assist in physical examinations. Take the time to understand the various methods of obtaining vital signs as well as the proper functioning of all equipment. Accuracy and precision in measurements is essential, as vital signs and body measurements will guide the physician's assessment and plan for the patient's health care.

Learning Assessment Questions

1. Which of the following is an example of a symptom?
   A. Blood pressure of 135/85mmHg
   B. Lower back pain
   C. Allergy to penicillin
   D. Bleeding from a laceration

2. Which of the following is *not* a category of the past medical history?
   A. Surgical history
   B. Psychiatric history
   C. Chronic conditions
   D. Tobacco use

3. Which of the following pairs correctly matches the attribute of a symptom with its description?
   A. Severity: How bad is the symptom?
   B. Location: Where are you when the symptom occurs?
   C. Setting: Where it is located?
   D. Quality: What makes it worse?

WRAP UP

4. Which of the following is an example of an open-ended question?

   A. "Are you feeling chills?"

   B. "How would you describe your health?"

   C. "Do you take a multivitamin?"

   D. "Are you married?"

5. What body systems or areas can be evaluated through inspection?

   A. The lungs

   B. The reflexes

   C. The heart

   D. The skin

6. Which of the following is *not* an example of mensuration?

   A. Temperature

   B. Chest circumference

   C. Date of last dental examination

   D. Limb length

7. What body systems or areas can be examined when the patient is in the Fowler's position?

   A. The head and upper body

   B. The back and spine

   C. The genitals and urinary system

   D. The abdominal organs

8. Which of the following positions is *not* routinely used during physical examinations?

   A. Sims' position

   B. Trendelenburg position

   C. Fowler's position

   D. Supine position

9. Which of the following is *not* considered a vital sign?

   A. Pulse

   B. Temperature

   C. Respiratory rate

   D. Weight

10. Which of the following correctly describes "white-coat syndrome"?

    A. A healthcare provider experiences elevated blood pressure due to the stress of his or her job.

    B. An auscultory gap is heard when assessing blood pressure in an office setting.

    C. A patient experiences abnormal blood pressure due to the anxiety associated with being in a physician's office.

    D. A healthcare provider is trained to treat patients with less personal attention and a more clinical perspective.

11. Which method for measuring temperature will lead to the highest reading?

    A. Oral

    B. Temporal artery

    C. Axillary

    D. Tympanic membrane

12. What evaluation technique(s) is (are) used to evaluate the chest during a physical examination?

    A. Inspection and palpation

    B. Auscultation

    C. Percussion and manipulation

    D. Mensuration

13. What position is used to examine female pelvic organs?

    A. Sims'

    B. Trendelenburg

    C. Lithotomy

    D. Fowler's

14. What color probe should be used to measure an oral temperature with an electronic thermometer?

    A. Red

    B. Blue

    C. Orange

    D. Green

WRAP UP

15. What position is used to obtain a rectal temperature?

    A. Prone

    B. Dorsal recumbent

    C. Lithotomy

    D. Sims'

16. What factor can influence a temperature reading obtained from a temporal artery thermometer?

    A. Perspiration on the forehead

    B. Excess earwax

    C. Drinking a caffeinated beverage

    D. Eating a hot food item

17. Which two vital signs are often obtained simultaneously?

    A. Height and weight

    B. Apical pulse and temperature

    C. Radial pulse and respiratory rate

    D. Head circumference and temporal artery temperature

18. What two pieces of equipment can you use to measure blood pressure?

    A. A tuning fork and a watch with a second hand

    B. An otoscope and an ophthalmoscope

    C. A thermometer and a pulse oximeter

    D. An aneroid sphygmomanometer and a stethoscope

19. How high should you inflate a blood-pressure cuff when measuring blood pressure?

    A. Until the brachial pulse disappears

    B. 30mmHg higher than the peak inflation level

    C. 10mmHg lower than the auscultory gap

    D. Until you hear Korotkoff sounds

20. What is the result of deflating a blood-pressure cuff too quickly?

    A. A low systolic blood-pressure reading

    B. A low diastolic blood-pressure reading

    C. Patient discomfort

    D. An auscultory gap will be heard

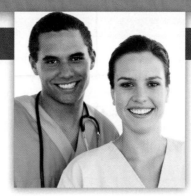

Dosage Calculations

OBJECTIVES

After reading this chapter, you will be able to:

- Understand ratio and proportion.
- Use the metric, household, and apothecary systems of measurement and convert between metric and apothecary systems.
- Understand units of medication dosage.
- Correctly calculate dosages for adults and children.

KEY TERMS

Accuracy	Equivalent ratios	Means
Apothecary system of measurement	Extremes	Meter (m)
	Gram (g)	Metric system
Body-surface area (BSA)	Household system of measurement	Nomogram
Cross multiplication		Precision
Dosage	International unit (IU)	Proportion
Dose	Liter (L)	

Chapter Overview

This chapter covers important topics relating to pharmaceutical measurements and basic dosage calculations necessary to ensure that a patient receives the correct dose or amount of medication. A mistake in a calculation or measurement will lead to under-dosing or overdosing. This could then lead to inadequate treatment or drug toxicity. Many dosage-related tasks performed by a medical assistant will relate to mathematics and calculations, and these tasks require proficiency in basic arithmetic skills.

Ratio and Proportion

Basic math skills are necessary for calculating and verifying medication dosages. The ratio and proportion method can be used to calculate dosages.

Ratios

A ratio is a representation of how two similar quantities are related to each other. A ratio may express either the relationship between two parts of one whole or between one part and the whole. Simply, a ratio is a comparison. Traditionally, ratios are expressed in odds notation, using a colon to separate the numbers, such as 1:2. A ratio can also be expressed as a fraction, such as $\frac{1}{2}$.

> A fraction, like a decimal, indicates part of a whole number. For example, $\frac{1}{2}$, $\frac{2}{3}$, and $\frac{7}{10}$ are all fractions. The top number of the fraction is called the numerator and the bottom number of the fraction is called the denominator.

In clinical practice, ratios are often used to express the concentration of a drug in solution or the weight or dose of a drug in a delivery unit or volume. For example, a tablet that contains 50mg of active ingredient can be expressed as 50mg:1 tablet or 1 tablet:50mg. Similarly, this value can be expressed as a fraction: $\frac{50mg}{1\ tablet}$ or $\frac{1\ tablet}{50mg}$. A solution that contains 1g of drug per 100mL of solution can also be expressed as a ratio (1g:100mL) or a fraction (1g/100mL).

When two ratios have the same value, they are equivalent. You can find **equivalent ratios** by multiplying or dividing both sides of the ratio by the same number. This is the same process as finding equivalent fractions.

You can find equivalent ratios by multiplying both sides of the ratio by the same number. For example, to find an equivalent ratio for 1:2, you can multiply both sides by 2 to get 2:4: $(1 \times 2):(2 \times 2) = 2:4$. To find another equivalent ratio for 1:2, you can multiply both sides by 4 to get 4:8: $(1 \times 4):(2 \times 4) = 4:8$. To find yet another equivalent ratio for 1:2, you can multiply both sides by 50 to get 50:100: $(1 \times 50):(2 \times 50) = 50:100$.

You can also find equivalent ratios by dividing both sides of the ratio by the same number. This number should be a common factor of both numbers of the ratio. For example, to find an equivalent ratio for 50:200, you can divide both sides by 25 to get 2:8: $(50 \div 25):(200 \div 25) = 2:8$. To find another equivalent ratio for 50:200, you can divide both sides by 50 to get 1:4: $(50 \div 50):(200 \div 50) = 1:4$.

When two ratios are equivalent and expressed as fractions, the product of the first numerator multiplied by the opposite denominator is equivalent to the product of the first denominator multiplied by

A ratio is written as 1:10. The same ratio is spoken as "one to 10." The same ratio expressed as a fraction would be $\frac{1}{10}$, and expressed as a decimal would be 0.1.

the opposite numerator. For example, 2:5 and 4:10 are equivalent ratios and can also be expressed as $\frac{2}{5} = \frac{4}{10}$. The product of the first numerator multiplied by the opposite denominator is equivalent to the product of the first denominator multiplied by the opposite numerator. For example:

$$\frac{2}{5} = \frac{4}{10}$$
$$2 \times 10 = 4 \times 5$$
$$20 = 20$$

Proportions

A **proportion** is an equation that states two ratios are equal. When the terms of a proportion are multiplied, the cross products are equal.

Example: $\frac{2}{8} = \frac{5}{20}$

Here, the product of the first numerator multiplied by the opposite denominator is equivalent to the product of the first denominator multiplied by the opposite numerator:

$$\frac{2}{8} = \frac{5}{20}$$
$$2 \times 20 = 8 \times 5$$
$$40 = 40$$

In the preceding example, this proportion is spoken aloud as "two is to eight as five is to 20."

Cross multiplication is frequently used within medical practice to determine correct doses and amounts of drugs needed to mix medications or to make specific doses for administration to a patient. **Cross multiplication** is the multiplication of the numerator of the first fraction by the denominator of the second fraction, and the multiplication of the denominator of the first fraction by the numerator of the second fraction FIGURE 7.1.

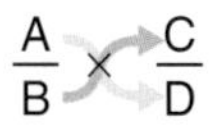

$$\frac{A}{B} \times \frac{C}{D}$$
$$AD = BC$$

FIGURE 7.1 Cross multiplication.
© Jones & Bartlett Learning

If one term of the proportion is unknown—meaning that three of the four values are known—cross multiplication can be used to find the value of the unknown term. The product of the first numerator multiplied by the opposite denominator is equivalent to the product of the first denominator multiplied by the opposite numerator.

Example $\frac{x}{8} = \frac{5}{20}$

This is the same as x is to 8 as 5 is to 20.

$$\frac{x}{8} = \frac{5}{20}$$
$$20x = 8 \times 5$$
$$20x = 40$$
$$\frac{20x}{20} = \frac{40}{20}$$
$$\frac{1}{1}\frac{20x}{20} = \frac{40}{20}\frac{2}{1}$$
$$x = 2$$

Cross multiplication is the multiplication of the numerator of the first fraction by the denominator of the second fraction, and the multiplication of the denominator of the first fraction by the numerator of the second fraction.

Means

$$1:5 = 2:10$$

Extremes

$$1 \times 10 = 2 \times 5$$

FIGURE 7.2 Means and extremes.

© Jones & Bartlett Learning

A practical application of ratios comes in the form of a proportion. A proportion is the expression of equality between two equivalent ratios. A proportion is designated by a double colon (::) between two ratios or as a fraction—for example, 3:5::6:10 or $\frac{3}{5} = \frac{6}{10}$. The values within a proportion are called means and extremes. The **means** are the numbers directly to the left and right of the equal sign and the **extremes** are the two outer numbers. As with equivalent ratios expressed as fractions, the product of the means always equals the product of the extremes in a proportion **FIGURE 7.2**.

Calculating the Value of a Missing Term in a Proportion

Understanding proportion is important because it enables you to calculate the value of a missing term in a proportion. This concept is critical to determining dosage calculations. For example, if a:b::c:d, then $\frac{a}{b} = \frac{c}{d}$ and a × d = b × c. Therefore, if any one of the variables is unknown, you can use the three known variables and solve for the unknown using basic algebra.

Example: $5:15 = x:45$

Step 1:   Multiply the means: $15 \times x = 15x$

Step 2:   Multiply the extremes: $5 \times 45 = 225$

Step 3:   Set up the equation (remember, the means equal the extremes): $15x = 225$

Step 4:   Divide both sides of the equation by 15 to find the value of x:
$15x \div 15 = 225 \div 15$
$x = 15$

Step 5:   Replace the x in the proportion with 15:
$5:15 = 15:45$ (five is to 15 as 15 is to 45)

The ratio-proportion method is based on comparing a known ratio with an unknown ratio.

Ratio-Proportion Method for Dosage Calculations

The ratio-proportion method is commonly used to calculate drug doses. For example, the concentration of a stock solution (a solution of known concentration) and the dose needed for administration are often known. The volume of the dose is the unknown. A ratio or proportion can be established to solve for the missing value. The ratio and proportion formula is as follows:

Dosage on hand:Amount on hand = Dosage desired:Amount desired

Before using this formula, make sure all measurements are in the same system of measurement. Next, plug the numbers in the formula above and solve for the unknown value.

Example: A physician prescribes 1,000mg of acetaminophen suspension and all that is available is a stock suspension of 500mg/15mL. How many milliliters of acetaminophen suspension would you give to the patient to fulfill the order?

Step 1:   Because the supply dosage and the amount prescribed are the same units, no conversion is necessary.

Step 2:   Set up the equation and calculate solving for x.

$$500\text{mg}:15\text{mL} = 1,000\text{mg}:x\text{mL}$$

$$(15 \times 1,000) = (500 \times x)$$

$$15,000 \div 500 = 500x \div 500$$
$$30 = x$$

Step 3:   Insert the answer back into the proportion to identify the units.

Answer: 30mL

Converting Between Ratios and Percents

To convert a ratio to a percent, first convert the ratio to a fraction, selecting the first number as the numerator and the second number as the denominator. Next, multiply the fraction by a number such that the denominator of the product equals 100. Express the final value followed by a percent sign.

Example: 1:25

Step 1: $1:25 = \frac{1}{25}$

Step 2: $\frac{1}{25} \times \frac{4}{4} = \frac{4}{100}$

Step 3: $\frac{4}{100} = 4$ percent

Reverse the process to convert a percent to ratio. First, express the percent as a fraction, with a denominator of 100. Then reduce the fraction to its most simplified form, if possible. Finally, express the final value as a ratio, designating the numerator as the first number and the denominator as the second number.

Example: 4 percent

Step 1:   4 percent $= \frac{4}{100}$

Step 2: $\frac{4}{100} = \frac{2}{50} = \frac{1}{25}$

Step 3:   1:25

Systems of Measurement

Several systems of measurement are used to calculate dosages: the common household system, the metric system, and the apothecary system. Other notations of quantity and measurement include international units and milliequivalents. Medical assistants should be familiar with all these systems, and be able to use them interchangeably. However, the metric system is the most common, and the safest, system used in medical practice.

Household System of Measurement

The **household system of measurement** is the one most patients in the United States are familiar with. These measurements are approximate measurements. This system includes drops, teaspoons, tablespoons, fluid ounces, cups, pints, quarts, and gallons for measuring liquid. It also includes ounces and pounds for measuring weight (1 pound = 16 ounces).

Instructions to patients are often provided in the household measuring system. Household measuring devices can vary in actual capacity. When using these devices to administer medications, remember to use

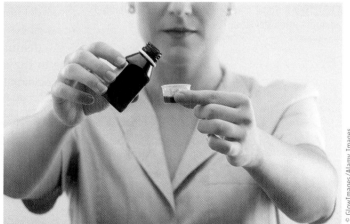

Stock solutions are often used to fill prescriptions.

© GlowImages/Alamy Images

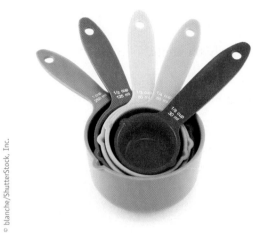

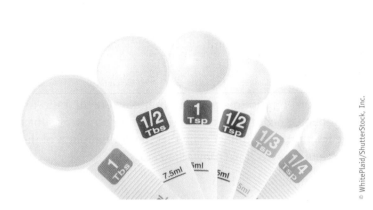

© blanche/ShutterStock, Inc.

© WhitePlaid/ShutterStock, Inc.

Household measuring devices.

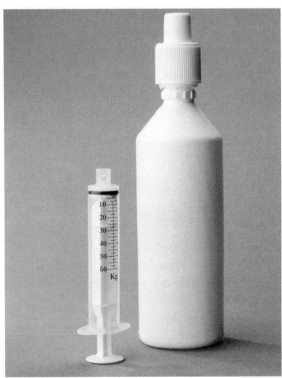

FIGURE 7.3 Some medications come with calibrated administration devices.
© Jupiterimages/Photos.com/Thinkstock

calibrated administration devices that come with medications **FIGURE 7.3**. Common household measurements are outlined in **TABLE 7.1**.

Apothecary System of Measurement

The **apothecary system of measurement** is an outdated system of measurement previously used in medicine and science. Unlike the household systems, the pound in the apothecary system is based on 12 ounces. The apothecary system consists of the grain to measure weight, and a quart, pint, fluid ounce, dram, and minim to measure volume. In general, the use of the apothecary system is discouraged because of safety concerns and inaccuracies. Two common exceptions are thyroid medications and phenobarbital dosing.

Metric System of Measurement

The **metric system** is by far the most commonly used system of measurement. The metric system is the legal standard of measurement for pharmacy and medicine in the United States. The metric system is based on the decimal system, and all units are described as multiples of 10. The correlations among units of measure are more distinct than in other systems of measurement, simplifying calculations and aiding in the **accuracy** (that is, how well a measurement represents the true value) and **precision** (that is, how well a series of measurements can be

Table 7.1 Common Household Measurements	
60 drops = 1 teaspoon	16 tablespoons = 1 cup
3 teaspoons = 1 tablespoon	2 cups = 1 pint
1 tablespoon = 15mL	2 pints = 1 quart
2 tablespoons = 1 ounce	4 quarts = 1 gallon
8 ounces = 1 cup	

reproduced or how close the measurements are to each other) of measurements.

Prefixes Used in the Metric System

In the metric system, prefixes are added to the base units to specify a particular measurement. When a metric prefix is combined with a root of physical quantity, you have multiples or submultiples of the metric system. Common prefixes and conversions used are provided in TABLE 7.2 .

The ladder method is a good way to convert from a larger unit to a smaller unit or from a smaller unit to a larger unit FIGURE 7.4 .

Help patients understand how to convert between the metric system and the household measuring system. Many patients will be more familiar with teaspoonfuls than milliliters.
© auremar/ShutterStock, Inc.

Fundamental Units Used in the Metric System

The basic units of measurement in the metric system are the **meter (m)**, for measuring length or distance; the **liter (L)**, for measuring liquid volume; and the **gram (g)**, for measuring dry weight. The gram is based on an actual cylinder of metal that is considered the kilogram. A cylinder locked away in Paris serves as the basis for all metric weight measurements.

Table 7.2 Common Prefixes and Conversions in the Metric System		
Prefix	**Meaning**	**Conversion**
Micro-	One millionth	Base unit × 10^{-6}
Milli-	One thousandth	Base unit × 10^{-3}
Centi-	One hundredth	Base unit × 10^{-2}
Deci-	One tenth	Base unit × 10^{-1}
Deka-	Ten times	Base unit × 10^{1}
Hecto-	One hundred times	Base unit × 10^{2}
Kilo-	One thousand times	Base unit × 10^{3}

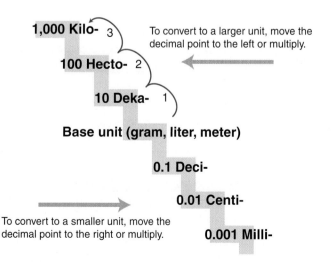

1,000 Kilo- 3

100 Hecto- 2

10 Deka- 1

To convert to a larger unit, move the decimal point to the left or multiply.

Base unit (gram, liter, meter)

0.1 Deci-

0.01 Centi-

0.001 Milli-

To convert to a smaller unit, move the decimal point to the right or multiply.

FIGURE 7.4 The ladder method.
© Jones & Bartlett Learning

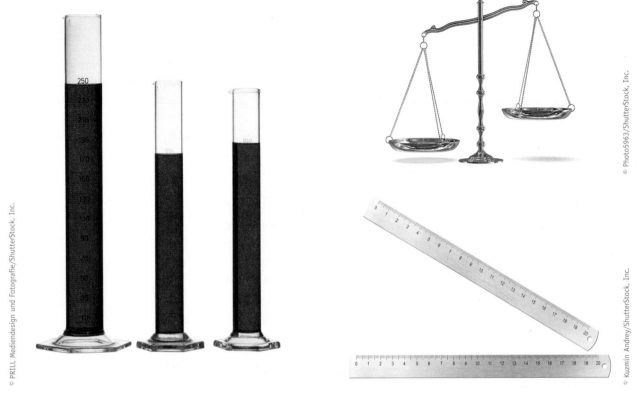

Measuring devices used in the metric system: cylinders (left), a balance scale (upper right), and rulers (lower right).

TABLE 7.3 outlines various length (meter) measurements.
TABLE 7.4 outlines various mass and weight (gram) measurements.
TABLE 7.5 outlines various volume (liter) measurements.

Converting Between Systems of Measurement

The base units and equivalents of the primary systems of measurement used for measuring weight and volumes are provided in **TABLE 7.6** and **TABLE 7.7**. In the metric system, changing from one unit to another involves multiplying or dividing by 10, 100, 1,000, and so on.

Table 7.3 Meter = Length	
1 millimeter (mm) = 0.001 meter	1 dekameter (dam) = 10 meters
1 centimeter (cm) = 0.01 meter	1 hectometer (hm) = 100 meters
1 decimeter (dm) = 0.1 meter	1 kilometer (km) = 1,000 meters
1 meter (m) = 1 meter	

Table 7.4 Gram = Mass and Weight	
1 microgram (mcg) = 0.000001 gram	1 gram (g) = 1 gram
1 milligram (mg) = 0.001 gram	1 dekagram (dag) = 10 grams
1 centigram (cg) = 0.01 gram	1 hectogram (hg) = 100 grams
1 decigram (dg) = 0.1 gram	1 kilogram (kg) = 1,000 grams

Table 7.5   Liter = Volume

1 microliter (mcL) = 0.000001 liter (L)	1 liter (L) = 1 liter
1 milliliter (mL) = .001L	1 dekaliter (daL) = 10L
1 centiliter (cL) = 0.01L	1 hectoliter (hL) = 100L
1 deciliter (dL) = 0.1L	1 kiloliter (kL) = 1,000L

Table 7.6   Household and Metric System Equivalents

Household Measurement	Metric Measurement
15 drops (gtt)	1mL
1 teaspoon (tsp)	5mL
1 tablespoon (tbsp or T) or 3 tsp	15mL
1 fluid ounce (fl oz) or 2 tbsp	30mL
1 cup	240mL
1 pint (pt) or 2 cups	480mL
1 quart (qt), 4 cups, or 2 pt	960mL
1 gallon, 16 cups, or 4 qt	3,840mL
1 ounce (oz)	30g
1 pound (lb) or 16 oz	454g
1 inch (in)	2.5cm
39.37 inches (in)	1m

Table 7.7   Apothecary, Metric System, and Household Measurement Equivalents

Apothecary Measurement	Metric Measurement	Household Measurement
1 minim	0.06mL	0.9 drops
1 fluidram or 60 minims	5mL	1 teaspoon (tsp)
1 fluidounce or 6 fluidrams	30mL	2 tablespoon (tbsp or T) or 1 fluid ounce (fl oz)
1 pint (pt)	480mL	2 cups
1 quart (qt) or 32 fluidrams	960mL	4 cups or 2 pints (pt)
1 gallon (gal), 8 pints (pt), or 4 quarts (qt)	3,840mL	16 cups, 8 pints (pt), or 4 quarts (qt)
1 pint (pt)	480mL	2 cups
1 quart (qt)	960mL	4 cups or 2 pints (pt)
1 grain (gr)	65mg	0.002 ounces
1 scruple or 29 grain (gr)	1.3g	0.05 ounces
1 dram or 60 grain (gr)	3.9g	0.14 ounces
1 ounce or 480 grain (gr)	30g	1 ounce
1 pound or 5,760 grain (gr)	373.2g	13.2 ounces

International Units

The **international unit (IU)** expresses drug amounts. Examples of drugs measured in international units include insulin, heparin, and vitamin D. The IU per milligram varies with each drug, so standard conversion factors are not possible. If necessary, the conversion factor will be provided by the drug manufacturer. To calculate medications that are ordered, use the ratio-proportion method.

Calculating Drug Doses, Dosages, and Quantities

A critical function of a medical assistant is ensuring that patients get the correct dose of a drug. There are many methods for accurately calculating drug quantity, as well as expressing and communicating the treatment regimen.

Dose and Dosage

A **dose** of a drug is the quantity that is intended to be administered, usually taken at one time or during one specified period such as per day. **Dosage** refers to the determination and regulation of the size, frequency, and number of doses. The dosage is the entire regimen or schedule of doses. Although often used interchangeably, dose and dosage have different meanings. The dose refers to the quantity of drug, while dosage refers to treatment duration and a cumulative effect. Doses can be expressed as a single dose, a daily dose, or a total dose. A daily dose, in turn, may be expressed as divided doses.

> Example: A dose of 100mg is prescribed twice daily for 10 days. The dose is 100mg, while the dosage is 200mg/day (100mg/dose × 2 doses/day = 200mg/day).

Doses and dosage regimens are highly variable among substances. Each is determined by a drug's biochemical and physical properties, the route of administration, and individual patient factors. A dose may be based on age, weight, body-surface area (BSA), liver or kidney function, or the specific illness being treated.

Determining Doses Based on Weight

The usual adult dose for most drugs is based on an average body weight of 70kg. However, some drugs act differently in the body depending on body size and composition and the concentration of drug desired at the site of action. Therefore some doses need to be increased or decreased for particularly lean or overweight persons. Also, body weight is often used to determine pediatric doses because age may not be a reliable indicator of body composition or function in children.

> The usual adult dose for most drugs is based on an average body weight of 70kg, or 154 lbs.

When drugs are intended to be dosed based on body weight, the dose will usually be expressed as a quantity of drug (usually in milligrams) per kilogram body weight. Therefore to determine the dose, multiply the patient's body weight by the dose required.

> Example: An antibiotic is dosed at 20mg/kg/day. Determine how many milligrams a 90kg patient will receive daily.
>
> Answer: Multiply the dose by the patient's weight: 20mg/kg/day × 90kg = 1,800mg/day

> Example: A pain medication is dosed at 35mg/kg/day. Determine how many milligrams a 75kg patient will receive daily.

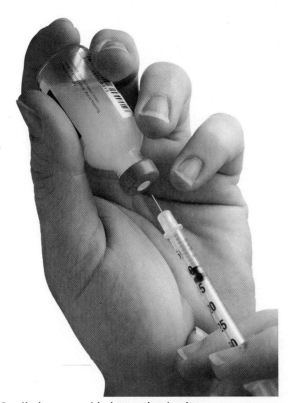

Insulin is measured in international units.

© Svanblar/ShutterStock, Inc.

Answer: Multiply the dose by the
patient's weight: 35mg/kg/day
× 75kg = 2,625mg/day

*When performing any calculation, make
sure the units are the same. If the units are
different, convert before proceeding with the
calculation.*
© auremar/ShutterStock, Inc.

Determining Doses Based on Body-Surface Area

Body-surface area (BSA) is a representation of a
patient's weight and height relative to each other.
Some patient populations or certain drugs require dosing based on BSA, such as cancer
patients receiving chemotherapy and pediatric patients who require special assessment
for drug response or adverse reactions.

BSA is calculated using the following equation:

$$BSA\ (m^2) = \left[\frac{Height\ (cm) \times Weight\ (kg)}{36,000}\right]^{1/2}$$

If inches and pounds are used to measure height and weight, respectively, the
following equation can be used:

$$BSA\ (m^2) = \left[\frac{Height\ (in) \times Weight\ (lb)}{3,131}\right]^{1/2}$$

The average adult has a BSA of $1.73m^2$. Using this value, a pediatric dose can be
calculated using the ratio-proportion method, defining the pediatric dose as a relative portion of the adult dose. Alternatively, to determine a pediatric dose based on
an adult dose and BSA, convert the child's BSA to a percent or fraction of usual adult
BSA and multiply the result by the adult dose.

Example: A child who is 40 inches tall and weighs 38 pounds has a BSA
of 0.7. If the average adult dose of a medication is 50mg, what
dosage should be given to this child according to the BSA
method?

Step 1: Remember that the average adult has a BSA of $1.73m^2$. Using
this value, a pediatric dose can be calculated using the ratio-
proportion method, defining the pediatric dose as a relative
portion of the adult dose.

Step 2: The ratio of the child's BSA to the adult BSA is $0.7:1.7m^2$.

Step 3: The adult dose is 50mg. The child's dose relative to the adult's
dose can be calculated using the following formula:
Child's BSA/Adult BSA × Adult dose/1 = Child's dose

Step 4: Plug the given values into the formula:
$\frac{0.7m^2}{1.7m^2} \times \frac{50mg}{1}$ = Child's dose

Step 5: Calculate the result: $\frac{0.7m^2}{1.7m^2} = 0.412$

Step 6: Multiply the result of the calculation (i.e., the child's relative
dose) by the adult dose: 0.412 × 50 = 20.5mg

Answer: The child's dose is 20.5mg.

The average adult has a BSA of $1.73m^2$. Usual adult doses are based on a weight of 70kg and a
BSA of $1.73m^2$.

Pediatric Patients

Patient age is often considered in calculating doses, particularly for very young or very
old patients. For example, both newborns and the elderly are especially sensitive to

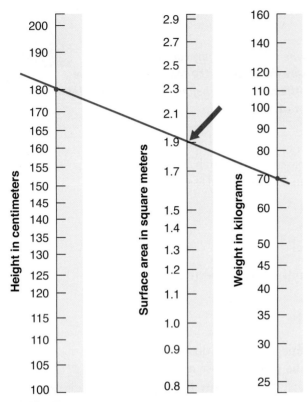

FIGURE 7.5 A nomogram is used to estimate the BSA of a pediatric patient based on height and weight.

Adapted from http://www.cecity.com/apha/rphguide/body_surface_area_nomogram_children .htm

the actions of certain drugs because of immature or abnormal liver or kidney function, which are required for healthy drug metabolism.

Several rules have been established to estimate the pediatric dose based on age or weight of the patient relative to the usual adult dose of a drug. However, these calculations are generally no longer used because age and weight are not always considered single reliable criteria for determining pediatric doses. Also, these calculations relate a pediatric dose to an adult dose, assuming that a child is simply a small adult. This is not always the case, however, because of different body composition and organ function between children and adults. Therefore, doses based directly on a child's BSA or body weight are the safest and most common choices to establish pediatric doses. The body weight method is generally the method of choice because it is easier to calculate. The BSA is an exact method, but you must use a formula and a **nomogram**, which is a graph that estimates the BSA of the patient based on height and weight **FIGURE 7.5**. Also, manufacturers often provide pediatric dosing tables with the drug information to aid in determining doses.

> For pediatric patients, doses based directly on BSA are the safest and most common choices to establish pediatric doses.

The BSA is determined by drawing a straight line from the patient's height to the patient's weight. Intersection of the line with the surface area column is the estimated BSA.

$$\frac{\text{BSA of child (m}^2)}{1.7 \text{ (m}^2)} \times \text{Adult dose} = \text{Child dose}$$

The BSA formula is based on an average adult who weighs 140 pounds and has a BSA of 1.7m^2.

Example: A five-year-old child who is 40 inches tall and weighs 38 pounds has just been prescribed an antibiotic for an infection. The average adult dose of antibiotic is 50mg/mL. What dosage should this patient receive according to the BSA method?

Step 1: Use the following formula:

$$\frac{\text{BSA of child (m}^2)}{1.7 \text{ (m}^2)} \times \text{Adult dose} = \text{Child dose}$$

Step 2: Plug the given values into the formula: $0.7\text{m}^2/1.7\text{m}^2 \times {}^{50\text{mg}}\!/_1 =$ Child dose

Step 3: $0.7 \times 50 \div 1.7 \times 1 = {}^{35}\!/_{1.7}$

Step 4: Simplify: 20.5mg

Step 5:   Use the ratio-proportion method:

$$\frac{50\text{mg}}{1\text{mL}} = \frac{20.\ 5\text{mg}}{x\text{mL}}$$

Step 6:   Cross multiply.

$$50\text{mg} \times x\text{mL} = 1\text{mL} \times 20.5\text{mg} = 50x = 20.5$$

Step 7:   Solve for x

$$\frac{50x}{50} = \frac{20.5}{50}$$

$$x = 0.41\text{mL}$$

Young's Rule

To determine pediatric doses based on age, Young's rule is used. It is as follows:

$$\text{Pediatric dose} = \frac{\text{Age of child (years)}}{\text{Age of child (years)} + 12} \times \text{Adult dose}$$

Example: Consider an 11-year-old girl who weighs 70 pounds. If the usual dose of a medication is 500mg, using Young's rule, what would the dose of medication be for the girl? (Remember that Young's rule uses age, not weight, to calculate pediatric doses.)

Step 1:   Use the following formula:
Pediatric dose = $\frac{\text{Age of child (years)}}{\text{Age of child (years)} + 12} \times$ Adult dose

Step 2:   Plug the given values into the formula: $\frac{11}{11+12} \times 500\text{mg}$

Step 3:   Convert both sides of the equation into fractions: $\frac{11}{23} \times \frac{500}{1}\text{mg}$

Step 4:   Multiply the numerators: $11 \times 500 = 5{,}500$

Step 5:   Multiply the denominators: $23 \times 1 = 23$

Step 6:   Divide the product of the numerators by the product of the denominators: $5{,}500 \div 23 = 239$

Answer: The pediatric dose is 239mg.

Clark's Rule

To determine pediatric doses based on weight, Clark's rule is used. It is as follows:

$$\text{Pediatric dose} = \frac{\text{Weight of child (pounds)} \times \text{Adult dose}}{150\ \text{lb}}$$

Note that here, the average weight of an adult is considered to be 150 lb. It is also important to note that Clark's rule uses weight in pounds, never in kilograms.

Example: Consider the same 11-year-old girl, who weighs 70 pounds. If the usual dose of a medication is 500mg, using Clark's rule, what would the dose of medication be for the girl? (Remember that Young's rule uses weight, not age, to calculate pediatric doses.)

Step 1:   Use the following formula:
Pediatric dose = $\frac{\text{Weight of child (pounds)} \times \text{Adult dose}}{150\ \text{lb}}$

Step 2:   Plug the given values into the formula: 70 lb × 500mg ÷ 150 lb

Step 3:   Calculate the product of the first part of the equation:
$70 \times 500\text{mg} = 35{,}000\text{mg}$

Step 4:   Divide the product by 150: $35{,}000\text{mg} \div 150 = 233\text{mg}$

Answer: The pediatric dose is 233mg.

Math Practice

Question: **What is the result of converting 2:1 to a percent?**

Answer:

Step 1: Convert the ratio to a fraction: 2:1 = $\frac{2}{1}$

Step 2: Multiply the fraction by 100: $\frac{2}{1} \times 100 = 200\%$

Question: **What is the result of converting 70% to a ratio?**

Answer:

Step 1: Express the percentage as a fraction: 70% = $\frac{70}{100}$

Step 2: Simplify the fraction: $\frac{70}{100} \div \frac{10}{10} = \frac{7}{10}$

Step 3: Express the fraction as a ratio: $\frac{7}{10}$ = 7:10

Question: **What is the result of converting 25% to a ratio?**

Answer:

Step 1: Express the percentage as a fraction: 25% = $\frac{25}{100}$

Step 2: Simplify the fraction: $\frac{25}{100} \div \frac{25}{25} = \frac{1}{4}$

Step 3: Express the fraction as a ratio: $\frac{1}{4}$ = 1:4

Question: **What is the result of converting 1:5 to a percent?**

Answer:

Step 1: Convert the ratio to a fraction: 1:5 = $\frac{1}{5}$

Step 2: Multiply the fraction by $\frac{20}{20}$ so the denominator equals 100: $\frac{1}{5} \times \frac{20}{20} = \frac{1 \times 20}{5 \times 20}$

Step 3: Express the fraction as a percent: $\frac{20}{100}$ = 20%

Question: **If each dose is 5mL, and the total amount of drug to be administered is 150mL, what is the total number of doses available?**

Answer: The total number of doses available is 150mL ÷ 5mL = 30

Question: **If the dose is 25mg, and the duration of therapy is seven days, what is the total amount of drug needed to complete the course of therapy?**

Answer: The total amount of drug needed to complete therapy is 25mg × 7 days = 175mg

---

Question: **If the dose is 500mg, and the total amount to be administered is 4g, what is the total number of doses available?**

Answer:

Step 1: Convert the quantities to the same unit. 1g = 1,000mg, so using the ratio and proportion method, set up the equation to solve for *x*: 1g/1,000mg = *x*g/500mg

Step 2: Cross multiply and solve for x: $1 \times 500 = 1,000 \times x$

$500 = 1,000x$

$\frac{500}{1000} = \frac{1,000x}{1,000}$

$\frac{1}{2} = x$

$0.5 = x$

Step 3: The total number of doses to be administered is $4g \div 0.5g = 8$ doses

---

Question: **What is the total amount of drug to be administered if each dose is 15mg and the total number of doses is 40?**

Answer: Multiply the number of doses by the quantity of each dose: 15mg/dose × 40 doses = 600mg

---

Question: **What is the total dose for a child weighing 15kg and requiring a dose of 0.5mg/kg?**

Answer: The total dose is 15kg × 0.5mg/kg = 7.5mg

Question: **What is the total dose for a man weighing 85kg and requiring a dose of 50mg/kg?**

Answer: The total dose is 85 kg × 50mg/kg = 4,250mg

Question: **In the equation $\frac{x}{5} = \frac{18}{45}$, solve for x.**

Step 1: $\frac{x}{5} = \frac{18}{45}$ is the same as x is to 5 as 18 is to 45, so the following applies:

$\frac{x}{5} = \frac{18}{45}$

$45x = 18 \times 5$

$45x = 90$

$\frac{45x}{45} = \frac{90}{45}$

$\frac{1}{1}\frac{45x}{45} = \frac{90}{45}\frac{2}{1}$

$x = 2$

Question: **Using the proportion 2:14 = x:42, solve for x.**

Answer: 2:14 = x:42

Step 1: Multiply the means ($14 \times x = 14x$)

Step 2: Multiply the extremes ($2 \times 42 = 84$)

Step 3: Set up the equation (remember, the means equal the extremes): $14x = 84$

Step 4: Divide both sides of the equation by 14 to find the value of x: $14x \div 14 = 84 \div 14$; $x = 6$

Step 5: Replace the x in the proportion with 6: 2:14 = 6:42

Question: **How many milliliters are in 20L?**

Answer: 1L = 1,000mL, so 20L = 20L × 1,000mL ÷ 1L = 20,000mL

Question: **How many grams are in 1,500mg?**

Answer: 1g = 1,000mg, so 1,500mg = 1,500mg × 1g ÷ 1,000mg = 1.5g

WRAP UP

Chapter Summary

- An understanding of basic mathematics and calculations is essential to ensure safe, accurate, and effective drug administration.
- A ratio represents how two quantities are related to each other. A ratio may also be expressed as a fraction, and vice versa.
- Proportions are equivalent ratios, often used to calculate unknown quantities or concentrations in pharmacy.
- Percents are the number of parts per 100 total parts. A percent can also be expressed as a fraction or ratio.
- The metric system is the most accurate, and preferred, system of measurement. Prefixes are added to base units of measurement in the metric system to denote larger or smaller quantities.

- The apothecary system is not used frequently because of inaccuracies and safety concerns. However, thyroid medications and phenobarbital are often dosed in grains, the base unit of weight in the apothecary system.
- Doses of drugs are highly variable and can be based on the drug's chemical composition or physical properties, the route of administration, or the condition being treated. Alternatively, patient factors such as age, body weight, body-surface area, and organ function may be used to calculate the correct dose.
- Pediatric patients require special consideration when determining doses because children have immature organ function and a different body composition than adults.

Learning Assessment Questions

1. Which system of measurement is most commonly used in the healthcare setting?
   - A. Apothecary
   - B. Household
   - C. Metric
   - D. Common

2. The prefix milli- means what?
   - A. 1/10
   - B. 1/1,000
   - C. 10
   - D. 100

3. The prefix hecto- means what?
   - A. 100
   - B. 1/10
   - C. 1,000
   - D. 1/100,000

4. How many grams are there in 1 kilogram?
   - A. 10
   - B. 100
   - C. 1,000
   - D. 1

5. The metric system is based on multiples of _____.
   - A. 5
   - B. 10
   - C. 20
   - D. 100

6. In the apothecary system, 1 pint is equal to _____.
   - A. 2 cups
   - B. 4 cups
   - C. 6 cups
   - D. 8 cups

7. A physician orders a drug at a dose of 2mg/kg. The patient weights 50kg. What is the correct dose?
   - A. 10mg
   - B. 1g
   - C. 25mg
   - D. 100mg

8. The ratio 6:25 is equivalent to what percent?
    A. 6 percent
    B. 24 percent
    C. 25 percent
    D. 90 percent
9. The ratio 10:25 is equivalent to what percent?
    A. 1 percent
    B. 25 percent
    C. 4 percent
    D. 40 percent
10. Percents are the number of parts per ____
    total.
    A. 50
    B. 100
    C. 1,000
    D. 1
11. A doctor prescribes 40mg of Zocor. You have
    80mg tablets on hand. How many tablets for
    one dose will you give to your patient?
    A. ½
    B. 1
    C. 2
    D. ¼
12. A doctor prescribes 120mg of a medicine. You
    have 40mg tablets on hand. How many tablets
    for one dose will you give to your patient?
    A. 1
    B. 2
    C. 3
    D. 4
13. Match the following prefixes with their
    corresponding measurement:
    A. Kilo-   1. One thousandth
    B. Hecto-   2. One millionth
    C. Deci-   3. One tenth
    D. Centi-   4. One hundred
    E. Milli-   5. One thousand
    F. Micro-   6. One hundredth

14. Which unit of the metric system measures
    volume?
    A. Meter
    B. Liter
    C. Gram
    D. Cup
15. Which unit of the metric system measures
    mass and/or weight?
    A. Meter
    B. Gram
    C. Ounce
    D. Pint
16. Which of the following shows how two similar
    quantities are related to each other?
    A. Ratio
    B. Fraction
    C. Numerator
    D. Denominator
17. Which of the following is an equation that
    states two ratios are equal?
    A. Ratio
    B. Fraction
    C. Proportion
    D. Numerator
18. The apothecary system uses which of the
    following to measure weight?
    A. Grain
    B. Gram
    C. Ounce
    D. Milligram
19. What are the two outer numbers in a
    proportion called?
    A. Means
    B. Equivalents
    C. Extremes
    D. Variables
20. Which rule determines pediatric doses based
    on age?
    A. Clark's rule
    B. Smith's rule
    C. Kepler's rule
    D. Young's rule

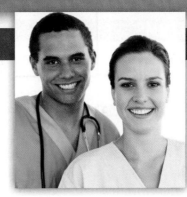

Integumentary System

OBJECTIVES

After reading this chapter, you will be able to:

- Identify combining word forms of the integumentary system and their role for the formation of medical terms.
- Define the structures and functions of the integumentary system.
- List abbreviations related to the integumentary system.
- Identify the most common diseases and disorders of the integumentary system.
- Discriminate among first-, second-, and third-degree burns.
- List rules to follow to protect sterile areas.
- Given a variety of surgical instruments, be able to identify each and describe the intended use of each one.
- Demonstrate the ability to select the most appropriate type of dressings for a given situation.
- List preoperative concerns to be addressed in patient preparation and education.
- List postoperative concerns to be addressed with the patient and the caregiver.
- Demonstrate the application of sterile gloves.
- Demonstrate setting up a surgical tray, including laying the field, applying supplies and instruments, pouring a sterile solution, using transfer forceps, and covering the sterile tray.
- Identify and care for different types of wounds.
- Understand the basics of bandage application.

KEY TERMS

Adipose tissue	Germinative layer	Scabies
Apocrine glands	Hair follicle	Seborrheic keratosis
Asepsis	Herpes simplex virus	Second-degree burn
Basal cell carcinoma	Herpes zoster	Shingles
(BCC)	Hives	Squamous cell
Candidiasis	Human papillomavirus	carcinoma (SCC)
Carbuncle	(HPV)	Squamous epithelial cells
Cellulitis	Impetigo	Sterile
Cerumen	Laceration	Stratum corneum
Collagen	Lice	Sweat
Comedone	Melanin	Third-degree burn
Cyst	Melanocytes	Thrush
Dermatitis	Melanoma	Tinea barbae
Dermatology	Nevus	Tinea capitis
Dermatophytoses	Papule	Tinea corporis
Eccrine glands	Pediculosis	Tinea cruris
Eczema	Perionychium	Tinea manuum
Emollients	Pimple	Tinea pedis
Fenestrated drape	Pruritis	Tinea unguium
First-degree burn	Psoriasis	Urticaria
Folliculitis	Pustule	Verrucae
Furuncle	Rule of nines	Warts

Chapter Overview

The integumentary system includes the skin and its accessory organs: the hair, nails, glands, and nerve receptors. The skin is the largest organ in the body and accounts for more than 10 percent of total body weight. The primary function of the skin is to act as a barrier between humans and the environment. Skin protects the body from loss of water, salt, and heat. Skin also protects the body from chemical, physical, and microbial injury. TABLE 8.1 lists word roots and terms used in the study of the integumentary system.

Disorders and diseases of the skin are a frequent cause for patients to visit a healthcare provider. As a medical assistant, you will have the opportunity to interact with many of these patients. Often, skin conditions are associated with shame and embarrassment on the part of the patient, and you have a critical role in maintaining the comfort of the patient.

The skin is the largest organ in the body and can weigh over 20 pounds in an adult.

© auremar/ShutterStock, Inc.

You may also have the opportunity to assist the physician in procedures and examinations related to the integumentary system. In this role, you must strive to maintain a positive attitude and ensure that the patient is confident in the treatment he or she is receiving. Ensuring that the patient understands his or her skin condition and its causes and consequences and that he or she is knowledgeable and comfortable with the treatment routine is essential to optimal patient care.

Dermatology is the study of the skin.

Table 8.1 Word Roots of the Integumentary System

Word Root or Term	Meaning	Example
Adip/o	Fatty	Adipoma (fatty tumor)
Albin/o	White	Albino (a person who is not able to produce melanin and has characteristic white skin and eyes)
Cutane/o	Skin	Subcutaneous (under the skin)
Cyan/o	Blue	Cyanosis (blue condition of skin or lips)
Derm/o or dermat/o	Skin	Dermatology (the study of skin)
Erythem/o	Flush	Erythema (redness)
Hidr/o	Sweat	Hyperhidrosis (excessive sweating)
Ichthy/o	Dry, scaly, or fishy in appearance	Ichthyosis (dry, scaly condition)
Kerat/o	Hard, horny	Keratosis (skin condition characterized by thick, horny growth)
Leuk/o	White	Leukoderma (white skin)
Lip/o	Fat	Lipocytes (fat cells)
Macul/o	Stain, spot	Maculopapular rash (rash characterized by small, flat discolored spots and red, raised bumps)
Melan/o	Black	Melanoma (black tumor)
Oncych/o	Nail	Schizonychia (condition characterized by splitting of the nail)
Papul/o	Pimple	Papule (small, elevated inflammation on the surface of the skin)
Pil/o	Hair	Depilatory (the process of removing hair)
Scler/o	Hard	Scleroderma (hardening of the skin)
Seb/o	Sebum, oil	Sebborrhea (excessive discharge of sebum)
Ungu/o	Nail	Ungual fibroma (fleshy papules in the nail bed)
Vit/o	Blemish	Vitiligo (a condition characterized by the loss of brown pigment from irregular patches of skin)
Xer/o	Dry	Xeroderma (dry skin)

Abbreviations Related to the Integumentary System

The following are abbreviations related to the integumentary system:

BCC—Basal cell carcinoma
BX—Biopsy
Ca—Cancer
DSD—Dry sterile dressing
HPV—Human papillomavirus
I&D—Incision and drainage
ID—Intradermal
NS—Normal saline
SOL—Space occupying lesion
Surg—Surgery
UV—Ultraviolet

Anatomy and Physiology of the Skin

Skin is composed of three layers: the epidermis, the dermis, and the subcutaneous tissue. Each region has distinct components and functions. **FIGURE 8.1** illustrates each of these layers.

Structure of the Skin

The epidermis is the thin, outermost layer of skin and contains compact, stratified (layered) squamous epithelial cells. **Squamous epithelial cells** are flat and scale-like. The epidermis contains part of the hair and nails. The epidermis lacks blood supply, connective tissue, and lymphatic vessels. The epidermis depends on deeper layers of skin for nourishment and hydration.

The epidermis is constantly shedding dead, dry skin cells and producing new ones. The new cells are produced in the **germinative layer**, the innermost layer of the epidermis. The germinative layer contains **melanocytes**, which produce melanin. **Melanin** is responsible for giving skin its pigmentation, or coloring, and protects the skin from damage caused by ultraviolet (UV) rays.

The outermost layer of the epidermis is the **stratum corneum**, which is the layer of cells exposed to the environment. The stratum corneum contains 10 to 20 percent water by weight; the high water content accounts for its flexibility. Water content is affected by heat, humidity, and skin trauma. If the water content of the stratum corneum falls below 10 percent, the stratum corneum becomes dry, brittle, and chapped and breaks easily. This loss of integrity of the skin structure increases the risk of infection and contamination.

The dermis is the second layer of skin, lying beneath the epidermis. The dermis is approximately 40 times thicker than the epidermis. The dermis provides structural and nutritional support to the epidermis. The dermis is composed of connective tissue and contains a rich supply of blood vessels, lymph vessels, nerves, sweat glands

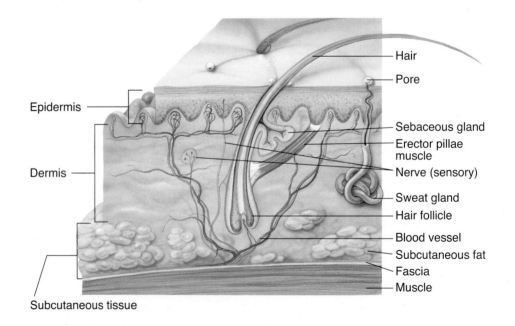

FIGURE 8.1 Illustration of the layers of human skin.
© Jones & Bartlett Learning

(also known as sudoriferous glands, which are small, tubular structures that produce sweat), and sebaceous glands (small structures that produce an oily substance and secrete it to the hair follicle). The dermis also contains most of the collagen found in the body. **Collagen** is a protein fiber found in the connective tissue of most organs and provides strength and elasticity to skin.

Hair turns gray as people age, when they no longer produce melanin. This is a normal part of aging.
© auremar/ShutterStock, Inc.

The dermis contains sensory receptors that convey information from the external environment to the central nervous system. The central nervous system then acts to protect the body from damage, such as becoming too hot or too cold.

The subcutaneous tissue is the innermost layer of skin. It contains loose connective tissue and **adipose tissue** (a type of connective tissue that contains stored fat) that is anchored to the dermis. The fat of the subcutaneous tissue provides cushioning for the body, maintains food reserves, and facilitates temperature control. The amount and distribution of adipose tissue in the body is largely determined by gender. Women tend to have an overall higher percentage of adipose tissue than men, which is generally distributed to the hips, upper thighs, breasts, and abdomen. Men tend to store excess fatty tissue in the abdomen. On average, approximately half of the body's total fat is contained in the subcutaneous tissue.

Function of the Skin

The skin is the body's primary defense mechanism. Healthy skin is essential for maintaining a healthy body. Age, health status, and environmental exposures are all important factors in maintaining skin in its optimal condition. In addition to working as a protective barrier, the skin contributes to sensory input, temperature regulation, skin pigmentation, emotional expression, the production, or synthesis, of vitamin D, and maintaining the moisture content of the body.

The skin produces two types of fluids: sebum and sweat. The sebaceous glands, located in the dermis, secrete sebum, an oily substance that prevents hair and skin from becoming too dry. Sebum is toxic to some bacteria and therefore also acts to protect the skin from infection. Too much sebum results in oily hair and skin, and too little sebum results in dry hair and skin.

Sweat glands, also located in the dermis, produce **sweat**, which primarily functions to maintain body temperature. Sweat is released from the sweat glands in response to an elevated body temperature; it evaporates off the skin into the air, thus cooling the body. Sweat glands are located throughout the entire body, but are concentrated in the forehead, underarms, palms of the hands, and soles of the feet.

Sweat is composed mainly of water. **Eccrine glands** produce sweat containing water and salt. **Apocrine glands**, located deeper in the skin, produce sweat containing water and organic material. An odor is produced when this organic material is broken down by bacteria on the skin. Apocrine glands in the skin of the ear produce **cerumen**, or earwax, which protects the ear from damage caused by pathogens and toxins.

The nail bed contains a rich blood supply. To test a patient's circulation using the capillary nail refill test, press down on the edge of the fingernail until the nail appears white. With proper circulation, the nail will immediately return to its normal color when the pressure is released.
© auremar/ShutterStock, Inc.

Hair and nails are appendages of the skin that protect the skin from damage. **Hair follicles** are located in the dermis, near sebaceous glands that provide lubrication for the hair. The follicles also contain

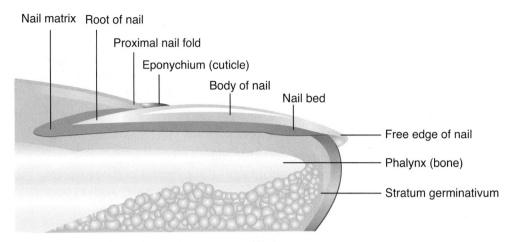

Nail matrix   Root of nail

Proximal nail fold

Eponychium (cuticle)

Body of nail

Nail bed

Free edge of nail

Phalynx (bone)

Stratum germinativum

FIGURE 8.2 Illustration of the parts of a human fingernail.
© Grei/ShutterStock, Inc.

melanocytes, which give hair its pigmentation. As hair grows from the follicle out of the scalp, it is composed of dead and hardened skin cells that have become filled with a protein called keratin.

Fingernails and toenails are also composed of keratinized skin cells that grow from a nail root. The **perionychium** is the soft tissue that surrounds the nail. The entire structure of the human nail is shown in **FIGURE 8.2**. Nails grow continuously, provided disease or trauma does not affect the nail root. Nails protect the sensitive ends of the fingers and toes and make gripping things easier. The size, shape, color, and growth patterns of the nails can provide clues to certain illnesses and medical conditions.

Diseases and Disorders of the Skin

Lesions are any type of disorder, damage, or abnormality of the skin. Lesions may appear as signs or symptoms of medical conditions or injuries or may be normal variations in the appearance of skin. Observation of the lesion, including attention to color, shape, and size, is valuable in characterizing and diagnosing the lesion. **TABLE 8.2** and **FIGURE 8.3** provide features and examples of common types of skin lesions.

Acne Vulgaris

Acne vulgaris is a common skin disorder, often appearing in adolescence, but which may extend through adulthood. Acne is not contagious and is not caused by poor personal hygiene. It does not signify poor physical health, but acne can be devastating to mental and psychosocial health.

Signs and Symptoms of Acne Vulgaris

Acne vulgaris results from the overactive production of sebum in the sebaceous glands, which gives the skin an oily appearance. When the ducts of the sebaceous glands become plugged, a blackhead or **comedone** forms. The gland and surrounding hair

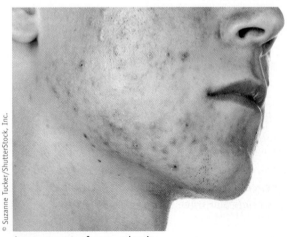

A severe case of acne vulgaris.

Table 8.2 Characteristics of Common Skin Lesions

Type of Lesion	Characteristics	Size	Example
Bulla (blister)	Fluid-filled area	Greater than 5mm across	Contact dermatitis or second-degree burns
Crust	A collection of dried serum and debris	Varies	Impetigo or eczema
Cyst	Encapsulated fluid-filled or semisolid mass in the subcutaneous tissue or dermis	Varies	Sebaceous cyst or epidermoid cyst
Excoriation	A missing area of the epidermis	Varies	Scrape or burn
Fissure	Linear crack from epidermis to dermis	Varies	Tinea pedis (athlete's foot)
Keloid	Enlarged scar past wound edges due to excess collagen formation	Varies	Burn scars
Macule	Round, flat, discolored area that is flush with the skin surface	Smaller than 1cm across	Freckle
Nodule	Elevated solid area; deeper and firmer than a papule	Greater than 5mm across	Wart
Papule	Elevated solid area	5mm or less across	Mole
Patch	Round, flat, discolored area that is flush with the skin surface	Greater than 1cm across	Vitiligo
Plaque	Solid, elevated lesion	Greater than 0.5cm across	Psoriasis
Pustule	Discrete, pus-filled area	Varies	Acne lesions
Scales	Flaking of the skin surface	Varies	Dandruff
Ulcer	Deep loss of skin surface; may extend into dermis and may bleed periodically	Varies	Bed sores (decubitus ulcers)
Tumor	Solid abnormal mass that may extend through cutaneous tissue	Greater than 1–2cm	Basal cell carcinoma
Vesicle	Fluid-filled raised area	5mm or less across	Chicken pox or herpes simplex
Wheal	Itchy, elevated area with irregular shape	Varies	Hives or insect bites

follicle become enlarged with sebum, forming a **papule**. If the papule becomes infected with a **pustule**, a whitehead will form, surrounded by redness and inflammation. **Pimples**, raised red lesions, and **cysts**, fluid-filled sacs surrounded by inflammation, may also appear as a result of plugged sebaceous glands.

The skin lesions of acne vulgaris most often appear on the face, but can also appear on the chest and back. If the pustules or papules break open, they often become infected. Inflammatory papular and pustular eruptions commonly occur in acne. In severe cases, scarring and pitting of the skin can occur as a result of acne.

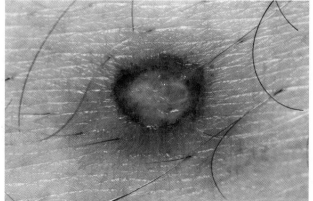

Ulcers extend deep into the skin.

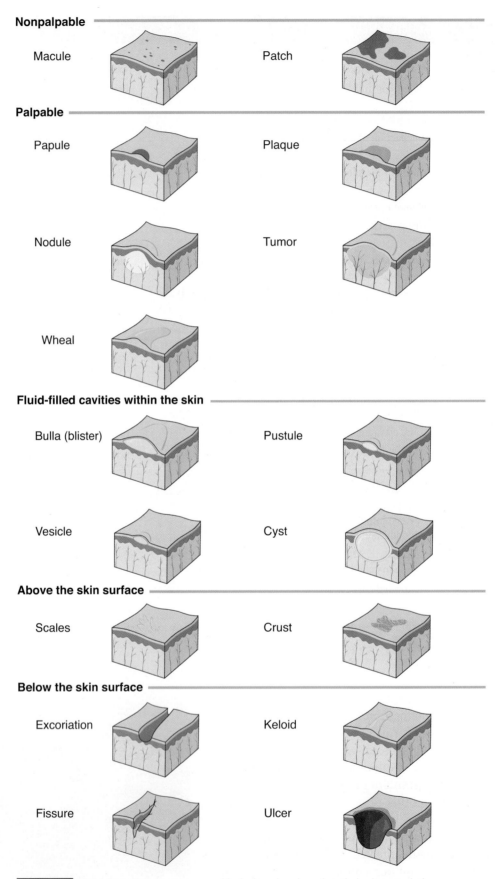

Nonpalpable

Macule   Patch

Palpable

Papule   Plaque

Nodule   Tumor

Wheal

Fluid-filled cavities within the skin

Bulla (blister)   Pustule

Vesicle   Cyst

Above the skin surface

Scales   Crust

Below the skin surface

Excoriation   Keloid

Fissure   Ulcer

FIGURE 8.3 Physicians diagnose common skin lesions by observing their characteristics.

Treatment of Acne Vulgaris

The goal of acne treatment is to alleviate the blockage of the glands to allow them to function properly, reduce the amount of oil produced by the glands, reduce inflammation, and prevent the ducts of the sebaceous glands from becoming blocked again. Gentle cleansing of the skin at least twice daily with mild soap or cleanser is the simplest form of acne treatment. A topical astringent may reduce the oiliness of the skin, and may be used throughout the day.

Moderate to severe acne that does not respond to simple cleansing routines may require antibiotic treatment to prevent the growth of *Propionibacterium acnes*. Several antibiotics are available to treat *P. acnes*, including tetracyclines, erythromycin, and sulfamethoxazole/trimethoprim. Because hormone fluctuations may exacerbate the signs and symptoms of acne, birth control pills are sometimes prescribed as part of an acne treatment regimen in girls and women.

Eczema and Dermatitis

Most common skin conditions and disorders can be classified as eczema or dermatitis. The two terms are often used together, and interchangeably. **Dermatitis** denotes any inflammation of the epidermis, and **eczema** is often used to denote chronic dermatitis. Broadly, the conditions are the same, and the characteristics and treatment of eczema and dermatitis are indistinguishable.

Dermatitis can result from an allergy, a reaction to excessive hot or cold temperatures, or emotional stress. Family and medical history are also significant factors in assessing dermatitis and eczema.

Signs and Symptoms of Eczema and Dermatitis

Most cases of eczema or dermatitis are caused by allergic or hypersensitivity reactions. The conditions may appear as early as a few weeks after birth and present as redness and chapping of the skin. Edema, or swelling from fluid accumulation around the lesions, may or may not be present. Often, tiny blisters that crust and weep appear, along with papules and scaling. Patients complain of **pruritus** (itching) and a burning sensation. Secondary infections due to scratching and breaking the skin are common complications of eczema and dermatitis.

Chronic conditions of dermatitis involve red, dry, thickened patches of skin. The lesions are usually symmetrical and appear most commonly at the flexor surfaces (knees, elbows, and collar area of the neck).

Treatment of Eczema and Dermatitis

Ideally, the source of the irritant or allergen causing the dermatitis or eczema can be identified and removed.

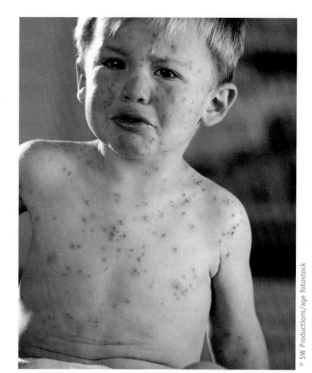

Chicken pox lesions are red, raised, fluid-filled vesicles.

© SW Productions/age fotostock

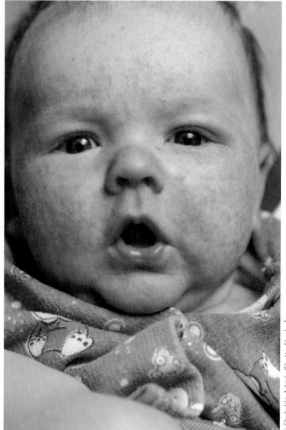

Eczema is characterized by redness and chapping of the skin, with lesions that crust along the border.

© Chubykin Arkady/ShutterStock, Inc.

What Would You Do?

A 14-year-old female presents to the physician's office where you work. She is experiencing severe acne that has not responded to over-the-counter cleansers and astringents. She is visibly anxious and mentions that her skin problems are affecting her friendships at school. What advice can you give the patient?

However, in most cases, no specific cause can be identified. Symptom relief is the primary goal of treatment. Antihistamines can be administered to relieve itching, and moist compresses may be used to cool the skin and aid in removal of the crusts. Steroid creams may also be applied topically to decrease inflammation associated with eczema and dermatitis.

Patients with eczema or dermatitis should take care to use gentle skin cleansers, avoid exposure to harsh chemicals and cleaners, and use proper infection-control practices to reduce the risk of infection if the skin is broken. The patient should also avoid extreme hot or cold temperatures and emotionally stressful situations, which can aggravate symptoms of eczema and dermatitis.

Urticaria (Hives)

Urticaria, or **hives**, is an acute allergic reaction of the dermis. Hives may appear following exposure to a certain food, medication, or psychological stressor. Hives may also appear as part of a chronic condition in which the trigger cannot be identified.

Signs and Symptoms of Urticaria

The lesions of urticaria are characterized by edema, redness, and pruritus. Typically, the center of the lesion becomes pale and the outer edges are red. In most cases, the lesions last a few hours, and often disappear without treatment if the exposure to the offending agent is stopped. The hives may worsen in severity with each exposure to the allergen.

Treatment of Urticaria

Ideally, removal and avoidance of the offending allergen, thus preventing urticaria, is superior to treatment of hives. When hives do occur, symptomatic treatment is

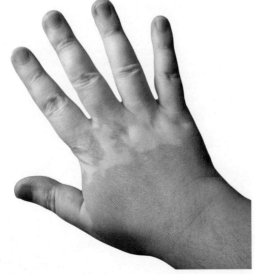

Vitiligo is characterized by irregular patches of discoloration.

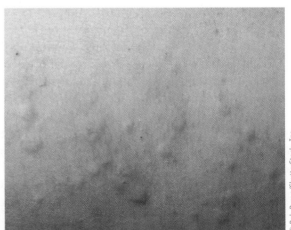

Hives appear as red, raised wheals on the skin.

aimed at relieving the discomfort and itching associated with the hives. Cold compresses may relieve the pain, and antihistamines and corticosteroids can relieve the itching and swelling.

Psoriasis

Psoriasis is a chronic inflammatory condition of the skin characterized by crusty papules that form patches with circular borders. The scales shed constantly and can cause embarrassment for the patient. The exact cause of psoriasis is unknown, but it is believed to be associated with an increased growth rate in the germinative layer of the skin.

Psoriasis is often a familial disease that first appears during puberty. The disease is not contagious and does not signify poor physical health. However, psoriasis can cause immense psychosocial and economic burden.

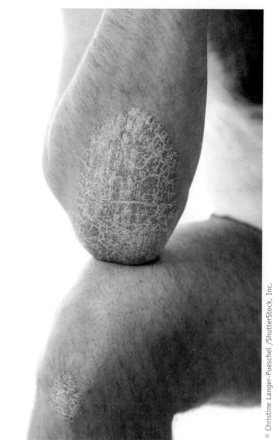

Psoriasis lesions are covered with thick, silvery scales.

Signs and Symptoms of Psoriasis

Psoriatic lesions are dark red and are covered with thick, silvery scales. The most common site for lesions are the elbows, palms of the hands, soles of the feet, and scalp. Psoriasis lesions are often localized, but may become generalized over large areas of the body. The lesions may result in disabilities and deformities that impair quality of life and impede normal functioning. Remissions and exacerbations of psoriasis are often unpredictable.

Treatment of Psoriasis

The goal of psoriasis treatment is to control or eliminate the signs and symptoms (scaling, itching, and inflammation) and prevent or minimize the likelihood of disease flares. Treatment for psoriasis is highly individualized. Many attempts of trial and error may be required before an effective treatment is discovered for a given patient.

An **emollient**, a softening and soothing cream, can be used to remove excess scales from the lesions. Tar-based compounds and salicylic acid products can be applied to soothe the lesions and decrease the rapid turnover of the epidermis. Topical corticosteroids can decrease swelling and discomfort associated with psoriasis. Biological agents that block the action of specific components of the immune system are relatively new options in the systemic treatment of psoriasis. These biological agents, which include etanercept (Enbrel), adalimumab (Humira), infliximab (Remicade), golimumab (Simponi), and ustekinumab (Stelara), are administered by IV injection or infusion. Lesions should be dressed with an occlusive dressing to prevent the lesion from drying out.

Bacterial Infections of the Skin

Bacterial infections can occur in the skin when there is a disruption in the integrity of the skin as a protective mechanism, occurring from improper wound healing or primary infectious disease. Some bacterial infections are mild, localized, and easily treatable, while others can progress to serious, systemic infections requiring antibiotic therapy.

Impetigo

Impetigo is a superficial infection of the skin. It is caused by the *Staphylococcus* or *Streptococcus* bacteria, which are present nearly everywhere and can live and thrive in almost any environment, and is highly contagious. It is common among children, the elderly, and individuals with poor hygiene. Impetigo is especially prevalent in warm, humid climates, which facilitate microbial colonization on the skin. Minor trauma or scrapes on the skin allow bacteria to enter the superficial layers of the skin.

Signs and Symptoms of Impetigo

Impetigo presents as small, red macules that become papules. The lesions often appear pale or clear in the center and have crusts on the outer border. Impetigo most commonly appears on the face, and the lesions are often pruritic. Rarely, weakness, fever, and diarrhea accompany impetigo.

Treatment of Impetigo

The goals of impetigo treatment are to relieve symptoms, prevent the formation of new lesions, and prevent complications, including an infection of the deeper layers of the skin. Though it may resolve spontaneously, antibiotic treatment is indicated for impetigo. Penicillins and cephalosporins are the preferred antibiotics for most cases of impetigo. Soaking the lesions in soap and warm water may provide symptomatic relief of the itching and discomfort. The lesions should not be covered while they are healing.

Cellulitis

Like impetigo, **cellulitis** is often caused by *Staphylococcus* or *Streptococcus* bacteria. Cellulitis initially infects the epidermis and dermis, but spreads rapidly through the other layers of skin and soft tissue. Cellulitis usually occurs following an injury, abrasion, ulcer, or surgery to the skin. It is a particularly dangerous infection, owing to its rapid spread and its propensity to spread to the lymphatic system and bloodstream, which can lead to serious or even fatal infections.

Cellulitis often appears in patients with compromised immune systems and/or poor nutrition, with resulting low blood pressure, dehydration, and altered mental status.

Signs and Symptoms of Cellulitis

Cellulitis produces localized redness, warmth, swelling, and pain. Fever, chills, and general malaise are also common. The lesions may be extensive; they are not elevated and have poorly defined margins.

Treatment of Cellulitis

The goal of treatment of cellulitis is to eradicate the infection as quickly as possible to prevent further complications. Antibiotics should be directed at the offending agent, based on either culture and sensitivity results or local susceptibility data. Penicillins, cephalosporins, or aminoglycosides are frequently used to treat cellulitis.

Elevation and immobilization of the affected area decrease swelling, and cool, sterile saline dressings help to localize the infection. Surgical incision and draining of the lesion is indicated in complicated cellulitis.

Folliculitis, Furuncles, and Carbuncles

Folliculitis is an inflammation of the hair follicle. Most cases of folliculitis occur after abrasions or injuries to the skin, such as friction from clothing, blockage of the follicle, or shaving. If bacteria (usually *Staphylococcus* or *Streptococcus*) enter the damaged follicle, an infection can occur.

Signs and Symptoms of Folliculitis, Furuncles, and Carbuncles

Folliculitis produces a red nodule at the base of the hair follicle that is not usually associated with pain. Folliculitis commonly occurs on the neck, in the groin, and in the genital area.

A **furuncle**, also known as a boil, is an infection of the hair follicle, sebaceous gland, and surrounding tissue. Furuncles usually appear in areas of the skin that are subject to friction or perspiration. The furuncle is usually pea-sized with a white or yellow pustule at its center. A furuncle signifies a deeper and more widespread infection than folliculitis. Furuncles cause itching, swelling, and redness accompanied by local pain and pus formation. Fatigue and fever may occur.

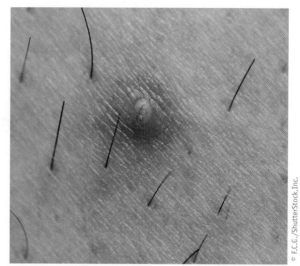

Furuncles are small pustules accompanied by redness and swelling.

A **carbuncle** is a group of infected hair follicles. They are broad, swollen, and deep follicular masses. They commonly occur on the back of the neck. Carbuncles signify a deeper and more widespread infection than a furuncle. Pain, redness, swelling, and tenderness are common symptoms of a carbuncle; drainage, fever, and systemic toxicity are possible. Spread of the infection into the bloodstream is common.

Treatment of Folliculitis, Furuncles, and Carbuncles

Mild folliculitis resolves on its own in most healthy individuals. Hot, moist compresses may help promote drainage of furuncles or carbuncles. In some cases, furuncle lesions drain and resolve spontaneously. Topical or systemic antibiotics or antifungal agents may be necessary to control the spread of the infection. Surgical incision and drainage of the furuncle or carbuncle may be necessary if it does not resolve on its own.

Viral Infections of the Skin

Like bacterial infections of the skin, viral infections of the skin occur when the integrity of the skin as a protective barrier is compromised due to injury or trauma to the skin or a compromised immune system. Warts and cold sores are the most common skin disorders caused by viruses.

Herpes Simplex

The **herpes simplex virus** is an infectious organism that can infect the skin and nervous system. Two types of herpes simplex viruses infect humans. Cold sores or fever blisters are caused by the herpes simplex virus 1 (HSV1). Most people are infected with HSV1 but rarely develop signs or symptoms of infection. An outbreak of the virus is triggered by stress, hormonal changes, environmental factors, illness, or sun exposure.

Another member of the herpes simplex virus family, HSV2, causes genital warts and is spread primarily through sexual contact. Both HSV1 and HSV2 are highly contagious and are spread from sharing personal items or from contact with the infected area during an outbreak.

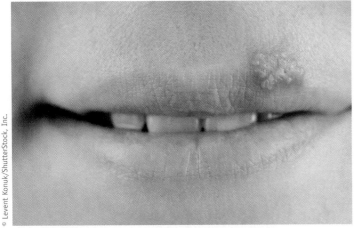

Cold sores are caused by the herpes simplex virus 1.

Signs and Symptoms of Herpes Simplex Virus

The lips and genitals are the most common sites of herpes lesions, but they may occur anywhere on the body. The lesions may be mild and cause little to no pain, or they may appear in severe outbreaks accompanied by fever and pain.

An itching, burning, or tingling sensation will often precede the outbreak of the herpes lesions. The lesion is a red macule that becomes a vesicle or a cluster of small vesicles.

Treatment of Herpes Simplex Virus

The goal of herpes simplex virus treatment is to relieve pain, reduce the redness and swelling of the lesion, and dry the vesicle. Herpes simplex virus is usually self-limiting and lesions will resolve in one to two weeks without treatment. Oral antiviral medications are available to prevent recurrent or severe outbreaks of herpes lesions. Topical antiviral agents are also available to treat cold sores.

Blindness may occur in infants born vaginally to women with an active herpes simplex infection of the genitalia.

Herpes Zoster (Shingles)

Herpes zoster, or **shingles**, occurs in adults and is caused by the varicella-zoster virus—the virus that causes chicken pox in children. After a chicken pox infection, the virus remains dormant in the body for many decades. Shingles is the result of the reactivation of the virus. The cause of the renewed activity is not known. Shingles does not normally occur more than once. Individuals over the age of 60 and those with compromised immune systems are most at risk for developing shingles.

If an adult or child has direct contact with the herpes zoster rash of shingles and has not had chicken pox or the varicella vaccine, he or she will develop chicken pox, not shingles.

Signs and Symptoms of Herpes Zoster

Shingles presents as a painful red rash characterized by groups of red papules or vesicles. The rash usually appears in a line or trailing pattern on the skin, generally following the distribution of a nerve or group of nerves. Pain often precedes the rash, and itching accompanies the lesions.

Treatment of Herpes Zoster

The goal of herpes zoster treatment is to relieve pain. Oral analgesics and cool compresses can alleviate the pain and itching associated with shingles. Lotions can be used to prevent the lesions from becoming too dry.

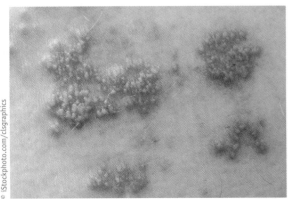

Shingles lesions on the torso.

In cases of severe pain, nerve-blocking agents are necessary to treat patients. Steroid injections to decrease inflammation or systemic antiviral agents can be administered to alleviate the symptoms of severe rashes.

Patients with an active shingles rash should avoid clothing that can cause friction or irritate the rash. They should also avoid dressing too warmly, as this can intensify the itching.

Postherpetic neuralgia is a painful condition that remains after resolution of the herpes zoster rash. The pain may persist for years and is difficult to treat.

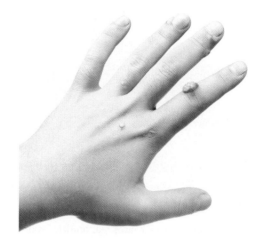

Warts commonly appear on the hand.

Verrucae (Warts)

Verrucae, more commonly known as **warts**, are common viral infections of the skin and mucous membranes. Warts occur when **human papillomavirus (HPV)** enters the skin through an abrasion or injury. Not everyone is susceptible to infection with HPV, which is why some people have warts and others do not. Warts may be spread from one part of the body to another, or from person to person, though the latter is rare.

Warts are not usually permanent, and many self-resolve within a few months. Most warts resolve within five years. Warts are not harmful, but are cosmetically unappealing and embarrassing.

Signs and Symptoms of Verrucae

Warts are small, rough growths on the skin. They are slightly scaly, rough patches of papules or nodules on the dermis with a characteristic cauliflower-like appearance. Warts are usually painless. They can appear on any skin surface, but most often appear on the hands.

Warts begin as small, smooth discolorations and change in appearance and size over time due to repeated irritation. Warts may itch or hurt, depending on their location.

Treatment of Verrucae

The goal of the treatment of warts is to remove the wart and prevent the spread of the infection. Warts require no treatment if they are unobtrusive and without pain. However, warts that are painful or irritating can be removed surgically or by freezing with liquid nitrogen. Small warts can be removed with products containing salicylic acid.

Fungal Infections of the Skin

Fungal infections are among the most common skin disorders. Superficial infections of the skin are called **dermatophytoses** and are caused by organisms that digest keratin in skin and hair. Fungal infections are highly contagious and very common, affecting nearly all children and adults at some point in their lives.

Fungal infections of the skin and mucous membranes can occur in association with compromised immune systems, steroid medications, long-term antibiotic use, and being very young or very old. Although some fungal infections may be mild and patients may be nonsymptomatic, treatment is essential to prevent the progression of the infection to more extensive or systemic disease.

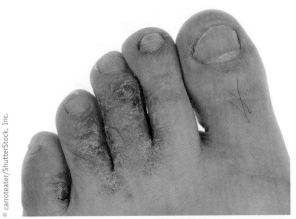

Tinea pedis, or "athlete's foot," causes red, pruritic lesions and fissures in the skin.

© carroteater/ShutterStock, Inc.

Tinea

Tinea refers to the collection of superficial fungal infections. Tinea infections infect nearly one-quarter of the United States population at any time. Brief exposure to the pathogen can lead to an infection; broken or damaged skin increases the likelihood of an infection.

Tinea infections are named for the area of the body that they affect: **tinea pedis** (feet), **tinea manuum** (palm of the hand), **tinea cruris** (thighs and buttocks), **tinea corporis** (trunk and extremities), **tinea capitis** (head), **tinea barbae** (beard and mustache), and **tinea unguium** (nails). Tinea infections are caused by one of three fungi: *Trichophyton*, *Epidermophyton*, or *Microsporum*.

Tinea pedis is commonly known as "athlete's foot."

Tinea cruris is commonly known as "jock itch."

Signs and Symptoms of Tinea

Each type of tinea has a characteristic presentation, but, generally, tinea lesions are pruritic and red and change the texture of the affected skin. The center of the lesion is often clear and the border is red, scaly, and elevated, thus also called "ringworm."

Treatment of Tinea

The goal of treatment of tinea infections is to provide symptom relief, cure the existing infection, and prevent future infections. The infected area should be kept clean and dry and exposure to the infected reservoir should be limited. Topical antifungal agents are the preferred treatment for most tinea infections and are available without a prescription for self-treatment. Oral antifungal medications are necessary for severe or extensive infections and when treating tinea capitis and tinea unguium.

Candidiasis

Candidiasis is a common fungal infection and can occur anywhere on the body, but primarily in warm, moist places such as underarms and folds of skin. When candidiasis occurs in the mouth, it is known as **thrush**; it can also occur in the vagina. It is caused by the fungus *Candida albicans* and can occur after the prolonged use of antibiotics or steroids or from wearing dentures, medication-induced dry mouth, smoking, malignancies, or nutritional deficiencies.

Signs and Symptoms of Candidiasis

Oral candidiasis appears as soft, yellowish-white plaques on top of red areas of the skin or mucous membrane. The lesions may be painful and sensitive and may lead to ulcers or fissures in the corners of the mouth.

Candidiasis of the vagina involves intense itching, soreness, irritation, and burning of the vulva and vagina. Redness, fissuring, edema, and a thick yellowish-white discharge are common signs of a fungal infection.

The name "ringworm" is a misnomer, as the tinea infection is caused by a fungus, not a worm. The name is derived from the red rings that look like worms under the surface of the skin.

© auremar/ShutterStock, Inc.

Treatment of Candidiasis

The goal of candidiasis treatment, regardless of the location of the infection, is to cure the infection and rid the body of signs and symptoms of infection. Topical treatment is effective for most *Candida* infections. Nystatin is frequently prescribed as a mouth rinse for oral candidiasis; topical creams and oral antifungal products are available for vaginal candidiasis.

Parasitic Infections of the Skin

External parasites can live on the outside of the body, often invading the hair and surface of the skin. External parasites are sometimes associated with poor hygiene and infections are transmitted by social and sexual contact.

Scabies

Scabies is a skin infection caused by the itch mite, *Sarcoptes scabiei*. Scabies can affect both humans and animals. Scabies infections usually occur in warm places of the body: between the fingers, the underside of the knee, the underarm, the umbilicus, and the scrotum.

In animals, mange is caused by the itch mite—the parasite responsible for scabies.
© auremar/ShutterStock, Inc.

Signs and Symptoms of Scabies

The incubation period of scabies is four to six weeks. During this time, the patient may complain of itching and an inability to sleep due to intense itching, as well as excoriations of the skin, which may lead to secondary bacterial infections. The mites may be seen under the skin as burrows or tracks, but these may be masked by the patient's self-inflicted scratching.

Only the female itch mite invades the skin.

Treatment of Scabies

The goal of scabies therapy is to eradicate the infection as quickly as possible and provide symptom relief. The entire body should be scrubbed thoroughly with soap and warm water using a soft brush to remove the mites. A permethrin lotion is then applied to the whole body (except the face, mucous membranes, and eyes) and the lotion is left in place for 8–14 hours. Anyone who has had close contact with the infected person should also be checked and treated for infection, even if no symptoms are present. Topical corticosteroids and antihistamines can be used to decrease the itching associated with scabies.

The patient may continue to have symptoms for several weeks after treatment. This is normal and does not mean that mites are still alive.

Pediculosis

Each year, an estimated 6–12 million people in the United States become infected with **pediculosis**, more commonly known as **lice**. Pediculosis may be caused by *Pediculus humanus capitis* (head lice), *Pediculus humanus corporis* (body louse), or *Phthirus pubis* (pubic or crab lice).

Lice are wingless insects with well-developed legs. They are 2–4mm in length. The female lice lay eggs, called nits, on the hair shaft of humans. They use the human as a host and receive nourishment from human blood. Lice are spread by direct contact with an infected individual or his or her belongings. Lice usually do not spread disease, but cause intense itching and discomfort. Abrasions caused by the lice or self-inflicted itching increases the risk for secondary bacterial infections.

Signs and Symptoms of Pediculosis

Intense itching of the infected body part is the hallmark symptom of pediculosis. The saliva of the louse causes the itching. In severe infections, a patient may have small, red macules and papules from the lice bites. Pediculosis can be confirmed by visual identification of the nits on the hair.

Treatment of Pediculosis

The goal of pediculosis treatment is to remove the adult lice and nits from the infected host. Nits cannot be removed easily; they are glued firmly to the hair shaft. A pediculicide, pyrethrum and piperonyl butoxide or permethrin, must be applied to the affected area, followed by combing or cleaning to remove the dead lice and eggs. The treatment should be repeated after 7–10 days to destroy any newly hatched lice.

Future and repeat infestations can be avoided by thoroughly washing all clothing, bedding, linens, and objects with which the infected person came in contact.

Tumors of the Skin

A **nevus** is a chronic, sharply demarcated lesion of the skin. Nevi are commonly called birthmarks or moles. Nevi vary in size, shape, elevation, and appearance, but most are harmless. Large nevi that are present at birth and nevi located at the junction of the dermis and epidermis are the most likely to undergo malignant or cancerous changes.

Frequent self-checks of the skin for new or changing nevi is an important early-detection tool for all types of skin cancer. Once skin cancer is diagnosed, it must be treated by an oncologist or dermatologist.

The ABCs of Skin Cancer

An easy-to-remember mnemonic can be helpful for patients to complete self-checks for skin cancer detection:

- **A is for asymmetry**—A skin-cancer lesion will vary in size, shape, and color. A benign mole is usually symmetrical and uniform.
- **B is for border**—The edges of a cancerous lesion will be blurry and uneven.
- **C is for color**—Cancerous lesions do not have a uniform or consistent color throughout the lesion.
- **D is for diameter**—Most melanomas are at least ¼ inch in diameter—roughly the size of a pencil eraser.
- **E is for evolving**—Cancerous lesions change over time. Patients may notice changes in the size, color, shape, or elevation of nevi, or the onset of bleeding, crusting, or itching.

Malignant Melanoma

Melanoma is a highly malignant cancer. Melanoma usually begins as a harmless junctional nevus, at the border between the epidermis and the dermis. Pigmented nevi of the palms of the hands, soles of the feet, and mucous membranes are nearly always junctional nevi and should be monitored carefully for signs and symptoms of a malignancy. Moles in areas of constant irritation are also at risk for malignant changes and can be removed prophylactically.

Malignant melanoma, which is capable of invading adjacent tissues and can be life threatening, has a hereditary component, as the disease tends to appear in families. Excessive or repeat sunburns are also a risk factor for the development of melanoma. Fair-skinned individuals and those with red or blond hair and blue, green, or gray eyes are at increased risk for melanoma.

Melanoma can be treated with a combination of surgery, immunotherapy, and chemotherapy. It is an aggressive form of cancer and is the leading cause of death from skin cancer.

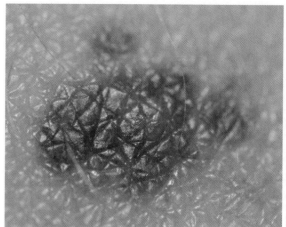

Melanoma on human skin.

© D. Kucharski & K. Kucharska/ShutterStock, Inc.

Basal Cell Carcinoma

Basal cell carcinoma (BCC) is a cancerous skin lesion that rarely metastasizes or spreads to other parts of the body to form new tumors. It is the most common type of skin cancer. It is particularly common in Caucasians because the major predisposing factor to BCC is fair skin. It is also frequent in males over the age of 50 whose occupation or leisure activities allowed prolonged exposure to UV light from the sun.

BCC lesions appear as red, scaly patches. The lesions may have a slightly depressed center and a raised, rolled border. Nearly all BCCs occur on the face, between the hairline and the lip. BCC is almost always curable with surgical excision or radiation therapy.

Squamous Cell Carcinoma

Squamous cell carcinoma (SCC) is the second most common type of skin cancer. SCC is a tumor of the epidermis that can occur anywhere in the body. It exhibits rapid growth and local invasion, and it has the ability to metastasize via the lymphatic and blood systems. Like BCC, repeat and excessive sun exposure is a risk factor for SCC. Actinic keratosis is a precancerous lesion caused by sun exposure that can lead to SCC.

SCC appears as a slightly raised, red, thickened macule or papule. SCC can often be treated effectively with prompt surgical excision and radiation therapy. SCC is rarely fatal but can decrease quality of life, impair daily functioning, and impose social and economic burdens.

Seborrheic Keratosis

Seborrheic keratosis is a benign skin tumor. Its cause is unknown, but it tends to run in families and most commonly appears after the age of 40 years. The lesions vary in appearance, size, and color, but are often rough and wartlike in appearance and can appear anywhere on the body. They are painless, though some may itch. They are harmless, but may cause cosmetic discomfort. If desired, lesions can be removed with products used for removing warts.

Trauma of the Skin

The skin is vulnerable to injury and trauma. Maintaining strong, healthy skin is essential to preventing secondary infections and fluid loss. The skin is only an effective barrier if it is intact.

Lacerations

A **laceration** is a cut, tear, or puncture in the skin. Lacerations can be small or large and can involve only superficial layers of the skin or multiple layers of skin and soft tissue. Depending on the extent of the trauma that caused the laceration, the injury to the skin may be accompanied by damage to underlying tissues such as muscles, nerves, tendons, or blood vessels.

Signs and Symptoms of Lacerations

Lacerations are characterized by broken skin and bleeding. Lacerations usually present with pain, as well as a loss of function or feeling in the area surrounding the injury.

Treatment of Lacerations

Treatment of lacerations begins with cleaning the wound and surrounding skin with an antiseptic cleanser. Irrigation of the wound with sterile water or saline may be necessary to remove debris or foreign bodies from the wound.

Small, superficial lacerations may be simply treated with an adhesive bandage to hold the edges of the laceration together. Deeper lacerations that involve several layers of skin require sutures to hold the skin together.

The laceration is usually covered with a sterile dressing to protect it from dirt. The wound should be monitored for signs of secondary infection: swelling, redness, fever, or pus. Antibiotic ointments may be used to relieve signs and symptoms of an infection.

Complications of Lacerations

The overall health of the patient dictates the healing process of a laceration. Systemic illnesses, poor circulation, and compromised immune systems place patients at risk for slow healing and increased chance of infection. A secondary infection resulting from a wound in the skin is the primary complication associated with lacerations.

Burns

Burns are one of the most serious traumas affecting the skin. A burn may result from exposure to fire, electricity, UV radiation, hot liquids, hot objects, or chemicals. The seriousness of a burn is determined by the amount of body-surface affected by the burn, as well as the depth of the burn or the number of skin layers or structures involved.

Commonly, healthcare workers use the **rule of nines** to estimate the amount of body-surface area affected by a burn. As illustrated in **FIGURE 8.4**, the body is divided into 11 sections, with each section accounting for 9 percent of total body-surface area. The genitals account for the remaining 1 percent.

Generally, if more than 2 percent of the body surface area is affected by a second-degree burn, medical attention is required. For burns affecting smaller areas, self-treatment may be indicated.

A mild burn can cause redness and discomfort to the outer layers of skin. A more serious burn can destroy all layers of skin and underlying body tissues. Burns are classified into three categories:

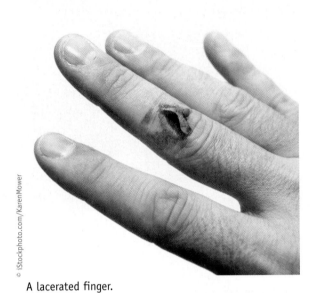

A lacerated finger.
© iStockphoto.com/KarenMower

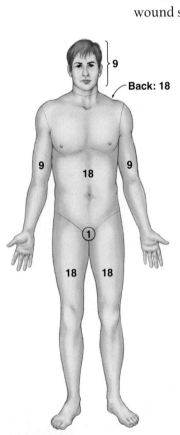

FIGURE 8.4 The "rule of nines" is used to estimate body-surface area affected by a burn.
© Jones & Bartlett Learning

- A **first-degree burn** involves the superficial layers of skin or the outer layers of the epidermis. They are the least serious and least damaging type of burn. The sun is the most common cause of first-degree burns. Generally, there is no scarring after a first-degree burn.

A suntan is the result of a gradual deposit of melanin in the skin, which protects skin from damage caused by UV rays.
© auremar/ShutterStock, Inc.

- A **second-degree burn** extends through the epidermis and into the dermis, causing blisters to form. Scarring may occur after a second-degree burn.

- A **third-degree burn** extends through all three layers of skin and into the underlying tissues. Infection and fluid loss are major complications of third-degree burns. Scarring will occur after a third-degree burn.

Signs and Symptoms of Burns

First-degree burns may cause only redness, minor swelling, and discomfort. The redness that appears as a result of a burn is the body's attempt to increase circulation to the damaged skin by dilating blood vessels. This increased circulation stimulates the melanocytes to produce melanin, which, in turn, protects the skin from further damage.

The blisters produced in response to a second-degree burn are a protective mechanism that adds an insulating layer of water between the epidermis and the dermis. The blisters of a second-degree burn should never be broken. If one breaks accidentally, care should be taken to keep the area clean because it is vulnerable to infection. Large blisters that break place a patient at risk for fluid and protein loss.

Third-degree burns often result in a charring of the skin. Such burns require hospitalization and careful monitoring to protect from infection and fluid and nutrient loss. Skin grafts and physical therapy are often required after third-degree burns to prevent loss of motion due to scarring.

Treatment of Burns

Each type of burn is treated differently, but the primary goal of treatment is to relieve pain and prevent infection. Superficial first-degree burns are not likely to become infected. In these cases, only pain relief is required. Cold compresses, skin protectants, external anesthetics, topical corticosteroids, and oral analgesics usually provide satisfactory pain relief. Dressings may be applied to first-degree burns for comfort of the patient, but physical protection to guard from infection is usually not required.

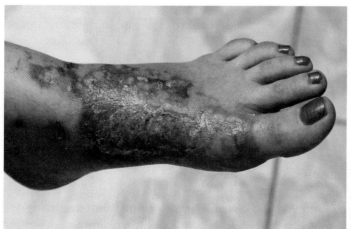

© OlegD/ShutterStock, Inc.

Second-degree burns are characterized by the formation of blisters.

Topical Pain Relief for the Treatment of Minor Burns

Local anesthetics
  Benzocaine 5–20%
  Dibucaine 0.25–1%
  Lidocaine 0.5–4%
  Tetracaine 1–2%

Counterirritants
  Camphor 0.1–3%
  Menthol 0.1–1%
  Phenol 0.5–1.5%

Antihistamines
  Diphenhydramine hydrochloride 1–2%
  Tripelennamine 0.5–2%

Corticosteroids
  Hydrocortisone 0.25–0.5%

If blisters have formed or if the surface of the skin is exuding a discharge of any kind, the skin is prone to infection. Dressings and skin protectants should be applied to prevent infection and promote healing. Counterirritants should not be applied to wounds that are blistered or weeping.

Skin Protectants for Use in Treating Minor Burns
  Allantoin 0.5–2%
  Cocoa butter 50–100%
  Petrolatum 30–100%
  Zinc oxide 10–40%

Complications of Burns

Burns to the eyes or ears should be promptly referred to a specialist, as damage to these structures may result in permanent loss of function. Facial burns may be associated with respiratory injuries. Burns over joint areas may result in loss of range of motion due to the formation of scar tissue. Individuals with compromised immune systems or those who are otherwise at risk for infection can develop serious infections as a result of burn injuries.

Repeat sunburns are a risk for melanoma. Excessive exposure to the sun can also cause damage to the eyes and premature aging of the skin.

Skills for the Medical Assistant

The medical assistant will have the opportunity to assist the physician with minor surgical procedures, which requires an understanding of sterile or aseptic technique. **Asepsis**, or being **sterile**, means that all instruments, surfaces, and environments are free from all infection-causing microorganisms.

Special techniques are used to ensure a sterile environment, including preparing yourself to handle sterile equipment and assembling, cleaning, and sterilizing the supplies needed for minor procedures or surgeries. You will learn and practice these skills here.

Rules to Protect a Sterile Area

- A sterile object may not touch a nonsterile object.

- Sterile objects must not be wet. Moisture can draw microorganisms into or onto the sterile object.

- An acceptable border between a sterile area and a nonsterile area is one inch. The portion of a drape that hangs over the edge is considered nonsterile, no matter what its size. Sterile articles should be placed in the center of the sterile field and away from the edge as much as possible.

- Do not turn your back on a sterile field. If you cannot see the field, you cannot be aware of what touched it.

- Anything below the waist is considered contaminated. Therefore, all surgery trays should be positioned above the waist. All articles are to be held above the waist.

- All sterile objects, including gloved hands, must be held in front of and away from the body and above waist level.

- Do not cough, sneeze, or talk over a sterile field. Airborne particles may fall onto a sterile area and contaminate it.

- Do not reach over a sterile area. Contaminants may fall onto the area or clothing may touch it, thereby contaminating the area. Spend as little time as possible reaching into the sterile area.

- Do not pass contaminated dressings or instruments into the sterile field. Arrange for the provider to place contaminated dressings or instruments into a separate container or area.

- Always be aware of your own and other people's actions to determine whether the sterile field has been contaminated. When in doubt, err on the side of safety.

- When opening sterile packages, the outer wrapper is considered contaminated. It should be opened without touching the inner contents, and the contents are then dropped into the sterile field. Double wrapping can be used to maintain sterility.

- Sterile solutions in bottles should be poured into sterile basins or cups on the sterile field without touching the rim of the bottle and without splashing solution onto the sterile field.

© auremar/ShutterStock, Inc.

Surgical Instruments

A typical soft tissue tray contains some or all of the following instruments. See FIGURE 8.5 for illustrations of common surgical instruments.

- **Scalpel handle and blade**—A small, sharp instrument used for incisions and surgical procedures

- **Scissors**—Used for cutting bandages or sutures and during surgical procedures; may have blunt/blunt, blunt/sharp, or sharp/sharp blades, depending on the intended use

- **Hemostats**—A clamp used to control bleeding during surgical procedures

- **A needle holder**—An instrument used to hold the needle for suturing

- **Gauze sponges or pads**—Disposable pads used for wound care and cleaning

- **A drape**—A disposable or nondisposable sheet or towel placed over a sterile field or around a surgical site to prevent contamination and maintain sterility

- **Cotton balls**—Used for cleaning and wound care
- **Sponge forceps**—An instrument for grasping surgical sponges and handling sterile dressings
- **Toothed forceps**—An instrument used for holding tissues; teeth on the tip of forceps grasp better than smooth forceps
- **Smooth forceps**—An instrument used for holding and tying sutures
- **Suture material**—A thread attached to a needle that is used to join edges of a wound back together

Aseptic Hand Washing

Aseptic technique and surgical asepsis require proper hand washing. Hand washing is the simplest and most effective way to reduce the transmission of pathogens. Aseptic hand washing is essential to working in a sterile field. Aseptic hand washing is more vigorous and comprehensive than basic hand washing, but the goal is the same: to eliminate disease-causing microorganisms from the skin and reduce the risk of contamination by touch, the most common source of contamination.

Aseptic hand washing procedures remove contamination from the fingertips to the elbows. A minimum of 30 seconds is required to complete proper aseptic hand washing procedures, but a thorough cleansing requires several minutes. For the first hand washing of the day prior to sterile preparation, it is recommended to wash hands from the tips of the fingers up to the elbows for 2–4 minutes. The hands should be the cleanest part of the entire body.

In this exercise, you will learn how to complete aseptic hand washing.

Equipment Needed

- Sink suitable for aseptic hand washing
- Sterile surgical scrub sponge/brush containing antimicrobial solution
- Aseptic, lint-free paper towels

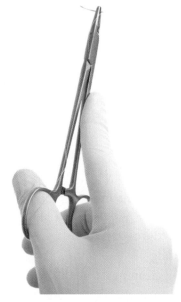

A needle holder is used to hold a needle for suturing.

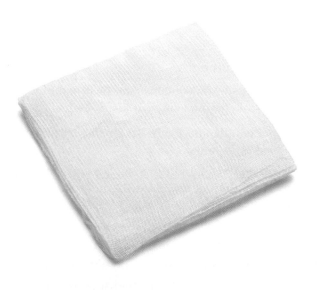

Use gauze pads for wound care and cleaning.

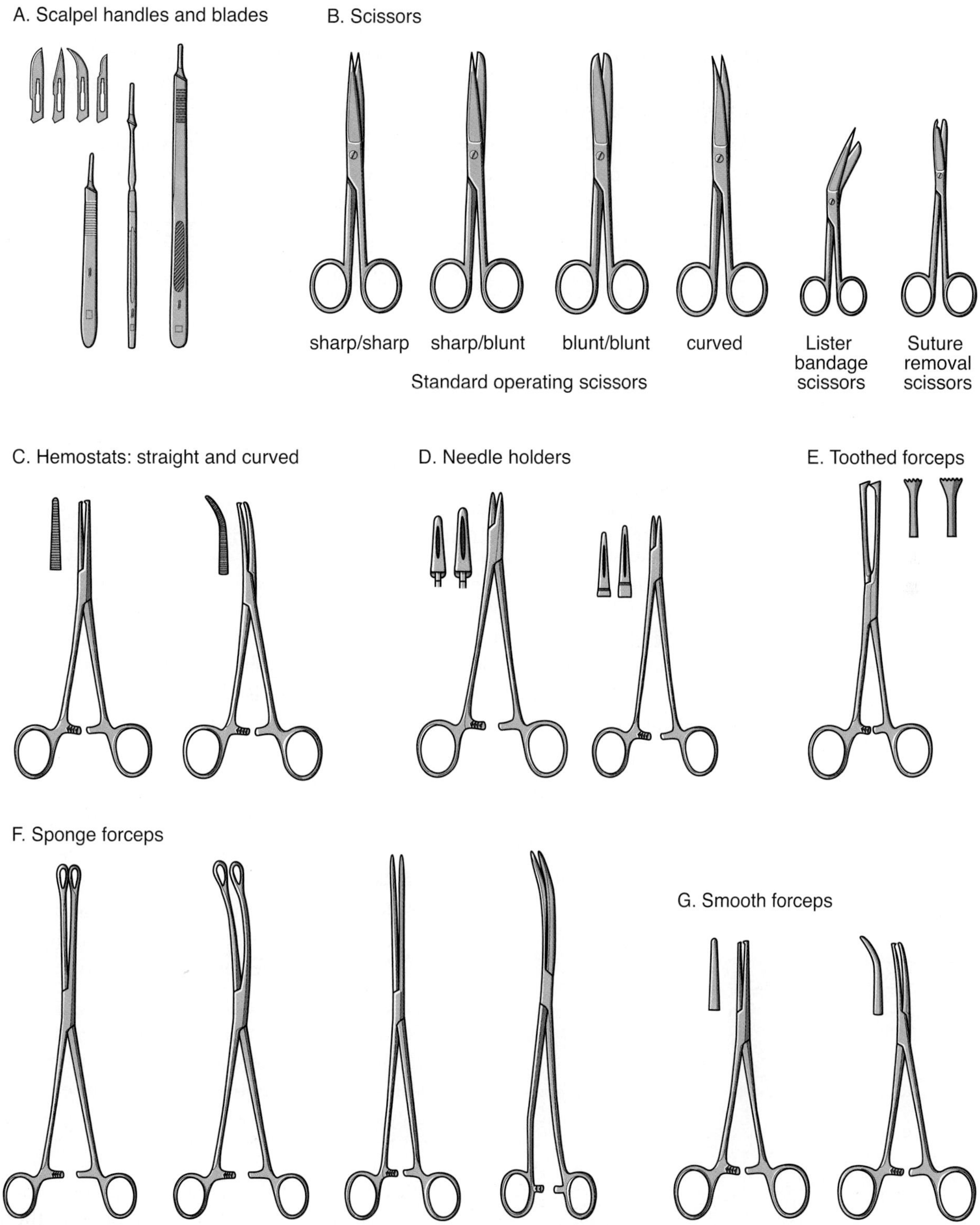

A. Scalpel handles and blades

B. Scissors

sharp/sharp   sharp/blunt   blunt/blunt   curved   Lister bandage scissors   Suture removal scissors

Standard operating scissors

C. Hemostats: straight and curved

D. Needle holders

E. Toothed forceps

F. Sponge forceps

G. Smooth forceps

FIGURE 8.5 Surgical instruments come in many different types and shapes.

© Jones & Bartlett Learning

Steps

1. Remove all jewelry from the hands and arms. Nail polish and artificial nails should not be worn in a sterile field. Roll up sleeves if necessary, exposing bare arms up to the elbows.

2. Squeeze the prepackaged surgical sponge inside the package to activate the soap. Open the package and discard the wrapper. Do not set the sponge down.

If you inadvertently drop the sponge or place it in the sink or on the counter, it must be discarded and you must begin the process of aseptic hand washing again.

---

3. Turn on the water and let it run until warm. Wet your hands and forearms. Use the nail pick provided with the sponge to clean under your fingernails. Discard the pick.

4. Wet the sponge and squeeze it several times until a rich, soapy lather appears.

If the sink you are using has foot-pedal controls, you may turn the water off after step 4. If the sink has hand controls, let the water run during the entire hand washing procedure.

---

5. Use the brush side of the sponge to clean under the thumbnail of the first hand **FIGURE 8.6**. When the thumbnail is clean, proceed to the index finger on the same hand, and scrub under its nail with the brush. Continue to remaining fingers, moving from thumb to pinky, until each nail is clean.

6. Switch to the opposite hand and clean under the nails with the scrub brush, beginning with the thumbnail.

7. Use the sponge to clean the fingers on the first hand. To begin, scrub the top, bottom, and two sides of the thumb. Clean the webbing between the thumb and index finger. Proceed to clean each finger and webbing in turn, taking care to scrub all sides of each finger **FIGURE 8.7**.

8. Repeat step 7 on the opposite hand, cleaning all the fingers and webbing. Move from the thumb to the pinky.

Do not use the brush to clean the skin. This may cause damage to the skin or cause contaminated skin to flake off into the clean environment. Use only the sponge to clean the skin.

---

9. Use the sponge to wash the palm of the first hand. When the entire palm of the first hand is clean, clean the palm on the opposite hand.

10. Use the sponge to wash the back of the first hand. Repeat on opposite hand.

11. Use the sponge to clean the forearm of the first hand. Begin at the wrist and clean in a circular pattern around the

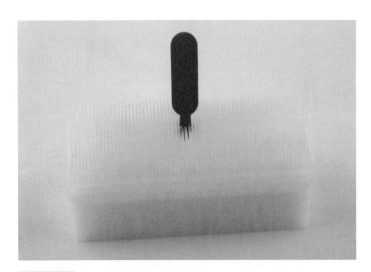

FIGURE 8.6 A disposable surgical scrub brush has a sponge on one side and a brush on the other. A nail pick is included to clean underneath the fingernails.
© Henry Adams/Fotolia

forearm, winding toward the elbow. Stop cleansing at the elbow. Repeat this pattern on the opposite hand.

> Because aseptic hand washing is designed to move contamination down the arm, from the fingers to the elbow, the fingers must always remain pointed up during hand washing and rinsing.

12. Throw the sponge away.

13. If the water is not on, turn it on with the foot pedals and let it run until warm. Rinse the hand and forearm of the first arm. Begin rinsing at the fingers, keeping the fingers pointed up through the entire rinse. The water should run down your elbow into the sink FIGURE 8.8.

14. Repeat the rinsing process on the opposite hand. If the sink has foot pedals, turn off the water. If the sink has hand controls, continue to let the water run.

15. Use aseptic, lint-free towels to dry your hands. Discard the towels. Use new aseptic, lint-free towels to dry your forearms. Discard the towels.

16. If the sink has hand controls, use a new, aseptic lint-free towel to grab the handle of the faucet and turn off the water. Discard the towel.

> Do not apply lotion or any other materials to your hands after completing aseptic hand washing procedures. This results in contamination.

Applying Sterile Gloves

Hand washing cannot eliminate all infectious organisms, so hands must be covered with sterile gloves during surgical procedures. Gloves are made of latex or vinyl, and both offer equal levels of protection. Gloves are disposable and are worn only once. In this exercise, you will learn how to apply sterile gloves while maintaining sterility.

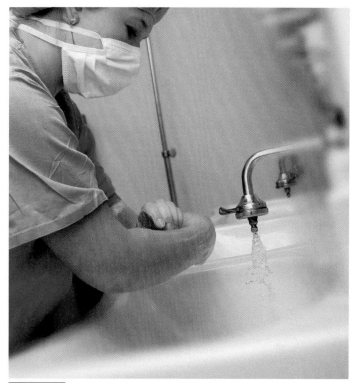

FIGURE 8.7 Wash all sides of each finger and the webbing between fingers.
© Digital Vision/Thinkstock

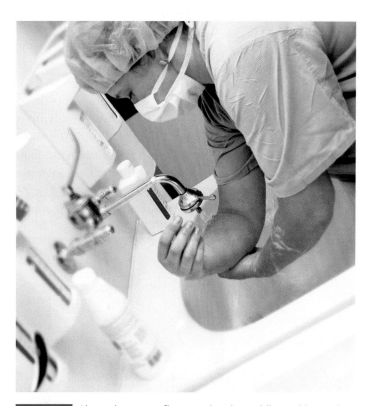

FIGURE 8.8 Always keep your fingers pointed up while washing and rinsing your hands to allow contamination to run down your arm, off your elbow, and into the sink.
© Photodisc/Thinkstock

Equipment Needed

- One pair of sterile gloves

Steps

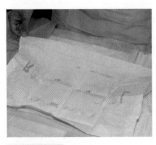

FIGURE 8.9 Carefully open the inner wrapper of the gloves.
© Jones & Bartlett Learning

1. Remove all rings, watches, and other jewelry from the hands and wrists. Wash hands using aseptic technique. Alternatively, sanitize hands with foamed alcohol sanitizer. Wash or sanitize the entire surface of the hand, including the palm of the hand, each finger, the backs of the hand, and the wrist. Dry hands using aseptic technique.
2. Inspect glove package for tears or stains, which indicate that the gloves are no longer sterile.
3. Place the package of gloves on a clean, dry, sterile surface.
4. Open the outer wrapper of the gloves, taking care not to touch the inner package. Carefully peel open the inner package. Take care not to touch the inside of the packaging or the gloves. The gloves should be opened with the cuffs toward you, palms up, and thumbs pointing outward **FIGURE 8.9**.

Sterile gloves are packaged to ease their application and decrease the need to handle or touch them.

---

5. With the index finger and thumb of your nondominant hand, grasp the inner cuffed edge of the opposite glove. Pick the glove straight up without dangling or dragging it off the package surface **FIGURE 8.10**.
6. With the palm of the dominant hand facing up, slide the glove onto the dominant hand. Do not allow the outside of the glove to come in contact with any surface or object. Hold the hands up and away from the body while applying gloves.
7. Pick up the remaining glove by sliding the four gloved fingers of your dominant hand under the outside of the cuff. This surface is sterile and may only be touched by another sterile object. Lift up the glove and keep it away from the body and other nonsterile surfaces **FIGURE 8.11**.
8. With the palm of the hand facing up, pull glove onto hand. Do not allow a sterile surface to touch a nonsterile one.
9. Adjust gloves as needed, but do not touch the wrist area. Hold gloved hands up and away from your body so you do not touch any nonsterile surfaces **FIGURE 8.12**.

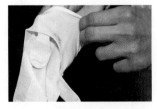

FIGURE 8.10 When applying the first glove, do not touch any part of the glove with the opposite hand, except the inner cuff.
© Jones & Bartlett Learning

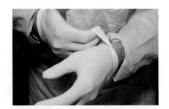

FIGURE 8.11 When applying the second glove, place fingers of the first gloved hand under the outside cuff.
© Jones & Bartlett Learning

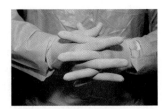

FIGURE 8.12 Adjust gloves as needed, but do not touch any nonsterile surfaces.
© Jones & Bartlett Learning

Preparing a Sterile Field

Disposable sterile field drapes or towels isolate and cover a sterile area. Many types of drapes and towels are available, and their use is determined by office or physician preference and economic considerations. For example, a **fenestrated drape** is a drape with a slitlike opening in the middle. In this exercise, you will learn how to set up and cover a sterile field for a minor surgical or office procedure.

> *If a patient is allergic to latex, do not wear latex gloves when preparing for or assisting in a surgical procedure. In this case, you should wear vinyl gloves.*
> © auremar/ShutterStock, Inc.

Equipment Needed

- Two disposable sterile field drapes or towels
- Mayo instrument stand/tray
- Sterile transfer forceps

Steps

1. Wash hands using aseptic technique.
2. Sanitize and disinfect the instrument tray.
3. Select a disposable drape and place it on a clean, dry, flat surface. Peel open the package to expose the fan-folded drape. Adjust the package so the cut corners of the drape are facing you. Alternatively, select a sterile cloth towel from a storage canister using transfer forceps.
4. With the thumb and index finger of one hand, grasp the top cut corner of the drape or towel, taking care not to touch the rest of the drape. Hold the drape high enough so it does not touch any other surface as you are lifting it out of the package and unfolding it **FIGURE 8.13**.
5. Hold the drape above waist level and away from your body. Grasp another corner of the drape so that you are holding both corners along the short edge of the drape.
6. Reach over the instrument tray with the drape, taking care not to let the drape touch any surfaces as it passes over the tray **FIGURE 8.14**.
7. Gently lay the drape over the field, beginning at the far edge of the tray and pulling toward you. If the drape needs adjustment, do not touch the center of the drape or reach over the sterile field, as this would contaminate the tray. Walk around the tray or reach underneath it to make adjustments.

> Once a drape is laid across a sterile field, the edges that hang over the tray are no longer considered sterile.

8. If a second field drape is desired or required, repeat steps 3–5. Next, instead of pulling the drape toward you as it is laid across the sterile field, apply the cover by holding the drape toward you with the lower edge even with the lower edge of the existing drape. Carefully lay the drape across the field using a forward motion.

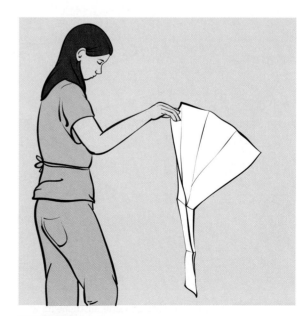

FIGURE 8.13 Grab only the top corner of the drape when removing it from its sterile packaging.
© Jones & Bartlett Learning

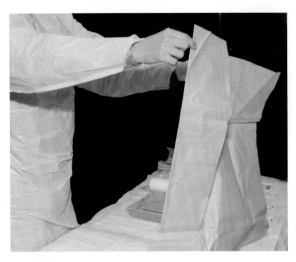

FIGURE 8.14 Reach over the instrument tray with the drape, but do not let the drape touch any nonsterile surfaces.
© Jones & Bartlett Learning. Courtesy of MIEMSS

Opening Sterile Packages of Instruments and Supplies

Instruments and supplies necessary for surgical procedures are presterilized and packaged in a manner that allows them to be opened and applied to the sterile field without compromising sterility. In this exercise, you will learn how to open sterile packages of instruments and supplies and place them on a surgical field using sterile technique.

Equipment Needed

- Mayo instrument stand/tray
- Two sterile field drapes or towels
- One pair of sterile gloves
- Sterile surgical instruments, wrapped twice
- Prepackaged sterile surgical supplies

Steps

1. Collect necessary supplies and instruments.
2. Wash hands and set up a sterile field, as described in previous exercises.
3. Place the package of surgical equipment on the palm of your nondominant hand with the outer flap facing up.
4. Grasp the taped end of the top flap and open it away from you. Do not touch the inside of the flap.
5. Grasp the folded-back tip of the right-sided flap and pull it to the right. Use the same technique to pull the left-sided flap to the left. Do not reach over the package.
6. Grasp the tip of the last flap and pull it toward you **FIGURE 8.15**.

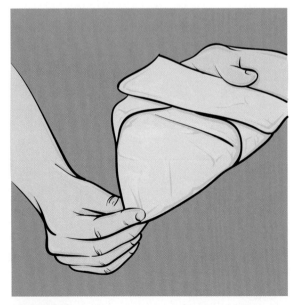

FIGURE 8.15 Hold the package of sterile instruments in your nondominant hand and unwrap carefully, taking care not to touch the inside of the packaging.
© Jones & Bartlett Learning

7. Gather the loose edges of the outer package to create a cover for your nondominant hand. Grasp the inner package with your covered hand and carefully place the inner package onto the sterile field. Discard outer wrapping **FIGURE 8.16**.
8. Open the peel-apart package by grasping both edges of the flaps and pulling them apart. Use a rolling-down motion and keep hands close together. Move slowly to gradually expose the sterile contents of the package. The sterile instrument or supply can then be offered to a gloved physician or applied to the sterile field using a flipping motion. Take care not to touch or contaminate the package contents or the sterile field. Discard the inner wrapping **FIGURE 8.17**.
9. Apply sterile gloves as described in previous exercises. Arrange instruments and supplies on the sterile field in an organized and logical manner according to the physician's preference. All handles should be positioned toward the user and instruments should be separated from each other as much as possible **FIGURE 8.18**.

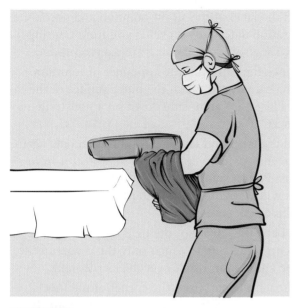

FIGURE 8.16 Gather the loose edges of the outer package underneath your hand and place the inner package on the sterile field.
© Jones & Bartlett Learning

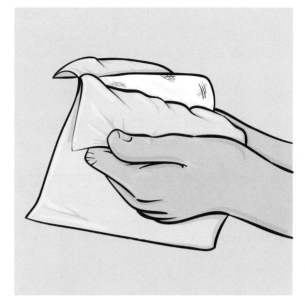

FIGURE 8.17 Open peel-apart packaging by keeping your hands close together and using a rolling-down motion.
© Jones & Bartlett Learning

> Usually, instruments and supplies are arranged in order of use from right to left, or from left to right for a left-handed physician. In all cases, physician preference dictates the exact placement and use of instruments and supplies.

10. Apply a sterile field cover, as described in previous exercises. A cover is needed if the tray will not be used immediately, if it needs to be moved, or if it will be left unattended.

Pouring a Sterile Solution into a Cup on a Sterile Field

In some procedures, sterile solutions will need to be poured into a sterile cup in the sterile field. The solution will be sterile, but the outside of the container will not be, so care must be taken not to contaminate the sterile field and its contents. The solution is always poured after the surgical tray has been moved and is in the surgical area to avoid spilling. In this exercise, you will learn how to pour a sterile solution into a cup on a sterile tray.

Equipment Needed

- Covered sterile surgical tray with sterile cup
- Container of sterile solution

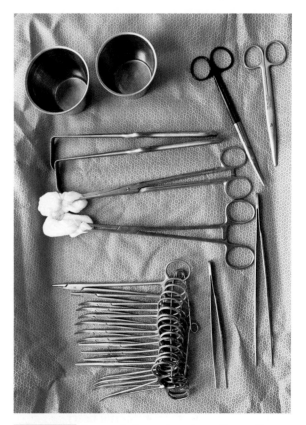

FIGURE 8.18 Arrange instruments and supplies on the sterile field in an organized and logical manner.
© Sielemann/ShutterStock, Inc.

Steps

1. Transport the surgical tray to the surgical area or set up a surgical tray for immediate use.

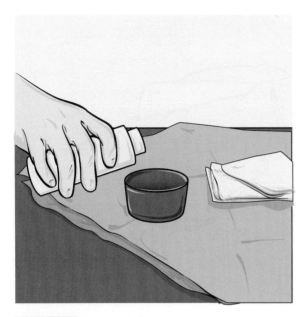

FIGURE 8.19 Do not reach over the sterile field when pouring solutions.
© Jones & Bartlett Learning

2. Read the label of the sterile solution and check the expiration date. This prevents you from pouring the wrong solution or using an expired product.
3. Remove the cap from the container of solution, taking care not to touch the inner surface of the cap. Place the cap upside down on a nonsterile surface.
4. Read the label and check the expiration date again. Place your palm over the label to protect it from stains. Pour a small amount of solution into a cup or bowl that is outside the sterile field to cleanse the lip of the container.
5. Pull back the corner of the field drape to expose the cup. Take care to touch only the corner of the drape and do not reach over the sterile field.
6. Approach the cup from the corner of the tray. Use the cleansed lip of the container to pour the desired amount of solution into the cup. Take care to avoid spilling or splashing the solution and reaching over or touching any sterile surfaces **FIGURE 8.19**.
7. Replace the cap of the solution. Avoid touching the inside of the cap.
8. Replace the corner of the drape. Avoid touching or reaching over any sterile surfaces.

Preparation of Patient Skin for Minor Surgery

The surface of the skin contains many microorganisms that can cause infection if allowed to enter the body through an incision. Therefore, it is important to clean the skin thoroughly prior to any surgical procedure to remove as many infection-causing organisms and contaminants as possible. Infections following surgical procedures are a significant complication, so infection prevention is essential. The skin surrounding the surgical site should be scrubbed, shaved, washed, and cleansed with an antiseptic solution. In this exercise, you will learn how to prepare a patient's skin for minor surgery.

Equipment Needed

- Absorbent pad
- Surgical drape
- Disposable prep kit that includes antiseptic soap, sponges, a razor, and a container for water
- Sterile water
- Antiseptic solution, such as Betadine
- Sterile bowl
- Two pairs of sterile gloves

Steps

1. Wash hands using aseptic technique, as described in previous exercises.
2. Collect necessary equipment and supplies near where you will be working.

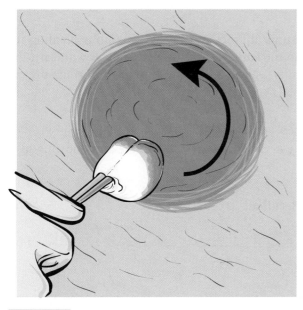

FIGURE 8.20 Wash the surgical site in a circular motion.
© Jones & Bartlett Learning

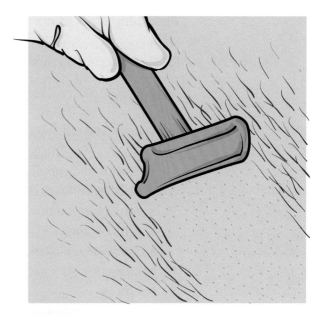

FIGURE 8.21 Shave in the direction of hair growth.
© Jones & Bartlett Learning

3. Identify the patient. Explain the procedure to him or her and provide privacy. Drape the patient if necessary.
4. Position the patient under a good light source with the surgical site exposed. Ensure patient comfort.
5. Place an absorbent pad underneath the site to protect the area and the patient.
6. Wash hands again and apply sterile gloves using aseptic technique, as described in previous exercises.
7. Apply antiseptic solution with gauze pads or sponges, beginning at the surgical site and moving outward in a circular motion **FIGURE 8.20**.

When cleaning a patient's skin, always move from the cleanest area to the least clean to prevent contamination.

---

8. Discard used sponges.
9. Hold the skin taut and use the razor to shave hair away from the surgical site, following the direction of hair growth **FIGURE 8.21**.

Shaving in the direction of hair growth prevents accidental abrasions to the skin, which could lead to infection.

---

10. After hair has been removed, scrub the area again with antiseptic solution using a circular motion, moving from the center of the site outward. Clean the area for two to five minutes.
11. Rinse the surgical site with sterile water and pat dry with a sterile 4 × 4 gauze sponge.
12. Cover the surgical site with a sterile towel and instruct patient not to touch the area.
13. Pour antiseptic solution into the sterile bowl. The physician will again wash the area immediately prior to beginning the procedure.

Assisting With Minor Surgery

Maintaining sterility during minor surgical procedures is essential to preventing infections and complications related to the surgery. In this exercise, you will learn the principles behind maintaining sterility as you assist the physician during surgical procedures.

Equipment Needed

- Mayo stand on which to create a sterile field that will include the following instruments and supplies:
  - Needles and syringe
  - Antiseptic solution, such as Betadine
  - Gauze sponges
  - Scalpel and blades
  - Operating scissors
  - Forceps
  - Two curved hemostats
  - Two straight hemostats
  - Thumb forceps
  - Suture material
  - Tissue forceps
  - Needle holder
  - Skin retractor
  - Transfer forceps
- Side table on which to create a nonsterile field that will include the following instruments and supplies:
  - Sterile gloves
  - Labeled biopsy containers with formalin
  - Appropriate laboratory requisition paperwork
  - Local anesthesia
  - Alcohol wipes
  - Dressing tape
  - Bandages
  - Biohazard container

Steps

1. First, check the room for readiness and equipment for cleanliness.
2. Wash hands.
3. Set up side table of nonsterile items.
4. Wash hands again using aseptic technique, as described in previous exercises.
5. Set up sterile field on Mayo stand, as described in previous exercises.
6. Apply sterile gloves, as described in previous exercises. Arrange all sterile instruments and supplies listed in the equipment list on the field. Cover the field if it will not be used immediately.
7. Identify the patient, explain the procedure, and prepare the patient's skin, as described in previous exercises.

8. If covered, remove the cover from the sterile field as the physician prepares for the procedure. Lift the drape by grasping the farthest corner from you and lifting back toward yourself. Do not allow arms or any other objects to pass over the sterile field FIGURE 8.22 .

9. Assist the physician during the procedure as necessary. You may be asked to hold vials of local anesthetic while the physician withdraws the necessary amount, adjust the instrument tray or equipment around the physician, adjust the light source in the room, or hold the specimen container into which the physician places the excised sample. You may also need to comfort the patient and provide emotional support.

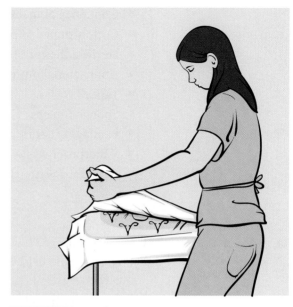

Always hand or accept instruments and supplies to and from the physician out of the patient's sight.

FIGURE 8.22 Uncover the sterile field.
© Jones & Bartlett Learning

10. After the procedure, handle the specimen container with gloved hands only. Tightly cover the container and label with the patient's name, date, type of sample, and source of specimen as recommended or directed by the laboratory.

11. After the procedure is complete and the patient has left the room, clean the room. Dispose of used sponges in a biohazard container and dispose of knife blades and any other disposable sharp objects in the puncture-proof sharps container. Rinse, soak, sanitize, and sterilize surgical instruments for future use. Remove gloves and other personal protective equipment and dispose of them.

12. Wash hands.

13. In the patient's chart, document that the specimen was sent to the laboratory. For example, write "0945: Specimen obtained from patient's right forearm and sent to AB labs for C&S; patient tolerated procedure well. J. Jones, CMA."

Dressing Application and Change

After surgical procedures or after trauma to the skin, wounds are often covered with a dry, sterile dressing (DSD). The dressing will need to be changed periodically so the wound can be checked or cleaned or the sutures can be removed. Another sterile dressing may then be applied. In this exercise, you will learn how to apply a dressing, either initially or as a dressing change.

Equipment Needed

- Sterile field containing the following instruments and supplies:
  - Several gauze pads and sponges
  - Sterile bowl with antiseptic solution, such as saline
  - Sterile dressing forceps
- Nonsterile field containing the following instruments and supplies:
  - Nonsterile gloves
  - Sterile gloves

- Container of hydrogen peroxide or sterile water
- Cotton-tipped applicators
- Sterile adhesive strips
- Antibacterial ointment or cream, as ordered by the physician
- Tape
- Sponge forceps
- Bandage scissors
- Waterproof waste bag
- Biohazard waste container

Steps

1. Wash hands.
2. Prepare sterile field with instruments and supplies listed, as described in previous exercises.
3. Pour antiseptic solution into a sterile bowl.
4. Identify the patient and explain the procedure. Position the patient so the wound is exposed and the patient is comfortable. Reassure the patient and provide emotional support as necessary. If the patient already has a dressing in place, continue with the following steps. If this is the first application of a dressing, skip to step 9.
5. Loosen tape on dressing or use scissors to cut off the bandage, if necessary.
6. Put on nonsterile gloves or use forceps to remove the bandage and place it in the biohazard container. Do not pass objects or instruments over the sterile field. Take care not to damage the wound as you remove the bandage. If the bandage is stuck to the wound, pour small amounts of sterile water or hydrogen peroxide over the dressing and allow it to soak for a short time. Remove the dressing completely when it loosens from the wound **FIGURE 8.23**.
7. Place the used dressing in the waterproof waste bag without touching the inside or outside of the bag.
8. Assess the wound and note any signs of infection or drainage. Remove and discard gloves in the waterproof bag.

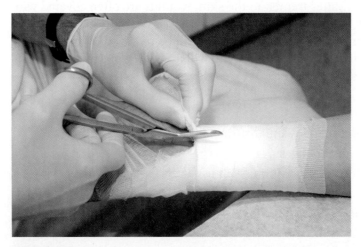

FIGURE 8.23 Remove the dressing without causing further pain or damage to the wound.
© iStockphoto.com/Wicki58

Signs of infection around a wound include discharge of yellow or green pus, redness around the wound, swelling or pain surrounding the wound, and red streaks appearing on the skin.

9. Wash hands using aseptic technique and apply sterile gloves, as described in previous exercises.

10. Dip a gauze sponge in antiseptic solution and clean the wound. Discard used sponges in the waterproof bag.

11. Use forceps to apply sterile gauze to the wound.

12. Remove gloves and dispose of them in the waterproof bag.

13. Secure dressing with adhesive tape or an appropriate bandage **FIGURE 8.24**.

14. Dispose of the waterproof bag in a biohazard container.

15. Wash hands.

16. Document the procedure in the patient's chart and describe the wound's appearance. For example, write "1320: Dressing changed on patient's right forearm; no sign of redness or swelling of lesion; patient tolerated procedure well. J. Jones, CMA."

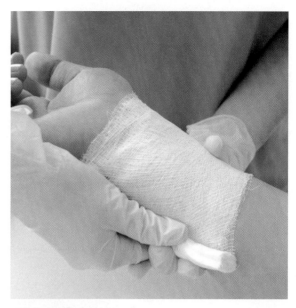

FIGURE 8.24 Place clean, dry gauze on the wound and secure with tape or bandage.
© sfam_photo/ShutterStock, Inc.

Assisting With a Laceration or Incision

If a wound is gaping, bleeding, extends deep into underlying tissue, or is located on the face, neck, or bend of a body part, suturing is recommended to bring the edges of the wound together and facilitate healing. Suturing decreases scarring and decreases the likelihood of infection. In this exercise, you will learn how to assist a physician in suturing a wound.

Equipment Needed

- Sterile surgical field containing the following instruments and supplies:
  - Syringe and needle for local anesthetic
  - Curved hemostats
  - Tissue forceps
  - Curved iris scissors
  - Suture material and needle
  - Needle holder
  - Gauze sponge
- Nonsterile side table containing the following instruments and supplies:
  - Local anesthetic, as ordered by the physician
  - Dressings, bandages, and/or tape
  - Sterile gloves

Steps

1. Wash hands.

2. Identify the patient and explain the procedure. Check for signed consent forms. Reassure the patient, and provide emotional support and comfort as needed.

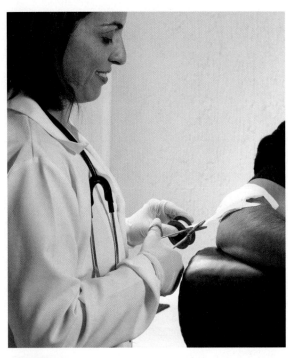

FIGURE 8.25 Dress the wound after sutures have been applied.
© sfam_photo/ShutterStock, Inc.

3. Obtain information on any known allergies, vaccination record (specifically note the date of last tetanus booster), and other health conditions that may complicate the healing process.

4. Clean and dry the wound as directed by the physician.

5. Position the patient in a comfortable, lying-down position.

6. Assist the physician with the suturing procedure and provide support to the patient as needed.

7. After the sutures are applied, apply sterile gloves and clean the area around the wound. Dress or bandage the wound according to the physician's direction **FIGURE 8.25**.

8. Remove gloves and wash hands.

9. Check the patient's vital signs.

10. Explain wound care and the signs and symptoms of infection. Also provide written instructions to the patient and to the caregiver, if present. Arrange for a follow-up appointment and medication as ordered by the physician.

11. Dispose of supplies and clean, sanitize, and sterilize the room for future use.

12. Document the procedure in the patient's chart. For example, write "1430: 6 sutures applied to incision on patient's left forearm by Dr. Bond; dressed wound with DSD and provided instructions for follow-up care and appointments with patient; patient tolerated procedure well and reported understanding of the instructions. J. Jones, CMA."

Suture or Staple Removal

Sutures used to promote healing of a wound may not be absorbable. Therefore, they need to be removed after the wound has healed. In this exercise, you will learn how to remove sutures.

Equipment Needed

- Gauze sponges
- Bandage scissors
- Biohazard waste container
- Tape
- Sponge forceps
- Suture-removal kit or suture-removal scissors or staple remover
- Thumb forceps
- Sterile gloves
- Antiseptic solution, such as Betadine

Steps

1. Identify patient and explain the procedure.
2. Wash hands.

3. Open the suture removal kit or gather supplies if kit is unavailable.

4. Apply sterile gloves, as described in previous exercises.

5. If removing sutures, using thumb forceps, gently pick up the knot of one suture. Gently pull toward the suture line. Using suture-removal scissors, cut one side of the suture as close to the skin as possible. Repeat the same procedure with the remaining sutures, noting the number of sutures to ensure you have removed all of them. Dispose of sutures on a gauze pad FIGURE 8.26 .

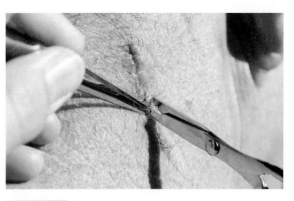

FIGURE 8.26 Gently pull up on the knot of the suture and cut it as close to the skin as possible.
© Carolina K. Smith, M.D./ShutterStock, Inc.

6. If removing staples, gently place staple remover on top of the staple. Squeeze the handle of the staple remover until the staple is pinched outward and upward. Gently pull up to remove staple.

7. Examine the wound, and ensure all sutures or staples have been removed.

8. Apply antiseptic solution to the area and apply a clean, dry dressing if directed by the physician.

9. Remove gloves. Dispose of used items. Wash hands.

10. Check the patient's vital signs. Explain wound care and the signs and symptoms of infection. Also provide written instructions to the patient and to the caregiver, if present. Arrange for a follow-up appointment and medication as ordered by the physician.

11. Document the procedure in the patient's chart. For example, write "1015: Removed 6 sutures from patient's left forearm; explained wound care instructions; patient tolerated procedure well and reported understanding of the instructions. J. Jones, CMA."

Application of Adhesive Skin-Closure Strips

If a wound is superficial, it will not require sutures to hold the skin in place as the wound heals. However, the edges of the wound must still be brought together and secured with sterile adhesive strips to facilitate healing. Or, adhesive strips may be used after sutures have been removed or at the same time as sutures, depending on the location and severity of the injury. In this exercise, you will learn how to apply sterile adhesive skin-closure strips.

Equipment Needed

- Sterile surgical field containing the following instruments and supplies:
  - Sterile adhesive skin-closure strips
  - Straight iris scissors
  - Tincture of benzoin
  - Sterile cotton-tipped applicators
- Nonsterile side table containing the following instruments and supplies:
  - Two pairs of sterile gloves
  - Dressings, bandages, and tape

Steps

1. Identify the patient and explain the procedure.
2. Position the patient comfortably with the wound exposed.
3. Wash hands and apply sterile gloves, as described in previous exercises.
4. Remove any bandages or dressings already in place, as described in previous exercises. Remove sutures, if indicated, as described in previous exercises.
5. Remove gloves and wash hands. Open the container of tincture of benzoin, cotton-tipped applicators, and skin-closure strips. Apply a new pair of sterile gloves.
6. Clean and dry at least two inches around the wound with antiseptic solution, as described in previous exercises.

Tincture of benzoin is used to protect the skin from allergic reaction or irritation to adhesive from skin-closure strips. It also helps the adhesive strips stay in place tighter and longer.

---

7. Apply tincture of benzoin to the edges of the wound, using cotton-tipped applicators. Do not let the tincture of benzoin come in contact with the actual wound.
8. Remove adhesive strips from the sterile packaging one at a time. Apply one end of the first strip to one side of the skin at the center of the wound. Using your hands or forceps, bring the edges of the wound close together and place the strip over the wound. Press down on the opposite side to secure it in place. The edges of the wound should be together, but not puckered. Apply the next strip in the same manner, placing it halfway between the first strip and the end of the wound. Repeat with remaining adhesive strips until the wound is secured **FIGURE 8.27**.
9. Dress and bandage the wound as directed by the physician.
10. Dispose of used items, remove gloves, and wash your hands.

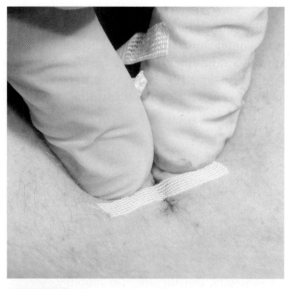

FIGURE 8.27 Apply adhesive strips to the wound to close the skin and facilitate healing.
© Life in View/Photo Researchers, Inc.

Preoperative and Postoperative Patient Concerns

When scheduling a surgical procedure, provide the patient with the following:

- Printed educational materials about the procedure in a language that the patient can understand
- The approximate length of time of the procedure
- The appropriate clothing to wear to the procedure
- The amount of time to fast and the medications from which to abstain prior to the procedure, if applicable
- Information about the need for transportation after the procedure
- The anticipated time off work and/or home care after the procedure

Before beginning the procedure, do the following:

- Verify patient allergies, including medications, latex, and adhesives.
- Provide written instructions regarding postoperative and follow-up care in a language that the patient can understand.

After the procedure, advise the patient to do the following:

- Keep the surgical site clean and dry.
- Place no stress on the area.
- Drink plenty of fluid.
- Get plenty of rest.
- Eat a sensible, balanced diet.
- Return for all scheduled follow-up appointments.
- Report any pain, burning, or discomfort at the site; swelling, redness, or discoloration at the site; bleeding or discharge from the site; fever, nausea, or vomiting; or any other problems or symptoms.

© auremar/ShutterStock, Inc.

11. Check the patient's vital signs. Explain wound care and the signs and symptoms of infection. Also provide written instructions to the patient and to the caregiver, if present. Arrange for a follow-up appointment and medication as ordered by the physician.

12. Document the procedure. For example, write "1720: Applied 4 steri-strips to laceration on patient's left shoulder; provided instructions for follow-up appointments and wound care; patient tolerated procedure well and expressed understanding of the instructions. J. Jones, CMA."

Math Practice

Question: What is the simplest form of the fraction $\frac{20}{60}$?

Answer: $\frac{1}{3}$

Question: **Which of the following quantities is the smallest:** $\frac{1}{2}$ **mL,** $\frac{3}{4}$ **mL,** $\frac{2}{5}$ **mL, or** $\frac{7}{10}$ **mL?**

Answer: $\frac{2}{5}$ mL

Question: **Which of the following quantities is the largest:** $\frac{7}{8}$ **mg,** $\frac{3}{4}$ **mg,** $\frac{6}{10}$ **mg, or** $\frac{1}{3}$ **mg?**

Answer: $\frac{7}{8}$ mg

Question: **What is the sum of** $\frac{4}{5} + \frac{3}{10}$**?**

Answer: $1\frac{1}{10}$

Question: **What is the sum of** $\frac{2}{7} + \frac{1}{4}$**?**

Answer: $\frac{15}{28}$

Question: **What is the difference of** $\frac{3}{4} - \frac{6}{11}$**?**

Answer: $\frac{9}{44}$

Question: **What is the difference of** $\frac{2}{3} - \frac{5}{18}$**?**

Answer: $\frac{7}{18}$

Question: **What is the product of** $\frac{1}{3} \times \frac{4}{5}$**?**

Answer: $\frac{4}{15}$

Question: **What is the product of** $\frac{2}{5} \times \frac{7}{8}$**?**

Answer: $\frac{7}{20}$

Question: **What is the quotient of** $\frac{3}{4} \div \frac{2}{3}$**?**

Answer: $1\frac{1}{8}$

Question: **What is the quotient of** $\frac{6}{7} \div \frac{4}{5}$**?**

Answer: $1\frac{1}{14}$

Question: **What is the sum of 2.87 + 1.2 + 9.1?**

Answer: 13.17

Question: **What is the sum of 4.62 + 7.185 + 2.3?**

Answer: 14.105

Question: **What is the difference of 8.52 − 6.9?**

Answer: 1.62

Question: **What is the difference of 13.7 − 4.89?**

Answer: 8.81

Question: **What is the product of 2.3 × 1.75?**

Answer: 4.025

Question: **What is the product of 5.3 × 2.1?**

Answer: 11.13

Question: **What is the quotient of 4.9 ÷ 0.7?**

Answer: 7

Question: **What is the quotient of 2.4 ÷ 0.6?**

Answer: 4

Question: **What is $3/60$ expressed as a percent?**

Answer: 5%

Question: **What is $2/5$ expressed as a percent?**

Answer: 40%

Question: **What is 25% expressed as a fraction?**

Answer: $1/4$

Question: **What is 60% expressed as a fraction?**

Answer: $3/5$

WRAP UP

Chapter Summary

- The integumentary system is composed of the skin and its accessory organs: hair, nails, glands, and nerve receptors.

- The skin is composed of three distinct layers, each with its own components and features: the epidermis, the dermis, and the subcutaneous tissue.

- The epidermis is the thin, outermost layer of skin. It lacks blood supply, connective tissue, and lymphatic vessels. The epidermis is constantly shedding old, dead cells and producing new ones. The stratum corneum is the outermost layer of the epidermis and the germinative layer is the innermost layer.

- The dermis is the thick, middle layer of skin that provides nutritional and structural support to the epidermis. It contains connective tissue and a rich supply of blood vessels, lymph vessels, nerves, and glands. The dermis also contains sensory receptors.

- The hypodermis, or subcutaneous tissue, is the innermost layer of skin. It contains loose connective tissue and fat.

- The skin's primary function is to protect the body from loss of water or nutrients and against invasion by a chemical or biological injury. The skin also maintains temperature and moisture content of the body and contributes to vitamin D synthesis and emotional expression.

- Lesions of the skin can be signs and symptoms of underlying medical conditions or exist as normal variations in skin. Skin diseases and disorders can provide significant emotional stress and embarrassment for patients.

- Acne vulgaris is caused by overactive sebaceous glands. This overactivity causes the glands to become blocked, forming papules. If the papules become infected, pustules appear along with cysts. Simple skin-cleansing routines may be effective treatment for some cases of acne, but others may require systemic therapy with antibiotics or hormone therapy.

- Eczema and dermatitis are inflammations of the skin, most often caused by exposure to an allergen or irritant, extreme temperatures, or emotional stress. Symptom relief is the primary goal of treatment and can often be achieved with antihistamines and steroid creams. Patients should be advised to avoid offending allergens or irritants and use only mild cleansers and cleaning products.

- Urticaria, or hives, is an acute allergic reaction of the dermis in response to exposure to a food, medication, or psychosocial stressor. Like eczema and dermatitis, antihistamines and steroid creams can provide effective symptom relief for hives.

- Psoriasis is a chronic inflammatory skin condition that appears as red patches covered with thick, silvery scales. The lesions may result in significant disability and deformity. Treatment is highly individualized and effectiveness varies among patients.

- Impetigo is a common bacterial infection caused by *Staphylococcus* or *Streptococcus* bacteria. It is highly contagious and often seen among children, the elderly, and individuals with poor hygiene. It is a superficial infection that responds well to antibiotic treatment.

- Cellulitis is also caused by *Staphylococcus* or *Streptococcus* bacteria. Cellulitis is an infection of the dermis and epidermis that spreads rapidly and has the ability to cause serious, life-threatening infections. Prompt antibiotic treatment is necessary for cellulitis.

- Folliculitis is the inflammation of a hair follicle. A furuncle occurs when the hair follicle becomes infected. A carbuncle is a group of furuncles. Mild folliculitis usually resolves on its own, but more severe cases of furuncles and carbuncles require antibiotic therapy to prevent the spread of the infection.

- Herpes simplex virus 1 (HSV1) causes cold sores or fever blisters. Most people are infected with HSV1, but the virus remains dormant until a physical, chemical, or biological stressor prompts an outbreak of lesions. Herpes simplex virus 2 (HSV2), a related virus, causes genital warts and is transmitted primarily by sexual contact. Herpes lesions are usually self-limiting and resolve without treatment in a few weeks. Antiviral medications can reduce the frequency and severity of recurrent outbreaks.

- Herpes zoster, or shingles, is an infection in adults caused by the varicella-zoster virus. The same virus causes chicken pox in children, and shingles is a result of reactivation of the virus after decades of dormancy. Treatment of herpes zoster infection consists of treating the symptoms of infection, as the virus itself cannot be treated. The rash associated with shingles is painful, and oral analgesics are appropriate for pain relief.

- Warts are a common skin condition caused by human papillomavirus. Warts are not harmful, are generally not painful, and resolve within a few months or years without treatment.

- Tinea infections are a group of fungal infections that can affect nearly every part of the body. Broken or damaged skin increases the likelihood of an infection. Topical antifungal agents are the preferred treatment for most tinea infections. Oral antifungal agents are required for tinea infections of the nail, head, and scalp.

- Candidiasis is a fungal infection, most often seen in the mouth or vagina. Intense itching, redness, and irritation are accompanied by a thick yellowish-white discharge. Topical antifungals are effective for candidiasis.

- Scabies is a parasitic infection of the skin. The itch mite burrows under the skin of the infected host and causes intense itching. Poor hygiene is a risk factor for scabies.

- Pediculosis, or lice, is a parasitic infection usually seen on the scalp, but can also be seen on other parts of the body. The female louse lays eggs (nits) that attach to the base of the hair. A pediculicide is necessary to remove lice and nits. The treatment must be repeated after 7–10 days to remove newly hatched lice.

- Nevi are generally harmless lesions on the skin. However, skin cancer can develop when nevi change in size, shape, or appearance. Melanoma is an aggressive form of cancer that can be fatal. Basal cell carcinoma is the most common form of cancer and rarely metastasizes. Squamous cell carcinoma is treatable if identified early, but has the ability to metastasize. Frequent self-checks of the skin can aid in early detection of cancerous skin lesions.

- A laceration is a cut, puncture, or tear in the skin. Lacerations vary in size and location and may involve superficial injury or deep tissue damage. Infection is the most worrisome complication of lacerations.

- Burns are one of the most serious traumas affecting the skin. Burns vary in severity and intensity, as well as the amount of body area and skin structures involved. If burns are large or severe, fluid and protein loss may occur. Pain relief and preventing infection are the primary goals of treating burns.

- Medical assistants have the opportunity to assist physicians in office and surgical procedures that require sterility. Maintaining a sterile surgical environment, and maintaining sterility when cleaning or dressing a wound, prevents infection and promotes healing.

Learning Assessment Questions

1. What is the largest organ in the body?
   A. The brain
   B. The hair
   C. The skin
   D. The blood

2. What is the correct term for the medical specialty that studies the skin and its diseases and disorders?
   A. Integumentary
   B. Dermatology
   C. Anatomy
   D. Scleroderma

3. What layer of the skin contains the sweat and sebaceous glands?

   A. Epidermis

   B. Dermis

   C. Hypodermis

   D. Stratum corneum

4. Where is most of the adipose tissue in the body found?

   A. Germinative layer

   B. Epidermis

   C. Dermis

   D. Subcutaneous tissue

5. What is the primary function of the skin?

   A. Protective barrier

   B. Lubricate the internal organs

   C. Calcium synthesis

   D. Support the skeleton

6. What is the cause of acne vulgaris?

   A. Staphylococcus infections

   B. Overactive sebaceous glands

   C. Chronic dry skin

   D. Long-term antibiotic use

7. Which of the following does *not* aggravate eczema and dermatitis?

   A. Extreme temperatures

   B. Emotional stress

   C. Steroid creams

   D. Harsh chemicals

8. Which of the following is the correct description of a psoriatic lesion?

   A. Dark red patches covered with thick, silvery scales

   B. Small, elevated inflammations on the surface of the skin

   C. Loss of pigment from irregular patches of skin

   D. Red, fluid-filled sacs surrounded by inflammation

9. Which of the following are risk factors for impetigo?

   A. Elderly, cold climates, and wearing dentures

   B. Altered mental status and vitamin deficiencies

   C. Warm climates, poor hygiene, and young age

   D. Dehydration, allergen exposure, and humid climates

10. What are the most common causes of cellullitis?

   A. Human papillomavirus

   B. *Staphylococcus* or *Streptococcus* bacteria

   C. Herpes simplex 2 virus

   D. Epidermophyton

11. Which of the following signifies the most serious, widespread infection: folliculitis, furuncles, or carbuncles?

   A. Folliculitis

   B. Furuncles

   C. Carbuncles

   D. All are equally serious and widespread.

12. The virus that causes shingles in the elderly also causes what childhood disease?

   A. Impetigo

   B. Chicken pox

   C. Influenza

   D. Measles

13. Which of the following infections is correctly matched with the affected body part?

   A. Tinea manuum: feet

   B. Tinea capitis: fingernails

   C. Tinea pedis: scalp

   D. Tinea cruris: thighs and buttocks

14. Oral candidiasis is more commonly known as what?

   A. Lice

   B. Thrush

   C. Scabies

   D. Psoriasis

15. Which of the following products can effectively treat pediculosis?

    A. Permethrin or piperonyl butoxide

    B. Coal tar

    C. Salicylic acid

    D. Topical corticosteroids

16. What mnemonic can patients use to conduct self-checks of moles for signs of skin cancer?

    A. 123s

    B. ABCs

    C. Four Cs

    D. Roy G. Biv

17. What type of skin cancer is the least likely to metastasize?

    A. Squamous cell carcinoma

    B. Melanoma

    C. Basal cell carcinoma

    D. Actinic keratosis

18. What is the most significant complication of a laceration?

    A. Secondary infection

    B. Keloid scarring

    C. Pitting of the skin

    D. Loss of range of motion

19. Which type of burn extends through all three layers of skin?

    A. First-degree burn

    B. Second-degree burn

    C. Third-degree burn

    D. Sunburn

20. Which of the following is *not* a complication of repeat and excessive sun exposure?

    A. Skin cancer

    B. Damage to the eyes

    C. Premature aging

    D. Decreased vitamin D synthesis

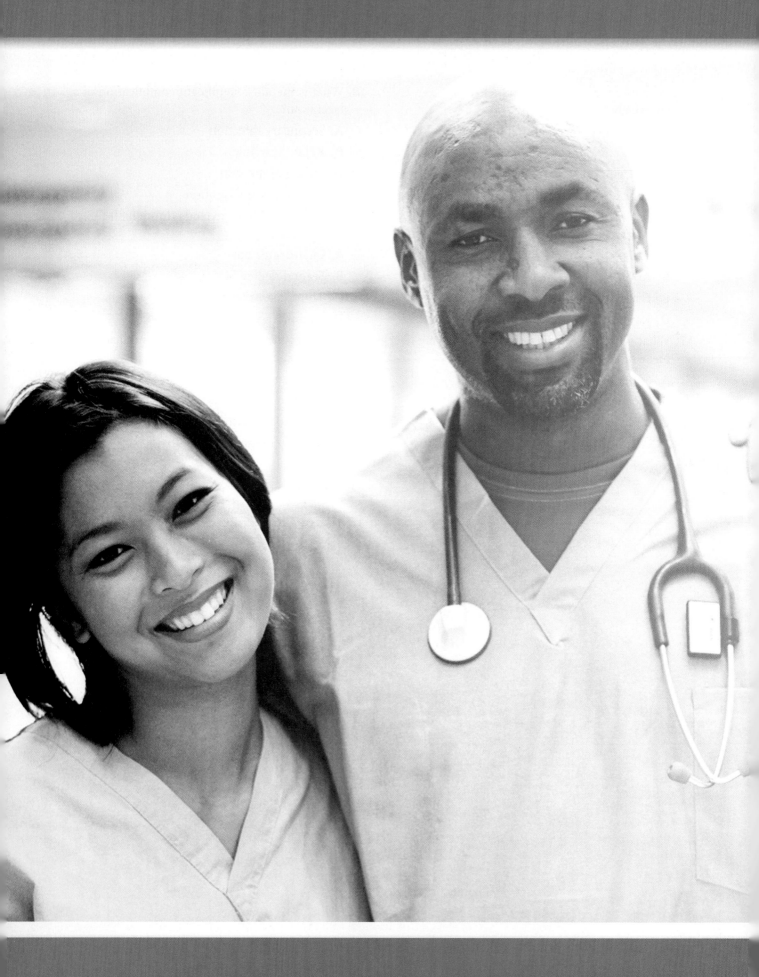

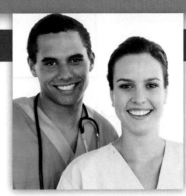

Respiratory System

OBJECTIVES

After reading this chapter, you will be able to:

- Identify key terms and root words related to the respiratory system and their role in the formation of medical terms.
- Define the structures and functions of the respiratory system.
- List common upper-respiratory diseases and breathing disorders and their treatment.
- Identify diagnostic procedures of the respiratory system.
- List abbreviations related to the respiratory system.
- Describe the proper use of a metered dose inhaler.
- Briefly discuss the role of the medical assistant during peak flow and pulse oximetry.
- Explain oxygen administration using a nasal cannula.
- Describe how to perform a nasal irrigation.
- Identify patient education information for sputum collections.
- Describe how to perform a throat culture.
- Perform dosage calculations relating to the respiratory system.

KEY TERMS

Alveoli	Bronchioles	Chronic obstructive
Antitussive	Bronchitis	pulmonary disease
Arterial blood	Bronchodilator	(COPD)
gases	Bronchoscopy	Cough
Asthma	Carbon dioxide	Cystic fibrosis
Bronchi	Chronic bronchitis	Diaphragm

Diluent	Mucus	Sinus cavities
Emphysema	Nose	Sinusitis
Expectorant	Otorhinolaryngology	Smoking cessation
Expiration	Oxidation	Spirometry
Forced expiratory volume	Oxygen	Sputum
Forced vital capacity	Peak expiratory flow	Sputum culture
Gas diffusion	Pharynx	Thoracic cavity
Gas transport	Pneumonia	Throat culture
Hypoxia	Protussive	Tonsillitis
Inspiration	Pulmonary function test	Tonsils
Laryngitis	Pulmonology	Total lung capacity
Larynx	Pulse oximetry	Trachea
Lower respiratory tract	Respiration	Tuberculosis (TB)
Lungs	Respiratory syncytial virus (RSV)	Upper respiratory tract
Lysozyme		Ventilation

Chapter Overview

The primary function of the respiratory system is gas exchange. The goal is to maintain normal pressures of **oxygen** and **carbon dioxide** in the arteries. This is accomplished by taking in oxygen from inspired air and removing carbon dioxide though expired air. This process of exchanging oxygen and carbon dioxide is known as **respiration**. Respiration is divided into two distinct but simultaneous processes: **inspiration** (breathing air in) and **expiration** (exhaling air out).

One respiratory cycle consists of one breath in and one breath out. In one minute, the average human adult completes 12 to 20 respiratory cycles.

Terminology

Because the respiratory system is highly integrated with other body systems, several medical specialties work with respiratory diseases and disorders. **Pulmonology** is the study of acute and chronic lung diseases. **Otorhinolaryngology**—more commonly called ear, nose, and throat—treats disorders of the upper respiratory tract. TABLE 9.1 provides common word roots used to describe the respiratory system.

Anatomy and Physiology of the Respiratory System

The respiratory system is a combination of organs that perform the mechanical and chemical processes of respiration. The respiratory system works closely with the cardiovascular system, including the heart and blood vessels. Respiration involves gas exchange, bringing oxygen into the lungs through inhalation and removing carbon dioxide from the body through exhalation. The respiratory system is important to the body's acid-base balance, which is an essential part of homeostasis. Thus respiration must be a continuous process. Even short interruptions in respiration can lead to brain damage or death.

Table 9.1 Word Roots of the Respiratory System

Word Root or Term	Meaning	Example
Bronchi/o	Bronchiole	Bronchiolitis (inflammation of the bronchioles)
Bronch/o	Bronchus	Bronchoscopy (technique for visualizing the inside of the lung's airways)
Laryng/o	Larynx, voice box	Laryngitis (inflammation of the larynx)
Nas/o	Nose	Nasal (concerning the nose)
Osmia/o	Smell	Anosmia (without a sense of smell)
Pector/o	Chest	Pectoralis (muscles of the chest)
Pharyng/o	Pharynx, throat	Pharyngitis (inflammation of the throat)
Phonia/o	Voice	Dysphonia (difficult or painful voice)
Pleur/o	Pleura, side	Pleurisy (inflammation of the lining surrounding the lungs and inside the chest)
-Pnea	Breathing	Dyspnea (difficult breathing) Tachypnea (fast breathing) Bradypnea (slow breathing)
Pneum/o	Lung, air	Pneumonia (infection of the air spaces in the lungs)
Pulmon/o	Lung	Pulmonologist (physician who studies chests and lungs)
Rhin/o	Nose	Rhinorrhea (nasal discharge or "runny nose")
Spir/o	Breathing	Spirometer (instrument used to measure breathing)
Trache/o	Trachea, windpipe, neck	Tracheotomy (surgical incision that opens the windpipe)
Thorac/o	Chest	Thoracentesis (surgical procedure to remove fluid from the space between the outside of the lungs and the chest wall)

Abbreviations Related to the Respiratory System

The following are abbreviations related to the respiratory system:

ABG—Arterial blood gases

A&P—Auscultation and percussion

CO_2—Carbon dioxide

DOE—Dyspnea on exertion

ENT—Ear, nose, and throat

FEV—Forced expiratory volume

FVC—Forced vital capacity

LLL—Left lower lobe

LRI or LRTI—Lower respiratory tract infection

LUL—Left upper lobe

O_2—Oxygen

PFT—Pulmonary function test

Pox or PulseOx—Pulse oximetry

RLL—Right lower lobe

RUL—Right upper lobe

SOB—Shortness of breath

T&A—Tonsillectomy and adenoidectomy

TLC—Total lung capacity

URI or URTI—Upper respiratory tract infection

The major organs of the respiratory system are the nose, pharynx, larynx, trachea, bronchi, and lungs. **FIGURE 9.1** illustrates the entire respiratory system.

Structure

The respiratory system is divided into two sections: the upper and lower respiratory tracts. The **upper respiratory tract** filters, warms, and humidifies inhaled air. The **lower respiratory tract** directs airflow and facilitates gas exchange.

Upper Respiratory Tract

The upper respiratory tract includes the **nose**, the sinus cavities, and the pharynx. **Sinus cavities** are hollow, air-filled pockets in the skull that decrease the weight of the skull, give resonance to the voice, and humidify and heat inhaled air. The **pharynx**, or back of the throat, contains three sets of **tonsils**, which are composed of lymphatic tissue and prevent infectious agents from entering the body through the upper respiratory tract: palatine tonsils, pharyngeal tonsils or adenoids, and lingual tonsils. The pharynx is also part of the digestive system.

The upper respiratory tract is lined with small, hairlike projections called cilia and a thin mucous membrane. **Mucus** is a slippery film produced by glands underneath the mucous membrane that helps trap foreign bodies and infectious organisms. Mucus also contains the enzyme **lysozyme**, which destroys many bacteria that come in contact with it.

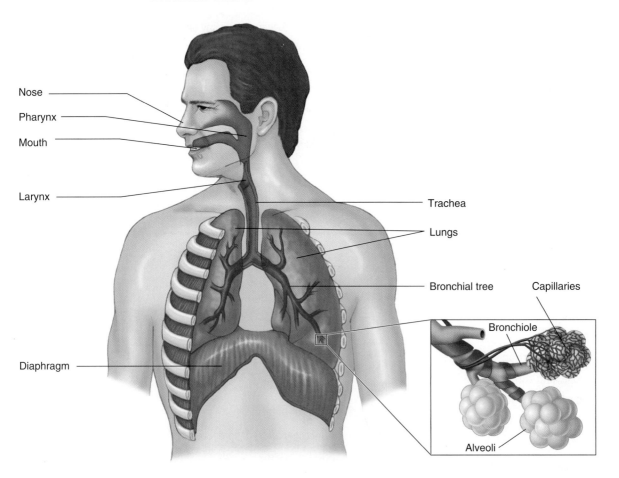

FIGURE 9.1 The respiratory system.
© Jones & Bartlett Learning

The cilia continuously move the mucus toward the pharynx and away from the lungs so it can be coughed out of the body. The cilia also help filter inspired air by trapping particles in the air.

The upper respiratory tract contains a rich blood supply to maintain enough heat and moisture to warm and humidify air to 35 to 37°C (95 to 98.6°F) and 75 to 80 percent humidity.

Lower Respiratory Tract

The lower respiratory tract includes the larynx, trachea, bronchi, and lungs. The **larynx**, or voice box, is composed of cartilage that is situated between the trachea and the pharynx. The **trachea** is a smooth, flexible tube that is approximately five inches long. It is supported by c-shaped pieces of cartilage. The trachea is lined with mucous membrane and cilia, just like the upper respiratory tract, which filters the air. The trachea divides into two primary **bronchi**, with one bronchus entering each lung. (The **lungs** are the major organs of the respiratory system where gas exchange takes place.) The right lobe consists of three lobes and the left lung consists of two lobes.

The primary bronchi branch into secondary bronchi that enter the separate lobes and segments of the lungs and conduct air into the lungs. The secondary bronchi branch into progressively smaller **bronchioles**, which ultimately conduct air into the **alveoli**, or air sacs, contained in the lungs. The alveoli are surrounded by a bed of capillaries supplied with blood from the pulmonary artery and the pulmonary vein. Oxygen and carbon dioxide diffuse between the capillaries and the alveoli. Unoxygenated blood from the pulmonary artery receives oxygen and travels back to the heart through the pulmonary vein. A more detailed description of circulation is provided in Chapter 13.

There are 10 secondary bronchi in the right lung and 8 secondary bronchi in the left lung. The right lung has three lobes and the left lung has two lobes.
The respiratory tract is like an upside-down tree, with the trachea at the base of the tree, the bronchi as the main branches, the bronchioles like smaller branches, and the alveoli like the fruit at the end of the branches.

Each lung contains millions of alveoli, equating to a total surface area of 60 inches for gas exchange.

Contents of Air

Inspired Air
    79% nitrogen
    20% oxygen
    0.04% carbon dioxide
    Trace amounts of other gases and water vapor
Expired Air
    79% nitrogen
    16% oxygen
    4% carbon dioxide
    Trace amounts of other gases and water vapor

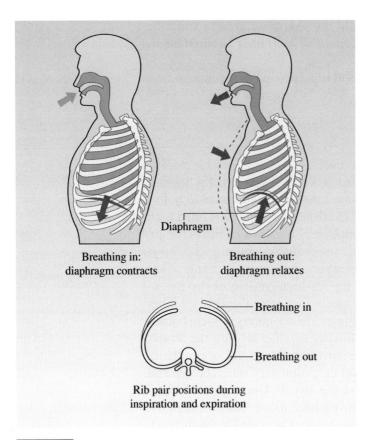

Diaphragm

Breathing in:
diaphragm contracts

Breathing out:
diaphragm relaxes

Breathing in

Breathing out

Rib pair positions during
inspiration and expiration

FIGURE 9.2 The action of the thoracic cavity during inspiration and expiration.

© Rob3000/ShutterStock, Inc.

Muscles of the Respiratory System

The **thoracic cavity** is a closed system that is shaped by the ribs. The muscles of each rib support the thoracic cavity. A heavy, dome-shaped muscle, called the **diaphragm**, separates the thoracic cavity from the abdominal cavity. As illustrated in **FIGURE 9.2**, during inspiration, the diaphragm contracts downward, drawing air into the lungs, which expands the thoracic cavity. The diaphragm relaxes and the abdominal muscles pull the ribs back down, which pushes the abdominal organs upward, shrinking the thoracic cavity and pushing air out of the lungs.

Function

The three main functions of the respiratory system are to support ventilation and the mechanics of breathing, transfer and transport gases, and control breathing. The first two functions are nearly completely involuntary, meaning they are almost entirely controlled by the autonomic nervous system and occur as automatic reflexes without conscious control. The third function, control of breathing, occurs at least in part by metabolic and voluntary activities. Voluntary actions of the respiratory system can be controlled by an individual.

Respiration takes place in two phases: gas exchange and cellular respiration. Gas exchange is the process of transferring oxygen and carbon dioxide between the atmosphere or external environment and the lungs. First, air is moved in and out of the lungs in a process called **ventilation** or internal respiration. Next, oxygen and carbon dioxide are transferred from the lungs to the pulmonary blood in a process called **gas diffusion** or external respiration. Last, the oxygen and carbon dioxide are carried throughout the body by the blood in a process called **gas transport**.

Cellular respiration is a complex series of metabolic processes that break down food into energy for cells. **Oxidation** (the combination of a substance with oxygen) is the final step of cellular respiration. The waste product of cellular respiration is carbon dioxide, which must be removed from the cells. This constant supply of oxygen to the cells of the entire body provides the energy for all metabolic activities. The respiratory system is remarkably efficient and the gas exchange and transport required for healthy cellular functioning rarely limits activity.

The lungs can increase gas exchange by more than 20 times to meet a body's energy demands.

Diseases and Disorders of the Respiratory Tract

Respiratory disorders are among the most common conditions for which people seek medical attention. Many conditions require only self-care, but others will require medical attention, both long-term and short-term care. Many symptoms of respiratory conditions overlap, so proper medical histories and examinations are necessary to determine the accurate diagnosis. Respiratory symptoms can also indicate diseases and disorders of other body systems.

Many patients with respiratory diseases will be very young or very old. As a medical assistant, you will have the opportunity to interact with each of these unique groups. You can work to establish a rapport with patients and their caregivers and offer support and reassurance during difficult or anxious procedures.

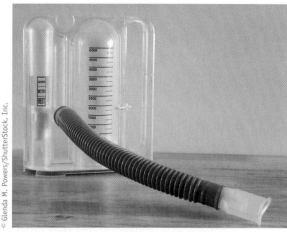

Pulmonary function is measured with a spirometer.

Cough

Infectious organisms, environmental factors, and chronic respiratory conditions can induce **cough**. The cough reflex is a defensive mechanism of the respiratory tract. During a cough, the abdominal and chest walls and the diaphragm forcefully contract, expelling air at a high velocity, taking with it mucus, cellular debris, or foreign bodies from the lower respiratory tract. Coughing, though a protective mechanism, can be bothersome, painful, and irritating to the chest and throat, and can interfere with work and sleep.

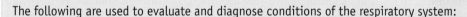

Evaluation and Diagnosis of Conditions of the Respiratory System

The following are used to evaluate and diagnose conditions of the respiratory system:

- **Arterial blood gases**—Tests to determine the presence of oxygen and carbon dioxide in the blood
- **Auscultation**—Listening to sounds of the body; usually performed with a stethoscope
- **Bronchoscopy**—Using a bronchoscope to visualize the bronchi; a bronchoscope can also be used to obtain specimens for a biopsy and remove foreign objects
- **Forced expiratory volume**—A spirometry parameter; the volume of air that can be forcibly exhaled in one second after a complete inhalation
- **Forced vital capacity**—A spirometry parameter; the volume of air, in liters, that can be forcibly exhaled after a complete inhalation
- **Peak expiratory flow**—A spirometry parameter; the maximum speed, in liters per minute, of a forced exhalation also known as a "peak flow"
- **Percussion**—Using the fingertips to tap on a body surface to determine the condition beneath the surface
- **Pulmonary function tests**—A group of tests used to determine respiratory function and measure lung volumes and gas exchange
- **Pulse oximetry**—A noninvasive test to measure the oxygenation of the blood
- **Spirometry**—A pulmonary function test that measures the breathing capacity of the lungs
- **Throat culture**—A method for removing tissue or material from the pharynx to determine bacterial growth
- **Total lung capacity**—A spirometry parameter; the total volume of air present in the lungs

Americans spend approximately $1 billion every year to treat cough.

Signs and Symptoms of Cough

Coughs are classified as productive or nonproductive. A productive cough is described as "wet" and expels mucus and other secretions from the lower respiratory tract. The secretions may be clear, discolored, or blood-tinged or have a bad odor. Each feature signifies a different etiology of cough, and a thorough description of the cough is helpful for an accurate diagnosis.

A nonproductive cough is a dry or hacking cough and serves no physiological purpose. Most nonproductive coughs are caused by viruses, cardiac disease, gastroesophageal reflux disease, or certain medications.

Cough is often a symptom of other conditions and may be accompanied by fever, sneezing, rhinorrhea, fatigue, breathlessness, wheezing, or chest tightness. Chronic cough can cause exhaustion, insomnia, musculoskeletal pain, hoarseness, and urinary incontinence.

Treatment of Cough

The goals of cough treatment are to relieve the symptoms of cough and improve patient comfort. Vaporizers and humidifiers moisten and soothe irritated airways and improve cough. Cool-mist vaporizers are preferred to warm-mist vaporizers, as the latter can harbor bacterial and mold growth and present a risk of burns.

Antitussives or cough suppressants eliminate cough and are the treatment of choice for nonproductive cough. Common antitussives include codeine, dextromethorphan, and diphenhydramine. Camphor, menthol, and eucalyptus are common topical antitussives available in ointments, creams, and lozenges.

Protussives or **expectorants** change the consistency of mucus, allowing it to be expelled with cough. Expectorants are the treatment of choice for productive coughs that expel thick secretions with difficulty. Guaifenesin is the most widely available commercial expectorant. However, drinking water is also an effective expectorant. Cough should resolve in 7 to 10 days.

Combination products that contain an expectorant and an antitussive are counterintuitive and should be avoided.

Asthma

Asthma is a chronic inflammatory condition of the airways. The pathophysiology of asthma is not well defined, but it is partially caused by abnormal activity of the immune system. There is a strong genetic link in asthma, as well, which likely interacts with environmental factors.

Signs and Symptoms of Asthma

Due to the broad definition of asthma, the disease's presentation can vary widely among individuals. Most people with asthma, however, experience recurrent episodes of wheezing, breathlessness, chest tightening, and coughing **FIGURE 9.3**. These episodes often include airway obstruction due to inflammation, bronchospasm, or excess mucous secretions, which may resolve spontaneously or after treatment. Symptoms usually worsen at night and early in the morning.

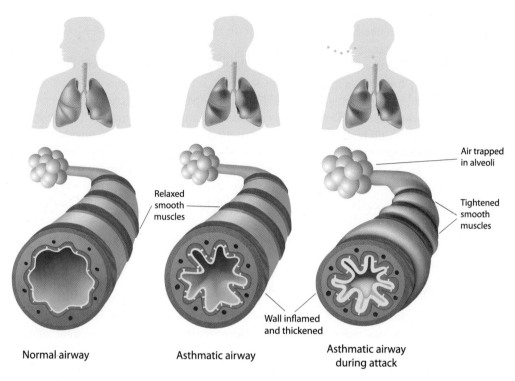

Air trapped in alveoli

Relaxed smooth muscles

Tightened smooth muscles

Wall inflamed and thickened

Normal airway   Asthmatic airway   Asthmatic airway during attack

FIGURE 9.3 The pathology of asthma.
© Alila Sao Mai/ShutterStock, Inc.

Many factors can trigger asthma symptoms: respiratory infection, allergens, environmental pollution, weather, emotional stress, exercise, certain drugs, and food chemicals. Symptoms will appear and/or worsen in response to a trigger and remain for days or weeks. Asthma is a disease of exacerbation and remission, so patients may remain symptom free for long periods of time.

What Would You Do?

A mother brings her six-year-old son to your office for follow-up related to his asthma. He was diagnosed with asthma three years ago and his symptoms have been fairly well controlled since that time. Today, she notes that he has been having an increase in the severity and frequency of his exacerbations, which is causing anxiety for the child and his mother. What would you recommend?
© NorthGeorgiaMedia/ShutterStock, Inc.

Treatment of Asthma

The goal of asthma treatment is to prevent symptom onset. Ideally, the patient will recognize triggers and avoid them, if possible. Otherwise, medications can be taken to prevent asthma attacks. These include corticosteroids or nonsteroidal anti-inflammatory drugs to decrease inflammation, **bronchodilators** to expand the airways, and immune modulators. Some medications are oral tablets or syrups, while others must be administered by a metered dose inhaler (MDI) or a nebulizer.

Patient education regarding self-management and trigger avoidance ensures compliance and optimal outcomes. A combination of short- and long-acting drugs is often used to control symptoms.

Chronic Obstructive Pulmonary Disease (COPD)

Chronic obstructive pulmonary disease (COPD) is one of the most common lung diseases, and its prevalence has increased dramatically in recent decades. Most cases of COPD are due to cigarette smoking.

COPD is a progressive disease characterized by airflow limitation. The airflow limitation is not fully reversible and the symptoms of COPD are associated with a hyperactive inflammatory response. COPD is divided into two conditions: chronic bronchitis and emphysema. **Bronchitis** is an inflammation of the lining of the bronchi and bronchioles, which leads to airflow obstruction on exhalation. **Chronic bronchitis** is caused by damage or trauma to the respiratory tract, while acute cases of bronchitis are caused by an infectious microorganism. **Emphysema** is characterized by the destruction of the alveoli, which leads to a loss of the alveoli's ability to expand and contract and remove carbon dioxide. People can have a combination of both types of COPD.

Pink Puffers Versus Blue Bloaters

The nicknames "pink puffer" and "blue bloater" are often used to describe patients with COPD. Blue bloaters have chronic bronchitis as the primary underlying etiology. Ventilation decreases and **hypoxia**, or low oxygenation of the blood, occurs. This decreased oxygenation leads to cyanosis, or blue discoloration of the lips and skin ("blue"). Increased pressure in the blood vessels surrounding the heart also leads to fluid retention in chronic bronchitis ("bloater"). Pink puffers have emphysema as the primary underlying etiology. Due to the destruction of the alveoli, ventilation increases to rapid, shallow breaths ("puffer"). Patients have to struggle for each breath, causing redness in their faces and necks ("pink"). Also, patients with emphysema experience less hypoxia than patients with chronic bronchitis, making them appear pink in contrast to blue bloaters.

© auremar/ShutterStock, Inc.

Signs and Symptoms of COPD

Patients with chronic bronchitis present with a productive cough that contains pus or blood and experience shortness of breath and excess mucus production. Patients with emphysema experience shortness of breath with only mild activity. All patients with COPD also experience fatigue, frequent respiratory infections, and wheezing **FIGURE 9.4**.

Treatment of COPD

COPD cannot be cured. However, the symptoms can be managed with chronic therapy. The goal of COPD treatment is to decrease the occurrence and severity of symptoms and improve quality of life. Like asthma, the symptoms of COPD can be managed with anti-inflammatory drugs, bronchodilators, and immune modulators. Anticholinergic agents, which relax the smooth muscles of the bronchioles, are also used in the treatment of COPD. If signs or symptoms of an active infection are present, COPD treatment may include antibiotics. In severe cases of COPD, oxygen supplementation may be necessary to maintain appropriate arterial levels of oxygen. If COPD patients are still active smokers, **smoking cessation** may slow the progression of COPD.

Pneumonia

Pneumonia is an infection in one or both lungs. Bacteria, viruses, and fungi can cause pneumonia. The infectious organism can come from contact with an infected person;

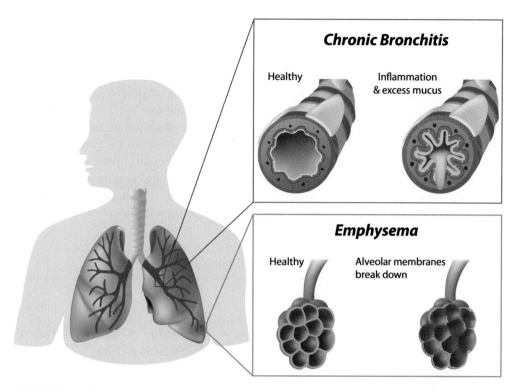

FIGURE 9.4 The pathology of COPD.
© Alila Sao Mai/ShutterStock, Inc.

normal microorganisms living in the nose, sinuses, or mouth; or inhaled food, fluids, or vomit that enter the lungs.

The most common cause of pneumonia in adults is the bacterium *Streptococcus pneumoniae*. Other causes of pneumonia include bacteria such as *Legionella pneumophila*, *Mycoplasma pneumoniae*, and *Chlamydophila pneumoniae*.

Smoking Cessation

Smoking is a risk factor for many acute and chronic respiratory conditions, including lung cancer and COPD, as well as cardiovascular, genitourinary, and endocrine disorders. Nicotine, the addictive chemical found in tobacco, leads to physical and psychological dependence. Many patients need medical assistance to quit smoking.

Cognitive behavioral therapy and pharmacological therapy are effective methods of smoking cessation. Common pharmacological agents include Bupropion, Varenicline, and controlled-release nicotine in patches, gums, lozenges, and sprays.

The "five As" provide a stepwise strategy for advising patients on smoking cessation:

- **Ask**—Identify tobacco users by asking about smoking at each visit.
- **Advise**—Urge tobacco users to quit by advising them regularly to quit smoking in a clear, personalized message.
- **Assess**—Determine a tobacco user's willingness to quit.
- **Assist**—Provide smoking-cessation support by assisting with setting stop dates, referring to support groups, or providing educational materials.
- **Arrange**—Schedule a follow-up and monitor progress and support.

© auremar/ShutterStock, Inc.

Pneumonia occurs year-round in all age groups. Patients with weakened immune systems or other chronic diseases are more susceptible to severe infections. Vaccines are available to reduce the risk of acquiring pneumonia for high-risk individuals. Currently, the pneumococcal conjugate vaccine (PCV13; Prevnar 13) is recommended for all children under 5 years of age. Additionally, pneumococcal polysaccharide vaccine (PPVSV; Pneumovax) is recommended for adults over the age of 65 years, as well as children over the age of 2 years who are at high risk for pneumonia, including those with sickle cell disease and those who have compromised immune systems. Adults who smoke, regardless of age, should also receive the vaccination. Most adults will need the pneumococcal vaccine only one time to receive protection for the rest of their life. The pneumococcal vaccines are inactivated bacterial vaccines and they do not entirely protect against acquiring pneumonia, but they do decrease the severity of the illness if it is acquired.

Pneumonia is the most common infectious cause of death in the United States.

Signs and Symptoms of Pneumonia

Cough is the most persistent symptom associated with pneumonia **FIGURE 9.5**. Patients also experience an abrupt onset of fever, chills, and shortness of breath. Chest pain may also be present. A sputum culture can be used to identify the causative agent of the infection.

Treatment of Pneumonia

The goal of pneumonia treatment is to alleviate symptoms and cure the infection. If the causative microorganism is known, antimicrobial agents will be administered to treat

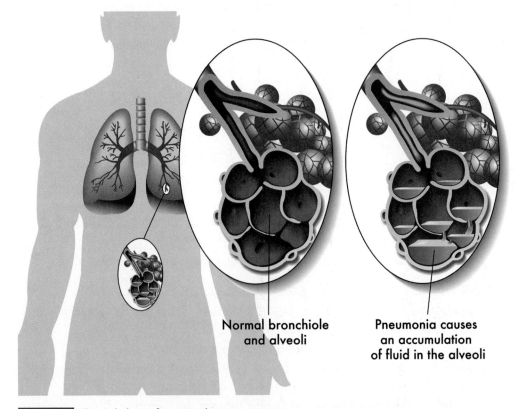

Normal bronchiole and alveoli

Pneumonia causes an accumulation of fluid in the alveoli

FIGURE 9.5 The respiratory pathology of pneumonia.
© Rob3000/ShutterStock, Inc.

Sputum Cultures: What the Patient Needs to Know

Sputum cultures identify infectious organisms in the respiratory tract. The patient must follow specific steps prior to sputum collection to ensure accurate results:

1. The sputum sample is usually collected in the morning, before the patient eats or drinks.

2. The patient should not use mouthwash prior to the collection because mouthwash may contain antibacterial agents that could alter the results of the culture.

3. The patient should cough deeply to loosen mucus in the lungs and spit the sputum into a collection container.

4. The patient can take several deep breaths to assist with coughing up sputum instead of saliva.

5. A bronchoscopy or catheterization may be used to collect a sputum sample if a patient is unable to cough on his own.

© auremar/ShutterStock, Inc.

the infection. If the causative microorganism has not been identified, broad-spectrum treatment—that is, treatment that is effective against a wide range of disease-causing bacteria—will be initiated based on local surveillance and susceptibility data.

Supportive treatment is often useful for pneumonia, which includes fluids, rest, and breathing humidified air. Symptoms often resolve within two weeks in most healthy individuals.

Cystic Fibrosis

Cystic fibrosis is a genetic disease characterized by thick, filmy secretions that build up in the respiratory and digestive tracts. It is commonly seen in children and young adults, and it is often diagnosed before the age of two years. Cystic fibrosis is the most common life-threatening genetic disorder among Caucasians.

In cystic fibrosis, thick mucus builds up in the lungs, making it difficult to breathe and easy to acquire frequent respiratory infections. In the early stages of cystic fibrosis, the small airways and bronchioles are blocked by mucus production; in later stages, the larger airways are affected.

Signs and Symptoms of Cystic Fibrosis

In newborns, cystic fibrosis is often evidenced by delayed growth, no bowel movement in the first 24 to 48 hours of life, and salty skin. (In cystic fibrosis, the cells of the body are unable to transport chloride ions, so sodium and chloride—the components of salt—are excreted by the body through sweat. This leads to salty tasting sweat and skin and, sometimes, visible deposits of salt on the surface of the skin. The sweat test is used diagnostically for cystic fibrosis.) Children with cystic fibrosis may not gain weight appropriately, and may experience abdominal pain, nausea, and loss of appetite. Pulmonary symptoms include coughing, fatigue, nasal congestion, recurrent episodes of pneumonia and other respiratory infections, and sinus pain or pressure. The repeated infections lead to pulmonary scarring or fibrosis.

Treatment of Cystic Fibrosis

There is no cure for cystic fibrosis. In the future, gene therapy may be applicable to cystic fibrosis, but current therapy aims at slowing or stopping the disease progression. Ideally, patients will receive an early diagnosis and be able to develop and grow normally and live active lifestyles.

Treatments include percussion, a tapping motion to induce cough and release mucus from the lungs; nebulizers to liquefy secretions; and bronchodilators to open the respiratory tracts. Antibiotics are used to treat recurrent infections.

All patients with cystic fibrosis must remain up to date on vaccines and work to prevent infections as much as possible. This includes staying away from sources of pollution and infection and remaining in optimal physical health through diet and exercise. The treatment for cystic fibrosis is multidisciplinary and long-term.

Tuberculosis

Tuberculosis (TB) is a contagious bacterial disease that causes an infection in the lining of the lungs. It is caused by the bacterium *Mycobacterium tuberculosis*, which is transmitted by contact with infected droplets containing the bacteria. Once inhaled, the bacteria spread through the blood and lymph systems.

TB develops slowly. It may take several weeks for symptoms to develop after exposure to the bacteria. In the United States and other developed nations, TB is usually confined to immunocompromised patients, elderly patients, and prison populations. However, TB remains the most communicable infectious disease on earth, occurring frequently and uncontrollably in underdeveloped nations. The treatment of TB lasts six to nine months. As with all antibiotic treatments, the patient should be encouraged to follow through with the therapy and take all the medication as scheduled and prescribed or be at risk for the TB to return.

Signs and Symptoms of Tuberculosis

Patients with TB experience weight loss, a productive cough, fever, and night sweats **FIGURE 9.6**. Blood in the **sputum** or mucus of the lower respiratory tract is often the first serious symptom that will prompt a patient to obtain medical treatment. A **sputum culture** is completed to confirm the presence of the infectious organism. Chest X-rays and skin tests are also used to diagnose TB. Chest X-rays can reveal current, active TB infections in the lungs, as well as fibrosis and scarring due to previous, inactive infections. To diagnose TB using a skin test, a small amount of purified protein from TB-causing bacteria is injected intradermally. If a person has TB, the site of administration will become red and swollen, known as a positive test. If no infection is present, there will be no reaction to the purified protein, known as a negative test. For more information on diagnostic skin tests and intradermal injections, see Chapter 11.

Treatment of Tuberculosis

The goal of TB treatment is to alleviate the symptoms of infection and eradicate the causative organism. First, a patient with TB will be isolated, often in a negative-pressure hospital room, to prevent the spread of the disease. The two most common antibiotics used to treat TB are Rifampin and Isoniazid, but bacteria resistant to these agents are becoming more common, decreasing their effectiveness and increasing the danger associated with TB infections.

The Common Cold and Other Infectious Conditions

Infectious microorganisms cause many common ailments of the respiratory system, including the common cold, laryngitis, bronchitis, tonsillitis, sinusitis, and respiratory syncytial virus (RSV). The symptoms of these conditions overlap extensively or the conditions may occur together. For many of these illnesses, prevention is the best medicine. Frequent hand washing and hygiene are essential to preventing the spread of infectious organisms.

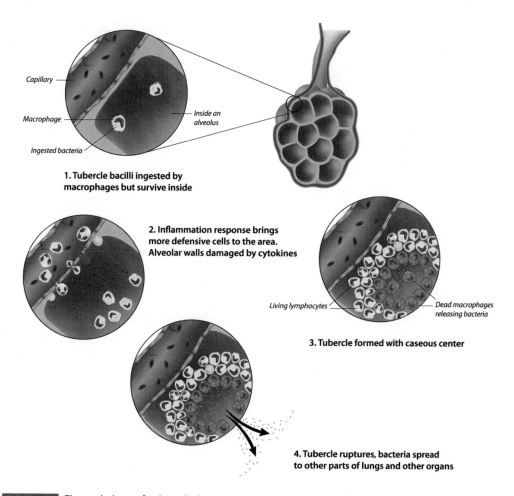

1. Tubercle bacilli ingested by macrophages but survive inside

Capillary

Macrophage

Inside an alveolus

Ingested bacteria

2. Inflammation response brings more defensive cells to the area. Alveolar walls damaged by cytokines

Living lymphocytes *Dead macrophages releasing bacteria*

3. Tubercle formed with caseous center

4. Tubercle ruptures, bacteria spread to other parts of lungs and other organs

FIGURE 9.6 The pathology of tuberculosis.
© Alila Sao Mai/ShutterStock, Inc.

Signs and Symptoms of the Common Cold and Other Infectious Conditions

The common cold is caused by one of hundreds of viruses. Symptoms often include sneezing, rhinorrhea (runny nose), nasal congestion, cough, and sore throat. A fever indicates a possible bacterial infection.

Laryngitis, an inflammation of the larynx, may occur independently as the result of an infection or chronic irritation or from inhaling irritants, such as smoke. Hoarseness is the most common symptom of laryngitis. Cough and sore throat are also common symptoms.

Bronchitis is an inflammation of the bronchi and bronchioles. Acute bronchitis is often caused by a virus and is characterized by a nonproductive cough that changes to a productive cough.

Tonsillitis, an inflammation of the tonsils, is often caused by the *Streptococcus* bacteria. The infection is most commonly seen in children. A sudden onset of sore throat or fever often accompanies chills, headache, loss of appetite, and lethargy. The tonsils will be visibly red and swollen.

Sinusitis is an inflammation of the lining of the sinuses. It may result from an acute infection or a chronic condition. The symptoms of sinusitis resemble those of a cold, but are more severe. Severe,

The respiratory symptoms of allergies are the same as those of a common cold. But, allergies are an immune reaction in response to a particular allergen, such as pollen or pet dander, instead of an infectious agent. The same medications can be used to treat the symptoms of allergies and the common cold. Trigger identification and avoidance also mitigate allergy symptoms.
© auremar/ShutterStock, Inc.

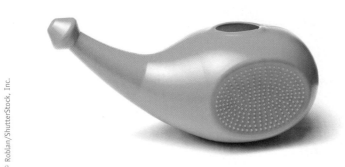

A neti pot can be used for nasal irrigation.

© Roblan/ShutterStock, Inc.

painful headaches, as well as facial and nasal pain, are symptoms of acute sinusitis. Patients also experience a nasal discharge and a sore throat and cough. In cases of chronic sinusitis, the symptoms are milder and are accompanied by a nonproductive cough and malodorous breath.

Respiratory syncytial virus (RSV) is one of the most common respiratory illnesses affecting children. Early symptoms are often confused with those of a common cold but progress to more serious symptoms that include shortness of breath, fever, wheezing, a barking cough, and decreased oxygenation. RSV can be life threatening to very young infants. Infants born prematurely, those with low birth weight, or those experiencing failure to thrive are at the highest risk for a serious infection.

Treatment of the Common Cold and Other Infectious Conditions

The goals of treatment of infectious diseases of the respiratory system are to eradicate the infection, if possible, and improve the patient's symptoms. In the case of viral infections, antibiotics are not effective, so treatment is entirely supportive. Patients should get plenty of rest and drink fluids. Pain relief, cough suppressants, expectorants, decongestants, and antihistamines are appropriate for treatment, depending on the patient's symptoms. Most viral infections are self-limiting and symptoms resolve in 7 to 10 days. Serious cases of RSV and other infections require hospitalization for administration of fluids and oxygen. If a bacterial agent is identified as the cause of the infection, antibiotics are effective. Symptomatic treatment is also appropriate.

Nasal irrigation is a symptomatic treatment that can be used for nasal congestion associated with the common cold, sinusitis, allergies, and other upper-respiratory conditions. Nasal irrigation cleanses the lining of the nose and nasal passages and removes excess mucus and debris. To irrigate the nasal passages, warm saline solution is flushed through the nostrils, either by inhaling water from cupped hands or pouring water into one nostril and letting it run out the other. Nasal cleansing can also be accomplished by employing topical saline spray delivered to the nostrils.

Salt water must be used for nasal irrigation. Ordinary tap water cannot be used because it increases the risk of infection and is uncomfortable and irritating to the mucous membranes of the upper respiratory tract.

Epistaxis

Epistaxis, or a nosebleed, can occur as the result of trauma to the nose, chemical irritants, a nasal infection, or the drying of the mucous membranes of the nose. Clotting disorders, hemorrhagic disease, high blood pressure, or nasal tumors can also cause nosebleeds. Certain medications, including blood thinners and topical decongestants, can cause or worsen nosebleeds. Although frightening and sometimes difficult to manage, nosebleeds are rarely serious or life threatening.

Topical decongestants, administered as nasal sprays, are effective symptomatic relief for nasal congestion, but these agents cannot be used for more than three consecutive days due to the occurrence of rebound congestion.

© auremar/ShutterStock, Inc.

Signs and Symptoms of Epistaxis

A nosebleed leads to blood loss from the nose. Bleeding usually occurs from only one side of the nose at a time. If bleeding continues for more than 20 minutes or is profuse and uncontrollable, patients should seek medical attention.

Treatment of Epistaxis

To stop a nosebleed, patients should sit comfortably and pinch the nostrils together gently. Lean slightly forward to avoid swallowing blood. Wait at least 10 minutes to check if bleeding has stopped. If needed, patients can apply ice or cold compresses to the bridge of the nose to slow or stop bleeding. Patients should not lie down during a nosebleed and they should avoid blowing or sniffling their nose for several hours after the bleeding has stopped. If a nosebleed is severe, a physician may choose to cauterize the bleeding area.

Skills for the Medical Assistant

As a medical assistant, you will have the opportunity to assist with respiratory examinations and procedures, including administering oxygen, administering nebulizer treatments, obtaining a throat culture and peak flow, instructing patients on how to use an inhaler, and performing a pulse oximetry test. These tests and procedures allow accurate diagnosis of acute conditions and evaluation of chronic conditions. Patients and their caregivers require a supportive environment and caring staff before, during, and after these procedures to ensure optimal health outcomes.

Administering Oxygen

Supplemental oxygen may be required to assist a patient with breathing. Oxygen can be administered through a nasal cannula or face mask connected by tubing to a portable oxygen container. Oxygen may be administered in a hospital or medical office setting during periods of acute respiratory distress, or patients may have portable oxygen containers for continuous oxygen supplementation. Caution should be exercised when administering oxygen to COPD patients. When more than two liters of oxygen is administered, there is risk of decreasing the drive to breathe. In this section, you will learn how to administer oxygen through a nasal cannula or face mask for minor respiratory distress.

Advise patients that oxygen is a highly combustible gas and fires are a hazard associated with oxygen use. Friction, static electricity, or a lighted cigarette can ignite a fire.

Equipment Needed

- Portable oxygen tank
- Disposable nasal cannula or face mask with tubing
- Flow meter
- Pressure regulator

Steps

1. Obtain the required equipment and supplies. Wash your hands.
2. Identify the patient and explain the procedure.
3. Open the container of oxygen by turning the knob one full counterclockwise turn.
4. Attach the nasal cannula or face mask to the tubing. Attach the tubing to the flow meter FIGURE 9.7 .

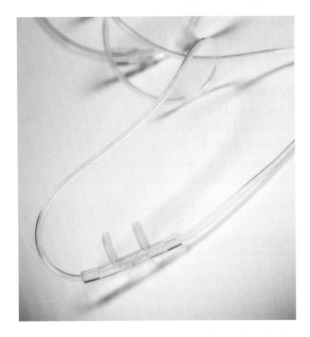

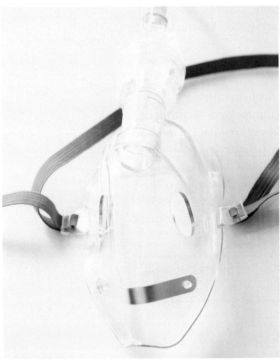

FIGURE 9.7 Nasal cannula (top) and face mask (bottom).
(Top) © GWImages/ShutterStock, Inc.; (Bottom) © 123RF

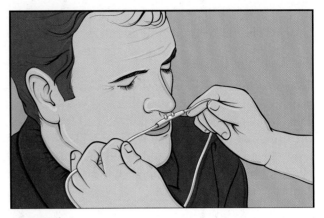

FIGURE 9.8 Insert the tips of the cannulas into the patient's nostrils.
© Jones & Bartlett Learning

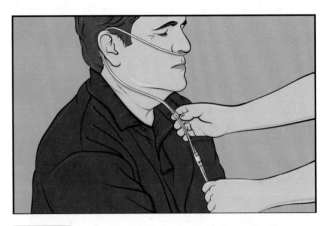

FIGURE 9.9 Secure the tubing underneath the patient's chin.
© Jones & Bartlett Learning

5. Adjust the flow rate according to the physician's orders. Check for oxygen flow through the cannula.

6. Place the tips of the cannulas into the nostrils or face mask over the mouth and nose of the patient. Take care not to insert the cannula more than one inch into the nostril FIGURE 9.8.

7. Drape the tubing behind the patient's ears and bring it forward toward the chin FIGURE 9.9.

8. Instruct the patient to breathe normally and comfortably. Monitor for signs of anxiety or distress.

9. Document the procedure in the patient's chart. For example, "1630: Administered O_2 3L/min via nasal cannula; Pulse 75, BP 130/80, PulseOx 98 percent. J. Jones, CMA."

Performing Pulse Oximetry Testing

Pulse oximetry is a simple, noninvasive test that measures the oxygen saturation levels of a person's blood.

Several respiratory conditions require routine monitoring of oxygen levels, including asthma, pneumonia, and other infections. Most pulse oximetry devices are small, handheld monitors that are clipped to a patient's finger. The sensor contains an infrared light that travels through the tissue of the patient's fingertip to a photo sensor on the opposite side. The monitor reports a percentage, which is interpreted as the percentage of oxygen saturation of the blood. A normal reading is 95 percent or higher. If the fingertip cannot be used for pulse oximetry, the clip can be placed on a toe, earlobe, or the bridge of the nose. In this section, you will learn how to perform a pulse oximetry test.

Equipment Needed

- Pulse oximeter
- Alcohol wipes

Steps

1. Obtain the required equipment and supplies. Wash your hands.
2. Identify the patient and explain the procedure.
3. Select a site to place the sensor. If the fingers are calloused, have poor circulation, are small (as in the case of a child), or have nail polish, select a site other than the finger.
4. Clean the sensor with an alcohol wipe.
5. Apply the sensor and read the results **FIGURE 9.10** .
6. Record the results, including the patient's pulse. Notify the physician immediately of abnormal results.
7. Document the test, including site of application and its results, in the patient's chart. For example, "1215: PulseOx test on right index finger; PulseOx 99 percent; patient tolerated well. J. Jones, CMA."

Administering Nebulizer Treatment

Nebulizers are used to deliver medication as a fine mist directly into the lungs. A nebulizer may be used instead of an MDI, particularly if patients have difficulty using an MDI. Nebulizer treatments are common in asthma, cystic fibrosis, and COPD. Compressed air and oxygen create an aerosol mist of medication placed in the machine, and a patient inhales the mist. In this section, you will learn how to administer a nebulizer treatment.

Equipment Needed

- Nebulizer
- Tubing
- Mouthpiece or face mask
- Medication

Steps

1. Obtain the required equipment and supplies. Wash your hands.
2. Identify the patient and explain the procedure. Instruct the patient to sit in a comfortable, semi-upright position.

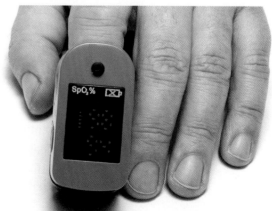

FIGURE 9.10 Applying a pulse oximeter, a normal reading is above 90 percent.
© RobByron/ShutterStock, Inc.

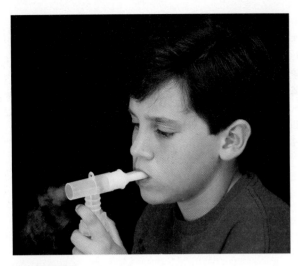

FIGURE 9.11 A nebulizer.
© iStockphoto/Thinkstock

3. Plug in the nebulizer and attach tubing to the machine **FIGURE 9.11**.

4. Measure and add the prescribed amount of medication and **diluent**, an inactive solution added to dry powder to prepare it for administration, or the liquid or solid medication as supplied, to the nebulizer cup.

5. Attach the tubing from the machine to the bottom of the nebulizer cup. Attach the mouthpiece to the top of the cup.

6. Place the mouthpiece in the patient's mouth (over the tongue and between the teeth) or place the face mask on the patient's face, covering the nose and mouth.

7. Turn the nebulizer on. Hold the nebulizer cup upright during the entire procedure. A fine mist should be seen emitting from the mouthpiece.

8. Instruct patients to breathe normally and comfortably through the face mask. If patients have difficulty breathing through their mouths when using a mouthpiece, a clip may be placed on the nose during the treatment.

9. Continue the treatment until all the medication has been administered, approximately 10 minutes.

10. Turn off the nebulizer and disassemble the tubing and mouthpiece or face mask. Place in the proper storage or cleaning receptacles.

11. Document the procedure in the patient's chart. For example, "1045: Administered Albuterol 2.5 mg via nebulizer; patient tolerated well. J. Jones, CMA."

Instructing Patients on the Use of an MDI

An MDI delivers a specific amount of medication in an aerosol form. MDIs are often used to treat asthma and COPD. A spacer should always be used to ensure the patient receives the full dosage. A spacer also helps to deliver the medication more slowly, allowing better penetration into the lungs. In this section, you will learn how to instruct a patient on the correct use of an MDI.

Equipment Needed

- Inhaler
- Spacer

Steps

1. Obtain the required equipment and supplies. Wash your hands.

2. Identify the patient and explain the procedure.

3. Teach the patient to prime the inhaler prior to use by shaking it for five seconds. Next, remove the cap and mouthpiece from the inhaler. Insert the stem of the inhaler into the flattened portion of the spacer. Expel the dose of medication from the inhaler into the spacer.

4. Instruct the patient to exhale fully and place the mouthpiece of the spacer in his or her mouth, biting gently with the teeth and closing the lips around

the mouthpiece or spacer FIGURE 9.12 . Alternatively, patients may use an open-mouth technique and hold the mouthpiece one to two inches from their mouth; this method may prevent medication from adhering to the back of the throat.

5. Instruct the patient to tilt his or her head back slightly and inhale the medication from the spacer slowly and deeply through the mouth. Continue to inhale until the lungs are full. For each dose administered from the inhaler, the patient should inhale two times from the spacer.

6. Instruct the patient to hold his or her breath for 10 seconds and then exhale slowly through pursed lips.

7. Repeat steps 3–6 if more than one dose has been ordered. Wait 30 to 60 seconds between inhalations.

8. Disassemble the spacer and the inhaler and rinse the mouthpieces with warm water. Place the cap on the inhaler and return the inhaler and spacer to its proper storage. Wash your hands.

9. Document the procedure in the patient's chart. For example, "1050: Instructed patient on use of MDI; patient tolerated well and demonstrated understanding. J. Jones, CMA."

The patient may gargle with normal saline solution or water after the administration of medication by MDI to remove any residual medication from the back of the throat.

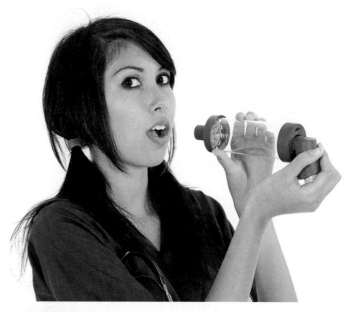

FIGURE 9.12 Demonstrate the use of an MDI to ensure the patient uses correct technique.
© iStockphoto.co/GordonsLife

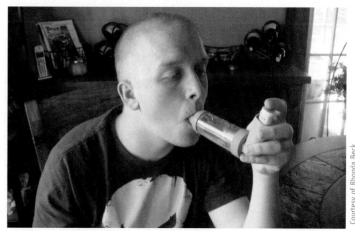

A spacer can help patients use an MDI correctly.

Courtesy of Rhonda Beck

Using a Peak Flow Meter

A peak flow meter measures the PEF of expired air. It is a routine test for asthma and other respiratory conditions, and can be used to assess the effectiveness of therapy, identify the triggers of respiratory distress, and indicate when medical care is needed for acute symptoms. A peak flow meter is a simple test and is appropriate for children and adults. In this section, you will learn how to assist a patient with the use of a peak flow meter.

An MDI contains a compressed gas as a propellant to expel the medication from the device. A dry powder inhaler (DPI) does not contain a propellant. If the patient is using a DPI, the procedure for administration of medication is the same, except that the patient should be instructed to inhale quickly.
© auremar/ShutterStock, Inc.

Equipment Needed

■ Peak flow meter
■ Mouthpiece

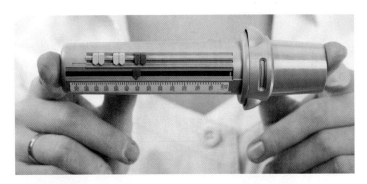

FIGURE 9.13 A peak flow meter.
© Dennis Mironov/ShutterStock, Inc.

Steps

1. Obtain the required equipment and supplies **FIGURE 9.13**. Wash your hands.
2. Identify the patient and explain the procedure. Instruct the patient to stand, if possible.
3. Ensure the red indicator is at the bottom of the scale on the meter.
4. Instruct the patient to hold the meter upright and not block the opening in the back.
5. Instruct the patient to inhale fully and place the mouthpiece of the meter in his or her mouth, biting gently with the teeth.
6. Instruct the patient to exhale one breath as hard and as fast as possible.
7. Record the reading on the meter. Slide the red indicator to the bottom of the scale.
8. Instruct the patient to repeat the test two more times, for a total of three readings.
9. Disassemble the peak flow meter and place the meter and the mouthpiece in the proper disposal or storage receptacle.
10. Document the test and record the highest reading in the patient's chart. For example, "1535: Completed peak flow test; PEF 430 L/min; patient tolerated well. J. Jones, CMA."

Obtaining a Throat Culture

A throat culture can be used to identify the organism causing an infection of the nasopharynx area or tonsils. The procedure may cause brief discomfort for the patient, so warn the patient that this may occur. Make sure you are in a well-lit area when performing this procedure. In this section, you will learn how to obtain a throat culture.

Equipment Needed

- Tongue depressor
- Culture tube with applicator stick (or commercially available culturette)
- Labels and requisition forms, as required
- Gloves and face shield
- Emesis basin and tissues

Steps

1. Obtain the required equipment and supplies **FIGURE 9.14**. Wash your hands.
2. Identify the patient and explain the procedure. Instruct the patient to sit comfortably.
3. Keep the emesis basin close to the patient throughout the procedure, as the process of obtaining the throat culture may initiate vomiting in some patients.
4. Wash your hands and apply gloves and the face shield.
5. Instruct the patient to open his or her mouth wide and say "ah."
6. Remove the swab from the culture tube or culturette using sterile technique.
7. Depress the patient's tongue with the tongue depressor and swab the back of the throat and the tonsils. Concentrate on red, swollen, or pus-filled areas. Do not touch the inside of the cheeks or the tongue.

8. Insert the swab into the culture tube using sterile technique and following the manufacturer's instructions.

9. Label the culture tube.

10. Discard contaminated supplies in a bio-hazard waste container.

11. Wash your hands and complete the required laboratory requisition paperwork.

12. Document the procedure in the patient's chart. For example, "0725: Throat culture specimen obtained and sent to AB labs for C&S; patient tolerated well. J. Jones, CMA."

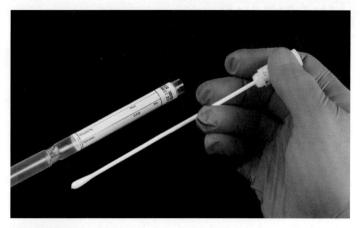

FIGURE 9.14 Culture tubes and swabs.
© Adam Fraise/ShutterStock, Inc.

Math Practice

Question: A physician prescribes amoxicillin 90mg/kg/day divided into three doses for a child diagnosed with pneumonia. The child is four years old and weighs 36 pounds. What is the total daily dose of amoxicillin?

Answer: 36 lb × 1kg ÷ 2.2 lb = 16.4kg

90mg/kg/day × 16.4kg = 1,476mg/day

Question: A physician prescribes albuterol syrup 4mg three times daily. What is the total daily dose of albuterol?

Answer: 4mg × 3 times/day = 12mg/day

Question: A six-year-old child is experiencing symptoms of a common cold. The parents are advised to administer the antihistamine diphenhydramine 25mg every six hours for symptom relief. What is the total daily dose of diphenhydramine?

Answer: 24 hours/day × 1 dose ÷ 6 hours = 4 doses/day

25mg/dose × 4 doses/day = 100mg/day

Question: A physician prescribes levalbuterol to be administered by nebulizer: levalbuterol 0.63mg/3mL, administer one 3mL vial three times daily. What is the total dose of medication in a 30-day supply?

Answer: 0.63mg × 3 doses ÷ 1 day × 30 days = 56.7mg

Question: A 17-year-old patient is allergic to penicillin. The physician prescribes azithromycin for pharyngitis caused by *Streptococcus* bacteria. He orders azithromycin 500mg on day 1, 250mg one time daily on days 2–5. What is the total dose of azithromycin in the five-day course?

Answer: 500mg/day + 250mg/day × 4 days = 1,500 mg

WRAP UP

Chapter Summary

- The primary function of the respiratory system is gas exchange. During respiration, oxygen is removed from inspired air and carbon dioxide is exhaled as a waste product in expired air. The respiratory system is highly integrated with other body systems and must be a continuous process.

- The major organs of the respiratory system are the nose, pharynx, larynx, trachea, bronchi, and lungs. The upper respiratory tract filters, warms, and humidifies air. The upper respiratory tract is covered with mucus and cilia that filter inspired air and protect the body from inhaling foreign objects and infectious organisms into the lungs. The lower respiratory tract facilitates gas exchange.

- Cough is a defensive, protective reflex that forces mucus, cellular debris, and foreign objects out of the lower respiratory tract. Cough can be triggered by infections, environmental contaminants, and chronic respiratory conditions. A productive cough expels secretions from the respiratory tract; a nonproductive cough is a dry cough that serves no physiological purpose. Antitussives eliminate the symptoms of a nonproductive cough, and protussives or expectorants facilitate the release of secretions in a productive cough.

- Asthma is a chronic inflammatory condition of the airways that is caused by a combination of environmental, genetic, and immune-mediated factors. Asthma symptoms include recurrent episodes of wheezing, breathlessness, chest tightening, and coughing. Ideally, patients will identify and avoid triggers of asthma exacerbations. Anti-inflammatory drugs, bronchodilators, and immune modulators can control the frequency and severity of asthma exacerbations.

- COPD is a progressive disease of airflow limitation. COPD is characterized by chronic bronchitis, an inflammation of the lungs, and emphysema, a destruction of the alveoli. Symptoms of COPD can be managed with anti-inflammatory drugs, bronchodilators, immune modulators, and anticholinergic agents.

Smoking cessation can slow the progression of COPD.

- Pneumonia is an infection in one or both lungs caused by bacteria, viruses, or fungi. Cough, fever, chills, and shortness of breath are symptoms of pneumonia. Antibiotics, as well as supportive treatment including rest, fluids, and breathing humidified air, alleviate the symptoms of pneumonia.

- Cystic fibrosis is a genetic disease that produces thick, filmy secretions in the respiratory and digestive tracts. The build-up of mucus blocks the airways, making breathing difficult and leading to recurrent respiratory infections. There is no cure for cystic fibrosis, but the disease can be managed with a healthy lifestyle and a multidisciplinary involvement.

- Tuberculosis is a contagious bacterial infection of the lungs. Symptoms of tuberculosis include a productive cough, fever, night sweats, and blood in the sputum. Antibiotics are used to treat tuberculosis, but their effectiveness is decreasing due to the emergence of bacterial resistance.

- The respiratory tract is susceptible to many contagious infections, including the common cold, laryngitis, bronchitis, tonsillitis, sinusitis, and respiratory syncytial virus. The symptoms of these conditions overlap and the conditions can also occur simultaneously. Infection control, including frequent hand washing and hygiene, can prevent these infections. Infectious conditions caused by bacteria can be treated with antibiotics, but those caused by a virus cannot. Treatment for all infectious illnesses should include supportive care and symptom relief.

- Epistaxis, or a nosebleed, is the loss of blood from the nose and can be caused by trauma, infection, irritation of the nose, drying of the mucous membranes, and other medical conditions and medications. Bleeding is normally minimal and controllable with self-care. If bleeding is excessive or continues for more than 20 minutes, patients should seek medical attention.

- Medical assistants have the opportunity to assist with respiratory examinations and procedures, as well as instruct patients on the use of respiratory devices for use at home. The procedures require a calm, confident attitude and the establishment of a rapport with the patient and caregivers because respiratory conditions are often sources of high anxiety for patients.

Learning Assessment Questions

1. What is the primary function of the respiratory system?
   A. Gas exchange
   B. Control heart rate
   C. Maintain blood pressure
   D. Remove waste from the body
2. How many respiratory cycles does the average human adult complete in one minute?
   A. 2 to 3
   B. 7 to 10
   C. 12 to 20
   D. 95
3. The function of the respiratory system is integrated with which other body system?
   A. The endocrine system
   B. The cardiovascular system
   C. The digestive system
   D. The musculoskeletal system
4. Which of the following structures is correctly matched with its function?
   A. Alveoli: direct air flow to larger branches of the respiratory system
   B. Larynx: filters air
   C. Upper respiratory tract: filters, warms, and humidifies inspired air
   D. Cilia: destroy bacteria with lysozyme
5. Which of the following structures in the respiratory system is the smallest?
   A. Bronchioles
   B. Bronchi
   C. Capillaries
   D. Alveoli
6. A bronchoscope can be used for all but which of the following?
   A. Administering nebulizer treatments
   B. Visualizing the bronchi
   C. Collecting a biopsy or sputum sample
   D. Removing foreign objects from the respiratory tract

7. Which of the following are common symptoms of an asthma exacerbation?
   A. Fever, chills, nausea, and vomiting
   B. Sore throat, nasal congestion, and sneezing
   C. Wheezing, breathlessness, chest tightening, and coughing
   D. Shortness of breath and frequent respiratory infections
8. Corticosteroids are used for what purpose?
   A. Decreasing inflammation
   B. Expanding the airways
   C. Increasing secretions
   D. Relaxing the muscles of the respiratory system
9. What is the most common cause of COPD?
   A. A genetic disorder
   B. Cigarette smoking
   C. Allergies
   D. A respiratory infection
10. What are the five As of smoking cessation?
    A. Acknowledge, analyze, arrest, allow, accept
    B. Ask, account, abide, abstain, accept
    C. Advise, agree, align, assist, allow
    D. Ask, advise, assess, assist, arrange
11. Which of the following lists the correct path of inspired air?
    A. Nose, pharynx, trachea, primary bronchi, secondary bronchi, bronchioles, alveoli
    B. Nose, pharynx, lungs, capillaries, pulmonary artery
    C. Sinus cavities, larynx, bronchi, lungs
    D. Trachea, alveoli, bronchioles, primary bronchi, secondary bronchi

12. All are true regarding cystic fibrosis *except* which of the following?
    A. It involves abnormalities of the respiratory and digestive tracts.
    B. It is usually diagnosed before the age of two years.
    C. It is caused by a viral infection.
    D. It causes scarring in the lungs due to recurrent infections.

13. What is the most common communicable infectious disease in the world?
    A. Pneumonia
    B. Respiratory syncytial virus
    C. Tuberculosis
    D. Common cold

14. What is the function of an antitussive?
    A. Suppress nonproductive coughs
    B. Decrease inflammation of the airways
    C. Decrease the volume of mucus in the lungs
    D. Relax the diaphragm

15. Which of the following is the most widely available expectorant?
    A. Dextromethorphan
    B. Isoniazid
    C. Eucalyptus
    D. Guaifenesin

16. When should a patient seek medical attention for epistaxis?
    A. If the bleeding does not stop in 20 minutes or is uncontrollable
    B. If the bleeding occurs from both nostrils
    C. If the bleeding is accompanied by a headache
    D. If the patient is also taking blood thinners

17. What is a hazard of oxygen administration?
    A. Decreased blood pressure
    B. Increased heart rate
    C. Fire
    D. Nasal irritation

18. What does pulse oximetry measure?
    A. Forced expiratory volume
    B. Total lung capacity
    C. Arterial blood gases
    D. Oxygenation of the blood

19. What is the function of a spacer?
    A. To allow for a larger dose of medication to be administered from a metered dose inhaler
    B. To deliver medication more slowly from a metered dose inhaler and allow better penetration into the lungs
    C. To prevent medication from a metered dose inhaler from adhering to the back of the throat
    D. To delay administration of medication from a metered dose inhaler

20. What does a peak flow meter measure?
    A. Rate of gas exchange
    B. Vital capacity
    C. Peak expiratory flow
    D. Volume of oxygen delivery

21. Difficulty breathing is called _____.
    A. Tachypnea
    B. Dyspnea
    C. Pleurisy
    D. Thoracentesis

22. A runny nose is also referred to as _____.
    A. Rhinorrhea
    B. Anosmia
    C. Dyphonia
    D. Sinusitis

23. The correct abbreviation for oxygen is _____.
    A. Ox
    B. POX
    C. O_2
    D. Oxy

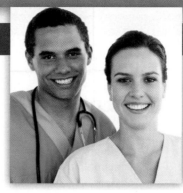

Pharmacology and Medication Administration

OBJECTIVES

After reading this chapter, you will be able to:

- Describe three types of drug names and give an example, for one drug, of all three names.
- Name the five controlled substances schedules and describe the appropriate storage of the substances.
- Describe the principal actions of drugs and three undesirable reactions.
- Describe routes of drug administration and drug forms.
- Describe handling and storing of drugs.
- List emergency drugs and supplies.
- Critique the legal role and responsibilities of the medical assistant.
- Discuss the legal and ethical implications of medication administration.
- Describe the medication order.
- Describe the parts of a prescription.
- Define drug dosage.
- Explain what information is found on a medication label.
- List the guidelines to follow when preparing and administering medications.
- Understand allergenic extracts.
- Describe inhalation medication and its administration.

KEY TERMS

Absorption	Elimination	Pharmacodynamic agent
Allergic reaction	Histamine	Pharmacology
Anaphylactic reaction	Hypoxemia	Prescription
Anaphylaxis	Indication	Prophylactic agent
Antineoplastic drugs	Isotope	Prophylaxis
Contraindication	Local effect	Route of administration
Controlled substance	Medication order	Side effect
Destructive agent	Metabolism	Synergistic effect
Diagnostic agent	Order	Systemic effect
Distribution	Over-the-counter drugs	Therapeutic agent
Dosage form	Parenteral	Therapeutic effect
Drug	Peroral (PO)	Transdermal patch
Drug dependence		

Chapter Overview

This chapter reviews basic fundamentals of pharmacology and medication administration. The legal form that a prescriber utilizes to order a medication, medical device, or piece of medical equipment to be dispensed to a patient is called a **prescription**. This chapter covers the legally required elements of a prescription and the information a medical assistant must know in order to administer a medication to the patient.

Pharmacology

During the 19th century, Claude Bernard, a French physiologist, used the laboratory to determine the relationship between drugs and their sites of action within the body. He established **pharmacology**—the study of drugs and their properties and how they interact with the body—as a discipline of study.

Pharmacology is the study of drugs and their properties and how they interact with the body.

Drugs

A **drug** is any substance used for the diagnosis, cure, treatment, or prevention of a disease or that is intended to affect the structure or function of any living system. Drugs can be made from a variety of sources. They can be derived from sources such as plants, animals, minerals, or chemicals. Drugs can also be produced by recombinant DNA technology. Most drugs available on the market today are synthesized from naturally occurring chemicals.

Drug Names

The manufacturer of each drug assigns a chemical name, a generic name, and a brand name (also called a trade name) to each drug:

- The chemical name describes the chemical structure of the drug.
- The generic name is often a shortened version of the chemical name. It is the drug's official name and is assigned to the drug by the U.S. Adopted Names

Council. It describes the drug without any indication to the name of the manufacturer.

- The brand name is the name under which the manufacturer markets the drug and is the name that is found on the product's official label. The brand name is protected by a patent; only the company that holds the patent has the right to market that product under that name. Once the patent expires, different manufacturers are allowed to market the same generic drug under different brand names, or by simply using the generic name.

TABLE 10.1 outlines various drugs' chemical names, generic names, and brand names.

Each drug is assigned a chemical name, generic name, and trade name by the manufacturer.

Drug Regulations and Classifications of Drugs

Medical practitioners who prescribe, dispense, or administer drugs must comply with federal and state laws. The laws govern the manufacture, sale, procurement, possession, administration, prescribing, and dispensing of all drugs. All legal drugs available for use are controlled by the Federal Food, Drug, and Cosmetic Act of 1938. This act called for the creation of the Food and Drug Administration (FDA) and required all drug manufacturers to provide evidence of a drug's safety before any drug could be approved for market. Manufacturers had to ensure the purity, safety, packaging, and strength of the medication. This act also prohibited the interstate commerce of adulterated and misbranded food, drugs, devices, and cosmetics.

Controlled Substances

The Controlled Substances Act (CSA) of 1970 required the pharmaceutical industry to keep records and implement security measures for certain medications. It was created to prevent and control drug abuse. This act divided controlled substances into five schedules, or classes, based on their potential for abuse. Schedule I drugs have the highest abuse potential, while Schedule V drugs have the least. A **controlled substance** is a drug with a potential for abuse or addiction. This act set limits on the number of refills allowed for each schedule. Schedule II drugs are not allowed any refills. Schedule III–IV drugs are allowed five refills, and the prescription is valid for six months from the date of issue. TABLE 10.2 outlines the five schedules under the Controlled Substances Act.

There are five schedules for controlled substances. They are classified based on their potential for abuse. No prescriptions can be written for Schedule I drugs.
© auremar/ShutterStock, Inc.

Table 10.1	Drug Names	
Chemical Name	**Generic Name**	**Brand Name**
N-acetyl-p-aminophenol	Acetaminophen	Tylenol
[R-(R*, R*)]-2-(4-fluorophenyl)-β, δ-dihydroxy-5-(1-methylethyl)-3-phenyl-4-[(phenylamino)carbonyl]-1H-pyrrole-1-heptanoic acid, calcium salt (2:1) trihydrate	Atorvastatin calcium	Lipitor
Acetylsalicylic acid	Aspirin	Bayer Aspirin
(±)-N-methyl-3-phenyl-3-[(α,α,α-trifluoro-p-tolyl)oxy]propylamine hydrochloride	Fluoxetine	Prozac, Sarafem

Table 10.2	The Five Schedules Under the Controlled Substances Act		
Schedule of Drug	**Manufacturer's Label**	**About These Drugs**	**Examples of Drugs**
I	C-I	Drugs have no accepted medical use in the United States; highest abuse potential.	LSD, heroin
II	C-II	Drugs have an accepted medical use; high abuse potential, with severe psychological or physical liability; no refill allowed.	Amphetamines, methadone, opium, morphine, codeine, oxycodone
III	C-III	Drugs have an accepted medical use; moderate abuse potential (less than those in Schedules I and II); five refills allowed.	Combination narcotics such as codeine/acetaminophen, hydrocodone/ acetaminophen, and anabolic steroids
IV	C-IV	Drugs have an accepted medical use; low abuse potential (less than those in Schedule III); five refills allowed.	Benzodiazepines, barbiturates
V	C-V	Drugs have an accepted medical use; lowest abuse potential (less than those in Schedule IV); some drugs may be dispensed over-the-counter if over 18 years of age in some states.	Liquid cough preparations with codeine

The Drug Enforcement Agency (DEA) of the U.S. Justice Department regulates all matters relating to controlled substances. Under federal law, anyone who prescribes, dispenses, or administers controlled substances must register with the DEA **FIGURE 10.1**. The DEA is a federal regulatory body that has published regulations for enforcing the acquisition, storage, dispensing, and documentation of all controlled substances. The DEA works with local and state agencies to ensure compliance with these regulations.

A copy of the federal law and a complete list of controlled substances are available online or from any DEA office.

Storing Controlled Substances

There are strict guidelines not only for prescribing controlled substances, but also for their storage. Federal regulations require that all controlled substances be kept separately from other drugs. They must be stored in a locked cabinet that has a double lock. Controlled substances should be protected from possible misuse, abuse, and diversion, and persons who administer them must keep records on a daily basis. Records of daily counts must be reconciled by two parties who have legally authorized access to controlled substances. These records must be submitted to the DEA every two years and kept for three years. Schedule II controlled substances must be counted at the end of each workday, and verified by two individuals. A record must be submitted to the DEA every two years.

All controlled substances should be kept in a secure, locked cabinet separately from other drugs.

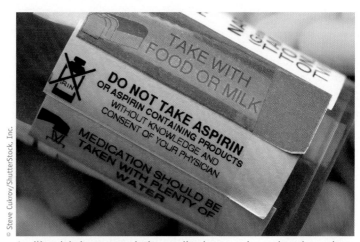

FIGURE 10.1 Form 224: Application for Registration with the Drug Enforcement Agency. The registration must be renewed at regular intervals.

Courtesy of the Drug Enforcement Administration

Medical Assistant Role and Responsibilities

Medical assistants must be well informed about the rules and regulations for controlled substances. Medical assistant responsibilities may include the following:

- Monitoring the healthcare practitioner's DEA registration renewal date
- Maintaining a record and inventory of all drugs and samples
- Keeping all drugs, especially controlled substances, in a secure location
- Keeping all prescription pads in a secure location
- Properly disposing of expired drugs and documenting their disposal
- Understanding federal and state laws that regulate drugs, including controlled substances

Medical assistants must also be able to recognize the symptoms of drug abuse in a patient or in other healthcare professionals. There are many programs available for treatment of drug abuse. The National Institute of Drug Abuse can provide information, treatment options, and programs for drug abuse.

Auxiliary labels on prescription medication containers alert the patient to precautions or special instructions.

© Steve Cukrov/ShutterStock, Inc.

Prescription Drugs

Prescription drugs are drugs that require an order by a licensed practitioner. These drugs can be noncontrolled or controlled substances, with the exception of Schedule I controlled substances.

Disposal of Drugs

All drugs have an expiration date. When that date has been reached, the drug must be removed from inventory and destroyed. Patients should be instructed to take their expired medications to their pharmacy, where pharmacists can arrange to have the medications incinerated. Controlled substances must also be returned to the pharmacy. Disposal of controlled substances must be witnessed and properly documented. For more information on disposal of controlled substances, contact your local DEA.

> Medical assistants must check the expiration date of the drug prior to administering it to the patient.

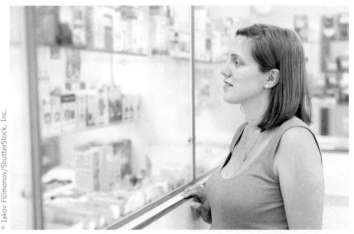

Over-the-counter drugs can be obtained legally without a prescription.

© auremar/ShutterStock, Inc.

Over-the-Counter Drugs

Over-the-counter drugs can be legally obtained without a prescription and are generally safe for use without medical supervision. These drugs are readily accessible to the public.

Although these drugs are generally considered safe, it would be useful for the medical assistant to offer patients some guidelines. Guidelines for patients include the following:

- Take all medication exactly as directed.
- Inform the medical assistant or provider of any side effects or adverse reactions.
- Inform the medical assistant or provider if you discontinue the medication.
- Check with your provider or the medical assistant before you take any new medications or herbal products.
- Store all medications away from children.
- Discard expired or unused medications properly. Many medications lose their potency after a period, while others can become toxic. Encourage patients to inspect their medicine cabinets yearly.

© Iakov Filimonov/ShutterStock, Inc.

Over-the-counter drugs are generally safe for use without medical supervision.

Handling of Drugs

There are three ways to handle drugs: by prescribing them, dispensing them, or administering them. A licensed practitioner with prescribing authority gives a written order to a patient to be taken to the pharmacist to be filled. A pharmacist dispenses the medication as ordered by the provider to the patient. Usually the pharmacist dispenses the medication; however, in some states medical assistants can also dispense samples of drugs under the provider's direction.

The patient or caregiver administers the drug as ordered by the provider. In some states, medical assistants can also prepare and administer medications under the supervision of a licensed prescriber. Although medical assistants work under the license of the physician, legally and ethically, medical assistants are responsible for their own actions and can be subject to legal action should harm come to a patient.

Anyone who has access to medications may be tempted to use them for personal gain. The personal use of medications intended for someone else is not ethical and is illegal. The law requires all medical assistants to know about the medications they are preparing and administering, and their side effects.

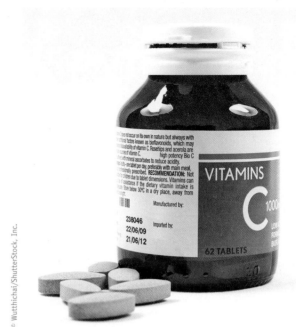

Vitamins are therapeutic agents that maintain health.

Storage of Medications

Many medications have specific storage requirements. Some medications must be stored in a dark container or in the refrigerator. Some must be kept in glass containers because plastic may alter the medication's chemical composition. The drug label will indicate the storage requirements for each drug.

Uses of Drugs

Drugs exert various actions on body organs and systems. Often, the quantity of a drug or how well it binds to the target cell receptor will determine the action of a drug. A drug's mechanism of action also determines how and where it works in the body. How the body affects a drug over a period of time is also crucial to understanding drug actions and disease management with medications.

Drugs can be classified according to their use or pharmacologic effect. Some medications may belong in more than one category.

- A **therapeutic agent** is any drug that relieves symptoms of a disease, stops or delays disease, or maintains health. Examples of therapeutic agents include vitamins, analgesics, antibiotics, and antidepressants.
- A **pharmacodynamic agent** is any drug that alters bodily functions. Examples include drugs used to increase or decrease blood pressure, general anesthetics to cause loss of consciousness, and caffeine to keep people awake.
- A **diagnostic agent** is any drug used in the diagnosis or identification of a disease. Examples include barium sulfate (an agent used commonly for imaging of the gastrointestinal system) and iodinated contrast agents (often used to visualize blood vessels or during a CT).

A therapeutic agent maintains health, relieves symptoms, combats illness, or reverses the disease process.

A pharmacodynamic agent alters bodily functions to elicit a desired response.

A diagnostic agent is any drug that is used for diagnostic purposes.

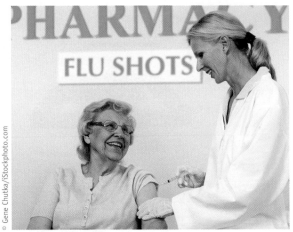

Prophylactic agents such as vaccines prevent an illness or disease from occurring.

Most diagnostic agents are chemicals that contain radioactive isotopes. An **isotope** is a form of a chemical element that contains the same number of protons as the regular element, but a different number of neutrons. Radioactive isotopes give off energy in the form of radiation, which can be used for diagnosis and treatment. One example of a radioactive isotope is iodine-131 (^{131}I).

A **prophylactic agent** is any drug that prevents a disease or illness from occurring. Examples of prophylactic agents include vaccines and antibiotics given for the prevention of disease. A **destructive agent** is a drug that destroys or kills abnormal and sometimes normal cells. Destructive agents can also kill bacteria, fungi, or viruses. Examples include penicillin, **antineoplastic drugs**, which are used to treat cancer, and radioactive iodine.

A prophylactic agent is used to prevent an illness from occurring.

A destructive agent destroys or kills abnormal or normal cells.

Drug Effects

A drug is administered to elicit a response in the body, either to prevent or manage a disease or to prevent or manage symptoms of a disease. Drugs can act like chemical messengers and stimulate certain receptors, causing the human body to react in a specific way. When the receptors are activated, they either trigger a particular response directly on the body or they trigger the release of hormones and/or other endogenous drugs in the body to stimulate a particular response.

The reactions to a drug, both therapeutic and adverse, vary from person to person. Response to drug therapy must be monitored to ensure that the therapy produces the desired effect and minimizes the chances of side effects.

In general, drugs can be grouped as follows:

- Drugs that act directly on the body
- Drugs that act on microorganisms
- Drugs that replace chemicals in the body

Understanding how the body affects a drug over a period of time is critical to understanding drug actions in the body. The four processes are as follows:

- **Absorption**—**Absorption** is the process by which a drug enters or passes through natural body barriers such as the skin, intestines, stomach, and blood-brain barrier and enters the bloodstream.
- **Distribution**—After a drug is absorbed into the bloodstream, it undergoes **distribution**, during which it is distributed to tissues, other body fluids, and ultimately to organs throughout the body.
- **Metabolism**—**Metabolism** is process of biochemical modification or degradation of a drug in the body.
- **Elimination**—**Elimination** is the removal of the drug from the body.

These factors depend on the individual patient, the drug, and the mode of administration.

Therapeutic Effects

A drug is given to produce a desired effect on the body, either to treat a disease or to relieve symptoms. This is referred to as a drug's **therapeutic effect**. Sometimes, drugs are administered to prevent the occurrence of an infection or disease. When a drug is administered in this fashion, its effect is referred to as **prophylaxis**.

The desired effect that a drug produces is called a therapeutic effect.

Drugs can have a local or systemic effect. When a drug has a **local effect**, the effect is confined to one area or organ of the body. An example of this would be local anesthesia, when an anesthetic medication is administered directly into one part of the body, such as procaine (Novocain) being administered into the gums during a dental procedure. When a drug has a **systemic effect**, the effect is on the entire body. An example of a system drug is a chemotherapy agent used to treat cancer. It affects all the cells in the body, not just cancer cells. Sometimes, drugs have a **synergistic effect**, meaning that one drug increases or counteracts the action of the other.

The healthcare professional must assess each individual patient to determine appropriateness of therapy. When a drug is given according to its labeling and is known to be of benefit for a given disease, symptom, or condition, that is an **indication** for that drug. Even if a drug is indicated for a specific patient, the physician must weigh the benefits of the drug for that disease or condition with the risks to the patient. When a patient has a certain condition, disease, or symptom for which the drug should *not* be used, it is a **contraindication** for that drug. When a drug is contraindicated for a particular patient, it should not be prescribed for that patient.

An indication for a drug is the disease, symptom, or condition that may be treated by using the drug (its FDA-approved use). When a drug is used off-label, it means it is being prescribed for a purpose other than that indicated on its label (non-FDA approved use).

A contraindication for a drug is a disease, condition, or symptom for which the drug is not indicated or will cause harm.

Side Effects

A **side effect** is an unintended response to a drug. A side effect may limit the usefulness of the drug. Examples of common side effects include nausea, diarrhea, vomiting, constipation, weakness, and drowsiness. Side effects can vary in severity, ranging from mild to serious. Some drugs have been marketed for use in one disease because of the side effects noted while using the same drug for treatment of another disease.

A side effect is any unintended response to the drug.

Allergic Reactions

An **allergic reaction** is a local or general response of the immune system to an antigen. An antigen is a molecule that stimulates an immune response. Allergic reactions can manifest in a variety of ways. The first response the body has to an allergen is usually little or no reaction. Upon subsequent exposure, the body remembers the antigen and responds with a more severe response. These responses can vary from mild to severe to life threatening. The reactions themselves could be immediate or delayed responses to the antigen.

Histamine is the chemical your body releases when you are having an allergic reaction. Examples of ways that an allergic reaction could manifest include rash, hives (urticaria), itching (pruritus), wheals (red, blistery areas), fluid accumulation in tissues, sneezing, wheezing, and swelling. A severe allergic response to an allergen is called an **anaphylactic reaction**. It is an immediate, life-threatening reaction that involves respiratory distress (difficulty breathing) followed by shock. Often, the response to a drug is unrelated to the dose of that drug.

Drug Interactions

One drug can exert an effect on another drug. Food, alcohol, herbal preparations, vitamins, and nicotine can also interact with prescription and over-the-counter drugs. Drugs can interact with other drugs by inhibiting (decreasing the activity) or inducing (increasing the activity) the enzymes responsible for the metabolism of the other drug. Drugs can also have an additive effect on each other. This means the combined effect of both drugs is additive.

Following are some common drug interactions:

- **Additive**—The combined effect of both drugs is equivalent to the sum of the effects of each drug taken alone.
- **Antagonism**—One drug blocks the action of another drug.
- **Synergism**—The combined effect of both drugs is greater than the sum of the effects of each drug taken alone.
- **Potentiation**—One drug increases the potency of the other drug.

Drug Dependence

Drug dependence means the body needs a drug to function normally, and that abruptly stopping the drug will lead to withdrawal symptoms and/or psychological symptoms.

Legal and Ethical Implications of Medication Administration

Healthcare professionals who prepare and administer medications are legally and ethically responsible for their own behavior. Federal and state laws require that these individuals be licensed or registered with the appropriate authorities or that they act under the supervision of a licensed physician.

Laws vary from state to state. Some states allow medical assistants to administer medications, while other states do not. Some states also have laws that determine the training needed to perform certain tasks. Therefore, it is important that medical assistants be familiar with the laws in the state in which they practice.

Under the law, those administering medications are expected to know about the drugs they administer and their side effects. Even if you are acting under the license of a physician, you could be held accountable for your actions.

Medical assistants must also act ethically. Healthcare professionals often have access to lots of different kinds of medications. Taking medications, including samples, without proper authorization is illegal.

Dosage Forms

Drugs are seldom administered in pure form. They are formulated into various dosage forms to facilitate ease of administration and ensure safety and efficacy. A **dosage form** is a system or device by which a drug is delivered to the body. In a dosage form, the active ingredient is combined with inert ingredients that facilitate administration of the drug.

The most common dosage forms are those that are administered orally. Taking an oral medication is the most convenient method to deliver medication. Some medications are not available in oral form because they cannot be properly absorbed in the GI tract. For instance, heparin is only available as an injectable because it is ineffective when administered orally. The route of administration and dosage form are also determined by other factors, including the age of the patient, the disease being treated, the area of the body that the drug needs to reach, and the characteristics of the drug.

Many top-selling drugs are available in several different dosage forms. Knowing the dosage form can ensure that the patient does not use a dosage form incorrectly.

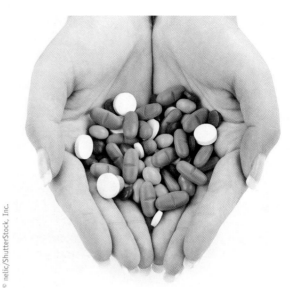

Tablets come in a variety of sizes, shapes, colors, and thicknesses.

A dosage form is the system or device by which a drug is delivered to the body.

Solid Dosage Forms

Solid dosage forms include tablets, capsules, lozenges/troches, pastilles, powders, and granules. Solid dosage forms offer several advantages:

- Increased stability
- Ease of packaging, storing, and dispensing
- Convenience
- Little or no taste or smell

Solid dosage forms also allow for accurate dosing because the entire dose is contained within the contents of the solid dosage form.

Tablets, capsules, and caplets (tablet that is shaped like a capsule, but smooth-sided like a tablet) come in a variety of shapes and sizes. Most tablets and caplets are designed to be swallowed whole and dissolve in the gastrointestinal tract, but some are also made to be administered sublingually (under the tongue), buccally, or vaginally. Tablets can also be designed to be chewed (chewable tablet) or to dissolve in the mouth without water (orally disintegrating tablet). They may also have a coating applied to mask unpleasant flavor or to protect the drug from stomach contents. Capsules may contain powders, granules, crushed tablets, or liquids. Tablets and capsules can also be designed to alter the rate of release of active drug.

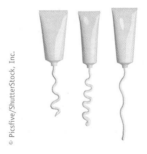

Semisolid Dosage Forms

Semisolid agents are different in their composition from liquids and solids. They are usually intended for topical application. They may be applied to the skin, placed on mucous membranes, or used in the nasal, rectal, or vaginal cavity. These dosage forms are too thick to be considered a liquid but not solid enough to be

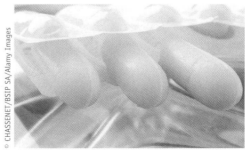

Semisolid dosage forms.

considered a solid. Examples include ointments, creams, lotions, gels, pastes, and suppositories.

Liquid Dosage Forms

Liquid dosage forms contain one or more active ingredients in a liquid vehicle. The drug may be dissolved in the vehicle or suspended as very fine particles. Examples of liquid dosage forms include solutions, suspensions, and enemas. They can be administered by many routes, but are often less stable than medications in solid dosage forms.

Liquid dosage forms offer several advantages:

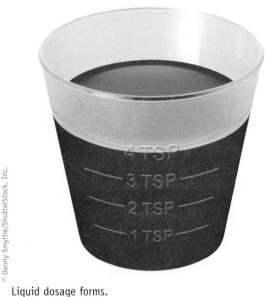

© Danny Smythe/ShutterStock, Inc.

Liquid dosage forms.

- They allow for easier dosage adjustments.
- They are easier to swallow.
- The onset of action is faster than that of solid dosage forms.

Inhalation Dosage Forms

Some patient populations, such as asthmatic patients, need their medications delivered to a specific site in the body, such as the bronchial tree. Gases, vapors, aerosols, powders, sprays, solutions, and suspensions intended to be inhaled via the nose or mouth are known as inhalations.

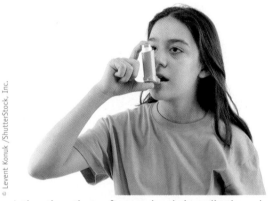

© Levent Konuk /ShutterStock, Inc.

Asthmatic patients often receive their medications via inhalation.

Transdermal Dosage Forms

A **transdermal patch** dosage is designed to hold a specific amount of medication to be released into the skin and absorbed into the bloodstream over time via a patch or disk. Patches can be applied to the arm, chest, back, and behind the ear, usually in a hair-free area. The patch consists of a backing, a drug reservoir, a control membrane, and an adhesive layer. The backing is removed and the adhesive layer is applied to the skin. The drug is slowly absorbed across the membranes of the skin and into the skin, where optimal absorption into the bloodstream will occur.

The duration of action for each transdermal formulation varies from one drug to another. Some patches should be changed daily, while others are changed every three to seven days. Localized heat from sun exposure, heating pads, electric blankets, hot tubs, and hot lamps should be avoided when using some transdermal formulations because it can increase absorption of the active drug into the bloodstream, resulting in an increase

© Custom Medical Stock Photo

Nitroglycerin is available in a transdermal patch formulation.

in adverse effects or toxicity. Transdermal formulations are convenient to use, and patient compliance is improved. Drugs such as nitroglycerin, fentanyl, scopolamine, and nicotine are administered in this manner.

Implantable Devices

Implantable devices are positioned beneath the skin near blood vessels that lead directly to the area to be medicated. An implantable device is used to provide a continuous supply of medication.

Routes of Administration

Medications can be administered by many different routes. A **route of administration** is a way to get a drug into or onto the body. Sometimes, combinations of routes are used at the same time. The route of administration is determined by a number of factors, including the age and condition of the patient, the desired effect, and the characteristics of the drug. The oral route is the most common route of administration.

Following is a list of routes of administration:

- **Buccal**—Administered inside the mouth on the mucosa of the cheek
- **Epidural**—Injection on or outside the dura mater of the spinal cord
- **Inhalation**—Drug administration into the lungs
- **Injection**—Injection by various routes
- **Intra-articular**—Injection into a joint
- **Intradermal**—Injection within the epidermis
- **Intramuscular**—Injection into a muscle
- **Intravenous**—Injection directly into a vein or into a venous line port
- **Nasal**—Administered via the nose
- **Ophthalmic**—Administered onto the surface of the eyeball or into the conjunctival sac
- **Oral**—Taken by mouth
- **Otic**—Administered into the external ear canal
- **Rectal**—Administered into the rectum
- **Subcutaneous**—Injection through the skin into the loose subcutaneous tissue under the skin
- **Sublingual**—Administered under the tongue
- **Transdermal**—Applied topically, with absorption through the skin for local or systemic effect
- **Vaginal**—Administered into the vagina

Peroral Route

The **peroral (PO)** route is commonly referred to as the oral route. It means that the drug is administered orally through the mouth and swallowed to reach the stomach. It must then undergo dissolution in the stomach, absorption in either the stomach or small intestine, activation in the liver, and distribution to the tissue before it exerts its therapeutic effect.

Advantages of the oral route are that it is safe, convenient, and easy to tolerate. In addition, oral medications are usually less expensive. Disadvantages include a delay between the administration of the drug and the onset of action, the possible interference of food and other drugs with absorption of the drug, and the possible degradation of the drug by the gastrointestinal fluids. Patients experiencing nausea or vomiting or who are sedated or otherwise unable to swallow should not take medications via the oral route.

Sublingual (under the tongue) and buccal (between the cheek and gum) routes of administration are used when a rapid onset of action is needed. The medication is absorbed directly by the blood vessels under the tongue or in the lining of the mouth. Drugs administered sublingually have a rapid onset of action because they enter the bloodstream directly.

To ensure that the correct medication is administered, follow these procedures:

1. Verify the provider's order.
2. Perform medical asepsis and proper hand washing procedures. See Chapter 5.
3. Follow the six rights of correct drug administration.
4. Work in a well-lit and clean area, away from distractions.
5. Obtain the correct medication.
6. Check the expiration date of the drug to make sure the expiration date has not been reached.
7. Compare the medication label with the prescriber's order. Make sure that the name of drug, dosage form, and strength of the drug ordered match that of the label.
8. If the strength ordered is different from that available, calculate the dosage needed.
9. Double-check and compare the medication label with the prescriber's order.
10. Transport the medicine to the patient.
11. Identify and, if needed, assess the patient.
12. Administer the medication and make sure the patient takes the entire dose required.
13. Monitor the patient for signs of an adverse or allergic reaction.
14. Document administration of the medication.
15. Store the medication properly as required by its labeling.

Parenteral Route

The **parenteral** route of administration bypasses the gastrointestinal tract. Drugs that are administered by this route can be given over a short (seconds to minutes) or extended (days) period. This route of administration distributes the drug systemically throughout the body to exert a systemic effect. Parenteral administration may be necessary when drugs are inactivated in the stomach. Drugs that are administered by this route are given via injection and must be sterile and free from particles.

Advantages of this route include that it can be used in patients who cannot take medications orally, it has a faster onset of action, and it can be used for drugs that are unstable in the acidic environment of the stomach. The IV route is the fastest route of drug administration. Disadvantages of this route include pain at the injection site, risk of infection, and the drugs are usually more expensive. Another disadvantage is that because injectable drugs exert their action quickly, there is little or no time to alter its effect if the wrong dose is given or an adverse reaction occurs.

When a drug is administered by injection into the muscle, it is called intramuscular (IM). The most

The IV route is the fastest route of drug administration.

common sites for IM injection are the upper arm, thigh, or buttock. When the drug is administered below the skin, it is called subcutaneous (SC or SQ).

Topical Route

Topical route of administration refers to the application of a drug to the surface of the skin or mucous membranes. Drug forms administered in this way include creams, ointments, gels, lotions, sprays, powders, and transdermal formulations. Topical agents can be used to fight skin infections, reduce inflammation, and protect the skin.

Advantages of topical agents include ease of application, fewer adverse effects than the same drug administered orally, and rapidity of action at the site of application. Most drugs that are applied topically are not well absorbed systemically, thereby reducing the incidence of side effects.

Drug Dosage

The dosage or dose of a drug is the amount of medicine that is prescribed for administration. It is determined by a licensed healthcare provider who considers important factors:

- **Age**—The usual adult dose is generally suitable for adults 20–60 years old. Infants, children, and the elderly often require a dosage adjustment.
- **Weight**—The average dose is based on a 70kg adult. Individuals who weigh more or less than this should have their dosage based on body-surface area (BSA) or kilograms of body weight.
- **Sex**—Many medications are contraindicated for use during pregnancy or while breast-feeding.
- **Other factors**—Patients with underlying conditions that may affect drug distribution or metabolism may also require dosage adjustments.

Emergency Drugs and Supplies

The ambulatory care setting should maintain drugs and supplies that may be needed in an emergency situation such as **anaphylaxis** or other form of shock. The drugs and supplies can be maintained in a tray, cabinet, or crash cart.

Examples of common emergency drugs include the following

- **Albuterol**—A bronchodilator
- **Atropine**—Used to restore heart rate
- **Benadryl**—An antihistamine used to relieve allergic symptoms
- **Dextrose**—Used for hypoglycemia
- **Diazepam**—Used to control seizures
- **Epinephrine**—A potent vasoconstrictor used for anaphylactic shock
- **Hydrocortisone**—A steroid used to suppress swelling and shock
- **Insulin**—Used for diabetic coma
- **Lidocaine**—Used to control ventricular arrhythmia
- **Narcan**—Used in narcotic overdose
- **Nitroglycerin**—Used for chest pain
- **Phenergan**—An antiemetic used to relieve nausea and vomiting

- **Valium**—Used to calm patients down
- **Verapamil**—Used for cardiac arrhythmia, stable and unstable angina

Supplies and equipment that should also be kept on the emergency cart include the following:

- IV fluids, tubing, syringes, alcohol wipes, tourniquet, and needles
- Stethoscope
- Sphygmomanometer
- Oxygen tank and mask
- Airways
- Defibrillator
- Personal protective equipment (PPE)

The Prescription

A prescription is a legal order for a specific product, to be dispensed to a patient by a licensed pharmacist. A prescription order can be made by any healthcare professional with prescribing authority. Although the most common issuer of prescription orders is a physician, prescription orders can also be issued by dentists, podiatrists, optometrists, physician assistants, nurse practitioners, and veterinarians. Some states have granted limited prescribing authority to clinical psychologists and pharmacists. Physicians have broad prescribing authority, which means there are no limitations to what prescription products they can prescribe. Other healthcare professionals may have limited prescribing authority, which means there are specific restrictions in place for these prescribers.

Prescription orders are sometimes given to patients by their prescriber. Other times, prescriptions are transmitted by the prescriber or an agent of the prescriber via mail, telephone, fax, or an e-prescribing service, which is a secure system that utilizes the Internet to deliver prescriptions directly to the pharmacy computer.

In an institutional setting, such as a hospital, the term prescription is not used. Instead, the prescriber's request is referred to as an **order** or a **medication order**. It is specific for the patient and denotes the name of the drug, form of the drug, frequency of administration, and route by which the drug is to be administered.

The Components of a Prescription

Although prescription components may vary from state to state, prescriptions typically contain the following information **FIGURE 10.2**:

- The prescriber's name, address, phone number, and DEA registration number
- The patient's name, date of birth, and address
- The date the prescription was written
- The name, strength, dosage form, and quantity of medication ordered
- Directions for use

Patient name   Prescription number

PHARMACY
WEGMANS FOOD MARKETS, INC.
1 MAIN STREET
ROCHESTER, NY 14624   AW-6116861

REFILLS: (123) 456-7890
Pharmacy # 123
Rx# 6000561
(123) 456-7890

SMARTFILL, MARY JANE   01/18/10
123 MAIN STREET, ROCHESTER, NY 14620
TAKE ONE TABLET BY MOUTH EVERY 8 HOURS AS NEEDED FOR PAIN.

IBUPROFEN 800 MG TABLET
QTY: 90

ANDREW SMITH
2 REFILLS BY 01/18/11

Number of refills remaining

FIGURE 10.2 The components of a prescription.

- The number of refills allowed
- If the prescriber requests "no generic substitution," a clear notation to that effect
- If it is a prescription for a controlled substance, the prescriber's Drug Enforcement Administration (DEA) number
- The prescriber's handwritten signature

The Components of a Patient Prescription Label

The components of a patient prescription label are as follows:

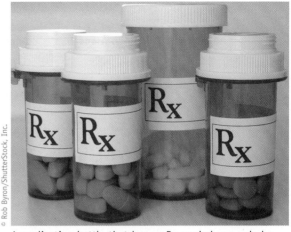

A medication bottle that has an Rx symbol can only be dispensed with a legal prescription.

- The name of the patient
- The name of the prescriber
- The date the prescription was filled
- The number of refills remaining
- The date the prescription expires
- The name, strength, dosage form, and quantity of product dispensed
- Directions for use
- The name, address, and phone number of the pharmacy
- The Rx number
- If it is a controlled substance, the required statement "Caution: Federal law prohibits the transfer of this drug to any person other than the patient for whom it was prescribed"
- Any necessary auxiliary labels

TABLE 10.3 lists abbreviations commonly used in prescriptions, while TABLE 10.4 lists problematic abbreviations found on prescription orders.

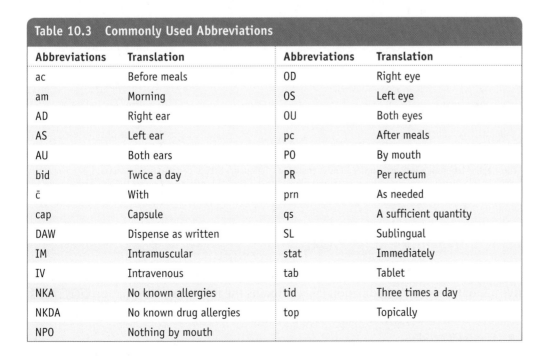

Table 10.3 Commonly Used Abbreviations

Abbreviations	Translation	Abbreviations	Translation
ac	Before meals	OD	Right eye
am	Morning	OS	Left eye
AD	Right ear	OU	Both eyes
AS	Left ear	pc	After meals
AU	Both ears	PO	By mouth
bid	Twice a day	PR	Per rectum
c̄	With	prn	As needed
cap	Capsule	qs	A sufficient quantity
DAW	Dispense as written	SL	Sublingual
IM	Intramuscular	stat	Immediately
IV	Intravenous	tab	Tablet
NKA	No known allergies	tid	Three times a day
NKDA	No known drug allergies	top	Topically
NPO	Nothing by mouth		

© Rob Byron/ShutterStock, Inc.

Abbreviations	Intended Meaning	Misinterpretation	Correction
QD and QOD*	Daily or every other day	Mistaken for one another	Write out daily or every other day
IU*	International unit	IV or ten (10)	Write out international unit
>	Greater than	Number 7	Write out greater than
<	Less than	Letter L	Write out less than
ūg	Microgram	mg	Use mcg
AD, AS, AU	Right ear, left ear, each ear	Mistaken as OD, OS, OU (right eye, left eye, each eye)	Write out right ear, left ear, each ear
OD, OS, OU	Right eye, left eye, each eye	Mistaken as AD, AS, AU (right ear, left ear, each ear)	Write out right eye, left eye, each eye
BT	Bedtime	BID	Write out bedtime
cc	cubic centimeters	u (units)	Use mL
D/C	Discharge or discontinue	Mistaken for one another	Write out discharge or discontinue
IJ	Injection	IV or intrajugular	Write out injection
IN	Intranasal	IM or IV	Write out intranasal
OD	Once daily	Right eye (OD)	Write out daily
q.d. or QD or Q.D. or qd*	Every day	qid	Write out daily
qhs	Nightly at bedtime	qh (every hour)	Use nightly
q.o.d. or qod or QOD or Q.O.D*	Every other day	q.d. or q.i.d.	Use every other day
SSRI	Sliding scale regular insulin	Selective serotonin reuptake inhibitor	Write out sliding scale insulin
U or u*	Unit	Number 0 or 4	Write out unit
UD	As directed	Unit dose	Write out as directed
Trailing zero after decimal point (e.g., 1.0mg)*	1mg	10mg	Do not use trailing zeros for doses expressed in whole numbers
No leading zero before decimal point (e.g., .5mg)*	0.5mg	5mg	Use zero before a decimal point when the dose is less than a whole unit

Table 10.4 Problematic Abbreviations Found on Prescription Orders

*These abbreviations are included on the Joint Commission's "minimum list" of dangerous abbreviations, acronyms, and symbols that must be included on an organization's "Do Not Use" list, effective January 1, 2004. Visit www.jcaho.org for more information about this requirement.

Medication Labels

Medication labels contain valuable information that is important for the safe and effective use of the drug. A medication label contains the following information FIGURE 10.3 :

- The brand and generic name of the product
- The NDC code

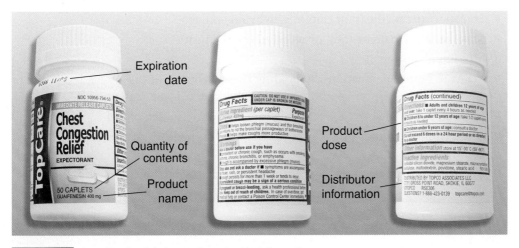

FIGURE 10.3 A medication label contains valuable information.
© Jones & Bartlett Learning

- The formulation
- The strength of the dose
- The product expiration date
- The net quantity
- The name and address of the manufacturer
- A list of active ingredients
- Indications for use
- Warning statements
- Directions for use
- Route of administration
- Other information

Medication Administration

Proper care must be taken to ensure that medications are administered properly. Regardless of the dosage form, certain guidelines must be followed. These guidelines are as follows:

- Always practice medical asepsis. See Chapter 5.
- Follow the rights of correct drug administration.
- Work in a well-lit area.
- Be knowledgeable about the drug you are administering.
- Always check allergies before administering any medication.
- Never give a medication without authorization from a licensed prescriber.
- Always check the expiration date of the drug prior to administration.
- Never give a medication that has been altered in any way.
- Administer only those medications that you have prepared for administration.
- Always verify the order prior to administration. Do not rely on your memory.
- Administer the prepared medication immediately. Do not leave it unattended.

- Transport the medication carefully to avoid spillage.
- Make sure the patient took or received the medication.
- Mix liquid suspensions.
- Measure liquid medications by holding the measuring device at eye level. The amount of medication should be read at the lowest level of the meniscus.
- Keep all drugs in a secure area and store according to drug label.
- Always follow proper procedures for the type of medication you are administering.
- Use standard precautions when necessary. See Chapter 5.

The Rights of Correct Drug Administration

The rights of a patient to medication safety are as follows:

- **The right patient**—Verify that the medication prescribed is for the correct patient. Use at least two patient identifiers such as the name of the patient and his or her date of birth.
- **The right drug**—Check that the right drug has been selected. Compare the medication order to the label on the bottle.
- **The right dose**—Check the order to make sure the right strength of medication is given. If the dose ordered and the dose on hand are not the same, determine the correct dose using mathematical calculations.
- **The right route**—Check the medication order to make sure it agrees with the drug's specified route of administration.
- **The right time**—Check the medication order to make sure you are medicating the patient at the proper time, with the correct frequency and duration.
- **The right documentation**—The recording process is the vital link between the provider, patient, and medical assistant. Document administration *after* giving the ordered medication. Note the time, route, and any other specific information as necessary—for example, the site of an injection or any laboratory value or vital sign that needed to be checked before giving the drug.

Allergenic Extracts

Medical assistants may have to administer allergenic extracts. Following are some guidelines:

- Allergenic extracts must be given in subcutaneous tissue, never in muscle.
- Use a tuberculin syringe with a 25-gauge, $\frac{5}{8}$-inch needle; 26-gauge, $\frac{3}{8}$-inch needle; or 27-gauge, $\frac{1}{2}$-inch needle or 1mL allergist syringe.
- Rotate site of administration for each allergenic extract.
- Document the allergenic extract, procedure followed, and dose administered.
- Allergenic extracts should be refrigerated. Discard when the expiration date has been reached.
- Adverse reactions such as rash, itching, swelling, redness, and difficulty breathing should be reported immediately to the physician.
- Severe allergic reactions such as anaphylactic shock must be treated immediately. Emergency equipment must be readily available for use.

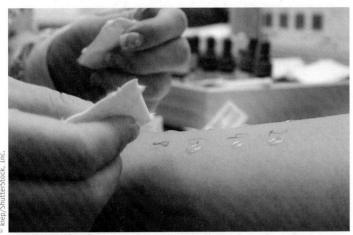

Allergenic extracts.

- Allergy testing should always be performed when the physician is present.
- Patients should be observed for at least 30 minutes after injection to make sure there is no reaction.

Inhaled Medications

Medications can be administered via inhalation. Inhalation refers to the act of drawing vapor, gas, or breath into the lungs. Inhalation therapy can be used to deliver medications, water vapor, or oxygen to the lungs. This route delivers medication from the mouth to the respiratory system. Proper administration of inhaled medications is necessary to ensure that the medication reaches the lungs. Some medications require that patients rinse their mouths thoroughly after each dose. This not only removes the aftertaste, but more importantly, it helps the patient to avoid fungal infection.

Patients should be advised to avoid overuse of an inhaler because it can lead to tolerance or rebound bronchospasm.
© auremar/ShutterStock, Inc.

An inhaler is often used to deliver medication to the lungs. An inhaler is a small device that, when activated, produces a fine mist or spray containing the medication. An inhaler is used for the treatment of chronic obstructive pulmonary disease (COPD) and asthma. There are two types of inhalers: those that use a propellant to push the drug into the lungs (metered-dose inhaler), and those that use a dry powder to release the medication as the patient takes a deep, quick breath. The type of inhaler needed depends on the medication and the level of convenience required. Advantages of inhalants include convenience and portability. The onset of action is usually quick, but when used incorrectly, the medication will not be able to reach the lungs.

When the body does not have enough oxygen, a state of **hypoxemia** (lack of oxygen in the blood) develops. This can lead to irreversible damage of body organs. In such cases, supplemental oxygen must be prescribed and administered immediately. Arterial blood gases should be measured after treatment has started. If the situation is not life threatening,

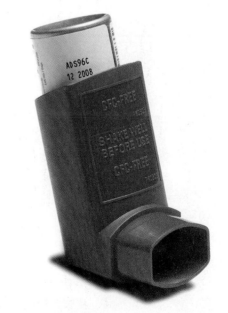

A metered-dose inhaler delivers a specific amount of medicine in aerosol form.

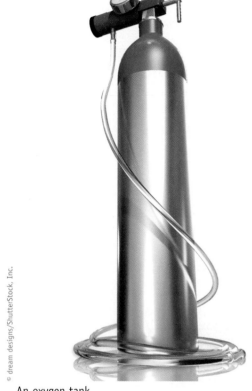

An oxygen tank.

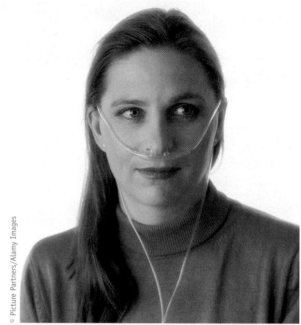

The nasal cannula is generally the preferred method for oxygen delivery.

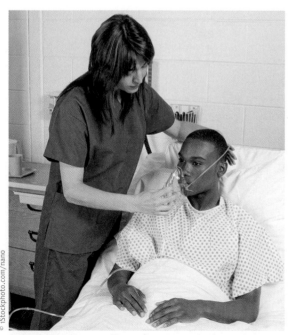

A medical assistant adjusts the oxygen mask.

some prescribers may measure it prior to starting oxygen therapy. The normal range for oxygen in the arterial blood is 80–100mm Hg (millimeters mercury). Oxygen can be supplied in tanks or in the hospital through a wall pipe system.

The physician will determine the flow rate, concentration, method of delivery, and duration of administration of oxygen. Oxygen is ordered as liters per minute and as a percentage of oxygen concentration.

The medical assistant must follow the provider's orders and follow proper procedures for administration of oxygen. Carefully observe the patient for signs of improvement or for toxicity. Oxygen toxicity can develop. Symptoms of oxygen toxicity include nausea, vomiting, malaise, fatigue, numbness, dizziness, and tingling of the extremities.

Oxygen can be delivered through a variety of methods. When a low concentration of oxygen is needed, a nasal cannula is the easiest and most convenient method of administration of oxygen. A nasal cannula has two hollow plastic prongs through which the oxygen passes. A strap or other device is used to attach it to the patient's head. The nasal cannula is generally the preferred method for oxygen delivery. Masks can also be used for inhalation therapy. They are used when the patient requires high humidity and a precise amount of oxygen.

Math Practice

Question: A patient needs to take 3.75mL daily for 30 days. What is the total number of milliliters needed?

Answer: 3.75mL × 30 days = 112.5mL for 30 days

Question: The physician asks you to give the patient 100mg of an antibiotic. The label on the bottle says that the strength of the antibiotic is 25mg/mL. How many milliliters should this patient receive?

Answer: 100mg ÷ 25mg/mL = 4mL

Question: A physician asks you to calculate the quantity of medication needed for a seven-day course of therapy. The prescription calls for 11mL of medication twice daily. How many milliliters will this patient need to complete the course of therapy?

Answer: Step 1: 11mL/dose × 2 doses/day = 22mL/day

Step 2: 22mL/day × 7 days = 154mL for 7 days of therapy

Question: A drug is available as 250mg/5mL. How many milliliters represent a dose of 375mg?

Answer: Step 1: xmL/375mg = 5mL/250mg

Step 2: xmL × 250mg = 375mg × 5mL

Step 3: xmL = 1,875mL/250

Step 4: x = 7.5mL

Question: A drug is available as 50mg/mL. The order calls for 150mg. How many milliliters will you prepare?

Answer: 150mg ÷ 50mg/mL = 3mL

Question: A dose of 60mg of famotidine is ordered. The drug is available as 40mg/4mL. How many milliliters need to be prepared to provide the ordered dose?

Answer: 60mg ÷ 40mg/4mL = 6mL

Question: What is the total dose for a man weighing 70kg and requiring a dose of 0.5mg/kg?

Answer: 70kg × 0.5mg/kg = 35mg

Question: What is the total dose for a woman weighing 110 lb and requiring a dose of 2mg/kg?

Answer: Step 1: Convert her weight to kilograms: 110 lb × 1kg/2.2 lb = 50kg

Step 2: 50kg × 2mg/kg = 100mg

WRAP UP

Chapter Summary

- Most drugs have three types of drug names: the chemical name, generic name, and brand name.

- Federal laws protect the public by ensuring the safety and efficacy of drugs brought to the market.

- The FDA sets regulations that require manufacturers to provide evidence of a drug's safety and efficacy before it can be approved for marketing.

- A drug's active ingredient is responsible for the drug's therapeutic effect.

- Drugs can be categorized as therapeutic, pharmacodynamic, diagnostic, or prophylactic, depending on their use.

- There are five categories of controlled substances. Dispensing, procurement, and administration of all controlled substances are regulated by the Drug Enforcement Administration.

- Drugs have therapeutic effects, adverse reactions, and side effects.

- A prescription is a written or verbal request for a medication.

- The rights for correct drug administration offer useful guidelines when administering medications.

- Drugs can be administered in a variety of dosage forms. The choice of dosage form will depend on the patient, the desired effect, the dose required, the duration of desired effect, and the properties of the medication.

- Routes of administration include oral, topical, and parenteral. The decision of which route to use will depend on the site, medication, desired effect, and duration of action.

- Parenteral administration includes IV, IM, and SC routes of administration.

- Administering medications is an important responsibility that the medical assistant performs.

- Medical assistants must become familiar with the laws of the state in which they are employed before administering any medication. Medical assistants have a legal and ethical responsibility and are expected to be knowledgeable about the drugs they administer and the effects the drug may have on the patient.

- Emergency drugs and supplies should be available on a crash cart or tray or cabinet for use during medical emergencies.

Learning Assessment Questions

1. The prescription label of a drug container will usually have two names on it: the generic name and the brand name. What is the trade or brand name?

   A. The chemical name of the drug

   B. The name of the drug given by the manufacturer

   C. The abbreviated generic name of the drug

   D. The common name

2. According to the Controlled Substances Act, a Schedule II drug is allowed how many refills?

   A. One refill

   B. Five refills

   C. No refills

   D. No limit as long as they are within six months from the date of issue

3. Questions involving controlled substances should be directed to which regulatory agency?

   A. The FDA

   B. The American Medical Association

   C. The DEA

   D. The Department of Health

4. An active ingredient exerts which of the following?
   A. The therapeutic effect
   B. The inert effect
   C. The placebo effect
   D. No physiologic effect

5. A therapeutic agent does which of the following?
   A. Maintains health
   B. Relieves symptoms
   C. Stops or delays the disease
   D. All of the above

6. A severe allergic reaction is called which of the following?
   A. Antigen
   B. Allergen
   C. Anaphylactic reaction
   D. Dependence

7. Which of the following drugs is commonly used in an emergency situation?
   A. Lomotil
   B. Aspirin
   C. Epinephrine
   D. Prozac

8. Which of the following did the Federal Food, Drug, and Cosmetic Act require all drug manufacturers to ensure?
   A. Purity
   B. Safety
   C. Packaging
   D. All of the above

9. A written legal document that gives directions for dispensing and administering medication to a patient is a _____.
   A. Prescription
   B. Subscription
   C. Medication note
   D. Notation

10. Which abbreviation means twice a day?
    A. tid
    B. bid
    C. NKA
    D. stat

11. Which of the following must be on a hard-copy prescription?
    A. Patient's name
    B. Date the prescription was written
    C. Name, strength, dosage form, and quantity of medication ordered
    D. All of the above

12. Which of the following routes of administration has the fastest onset of action?
    A. Oral
    B. Intravenous
    C. Transdermal
    D. Sublingual

13. To what does the abbreviation PO refer?
    A. By mouth or orally
    B. Rectally
    C. Intradermally
    D. Subcutaneously

14. Which of the following is *not* a solid dosage form?
    A. Solution
    B. Capsule
    C. Tablet
    D. Powder

15. A prescription label must have which of the following?
    A. The patient's name
    B. The name of the drug
    C. The expiration date
    D. All of the above

16. Advantages of transdermal patches include which of the following?
    A. Convenience
    B. Ease of administration
    C. Improved patient compliance
    D. All of the above

17. The abbreviation TID means which of the following?

    A. Twice daily

    B. Three times a day

    C. Take as directed

    D. Four times a day

18. Rights of correct drug administration include which of the following?

    A. Right dose

    B. Right route

    C. Right time

    D. All of the above

19. Advantages of solid dosage forms include which of the following?

    A. Increased stability

    B. Convenience

    C. Little or no taste or smell

    D. All of the above

20. Drugs administered between the cheek and gum are given by what route?

    A. Sublingual

    B. Otic

    C. Buccal

    D. Intramuscular

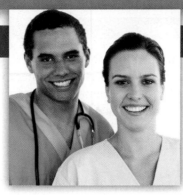

Administering Injections and Immunizations

OBJECTIVES

After reading this chapter, you will be able to:

- Safely dispose of syringes, needles, and biohazard materials.
- State the relationship between the diameter and the gauge of the needle.
- Describe the site selection for administration of injections.
- Demonstrate intradermal, subcutaneous, intramuscular, and Z-track injections.
- Document administration of therapeutic injections ordered by the provider and administered by the medical assistant.

KEY TERMS

Ampule	Needle gauge	Vastus lateralis
Biohazard materials	Needle length	Ventrogluteal
Deltoid	Needlestick	Z-track method
Dorsogluteal	Parenteral product	
Intradermal (ID)	Reconstitution	
Intramuscular (IM)	Scoop method	
Intravenous (IV)	Subcutaneous (subQ)	
Needle	Syringe	

Chapter Overview

Parenteral products are medications or other preparations intended for administration by injection, either through the skin or other external tissue, rather than through the gastrointestinal (GI) tract. Parenteral administration allows the active ingredient to be delivered directly to an organ, a lesion, a muscle, a nerve, or other body tissue. In addition to medication, fluids, electrolytes, and nutrients may be administered parenterally.

Because parenteral products are administered as liquids, the dose is usually expressed as the weight of the drug or active ingredient (milliequivalents, micrograms, milligrams, grams, or units) per volume (milliliters or ounces). Double-check all math calculations to maintain accuracy when converting units and determining doses or ask another medical assistant to do this for you.

© auremar/ShutterStock, Inc.

Parenteral administration is preferred over oral administration when a patient is unable to take medication by mouth, when a patient is unconscious, or when a patient is vomiting. Parenteral administration is also appropriate when drug action is required immediately or when a drug is not therapeutically active after oral administration. Parenteral products also allow for a rapid response to medication, accurate doses, and concentrating a medication in a small body area.

Parenteral products are typically more expensive than oral products, and their preparation and administration require specially trained staff. Parenteral products and their administration can also pose risks to the patient. After a parenteral product is administered, it cannot be removed. Steps to minimize errors and maximize safety are paramount when administering parenteral products.

Abbreviations Related to Injections and Immunizations

The following are abbreviations related to injections and immunizations:

- 1/2 NS—Half normal saline, 0.45% sodium chloride
- HBIG—Hepatitis B immune globulin
- ID—Intradermal
- Ig—Immunoglobulins
- IM—Intramuscular
- IV—Intravenous
- IVP—IV push
- IVPB—IV piggyback
- mL—Milliliters
- subQ—Subcutaneous
- SWI or SWFI—Sterile water for injection
- TB—Tuberculosis

Types of Injections

Drugs can be administered into almost any part of the body, including a vein (**intravenous [IV]**), a muscle (**intramuscular [IM]**), the skin (**intradermal [ID]**), or under the skin (**subcutaneous [subQ]**). Less commonly, drugs are injected directly into a joint (intra-articular), the fluid surrounding the joint (intrasynovial), the spinal column (intraspinal), spinal fluid (intrathecal), an artery (intra-arterial), or the heart (intracardiac). **FIGURE 11.1** illustrates the proper sites and techniques for common types of injections.

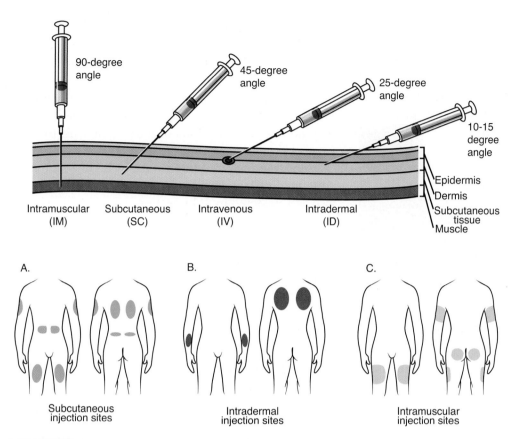

FIGURE 11.1 Drugs can be administered into almost any part of the body.

© Jones & Bartlett Learning

Medical assistants are not permitted to administer IV injections or initiate IV access. However, you may see patients with existing IV access in an office, hospital, or long-term care setting. Document infusing IV medications and fluids when assessing these patients; monitor the area around the site of access for redness, swelling, or discomfort; and immediately report these to the physician or other supervisor.

Intramuscular

IM injections are administered deep into a skeletal muscle. The common locations are usually the **deltoid** (upper arm), **dorsogluteal** (back hip), **vastus lateralis** (top of the leg), or **ventrogluteal** (side hip). Proper administration of IM injections requires insertion of the needle at a 90-degree angle to the muscle. IM injections are appropriate for nonirritating drugs. Nonirritating drugs include hormones, biologic agents, vaccines, and antibiotics. Drugs that may irritate or stain the skin include iron, haloperidol, and hydroxyzine. IM injections do not result in a rapid onset of action but do lead to a prolonged duration of effect. Injuries relating to IM injections usually result from the point of entry of the needle or the deposition of drug solution. Fluid or pus accumulation, blood clots, bruising, and scarring occur rarely following IM injections.

The volume of drug administered by IM injection is limited by the size of the muscle. In adults, up to 2mL can be administered in the deltoid, and 5mL can be administered to the dorsogluteal (back hip). However, the upper limits of injection volumes may cause discomfort and pain. Therefore, IM injections

"Subcutaneous" should not be abbreviated "SQ" or "SC," as these abbreviations can easily be misinterpreted. Instead, use "subQ," "sub-Q," or "subcutaneous."

© auremar/ShutterStock, Inc.

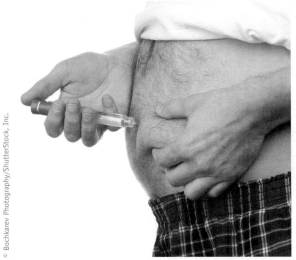

Insulin is often administered by subcutaneous injection.

are usually limited to half the maximum volume: 1mL for the deltoid and 2 to 2.5mL for the dorsogluteal.

The vastus lateralis is the preferred site for injection for IM injection in children because it is the largest muscle in children's bodies and has no major nerves or blood vessels. Children under the age of three years old may not receive injections of more than 1mL into the vastus lateralis.

Most vaccines are administered by IM injection. Narcotic medications and loading doses of antibiotics are also administered by IM injection.

> If a large volume of solution is required for IM injection, the dose may be divided into two syringes and injected into separate injection sites.

Subcutaneous

The subQ route of administration is used for small volumes of medication. Drug solutions are administered into the subcutaneous layer of fat beneath the surface of the skin between the dermis and the muscle, usually on the outer surface of the upper arm, the anterior surface of the thigh, or the lower portion of the abdomen. Proper administration of a subQ injection requires needle insertion at a 45-degree angle to the surface of the skin. An exception to this rule is the administration of insulin by the subQ route. In this case, the injection is made at a 90-degree angle to the skin surface. The site of injection should be rotated when frequent injections are administered, such as daily insulin injections. The maximum volume of drug that can be administered by the subQ route is 2mL. However, volumes greater than approximately 1.3mL cause painful pressure at the site of administration, so, as a matter of practice, subQ doses should be limited to 1mL if possible. Thick suspensions are not appropriate for subQ administration. Insulin administration is discussed in more detail in Chapter 15.

Intradermal

ID injections are administered into the vascular layer of the skin between the dermis and the epidermis. The usual site of ID administration is the anterior portion of the forearm. Proper administration of an ID injection requires needle insertion at a 10- to 15-degree angle to the surface of the skin. This route is frequently used for diagnostic skin tests such as tuberculosis testing or allergy desensitization, in which systemic absorption would be dangerous. ID injections are limited to very small volumes, often less than 0.1mL, but can range from 0.02mL to 0.5mL.

Equipment for Sterile Product Administration

To properly administer parenteral injections, personnel must have a working and usable knowledge of the equipment employed for such injections. Most notably, this includes syringes and needles. **FIGURE 11.2** shows the parts of a syringe and needle.

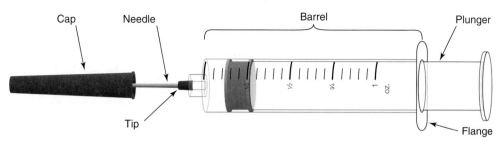

FIGURE 11.2 Most syringes are made of plastic or glass. Needles are made of aluminum or stainless steel.
© Jones & Bartlett Learning

Syringes

Syringes are used for the preparation and administration of sterile pharmaceutical products. Syringes are also employed in nonsterile environments for oral use and irrigation. The term *syringe* refers to the calibrated reservoir and plunger of a device intended to deliver medication to a body or introduce it to another delivery system.

Most syringes are made of plastic, but some are made of glass. Glass syringes are expensive and are used only for medications that are absorbed by plastic. Plastic syringes are available from manufacturers as sterile products, individually wrapped for convenience and storage. Plastic syringes are inexpensive and disposable.

A syringe consists of several parts:

■ **Barrel**—The barrel or reservoir holds the medication and has graduated markings or calibrations for measuring volumes.

■ **Plunger**—The plunger is a movable cylinder inside the barrel that provides the mechanism by which fluids are drawn into or pushed out of the barrel.

■ **Flange**—The flange is located at the end of the barrel, where the plunger is inserted. It has appendages where you can grasp the syringe.

■ **Tip**—The tip is at the end of the barrel where the needle attaches.

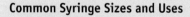

Common Syringe Sizes and Uses

A hypodermic syringe, calibrated in milliliters, is used for administering IM injections. The most common sizes of hypodermic syringes for parenteral administration are 1mL, 3mL, and 5mL. A tuberculin syringe has a capacity of only 1mL, calibrated in tenths of a milliliter, and is used for ID tuberculosis and allergy skin tests. An insulin syringe has a capacity of 100 units or 1mL, calibrated in units, and is used to administer subQ insulin.
© auremar/ShutterStock, Inc.

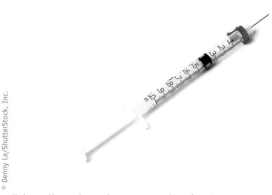

Tuberculin syringes have a capacity of 1mL.
© Denny Le/ShutterStock, Inc.

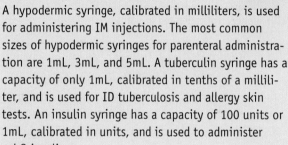

Most syringes are calibrated in milliliters.
© Valentyn Volkov/ShutterStock, Inc.

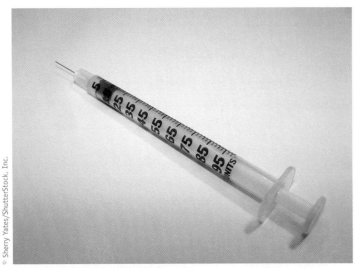

Insulin syringes are calibrated in units.

The plunger and the tip of the syringe must remain sterile to ensure asepsis. These components must not be touched. Only the flange and the barrel may be touched.

Syringes are available in a variety of sizes for medical use, ranging from 0.25mL to 60mL. When manipulating solutions with a syringe, choose the smallest size syringe that will measure the desired volume.

Needles

A **needle** is attached to a syringe and is the part that actually enters the medication vial, the container to hold medication for dispensing, or the body. Needles are made of aluminum or stainless steel. Needles vary in gauge and length. **Needle gauge** refers to the diameter of the needle. The larger the diameter, the smaller the gauge. For example, a 28-gauge needle has a smaller diameter than a 25-gauge needle. Needles for medical use are available in gauges ranging from 33 to 13. Common **needle lengths** range from $\frac{3}{8}$ to 2 inches. Needle gauge and length are important considerations for patient administration, mostly due to patient comfort and site of administration. In general, deltoid injections are administered with a 23- to 25-gauge needle that is 1 inch in length. Dorsogluteal injections are administered with a 20- to 22-gauge needle that is $1\frac{1}{2}$ inches in length. Vastus lateralis injections are administered with a 20- to 22-gauge needle that is $1\frac{1}{2}$ inches in length. For dorsogluteal and vastus lateralis injections, a 2-inch needle may be used for obese patients. Intradermal injections are administered with a 25- to 27-gauge needle that is $\frac{1}{4}$ to $\frac{5}{8}$ inches in length. A 1-inch needle may be used for obese patients. A subQ injection is administered with a 24- to 26-gauge needle that is $\frac{3}{8}$ to $\frac{5}{8}$ inches in length. SubQ insulin injections are administered with a 26- to 30-gauge needle.

A needle consists of several features:

- **The point**—The point is the sharp end of the needle.
- **The bevel**—The bevel is the flat, slanted surface near the point.
- **The lumen**—The lumen is the hollow core of the needle that forms an oval-shaped opening at the beveled point.
- **The shaft**—The shaft is the hollow steel tube that runs the entire length of the needle.
- **The hub**—The hub is the end of the needle that attaches to the syringe.
- **The hilt**—The hilt is the location where the hub attaches to the shaft.

A smaller needle gauge indicates a larger diameter and a larger needle gauge indicates a smaller diameter.

Hazards Associated With Parenteral Products

Administering injections requires caution—both for the patient and the healthcare worker. Care should be taken to avoid **needlesticks** (accidental punctures of the skin caused by a needle or other sharp object) and exposure to hazardous chemicals or

The "Seven Rights of Drug Administration"

The "Seven Rights of Drug Administration" have been developed to help healthcare professionals ensure proper administration of any drug. These seven rights should be routinely checked before, during, and after medication administration:

- **Right drug**—Ensure that the correct drug is used. Compare the medication order with the label on the medication bottle or vial. Make it a habit to read the medication label at several steps during medication administration.
- **Right dose**—Ensure that the patient receives the right dose. Verify the dose ordered and the dose dispensed. If the dose requires calculation, have a second person double-check the accuracy of your math.
- **Right route**—Ensure that the drug is administered by the route ordered.
- **Right time**—Ensure that the patient receives the medication at the right time. Time intervals are ordered to maintain safety and effectiveness of drug therapy, and accuracy in timing is important.
- **Right patient**—Ensure that the correct patient receives the medication. Before administering any medication, verify the patient's identity with at least two means of identification such as patient name, date of birth, telephone number, assigned identification number, or other person-specific identifier.
- **Right technique**—Ensure that the right technique is used to administer medication. This minimizes the risk of adverse reactions and patient discomfort and increases the effectiveness of the drug.
- **Right documentation**—Complete the required documentation after medication administration. The patient chart is a link among all healthcare providers and is a legal documentation of all procedures relating to the patient's medical care. Accurately and clearly record information, including the date and time of administration, the drug and dose, the route of administration, unusual reactions or complications following administration, patient data and vital signs, and your name.

bodily fluids, as well as to minimize pain and discomfort for the patient. Other dangers of parenteral administration include allergic reactions; injury to bones, nerves, or blood vessels; breaking of a needle in tissue; and injecting into a blood vessel rather than tissue.

Needle Safety

Needlesticks and other sharps-related injuries are dangerous and expose healthcare workers to hazardous chemicals and infectious agents. Nearly 1,000,000 needlesticks occur among healthcare workers annually in the United States. They occur in every healthcare setting, including hospitals, medical offices, ambulatory care centers, long-term care facilities, and home health settings. Every worker who comes in contact with sharp objects—syringes with needles, IV catheters, suture needles, scalpels, or lancets—is at risk for a needlestick.

For improved safety, needles are available with needle guards that remain on the needle until immediately before the injection is administered. Safety mechanisms are also available that can be activated immediately after administration that minimize the risk of accidental needlesticks.

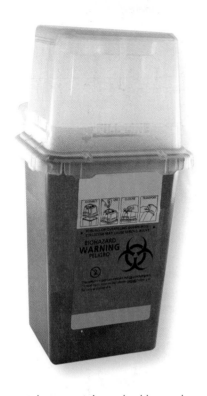

A sharps container—containers should never be reused and should never be discarded in the regular trash.

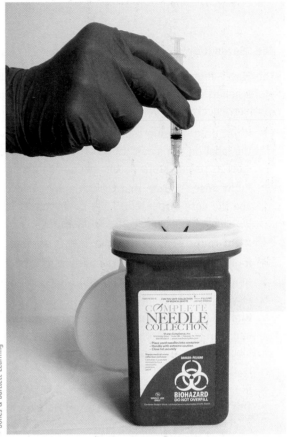

Dispose of used syringes capped and point-side down into a sharps container.

Needles should never be recapped after use. Needles and syringes should be immediately discarded, intact and point-side down, into a hard-sided biohazard sharps container. The container should never be overfilled and should be properly sealed before being destroyed. Sharps containers should never be reused and should never be discarded in the regular trash.

You can also avoid needlesticks and other occupational safety hazards by obtaining the proper safety training and understanding safe practices within the scope of your practice. Always use safety devices that are available. Keep a sharps disposal container close to where you are working and never overfill the container. Limit interruptions and congestion in your work area when working with needles or other potentially hazardous objects or materials.

If a needlestick occurs before a medication is administered, the needle and syringe should be discarded and a new dose of medication prepared. When exposure to a needlestick or any potentially infectious material occurs, immediately flush the area with water and wash the wound or exposed area with soap and water. Immediately report the incident to your supervisor and seek medical attention. Depending on the type of medication in the syringe and other circumstances surrounding the needlestick, a physician or other healthcare provider will determine the appropriate course of action following the needlestick or injury.

Needlesticks can happen easily when recapping a needle. Never recap a needle after giving an injection.

Occupational Safety

Needlesticks are an occupational hazard within the medical community. Most of the fear and concern about needlesticks and other sharps-related injuries is due to the risk of transmission of blood-borne pathogens, including hepatitis B virus, hepatitis C virus, and human immunodeficiency virus. The Occupational Safety and Health Administration established guidelines to protect healthcare workers who are at risk of coming in contact with blood-borne pathogens. Additionally, in 2001, the Federal Needlestick Safety and Prevention Act was passed, which requires employers to provide safer medical devices to reduce accidental needlesticks.

In general, employers are required to:

- Establish an exposure control plan, including ways to minimize occupational exposure to blood-borne pathogens, and update the plan annually.
- Implement the use of standard precautions.
- Identify and use controls such as sharps containers and needle-less systems when available.
- Identify and use work practice controls by updating policies and procedures for handling potentially hazardous products or devices.
- Provide personal protective equipment to employees.
- Make hepatitis B vaccinations available to employees with potential occupational exposure.
- Make available postexposure evaluation and care for employees who experience an exposure incident.
- Use labels and signs to communicate hazards.
- Provide safety information and training to employees.
- Maintain medical records, training documentation, and injury logs for employees.

© auremar/ShutterStock, Inc.

What Would You Do?

You have just administered a vaccine and you are attempting to recap the needle before disposing of it in the sharps container. You accidentally stick yourself on the tip of your index finger with the uncapped needle. What should you do?

© NorthGeorgiaMedia/ShutterStock, Inc.

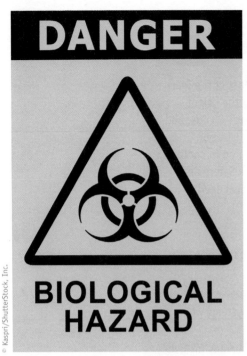

The universal biohazard symbol must appear on all bags and containers that contain potentially biohazardous material.

© Kaspri/ShutterStock, Inc.

Biohazard Materials

Biohazard materials are any infectious or dangerous bodily fluids, tissues, or other substances that pose a risk to the health or safety of humans or the environment. Proper personal protective equipment and biohazard disposal containers should always be used when handling potentially infectious or dangerous materials to decrease the exposure to blood-borne pathogens.

All infectious waste must be placed in a hazardous waste container. Any disposable material that contains even trace amounts of blood, tissue, or bodily fluid is considered biohazard waste and should be handled with caution. Red biohazard bags are used for biohazard waste. Biohazard labels should be affixed to the bag or container. Most disposable biohazardous items are destroyed by incineration.

Nondisposable items, such as bed linens or clothing, that contain potentially hazardous or infectious material should be placed and sealed in leakproof biohazard bags in the area in which they were soiled and transported directly to the laundry facility or laundry pickup site. Biohazard materials should never be disposed of with regular waste.

Surfaces and instruments that have been contaminated with potentially biohazardous materials should be sterilized, either by disinfecting with chemical sterilization or autoclaving.

Patient Safety

Parenteral administration delivers a drug or other substance directly into a patient's tissues or organs. Caution must be practiced and appropriate technique must be learned to ensure safe administration.

Before preparing to administer an injection, verify that you understand the medication, dose, and directions. Verify that the medication was ordered by a practitioner licensed to prescribe medication. Familiarize yourself with the medication by researching drug references. Never administer a drug that has expired or that has been altered or stored incorrectly. Never administer a medication if the order is unclear or questionable.

When the medication order is clear and you are confident with your duties, there are several things to remember to maintain patient safety:

- Disposable gloves should always be worn when administering injections.
- Injections should be administered only when emergency equipment is available, in case the patient experiences an adverse, allergic, or anaphylactic reaction. Check for known allergies prior to administering an injection and monitor the patient for distress after administration.
- The patient should be informed of all procedures and medication administrations. Be honest about the level of discomfort the patient may feel and ensure the patient has no questions before proceeding with the injection. Also ensure that all consent forms have been completed as necessary, and provide the patient with written information about the injections he or she is receiving.
- Choose the correct site of administration and use the correct technique for administration to maintain patient comfort and safety, as well as effectiveness of the medication. Do not choose an injection site that has any type of skin lesion, a burn, inflammation, trauma to the skin, scar tissue, moles or birthmarks, tumors

or hard nodules, large blood vessels, bones, swelling, or paralysis. Additionally, the arm on the same side as a mastectomy or lymphatic compromise should not be used for injection administration. Limbs that are disabled or that have poor circulation should also not be used to administer injections.

Skills for the Medical Assistant

Medical assistants are often responsible for administering medications. You will be responsible for ensuring the right patient receives the right dose of the right drug at the right time by the right route. You will also ensure that the right documentation is made of the procedure. Using appropriate techniques and practicing habits that minimize the risk of medication errors maintains patient safety and promotes optimal health outcomes.

Each state sets different rules and regulations regarding medication preparation and administration by healthcare personnel. You are responsible for maintaining appropriate licensure or certification in the state where you live and work. You are responsible for performing only those duties within your scope of practice.

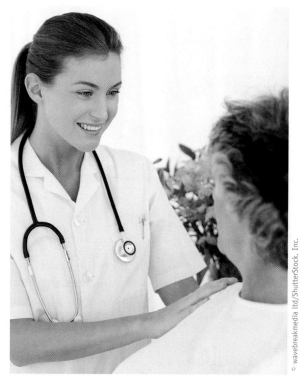

Ensure that both you and the patient are comfortable and well informed prior to any medication administration or procedure.

Reconstituting Sterile Powder for Injection

Some medications for parenteral administration are supplied as dry powder that requires **reconstitution** with a diluent prior to administration, or the process of adding a liquid to a dry powder to make it suitable for injection. Aseptic technique is required when reconstituting powders for injection. (A diluent is an inactive solution added to dry powder to prepare it for administration.)

Normal saline and sterile water for injection are the two most common diluents for reconstituting sterile powders for injection. In this exercise, you will learn how to reconstitute powder for injection.

Equipment Needed

- Medication supplied as sterile powder for injection
- Sterile water for injection
- Disposable gloves
- Syringe
- Regular needle, 25-gauge, 1-inch length
- Vented needle, 18-gauge, 1½-inch length
- Sharps container
- Alcohol wipes

Steps

1. Read the medication order, gather supplies, and ensure you have a clean work surface. Wash your hands and apply disposable gloves.

2. Select the appropriate syringe and needle size for the ordered volume and injection site.

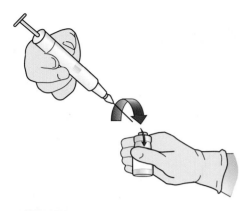

FIGURE 11.3 Gently press the needle into the rubber stopper while rotating your arm up.
© Jones & Bartlett Learning

3. Remove the metal cap from the vial of sterile water. Lift up on the pull tab to remove it from the top of the vial. Discard the cap. Wipe the vial's rubber stopper with an alcohol wipe.

4. Attach the needle to the syringe. Remove the cap from the needle and place it on the work surface.

5. Fill the syringe with an amount of air equal to the volume that will be withdrawn from the vial by pulling back on the plunger.

6. Hold the syringe between the thumb and forefinger of your dominant hand (similar to holding a dart or a pen). Securely hold the vial on the work surface with your nondominant hand. With the bevel of the needle facing up, lay the tip of the needle against the center of the rubber stopper of the vial.

7. Insert the needle into the vial by gently pressing into the rubber stopper and simultaneously rotating your arm up until the needle is perpendicular to the top of the vial and the tip of the needle has passed through the rubber stopper **FIGURE 11.3**.

Correct technique when inserting a needle into a vial prevents coring, or the breaking of small pieces of rubber into the vial. Correct technique requires that the bevel and the heel of the needle tip enter the rubber stopper in the same location.

---

8. Keep the syringe fully inserted into the vial and invert the vial. Hold the vial with your nondominant hand and hold the syringe with your dominant hand.

9. Press the plunger to dispense the air in the syringe into the vial. This creates a positive-pressure environment inside the vial and assists with withdrawing the solution. (A positive-pressure environment is one in which the pressure inside a system such as a glass vial is greater than the pressure outside the system.) Release the plunger and allow the syringe to fill with fluid.

10. Tap the syringe gently to move any air bubbles toward the hub of the syringe. Press the plunger to dispense the air bubbles back into the vial. Verify that the required amount of solution is in the reservoir of the syringe. If there is too much solution in the syringe, expel the excess solution into the vial. If there is not enough solution, withdraw the required amount from the vial, taking care to remove any excess air from the syringe before proceeding.

11. Invert the medication vial, with the needle and syringe still inserted. Place the vial on the work surface and continue to hold it with your nondominant hand. Hold the barrel of the syringe with your dominant hand and gently remove the needle from the vial by pulling it straight up out of the vial.

12. Use the scoop method to recap the needle **FIGURE 11.4**. The **scoop method** is a one-handed method for recapping syringes. Begin with the cap on a flat surface. Hold the barrel of the syringe in your dominant hand and move the tip of the needle inside the cap. When most

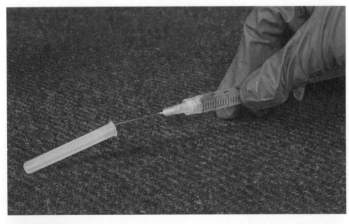

FIGURE 11.4 Use the scoop method to safely recap needles.
© Jones & Bartlett Learning

of the needle is inside the cap, lift the syringe, careful to lift the cap with the needle, and move it to an upright position. Use your nondominant hand to snap the cap in place. Do not touch the needle to the work surface, the outside of the cap, your hands, or your fingers while recapping the needle.

13. Use aseptic technique to remove the needle and replace it with a vented needle. Place the syringe and needle on the work surface.

14. Remove the cap from the vial containing the medication powder. Discard the cap. Wipe the rubber stopper with an alcohol wipe.

15. Pick up the syringe and needle and remove the cap. Discard the cap.

16. Hold the medication vial firmly on the work surface with your nondominant hand and hold the syringe directly above and perpendicular to the vial with your dominant hand. Apply direct downward pressure to insert the vented needle and its sheath through the rubber stopper of the medication vial.

17. Position the hub of the needle approximately ⅛ inch above the rubber stopper. Press the plunger of the syringe, releasing the diluent into the vial. There should be no pooling of fluid on top of the rubber stopper. If this happens, the needle is either inserted too far or not far enough into the rubber stopper.

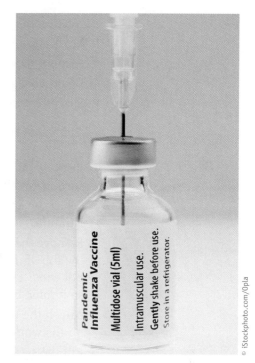

Apply direct downward pressure to insert the vented needle and its sheath through the rubber stopper of the medication vial.

Vented needles can only be used to inject diluents into a vial. They are not used to withdraw fluid.

---

18. Hold the barrel of the syringe in your dominant hand and pull straight up to remove the needle from the vial. Discard the syringe and needle into the sharps container.

19. Roll or gently shake the medication vial to dissolve the entire quantity of powder in the sterile water. Allow the vial to rest on the work surface until the foam or bubbles have disappeared. The medication is now ready for administration according to the prescriber's instructions.

Withdrawing Medication From a Vial

Medications are supplied in a variety of packages, including vials of solution. Vials are available in single- and multiple-dose varieties. Once opened, single-dose vials must be used within one hour or discarded. Once opened, a multiple-dose vial can usually be used for 28 days when stored under the proper conditions. Always note this date and your initials on the outside of the vial.

Vials are closed systems, so fluid cannot be withdrawn unless an equal amount of air is added to the vial. The needle and syringe are used to introduce air into the vial and to withdraw the required amount of fluid. Withdrawing medication from a vial requires a special technique to maintain sterility and ensure an accurate dose. In this exercise, you will learn how to withdraw medication from a vial.

Equipment Needed

- Medication order
- 3mL syringe

- Needle, 25-gauge, 1-inch length
- Medication vial
- Alcohol wipes
- Disposable gloves
- Sharps container

Steps

1. Read the medication order, gather supplies, and ensure you have a clean work surface. Wash your hands and apply disposable gloves.
2. Select the appropriate syringe and needle size for the dose and route of administration.
3. Remove the metal cap from the vial. Lift up on the pull tab to remove it from the top of the vial. Discard the cap. Wipe the vial's rubber stopper with an alcohol wipe. The hard rubber stopper on top of the vial can harbor contaminants, so it must be cleaned with isopropyl alcohol before the solution is withdrawn.
4. Attach the needle to the syringe. Remove the cap from the needle and place it on the work surface.
5. Fill the syringe with an amount of air equal to the volume that will be withdrawn from the vial by pulling back on the plunger.
6. Hold the syringe between the thumb and forefinger of your dominant hand (similar to holding a dart or a pen). Securely hold the vial on the work surface with your nondominant hand. With the bevel of the needle facing up, lay the tip of the needle against the center of the rubber stopper of the vial.
7. Insert the needle into the vial by gently pressing into the rubber stopper and simultaneously rotating your arm up until the needle is perpendicular to the top of the vial and the tip of the needle has passed through the rubber stopper.
8. Keep the syringe fully inserted into the vial and invert the vial. Hold the vial with your nondominant hand and hold the syringe with your dominant hand.
9. Press the plunger to dispense the air in the syringe into the vial to create a positive-pressure environment inside the vial. Release the plunger and allow the syringe to fill with fluid **FIGURE 11.5**.
10. Tap the syringe gently to move any air bubbles toward the hub of the syringe. Press the plunger to dispense the air bubbles back into the vial. Verify that the required amount of solution is in the reservoir of the syringe. If there is too much solution in the syringe, expel the excess solution into the vial. If there is not enough solution, withdraw the required amount from the vial, taking care to remove any excess air from the syringe before proceeding.
11. Invert the medication vial, with the needle and syringe still inserted. Place the vial on the work surface and continue to hold it with your nondominant hand. Hold the barrel of the syringe with your dominant hand and gently remove the needle from the vial by pulling it straight up out of the vial.

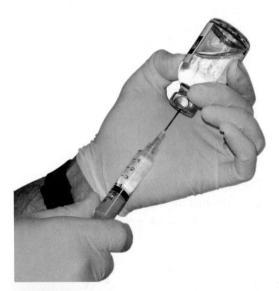

FIGURE 11.5 Invert the vial and allow the syringe to fill with fluid.
© Michael G. Smith/ShutterStock, Inc.

12. Administer medication according to the prescriber's instructions. Alternatively, replace the cap using the scoop method and place it on a medication tray for later administration.

13. Discard the syringe and needle into the sharps container. Remove the gloves and dispose of them in a biohazard container. Discard the medication vial in a trash container or store it appropriately.

14. Wash your hands and document the medication administration in the patient's chart.

Using an Ampule

An **ampule** is a glass container with a single dose of medication or active ingredient, usually in a volume of no more than 2mL **FIGURE 11.6**. An ampule contains no preservatives. An ampule is often used when the medication is incompatible with plastic or rubber used in medication vials. The glass of the neck of an ampule must be broken to withdraw the solution. This presents a challenge for maintaining sterility as well as safety. You must use a filter needle to withdraw the solution from the ampule to remove any fragments of glass, paint, or dust that entered the ampule. In this exercise, you will learn how to withdraw medication from an ampule.

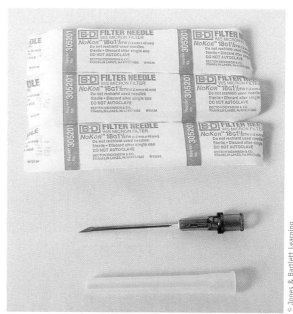

You must use a filter needle to withdraw a solution from an ampule.

Equipment Needed

- Medication order
- Ampule containing medication
- 3mL syringe
- Filter needle, 18-gauge, 1½-inch length
- Regular needle, 25-gauge, 1-inch length
- Alcohol swabs
- Trash container
- Sharps container

Steps

1. Read the medication order, gather supplies, and ensure you have a clean work surface. Wash your hands and apply disposable gloves using aseptic technique.

2. Gently tap or swirl the ampule to move fluid from the top of the ampule down into the body. Wipe the neck of the ampule with an alcohol swab.

3. Hold the body of the ampule with your nondominant hand. Hold the head of the ampule with the thumb and index finger of your dominant hand. You may wrap a small cotton square or alcohol swab around the neck of the ampule to protect your fingers from the sharp edges of the broken glass.

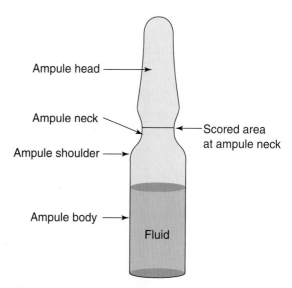

FIGURE 11.6 The parts of an ampule: Ampules are often used when the medication is incompatible with plastic or rubber used in medication vials.
© Jones & Bartlett Learning

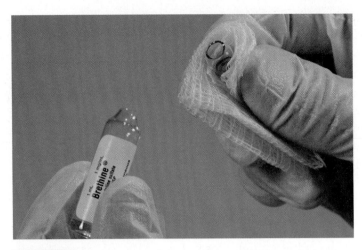

FIGURE 11.7 Snap the head of the ampule away from your body.
© Jones & Bartlett Learning.

Quickly snap the head of the ampule back, snapping your wrist away from your body **FIGURE 11.7**.

4. Discard the head of the ampule in the sharps container. Place the body of the ampule on your work surface. The broken edges of the ampule will be sharp; take care not to touch the broken surfaces to avoid cutting yourself or contaminating the edge of the ampule.

5. Attach a filter needle to a syringe. Remove the cap and place it on the work surface.

6. Hold the barrel of the syringe with your dominant hand. Hold the ampule on the work surface with your nondominant hand. Angle the ampule so the solution flows toward the neck of the ampule. Turn the syringe so the bevel of the needle faces down and insert the needle into the solution in the ampule **FIGURE 11.8**. Take care not to touch the edges of the ampule with the needle or with your fingers.

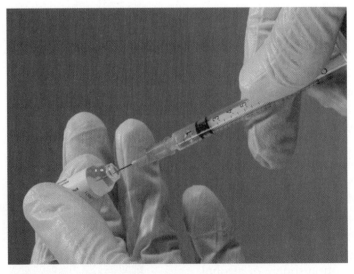

FIGURE 11.8 Tilt the ampule gently to move the solution toward the neck of the ampule.
© Jones & Bartlett Learning.

7. Use your dominant hand to pull the plunger of the syringe back to slightly more than the desired volume of solution.

8. Remove the needle from the ampule. Replace the cap on the needle using the scoop method.

9. Hold the needle upright and push up on the plunger to remove any excess air from the reservoir of the syringe. Tap the barrel of the syringe to move air bubbles toward the hub of the syringe. Pull down on the plunger to remove any fluid from the needle. Gently push up on the plunger again until fluid enters the needle hub. All of the air should now be removed from the reservoir of the syringe.

10. Remove the filter needle and replace it with a regular needle.

11. Administer medication according to the prescriber's instructions. Alternatively, place it on a medication tray for later administration.

12. Discard the syringe and needle into the sharps container. Remove the gloves and dispose of them in a biohazard container.

13. Wash your hands and document the medication administration in the patient's chart.

Preparing to Administer Injections and Immunizations

Regardless of the route of administration, administering injections and immunizations requires attention to detail and the completion of several steps to prepare the patient and the work area. In this exercise, you will learn the steps to prepare for the administration of an injection or immunization. You will complete these basic steps prior to any parenteral medication administration.

Equipment Needed

- Medication order
- Medication vial or ampule
- Appropriately sized syringe and needle
- Alcohol wipes
- Disposable gloves
- Sharps container
- Cotton ball
- Adhesive strip

Steps

1. Read the medication order, gather supplies, and ensure you have a clean work surface. Wash your hands.

2. Review the seven rights of medication administration.

3. Compare the medication label with the medication order. Check the expiration date on the medication. Calculate the dose if necessary.

4. Prepare the syringe and needle for use and withdraw the medication, as described in previous exercises.

5. Compare the medication label with the medication order for a second time.

6. Place the syringe and needle on a medication tray, along with the medication vial or ampule and the medication order. Compare the medication label with the order for a third time.

7. Transport the medicine to the patient.

8. Identify the patient and explain the procedure.

9. Put on a clean pair of disposable gloves.

10. Select the administration site. Place the patient in the correct position for administration, depending on the route and site of administration.

11. Cleanse the injection site with an alcohol wipe. Begin wiping at the injection site and work out, in a circular motion, cleansing approximately 2 inches outside the injection site.

12. Allow skin to dry.

13. Inject the medication according to the proper technique for each injection site.

14. Activate the safety mechanism on the syringe and dispose of the syringe in the sharps container.

15. Massage the injection site with a cotton ball, unless contraindicated.

16. Observe the patient for signs of difficulty or bleeding from the injection site. Apply an adhesive strip if necessary.

17. Dispose of the gloves and supplies in a biohazard waste container.

18. Wash your hands. Document the medication administration in the patient's chart. For example, write "0930: Administered pneumococcal vaccine (Prevnar-13), 0.5 mL, in right deltoid. Patient tolerated well. J. Jones, CMA."

Administering Intradermal Injections

The most commonly administered ID injection is the purified protein derivative (PPD) injection to diagnose tuberculosis. Allergy testing and desensitization are also performed using ID injections. Due to the small volumes that can safely be injected intradermally, medications are not often administered by this route. In this exercise, you will learn how to administer an ID injection.

Equipment Needed

- Medication order
- Medication vial or ampule
- Needle, 27-gauge, ½-inch length
- Alcohol wipes
- Disposable gloves
- Sharps container
- Adhesive strip
- Medicine tray

Steps

1. Complete steps 1–12 in the exercise "Preparing to Administer Injections and Immunizations."

2. Pull the skin at the injection site taut.

3. Carefully insert the needle at a 10- to 15-degree angle with the bevel facing up. Insert the needle approximately ⅛ inch. Do not aspirate **FIGURE 11.9**.

4. Release the skin and steadily inject the medication to form a wheal (a small, round, raised area of the skin).

5. Wait briefly, then remove the needle and activate the safety mechanism. Dispose of the syringe and needle in the sharps container.

6. Blot the injection site with a cotton ball. Do not massage.

7. Observe the patient for signs of difficulty or bleeding from the injection site for 15 to 20 minutes. Apply an adhesive strip if necessary.

8. Dispose of the gloves and supplies in a biohazard waste container.

9. Wash your hands. Document the medication administration in the patient's chart. For example, write "1045: Administered PPD 0.1 mL to left forearm. Patient instructed to return to clinic in 48–72 hours to observe test results. Patient tolerated injection well. J. Jones, CMA."

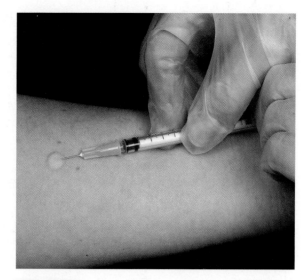

FIGURE 11.9 In an intradermal injection, you carefully insert the needle at a 10- to 15-degree angle with the bevel facing up.

Courtesy of Greg Knobloch/Gabrielle Benenson/CDC

Administering Subcutaneous Injections

SubQ injections are most commonly used for administering certain narcotics, reproductive hormones, and insulin. You may be required to help educate diabetic patients on self-administration of insulin. In this exercise, you will learn how to administer a subQ injection.

Equipment Needed

- Medication order
- Medication vial or ampule
- 1mL syringe
- Needle, 25-gauge, ½-inch length
- Alcohol wipes
- Disposable gloves
- Sharps container
- Adhesive strip
- Medicine tray

Steps

1. Complete steps 1–12 in the exercise "Preparing to Administer Injections and Immunizations."
2. Grasp the skin at the injection site to form a 1-inch fold.
3. Quickly insert the needle at a 45-degree angle with the bevel facing up **FIGURE 11.10**.

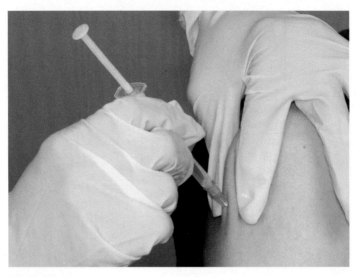

FIGURE 11.10 In a subcutaneous injection, you insert the needle at a 45-degree angle with the bevel facing up.
© Jones & Bartlett Learning

4. Slowly inject the medication.
5. Remove the needle and activate the safety mechanism. Release the skin. Dispose of the syringe and needle in the sharps container.
6. Massage the injection site with a clean cotton ball, unless contraindicated.
7. Observe the patient for signs of difficulty or bleeding from the injection site for 15 to 20 minutes. Apply an adhesive strip if necessary.
8. Dispose of the gloves and supplies in a biohazard waste container.
9. Wash your hands. Document the medication administration in the patient's chart. For example, write "1215: Administered 1,000 mcg vitamin B12 (1 mL) to the back of the left arm. Patient tolerated administration well. J. Jones, CMA."

Administering Intramuscular Injections

Many medications and vaccinations can be administered intramuscularly, including antibiotics, narcotics, hormones, steroids, and vitamins. In some cases, the medication has a rapid onset of action, but often the muscle acts as a depot for slowly releasing drugs, leading to infrequent dosing of medications. In this exercise, you will learn how to administer an IM injection.

Equipment Needed

- Medication order
- Medication vial or ampule
- 3mL syringe
- Needle, 25-gauge, 1-inch length
- Alcohol wipes
- Disposable gloves
- Sharps container
- Adhesive strip
- Medicine tray

Steps

1. Complete steps 1–12 in the exercise "Preparing to Administer Injections and Immunizations."
2. Depress and pull the skin taut with one hand. Hold the skin to the side of where you plan to inject the needle.
3. Using a dartlike motion, quickly insert the needle at a 90-degree angle. Insert the needle all the way to the hub. Release the skin **FIGURE 11.11**.
4. Slowly inject the medication.
5. Remove the needle and activate the safety mechanism. Dispose of the syringe and needle in the sharps container.
6. Massage the injection site with a clean cotton ball, unless contraindicated.
7. Observe the patient for signs of difficulty or bleeding from the injection site for 15 to 20 minutes. Apply an adhesive strip if necessary.
8. Dispose of the gloves and supplies in a biohazard waste container.
9. Wash your hands. Document the medication administration in the patient's chart. For example, write "1340: Administered leuprolide (Lupron Depot) 3.75 mg IM in patient's left deltoid. Patient tolerated procedure well. J. Jones, CMA."

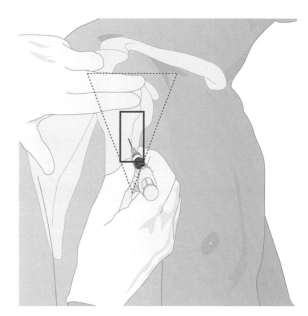

FIGURE 11.11 In an intramuscular injection, you insert the needle at a 90-degree angle.
© Peter Gardiner/Photo Researchers, Inc.

Administering Intramuscular Injections With the Z-Track Method

The **Z-track method** of IM injections is used to minimize leakage into the subcutaneous tissue and outer layers of skin and allows no method of exit for the medication. This method can also be used when administering dark-colored solutions that can stain the outer layers of the skin or those that are particularly irritating to the skin. In this exercise, you will learn how to administer an IM injection with the Z-track method.

Equipment Needed

- Medication order
- Medication vial or ampule
- 3mL syringe
- Needle, 25-gauge, 1-inch length
- Alcohol wipes
- Disposable gloves
- Sharps container
- Adhesive strip
- Medicine tray

Steps

1. Complete steps 1–12 in the exercise "Preparing to Administer Injections and Immunizations."

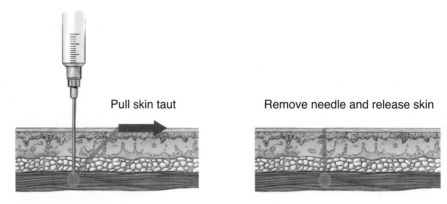

Pull skin taut   Remove needle and release skin

FIGURE 11.12 In an intramuscular injection using the Z-track technique, you pull the skin laterally 1½ inches from the injection site.
© Jones & Bartlett Learning

2. Pull the skin at the injection site taut, pulling skin laterally 1½ inches from the injection site.
3. Using a dartlike motion, quickly insert the needle at a 90-degree angle. Insert the needle all the way to the hub **FIGURE 11.12** .
4. Slowly inject the medication.
5. Wait 10 seconds to allow the medication to begin to absorb. Remove the needle and release the skin simultaneously. Activate the safety mechanism. Dispose of the syringe and needle in the sharps container.
6. Use dry gauze to apply very gentle pressure to the puncture site.
7. Observe the patient for signs of difficulty or bleeding from the injection site. Apply an adhesive strip if necessary.
8. Dispose of the gloves and supplies in a biohazard waste container.
9. Wash your hands. Document the medication administration in the patient's chart. For example, write "0850: Administered 0.5 mL iron dextran to patient's right deltoid using Z-track technique. Patient tolerated procedure well. J. Jones, CMA."

Math Practice

Question: A 12-year-old male patient weighs 95 pounds. His physician orders ceftriaxone (Rocephin) 75mg/kg/day divided into two daily doses for an infection. What is the total daily dose of ceftriaxone? How much ceftriaxone will be administered at each dose?

Answer: 95 lb × 1kg ÷ 2.2 lb = 43.2kg

43.2kg × 75mg/kg/day = 3,240mg/day
3240mg/day × 1 day ÷ 2 doses = 1,620mg/dose

Question: A man is prescribed 50 micrograms of octreotide to be administered subcutaneously three times daily for hormone therapy. The ampule of octretotide contains a 0.100mg/mL solution for injection. What volume of octreotide solution is needed for one dose?

Answer: 0.100mg/mL = 1mcg/1,000mg = 100mcg/mL; 100mcg/mL = 50 mcg/*x*; *x* = 0.5mL

Question: A diabetic patient needs to administer 40 units of insulin subcutaneously. If she has a 10mL vial of insulin containing 100 units/mL, what volume will she administer?

Answer: 100 units/mL = 40 units/*x*; *x* = 0.4mL

Question: A five-year-old boy is preparing to enter kindergarten. His pediatrician recommends the following immunizations prior to entering school:

Diphtheria-tetanus-acellular pertussis (DTaP): 0.5mL IM

Inactivated polio vaccine (IPV): 0.5mL IM

Measles-mumps-rubella vaccine (MMR): 0.5mL IM

Varicella vaccine: 0.5mL subQ

What is the total volume of medication that will be administered to the vastus lateralis?

Answer: 0.5mL DTaP + 0.5mL IPV + 0.5mL MMR + 0.5mL subQ = 2.0mL

Question: An adult weighing 215 pounds requires an IM injection of epinephrine 0.4mg for hypersensitivity reaction. Epinephrine is available in a solution for injection with a strength of 1:1,000. What volume of epinephrine is required for the patient?

Answer: 1:1,000 = 1g/1,000mL = 1,000mg/1,000mL = 1mg/1mL; 1mg/mL = 0.4mg/*x*mL; *x* = 0.4mL

WRAP UP

Chapter Summary

- Parenteral products are medications that are administered by injection rather than through the gastrointestinal tract. This allows an active ingredient to be directly delivered to an organ, lesion, muscle, nerve, or tissue. Parenteral administration is preferred when a patient is unable to take medication by mouth, when a patient is unconscious, or when a patient is vomiting.

- Most parenteral products are administered intravenously (IV, into a vein), intramuscularly (IM, into a muscle), intradermally (ID, into the skin), or subcutaneously (subQ, under the skin). Medical assistants are not allowed to administer medications intravenously, but you will likely prepare and administer other types of injections.

- IM injections are administered deep into a skeletal muscle, usually the deltoid, the dorsogluteal, or the vastus lateralis. IM injections are given at a 90-degree angle to the muscle. The volume that can be safely injected intramuscularly is limited by the size of the muscle.

- SubQ injections are used to administer small volumes of drugs underneath the skin, usually on the outer surface of the upper arm, the anterior surface of the thigh, or the lower portion of the abdomen. SubQ injections are given at a 45-degree angle to the skin. SubQ doses should be limited to 1mL, if possible.

- ID injections are used to administer very small amounts of diagnostic test materials or allergy desensitization products into the skin between the dermis and epidermis. ID injections are given at a 10- to 15-degree angle to the skin.

- Syringes and needles are the most common pieces of equipment used for preparing and administering parenteral medications. A syringe is a calibrated reservoir for measuring, preparing, and administering injections. A needle is the sharp component attached to a syringe that actually enters the body, medication vial, or container. Syringes and needles vary in size and length, depending on the intended use.

- Needlesticks are an occupational hazard related to preparation and administration of injections and immunizations. Needlesticks also expose healthcare workers to blood-borne pathogens and other hazardous materials. Safety mechanisms and proper handling, storage, and disposal techniques minimize the risk of injury related to needles and other sharp objects.

- Patient safety is a priority for parenteral medication administration. As the medical assistant, familiarize yourself with each medication you are asked to administer, and work to maintain patient safety and comfort as much as possible. Document all medication administrations, as well as details of patient reactions, concerns, or questions.

- Preparing and administering parenteral medications requires special training and technique to maintain sterility, patient comfort, and safety.

Learning Assessment Questions

1. Parenteral administration of a medication is preferred in all but which of the following situations?
   A. When a patient is unconscious
   B. When a patient is vomiting
   C. When a drug is inactivated by oral administration
   D. When a patient dislikes the taste of the oral medication

2. Which of the following are benefits of parenteral products?
   A. Rapid response to medication, accurate dosing, and concentrating medication in a small body area
   B. Long duration of action of medication and does not irritate tissues
   C. The ability to administer large doses in a short amount of time, increased activity of the medication compared with oral administration, and slow response to medication
   D. Increased drug concentration and decreased risk of side effects compared with oral administration

3. Which of the following is *not* considered a parenteral route of administration?
   A. Intramuscular
   B. Sublingual
   C. Intradermal
   D. Intrasynovial

4. Which of the following pairs correctly matches the injection site and the maximum volume for an IM injection for an adult?
   A. Vastus lateralis, 1mL
   B. Dorsogluteal, 6mL
   C. Deltoid, 1mL
   D. Dorsogluteal, 2mL

5. Which of the following medications is *not* administered intramuscularly?
   A. Antibiotics
   B. Narcotics
   C. Vaccines
   D. Insulin

6. Which of the following is true regarding subQ injections?
   A. The maximum volume for injection is 0.5mL.
   B. The injection should be made at a 10- to 15-degree angle to the skin.
   C. The injection delivers medication to the layer of skin between the dermis and epidermis.
   D. The injection site should be rotated when frequent administrations are required.

7. Which of the following parts of a syringe is correctly matched with its function?
   A. Flange: located at the end of the barrel; can be safely handled
   B. Barrel: the movable cylinder that draws fluid into the syringe
   C. Hub: the part that attaches to the needle
   D. Plunger: the component that contains calibrations for measuring fluid

8. Which of the following needles has the smallest diameter?
   A. A 13-gauge needle
   B. A 25-gauge needle
   C. A 28-gauge needle
   D. A 30-gauge needle

9. Why are needle gauge and needle length important considerations in parenteral product administration?
   A. For ease of medication preparation
   B. For drug compatibility
   C. For drug volume
   D. For patient comfort and safety

10. In what location are healthcare workers most at risk for needlesticks?
    A. Home healthcare settings
    B. Operating rooms
    C. Physician's offices
    D. All environments pose an equal amount of risk for injury.

11. Which of the following items does *not* pose a risk of needlestick or sharps-related injury?

    A. Suture needles

    B. Lancets

    C. IV tubing

    D. Scalpels

12. Which of the following injection sites is correctly matched with an appropriate needle gauge and length for administration?

    A. Deltoid: 27-gauge, 1-inch length

    B. Subcutaneous: 24-gauge, 1-inch length

    C. Intradermal: 30-gauge, ¼-inch length

    D. Dorsogluteal: 20-gauge, 1½-inch length

13. What should you do before administering a medication to a patient?

    A. Document the date, time, and appearance of the medication.

    B. Familiarize yourself with the medication and ensure a safe environment for the patient.

    C. Verify what time the patient prefers to receive medications.

    D. Assume that the prescriber has verified all allergies with the patient.

14. Which of the following is *not* a "right" of medication administration?

    A. Right drug

    B. Right patient

    C. Right time

    D. Right diagnosis

15. How do you create a positive-pressure environment when withdrawing solution from a vial?

    A. Withdraw excess air into the syringe.

    B. Core the rubber stopper on top of the vial.

    C. Dispense air into the vial equal to the volume of solution you need to withdraw.

    D. Use a filter needle.

16. What are the two most common diluents used for reconstituting sterile powders for injection?

    A. Dextrose and sterile water

    B. Sterile water and normal saline

    C. Lactated Ringer's and dextrose

    D. Half normal saline and dextrose

17. What is coring?

    A. A method for administering intramuscular injections to minimize leakage and tissue irritation

    B. A one-handed technique used for recapping needles

    C. The insertion of the needle into a vial of diluent

    D. The breaking of small pieces of the rubber stopper into a medication vial

18. What is the proper technique for using a vented needle?

    A. Use a vented needle to inject diluent into a vial; never use a vented needle to withdraw fluid.

    B. Press the hub of the needle all the way to the rubber stopper to ensure a tight seal with the vented needle.

    C. To insert the needle into the vial, begin with the needle and syringe in a horizontal position and apply downward pressure as you rotate your wrist and bring the syringe to a vertical position.

    D. Take care to insert the needle, but not its sheath, completely through the rubber stopper.

19. Which of the following is *not* a risk associated with using an ampule?

    A. Broken glass can injure the individual opening the ampule.

    B. Particles of dust or other contaminants can fall into the drug solution.

    C. Fragments of glass can cause injury if administered to a patient.

    D. The positive-pressure environment inside the ampule can cause the syringe to fill with excess fluid.

20. What is the final step in the administration of parenteral products?

    A. Document medication administration.

    B. Properly dispose of biohazard waste.

    C. Provide patient with follow-up care instructions.

    D. Wash your hands.

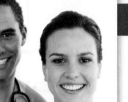

Muscular and Skeletal Systems

OBJECTIVES

After reading this chapter, you will be able to:

- Identify combining word forms of the muscular system and their role in the formation of medical terms.
- Define the structures and functions of the muscular system.
- List abbreviations related to the muscular system.
- Identify combining word forms of the skeletal system and their role in the formation of medical terms.
- Define the structures and functions of the skeletal system.
- Identify common diseases of the muscular and skeletal systems, diagnostic procedures, and their treatment.
- List abbreviations related to the skeletal system.
- Define rehabilitation medicine and explain its importance in patient care.
- Discuss the importance of correct posture and body mechanics and demonstrate how to safely transfer patients and lift or move heavy objects using proper body mechanics.
- Describe safety precautions and techniques used when helping a patient to ambulate and demonstrate how to assist the patient to safely stand and walk.
- Demonstrate how to safely care for a falling patient.
- Describe assistive devices and the importance of each in helping patients to ambulate.
- Demonstrate how to measure patients for a walker, crutches, and a cane, and how to help them ambulate safely with each device.
- Describe the ambulation gaits used with crutches.
- Discuss the safety precautions and techniques used when pushing a wheelchair.

- Explain the importance of joint range of motion and the method used to measure joint movement.
- Explain the importance of therapeutic exercise and the types of therapeutic exercises used in patient rehabilitation.
- Explain the body's physiological reactions to heat and cold therapeutic modalities.
- Identify and describe the various types of hot and cold modalities.
- Explain the medical assistant's role in cast application and cast removal and the guidelines for cast care.

KEY TERMS

Ambulation
Amphiarthrosis
Aponeurosis
Appendicular skeleton
Arthroscope
Arthroscopy
Articulation
Assistive devices
Axial skeleton
Axillary crutches
Body mechanics
Bunion
Bursa
Bursitis
Cancellous bone
Cane
Carpal tunnel
Carpal tunnel syndrome
   (CTS)
Cast
Closed fracture
Compact bone
Computed tomography
   (CT) scan
Condyle
Crepitus
Crutches
Cryotherapy
Diaphysis
Diarthrosis
Dislocation
Dual energy X-ray
   absorptiometry
   (DXA)
Epicondylitis
Epiphysis
Fibromyalgia

Fixed joint
Flat bones
Forearm crutches
Fracture
Gait belt
Goniometer
Goniometry
Gout
Hallux valgus
Herniated disk
Insertion
Irregular bones
Joint capsule
Kyphosis
Ligament
Long bones
Lordosis
Magnetic resonance
   imaging (MRI)
Massage therapy
Metaphysis
Open fracture
Origin
Orthopedics
Ossification
Osteoarthritis (OA)
Osteoblasts
Osteoclasts
Osteomyelitis
Osteopathy
Osteopenia
Osteoporosis
Patella
Pectoral girdle
Pelvic girdle
Periosteum

Platform crutches
Range of motion (ROM)
Reduction
Rehabilitation medicine
Rheumatoid arthritis
   (RA)
RICE protocol
Ruptured disk
Scoliosis
Sesamoid bones
Short bones
Skeleton
Skull
Spongy bone
Sprain
Strain
Striated muscle
Subluxation
Synarthrosis
Synovial cavity
Synovial fluid
Synovial membrane
Systemic lupus
   erythematosus (SLE)
Tendinosis
Tendonitis
Thermotherapy
Thoracic cage
Tophi
Trabecular bone
Ultrasound therapy
Vertebral column
Visceral muscle
Walker
Wheelchair
X-ray

Chapter Overview

The muscular and skeletal systems (known collectively as the musculoskeletal system) include bones, joints, muscles, and surrounding tissues that support and move the body. The 206 bones of the adult human body that make up the skeletal system provide structure and protection for the body's organs and are the points of attachment for muscles, ligaments, and tendons. The muscular system, including more than 600 muscles, tendons, and ligaments, coordinates the body's movements. The muscular system also gives the body shape and form.

Diseases and disorders of the musculoskeletal system are common and ranked among the top reasons people seek health care. **Orthopedics** is the medical field that studies disorders of the musculoskeletal system. **Osteopathy** is a holistic study of medicine that emphasizes the musculoskeletal system and the body as a whole. As a medical assistant, you will have the opportunity to interact with patients with a variety of acute and chronic disorders of the musculoskeletal system, as well as participate in diagnostic and treatment-related procedures.

Terminology

TABLE 12.1 lists word roots and terms used in the study of the muscular and skeletal systems.

Table 12.1 Word Roots of the Muscular and Skeletal Systems

Word Root or Term	Meaning	Example
Ankyl/o	Stiff joint	Ankylosis (abnormal stiffening)
Arthr/o	Joint	Arthroscopy (visual examination of a joint)
Brachi/o	Arm	Brachialis muscle (muscle of the upper arm that flexes the elbow)
Burs/o	Sac	Bursitis (inflammation of the fluid-filled sac in a joint)
Carp/o	Wrist	Carpal tunnel syndrome (symptoms resulting from pressure on the median nerve in the wrist)
Cephal/o	Head	Cephalocaudal (pattern of growth development from head to tail)
Cervic/o	Neck	Cervical spinal stenosis (narrowing of the spinal canal in the neck)
Chondr/o	Cartilage	Chondroplasty (corrective surgery of the cartilage, most often of the knee)
-Clasis	Break, fracture	Osteoclasis (bone break)
Cost/o	Rib	Intercostal space (space between two ribs)
Crani/o	Head, skull	Craniosynostosis (deformity of a baby's skull in which one or more sutures closes earlier than normal)
Femor/o	Femur, thigh bone	Patellofemoral syndrome (pain in the front of the knee where the patella meets the femur)
Ischi/o	Hip	Ischial bursitis (inflammation of the bursa surrounding the hip)
My/o	Muscle	Myalgia (muscle pain)
Myel/o	Bone marrow, spinal cord	Myelogram (X-ray of the spinal cord)
Orth/o	Straight	Orthodontia (related to straight teeth)
Oste/o	Bone	Osteomyelitis (inflammation of the bone and marrow)
Spondyl/o	Vertebrae, backbone	Spondyloarthropathy (any joint disease of the vertebral column)

Abbreviations Related to the Musculoskeletal System

The following are abbreviations related to the musculoskeletal system:

- ACL—Anterior cruciate ligament
- AP—Anteroposterior
- C1, C2, etc—First cervical vertebra, second cervical vertebra, etc.
- Ca—Calcium
- Fx—Fracture
- L1, L2, etc—First lumbar vertebra, second lumbar vertebra, etc.
- LAT—Lateral
- LE—Lower extremity
- LLE—Left lower extremity
- LUE—Left upper extremity

- PCL—Posterior cruciate ligament
- RLE—Right lower extremity
- RUE—Right upper extremity
- ROM—Range of motion
- T1, T2, etc—First thoracic vertebra, second thoracic vertebra, etc.
- THR—Total hip replacement
- TKA—Total knee arthroplasty
- TKR—Total knee replacement
- Tx—Traction
- UE—Upper extremity

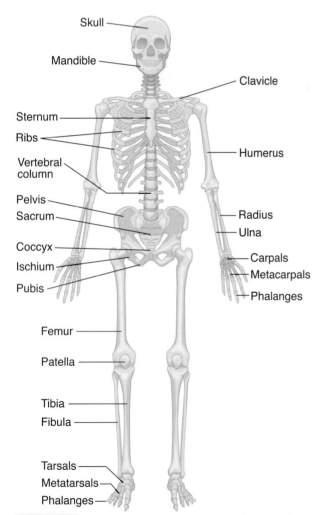

FIGURE 12.1 The human skeleton is the body's frame.

Skull
Mandible
Clavicle
Sternum
Ribs
Humerus
Vertebral column
Pelvis
Sacrum
Radius
Ulna
Coccyx
Ischium
Carpals
Metacarpals
Pubis
Phalanges
Femur
Patella
Tibia
Fibula
Tarsals
Metatarsals
Phalanges

Structure and Function of the Muscular and Skeletal Systems

Together, the bones make up the **skeleton**, which is the body's frame and provides protection to internal organs. The skeleton is divided into the **axial skeleton**, which has 80 bones, and the **appendicular skeleton**, which has 126 bones. The axial skeleton includes the **skull** and associated bones (the bones that encase the brain and support the face), the **thoracic cage** (the bones that surround the organs and soft tissues of the chest), and the **vertebral column** (the bones of the spinal column). The appendicular skeleton includes the **pectoral girdle** (the bones that connect the upper limbs to the axial skeleton), the upper limbs, the **pelvic girdle** (the bones that connect the lower limbs to the axial skeleton), and the lower limbs. **FIGURE 12.1** illustrates the major bones of the skeleton.

Muscles are attached to the bones, which enables the body to move. Like bones, muscles come in varying shapes and sizes, depending on their function and location. **FIGURE 12.2** illustrates the major muscle groups of the human body.

Bones

Each bone in the human body is a unique organ, with its own blood supply, nerves, and lymphatic system. Each bone contains two types of tissue: compact bone and cancellous bone. **Compact bone** is densely packed and forms a hard, protective shell around the **cancellous bone**, which is porous, less dense, and

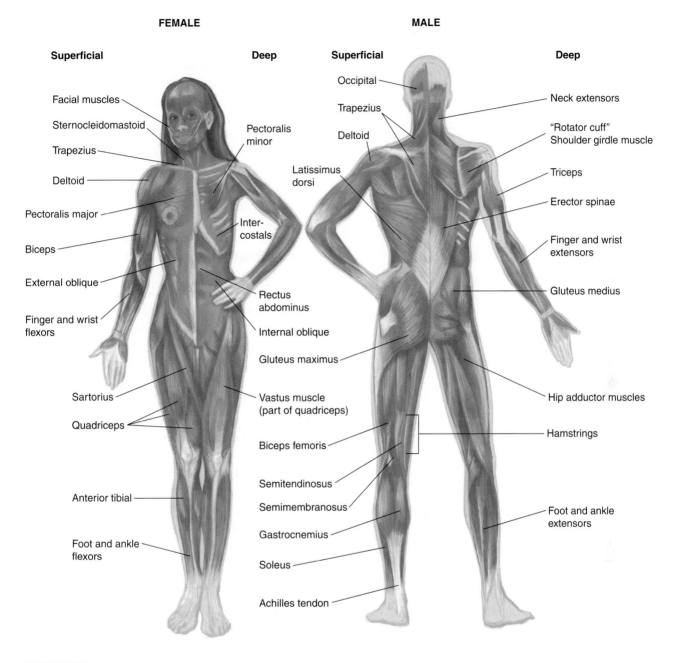

FIGURE 12.2 The major muscles of the adult human body enable the body to move.
© Jones & Bartlett Learning

resembles a sponge. Cancellous bone is also called **trabecular bone** or **spongy bone**. A thin membrane, called the **periosteum**, covers each bone and supplies the bone with lymph vessels, blood vessels, and nerves. In addition to providing support and protection for the body, bones also store minerals. Calcium and phosphorous are the two most prevalent minerals in bone.

To stay healthy, bone must undergo constant remodeling. **Osteoclasts** are cells that erode old bone and **osteoblasts** deposit new bone in its place. This process must remain balanced to maintain strong bones. A well-balanced diet that includes minerals such as calcium, phosphorous, and magnesium; protein; and regular exercise helps to maintain bone strength. Hormones also affect the rate of bone remodeling.

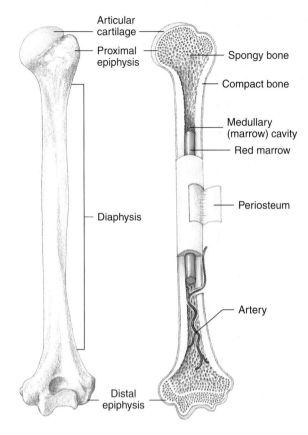

Articular cartilage
Proximal epiphysis
Diaphysis
Distal epiphysis

Spongy bone
Compact bone
Medullary (marrow) cavity
Red marrow
Periosteum
Artery

FIGURE 12.3 Anatomy of a bone.
© Jones & Bartlett Learning

Bones are classified by shape and function:

- **Long bones** consist of a shaft (the **diaphysis**) made of compact bone with a cavity in the middle that contains yellow bone marrow, which is composed of fat cells. The wide ends of long bones (called the **metaphysis**) contain cancellous bone that contains red bone marrow, which manufactures red and white blood cells and platelets. The **epiphysis** is the thick plate at each end of the bone. Growth plates are layers of cartilage between the epiphysis and diaphysis that expand as the bone elongates or grows. The **condyle** is the rounded portion at the end of a bone. **FIGURE 12.3** illustrates the main features of a long bone.

- **Short bones** are made of cancellous bone with a thin covering of compact bone. Short bones allow for greater flexibility than long bones.

- **Irregular bones** are shaped for a specific purpose or protective function. Vertebrae and the bones of the inner ear are examples of irregular bones.

- **Flat bones**, such as the plates of the skull and the ribs, are composed of cancellous bone between two layers of compact bone. Flat bones protect soft, vulnerable organs and structures such as the lungs, heart, and brain. They also provide flat surfaces for large muscle attachment.

- **Sesamoid bones**, such as the kneecap, or **patella**, are small, round bones that are embedded within a tendon. Sesamoid bones modify pressure, decrease friction, and increase the mechanical ability of a joint.

Joints

A joint is the point at which two or more bones meet. Joints are also called **articulations**. One type of joint, called a **synarthrosis**, allows no movement between the bones it connects. The bones are in almost direct contact with each other and are connected with thick, immovable connective tissue. Synarthroses are also called fibrous joints or **fixed joints**. The suture lines in the skull are examples of synarthroses **FIGURE 12.4**.

An **amphiarthrosis**, or cartilaginous joint, is a joint that allows very limited movement. An example of an amphiarthrosis is the pubic symphysis (or symphysis pubis), a small joint between pelvic bones **FIGURE 12.5**. Normally, this joint can only move 1–2mm and has 1 degree of rotation. In pregnancy, however, the joint allows for greater movement and flexibility, which aids in the birth process. The spot where the sternum and ribs connect is also an amphiarthrosis. In cartilaginous joints, discs of cartilage hold the bones together and act as cushions or shock absorbers.

The most common type of joint, a **diarthrosis** **FIGURE 12.6**, allows for free movement of the bones. In these joints, the bones do not touch each other. The bones are covered with cartilage and separated by a **synovial cavity**. The **synovial membrane** encapsulates the cavity and secretes **synovial fluid**, which lubricates the joint. The **joint capsule** surrounds the membrane and is strengthened by **ligaments**, which are bands

The humerus and the femur are examples of long bones. The bones in the hands and feet are examples of short bones.
© auremar/ShutterStock, Inc.

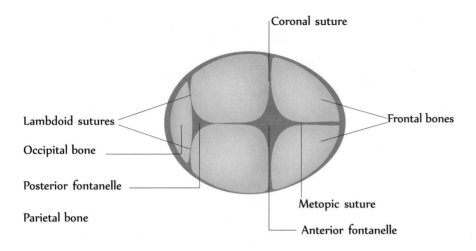

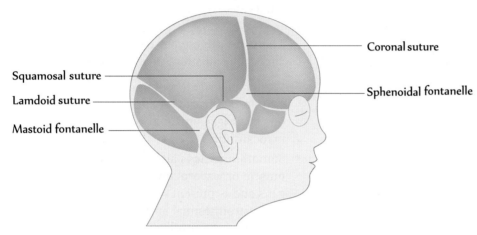

FIGURE 12.4 The sutures of the skull are fixed joints.
© Grei/ShutterStock, Inc.

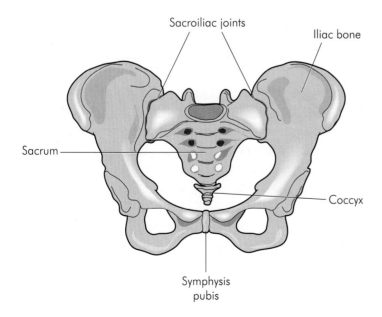

FIGURE 12.5 The pubic symphysis is a cartilaginous joint.
© Blamb/ShutterStock, Inc.

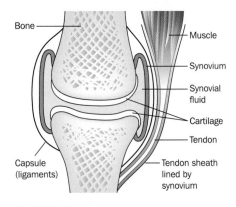

FIGURE 12.6 In a diarthrosis, or synovial joint, the bones do not touch each other.
© Blamb/ShutterStock, Inc.

The temporomandibular joints of the jaw are the most active joints in the body, opening and closing as many as 2,000 times each day.
© auremar/ShutterStock, Inc.

There are more than 400 skeletal muscles in the human body, accounting for nearly half of a person's body weight.
© auremar/ShutterStock, Inc.

of connective tissue that connect bone to bone. Ball and socket joints, hinge joints, and pivot joints are classified as diarthroses. Diarthroses are also known as synovial joints. Each synovial joint includes a **bursa**, or disk-shaped sac filled with synovial fluid that eases movement. The bursa lies between the skin and the surface of a bone or in areas where tendons or muscles rub against bone, ligaments, or other tendons or muscles.

Muscles

Muscle activity determines physical function. Muscles and joints work together to move body parts. Muscles work in pairs called flexors, which contract to bend a limb at a joint, and extensors, which contract to straighten the limb. **TABLE 12.2** includes terminology related to muscle movement. The muscular system is highly integrated with the nervous system, and motor neurons stimulate muscle contraction.

There are three types of muscle **FIGURE 12.7**, all of which differ in strength and function:

- Cardiac muscle is a unique muscle present only in the heart that allows for continuous beating. Cardiac muscle is also called myocardium.
- Smooth muscle is also called involuntary muscle or **visceral muscle**. It lines hollow organs and is present in body systems such as the gastrointestinal and urinary tracts. Smooth muscles are controlled solely by the nervous system and are responsible for activities such as digestion and respiration.
- Skeletal muscle is also called **striated muscle** because its fibers have horizontal stripes. It is attached to the skeleton. These muscles permit the voluntary movement of the body. Skeletal muscles are composed of muscle fibers that are

Table 12.2	Terminology Related to Muscle Movement
Term	**Definition**
Abduction	Movement away from the midline of the body
Adduction	Movement toward the midline of the body
Circumduction	Movement in a circular direction from a central point
Dorsiflexion	Bending backward
Eversion	Turning outward
Extension	Movement that makes limbs straight
Flexion	Bending
Inversion	Turning inward
Pronation	Rotation at the hand or ankle moving toward the midline of the body
Rotation	Movement around a central axis
Supination	Rotation at the hand or ankle moving away from the midline of the body

held together with connective tissue that contract and relax to produce movement. The bundles of fibers are grouped together and covered with another layer of connective tissue that supplies blood and oxygen to the muscles, as well as lymph vessels and nerves.

One end of a muscle attaches to the bone at a point called the **origin**. The origin remains stationary during muscle contraction. The opposite end of the muscle attaches to another bone at the **insertion**. The muscle flattens and broadens toward the points of attachment to the bone. A narrow cordlike structure of connective tissues, called a tendon, is one type of attachment. The other type of connection, an **aponeurosis**, is a flat band of connective tissue that connects muscle to bone. Muscles and joints work together to move body parts **FIGURE 12.8** .

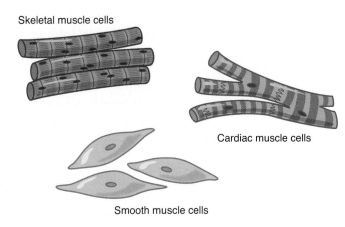

FIGURE 12.7 The types of muscle differ in strength and function.
© Jones & Bartlett Learning

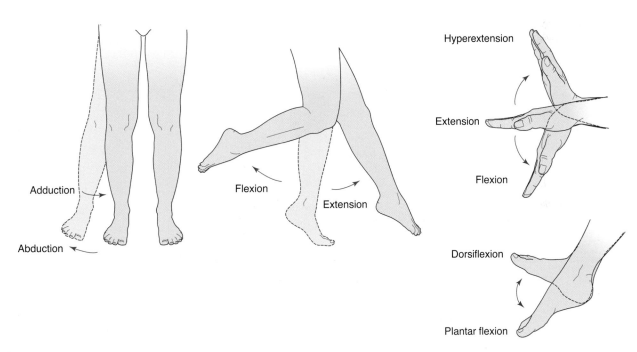

FIGURE 12.8 Muscles and joints work together to move body parts.
© Jones & Bartlett Learning

Diseases and Disorders of the Muscular and Skeletal Systems

Disorders of the muscular and skeletal systems vary in presentation, amount of pain, and level of care required. Any condition that disrupts the normal, integrated function of the skeletal and muscular systems impedes an individual's ability to move effectively and without pain. Some disorders that affect the musculoskeletal system also affect other body systems, making a definitive diagnosis difficult.

Musculoskeletal changes occur with age, including decreased power of skeletal muscles and diminished strength of ligaments, which also contribute to disability and impairment. Many patients with musculoskeletal complaints will require long-term care and follow-up, and many disorders are challenging to treat effectively. Often, treatment for musculoskeletal disorders will require immobilization of a joint or limb or significant lifestyle changes, both of which can make a patient uncomfortable, noncompliant, and irritable. A medical assistant who deals with orthopedic patients must be compassionate, understanding, and patient.

Bursitis and Tendonitis

Bursitis is a painful inflammation of the bursa. It occurs most frequently in the hip, shoulder, and knee. **Tendonitis** is an inflammation of a tendon. **Tendinosis**, or degeneration of a tendon, may accompany the inflammation **FIGURE 12.9**. Tendonitis frequently occurs in the wrist, heel, elbow, and shoulder. These conditions generally occur in middle age and result from recurring trauma, infection, or stress on a joint.

Signs and Symptoms of Bursitis and Tendonitis

Pain is the most common sign of bursitis and tendonitis. Pain occurs upon movement and limits the motion of the joint. Onset of pain may be gradual or sudden and can range in intensity from mild to severe depending on the joint involved and the underlying cause of the inflammation. Swelling, warmth, and redness may accompany

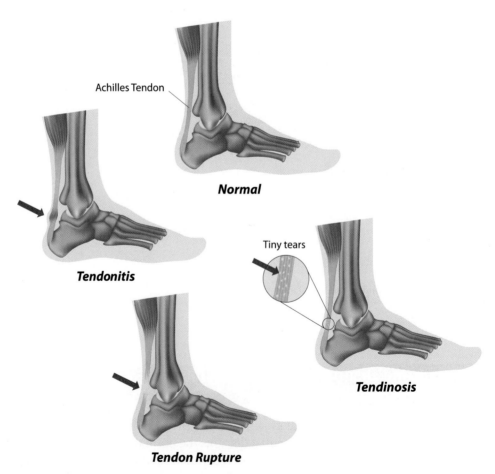

Achilles Tendon

Normal

Tendonitis

Tiny tears

Tendinosis

Tendon Rupture

FIGURE 12.9 Tendonitis, tendinosis, and rupture of the Achilles tendon can all cause foot pain.
© Alila Sao Mai/ShutterStock, Inc.

the inflammation. Recurrent episodes of bursitis and tendonitis can lead to chronic inflammation of the joint.

Treatment of Bursitis and Tendonitis

The goal of treatment of bursitis and tendonitis is to relieve pain and decrease inflammation. Joint rest is the mainstay of treatment for bursitis and tendonitis. Immobilization may be necessary to restrict the use of the affected joint. Pain medication can be administered to relieve discomfort associated with the inflammation. In severe cases, an injection of a steroid into the affected joint will relieve inflammation. Physical therapy to improve or preserve motion in the affected joints is advisable after the acute pain associated with bursitis or tendonitis is relieved. Stretching and strengthening the muscles around the affected joint can prevent future episodes of pain and inflammation.

Carpal Tunnel Syndrome

The **carpal tunnel** is a hollow tube in the wrist that contains nerves, blood vessels, and tendons **FIGURE 12.10**. When the sheaths of the tendons in the carpal tunnel become inflamed, swelling occurs and places pressure on the median nerve of the wrist, also found in the carpal tunnel.

Carpal tunnel syndrome (CTS) is a set of symptoms that occurs among people who use their hands on a regular basis, such as those who type, sew, clean, or do assembly-line work. Other conditions, including diabetes mellitus, pregnancy, menopause, hypothyroidism, and tumors, can cause swelling in the wrists, which can lead to symptoms of carpal tunnel syndrome.

Signs and Symptoms of Carpal Tunnel Syndrome

Pain, tingling, and numbness in the hands are symptoms of carpal tunnel syndrome. The thumb, index finger, and middle finger are most often affected. Patients with carpal tunnel syndrome will be unable to make a fist.

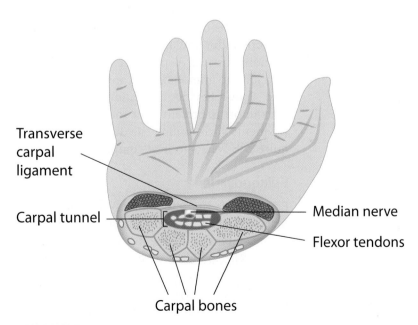

FIGURE 12.10 Carpal tunnel syndrome occurs among people who use their hands on a regular basis.
© Alila Sao Mai/ShutterStock, Inc.

Treatment of Carpal Tunnel Syndrome

The goal of treatment of carpal tunnel syndrome is to relieve pain and prevent future inflammation. Immobilization of the hand and forearm, often with a splint, can decrease the swelling and relieve the pressure on the nerves in the wrist. Systemic anti-inflammatory drugs or local injections of corticosteroids may be necessary to relieve the swelling. In severe cases of carpal tunnel syndrome, surgery may be necessary to relieve the pressure on the nerves.

Some sufferers of carpal tunnel syndrome may need to alter the patterns of use of their hands and wrists. Some must seek alternate employment if limiting the use of their hands is not feasible in their current job.

Dislocation

A **dislocation** is any displacement of a bone at a joint. When a dislocation occurs, surfaces that regularly articulate are no longer in contact with each other and motion at the joint is restricted. Fingers, shoulders, knees, and hips are the most frequent site of dislocations.

A **subluxation** is a partial or incomplete dislocation of a joint. Subluxations commonly occur at the shoulders, elbows, wrists, knees, fingers, toes, hips, and ankles. Dislocations and subluxations are caused by disease or trauma to the joint. Damage to surrounding nerves, blood vessels, ligaments, and soft tissues accompanies dislocations and subluxations. Dislocations can be caused by trauma or disease. Congenital dislocation of the hips is present at birth.

Signs and Symptoms of Dislocation

Dislocation and subluxation are painful and produce deformity in the joint. The deformity changes the length of the extremity, interferes with motion, and causes tenderness. The dislocation may also cause nerve impingement, which causes numbness and tingling in the extremity. A dislocation can often be recognized on visual examination, but an X-ray may be necessary to confirm the exact location and extent of the injury.

Treatment of Dislocation

Reduction, a relocation or realignment, of the joint is the only treatment for dislocation. Prompt reduction limits damage to the surrounding tissues. A splint or cast may be placed on a joint to immobilize the area after a dislocation. Pain-relieving medications can be used if discomfort is present after the reduction. The ligaments surrounding the dislocated joint require 2–8 weeks to heal completely.

Epicondylitis

Epicondylitis, more commonly known as tennis elbow, is an inflammation of the forearm extensor tendon at its attachment to the humerus **FIGURE 12.11**. Rarely, the inflammation occurs in the corresponding forearm flexor tendon. Epicondylitis begins as a small tear in the tendon after gripping objects tightly or twisting the forearm. Epicondylitis most often occurs in middle age.

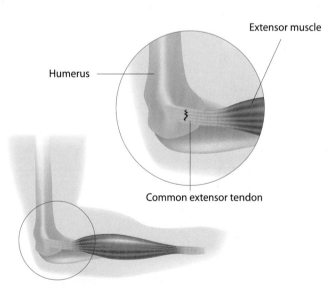

Humerus

Extensor muscle

Common extensor tendon

Right arm, lateral (outside) side

FIGURE 12.11 Epicondylitis is an inflammation of the forearm extensor tendon at its attachment to the humerus.
© Alila Sao Mai/ShutterStock, Inc.

Signs and Symptoms of Epicondylitis

Pain in the elbow is the hallmark symptom of epicondylitis. Tenderness occurs over the position where the radius articulates with the humerus.

Treatment of Epicondylitis

The goals of treatment of epicondylitis are to relieve symptoms and prevent their recurrence. Epicondylitis is most effectively treated with joint immobilization, a local steroid injection to relieve the swelling, systemic nonsteroidal anti-inflammatory drugs (NSAIDs) to relieve pain and reduce swelling, heat or cold therapy, and physical therapy. Usually, epicondylitis resolves, even without treatment. However, some cases, if left untreated, can progress into chronic, debilitating conditions.

Fibromyalgia

Fibromyalgia is characterized by diffuse, widespread pain. It affects people of all ages and both genders, but occurs more frequently in people with autoimmune diseases and arthritis disorders. The cause of fibromyalgia is unknown, but a genetic component likely plays a role in its development. Weather, stress, and poor physical fitness worsen symptoms of fibromyalgia. Symptoms may fluctuate in intensity, but fibromyalgia is a chronic, long-term condition for which there is no cure.

Signs and Symptoms of Fibromyalgia

Widespread pain and localized tenderness, without apparent trauma or injury, are the hallmarks of fibromyalgia. Typically, tenderness occurs at 18 points around the shoulders, hips, knees, low back, and elbows **FIGURE 12.12**. Persistent discomfort at 11 of the 18 points in considered definitive for the diagnosis of fibromyalgia. In addition to pain, fibromyalgia causes muscle stiffness, an inability to concentrate, sleep disturbances, dry eyes and mouth, frequent urination, irritable bowel syndrome, headaches, numbness in the extremities, bursitis, tendonitis, and depression.

Treatment of Fibromyalgia

The goals of fibromyalgia treatment are to reduce the frequency and severity of symptoms and improve quality of life. Massage, warm showers, low-impact exercise, and stress-reduction techniques can help manage fibromyalgia. Muscle relaxants and pain relievers are also appropriate for fibromyalgia treatment. Antidepressant and anti-epileptic drugs, usually given at lower doses than for their primary indications, are also used in the management of fibromyalgia.

Patients with fibromyalgia should be advised to make lifestyle choices that improve their symptoms, such as staying physically fit, maintaining a healthy body weight, and obtaining adequate restful sleep.

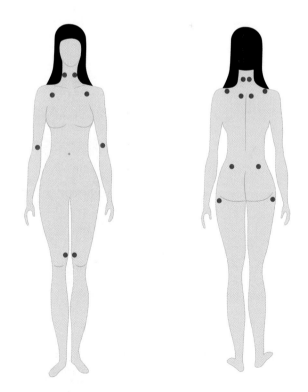

FIGURE 12.12 Common sites of tenderness and pain in fibromyalgia.
© Alila Sao Mai/ShutterStock, Inc.

Fracture

A **fracture** is a disruption of the continuity of the bone **FIGURE 12.13**. More simply, a fracture is a broken bone. Many terms can be used to define the type, location, and severity of a fracture. All fractures are classified as open or closed. An **open fracture** involves a break in the skin and, usually, bone protruding from this skin. In a **closed fracture**, the skin is not broken. An open fracture presents an increased risk for infection.

A bone breaks when more pressure is placed on it than it can tolerate. This pressure may be due to a fall, an impact, or repetitive force. Patients often report that they

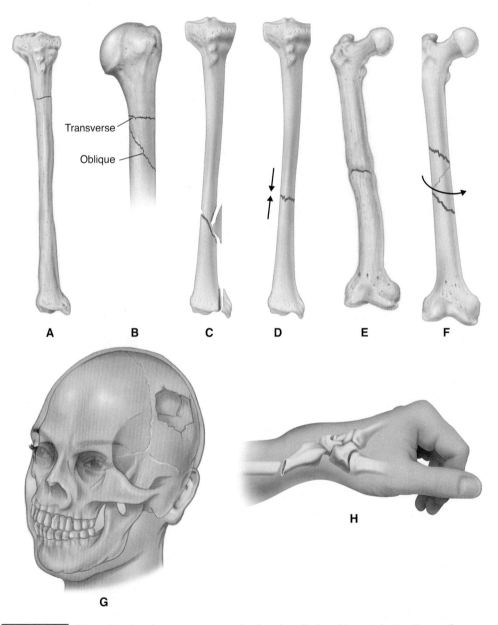

FIGURE 12.13 A bone breaks when more pressure is placed on it than it can tolerate. Types of fractures include: Incomplete (A), Transverse or Oblique (B), Comminuted (C), Impacted (D), Complete (E), Spiral (F), Depressed (G), and Colles (H).

© Jones & Bartlett Learning

heard the bone break or they sense a grating feeling at the site of the break.

Types of Fractures

- **Closed (simple)**—A fracture that has no break in the skin or surrounding muscle
- **Colles**—A fracture of the distal radius that results from falling with an outstretched hand; results in displacement and a bulging of the wrist
- **Comminuted**—A fracture in which the bone breaks into numerous pieces and more than one fracture line is present
- **Complete**—A fracture in which the bone breaks completely
- **Depressed**—A fracture of the skull in which the bone is pushed in
- **Greenstick**—A fracture occurring in childhood in which young, soft bones bend and partially break
- **Impacted**—A fracture in which the bone fragments are driven into each other
- **Incomplete**—A fracture in which the bone is still partially intact
- **Open (compound)**—A fracture that involves a break in the skin or soft tissues surrounding the bone
- **Spiral**—A fracture that occurs with a twisting motion and the break winds around a long bone
- **Stress**—A fracture that occurs after repeated or prolonged use, such as in running

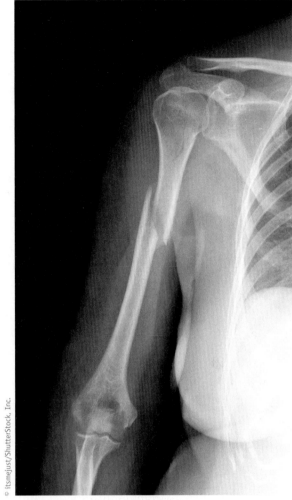

© itsmejust/ShutterStock, Inc.

A fracture of the humerus viewed in an X-ray.

Signs and Symptoms of Fracture

A fracture will often cause visible deformity in the affected limb or joint. However, some fractures, such as a closed simple fracture, may not cause a visible deformity. Pain is the most significant symptom of a fracture. The soft tissue surrounding the fracture immediately swells and a bruise may appear. Mobility will likely be affected by a break. If a nerve is damaged along with the fracture, numbness or tingling may occur. X-rays are often used to diagnose and assess a fracture, and to confirm whether a dislocation or subluxation is present.

Treatment of a Fracture

Reduction and immobilization are the proper treatments for a fracture. Reduction of the bone can be done in an office setting or may require surgery, depending on the severity of the break. Once reduced, the fractured bone is immobilized, often with a cast. The limb must remain immobilized until the bone has been allowed time to heal, which may be up to several months depending on the location and extent of the break. A patient with a broken bone should maintain a healthy diet high in vitamins, protein, iron, and calcium, which will facilitate healing.

Normal Bone Healing

After a fracture, bleeding from the ends of the fractured bones form a clot that fills in the space created by the break. Within 1 to 2 weeks of the fracture, the clot is replaced by a callus that is composed of cartilage and newly formed bone. Several weeks later, the callus is replaced by bone cells through a process called **ossification**, which is the layering of new bone by osteoblasts. The new bone is reshaped by osteoblasts.

Gout

Gout is a well-known and historic disease, with many notable historical figures known to be sufferers, including Hippocrates, Henry VIII, and Benjamin Franklin. Gout is sometimes referred to as gouty arthritis because its symptoms affect joints. The cause of gout is an accumulation of uric acid, caused by either an overproduction of uric acid or a failure to excrete uric acid. Uric acid is a product of the breakdown of the purine nucleotides, adenine and guanine. Excess uric acid leads to uric acid crystal deposits in the joints. The crystals lead to joint inflammation.

Gout affects men over the age of 30 and postmenopausal women. A metabolic defect is likely the cause of the overproduction of uric acid, and a family history of such metabolic defects is associated with gout. Gout can be associated with other diseases, such as leukemia, or treatments, such as chemotherapy or other drugs, that affect the production and excretion of uric acid.

There is a link between obesity and metabolic syndrome and gout. Increased weight and dietary intake of alcohol, meat, and fish contribute to the development of gout.

Signs and Symptoms of Gout

The symptoms of gout appear quickly and without warning, often leading to excruciating pain. The first metatarsophalangeal joint at the base of the big toe is the most commonly afflicted joint in gout. The toe becomes hot, red, and painful.

Fluid aspirated from a joint affected by gout is filled with uric acid crystals, called **tophi**, which can be seen under a microscope. Tophi are the definitive diagnostic feature of gout.

Gout is considered a long-term chronic disorder, with periods of remission and exacerbation. Early in the disease, symptom-free periods of remission generally last 6–24 months. Later exacerbations affect other joints of the feet and the legs, and exacerbations occur more frequently as the disease progresses.

Treatment of Gout

The goals of gout treatment are to eliminate the painful symptoms and improve quality of life. Historically, colchicine has been the treatment of choice for gout. Although effective at relieving the symptoms of gout, colchicine causes gastrointestinal upset in nearly all patients. Colchicine can be used to relieve acute attacks or prevent exacerbations. Anti-inflammatory drugs, including salicylates and corticosteroids, are also effective at relieving some of the symptoms of gout.

If failure to excrete uric acid is the cause of gout, drugs such as probenecid can be used to increase the kidney's excretion of uric acid. If overproduction of uric acid is the cause of gout, allopurinol can be used to prevent the formation of urates (uric acid salts).

Limiting alcohol intake, staying hydrated, and restricting purine-rich foods such as organ meat (liver,

Gout has been referred to as the "king of diseases" and the "disease of kings" due to its prevalence among affluent societies and cultures prone to overindulgence, gluttony, and intemperance.

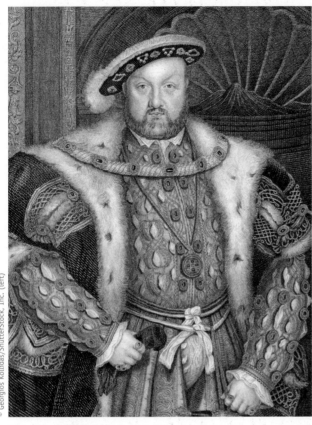

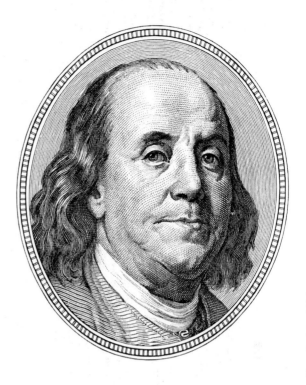

King Henry VIII of England and Benjamin Franklin are two of the most famous men who were afflicted with gout.

kidneys, and sweetbreads), legumes (dried beans and peas), anchovies, sardines, herring, oils, mushrooms, spinach, gravies, and yeast can aid in managing symptoms of gout. Maintaining a healthy weight is also advisable for patients with gout.

Hallux Valgus

Hallux valgus is a lateral deviation of the big toe, accompanied by the enlargement of the first metatarsal head. This **bunion** formation is the hallmark characteristic of hallux valgus. Bunions are often associated with painful bursa.

Hallux valgus occurs as the result of chronic, degenerative arthritis or prolonged pressure on the foot from narrow, high-heeled shoes. Due to this etiology, hallux valgus occurs most frequently in women. Over time, hallux valgus will alter the bone structure of the toes and feet and change a person's weight-bearing patterns.

Signs and Symptoms of Hallux Valgus

The bursa of the big toe becomes inflamed and swollen. The overlying skin will be red and tender. Severe deformities will be extremely painful.

Treatment of Hallux Valgus

Proper shoes (flat with a wide toe) and foot and leg exercises can correct hallux valgus if initiated early. A severe deformity requires surgical removal of the bunion. Hallux

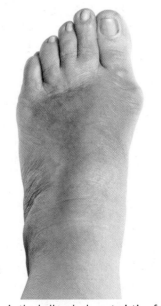

A formation is the hallmark characteristic of hallux valgus.

valgus can be prevented by avoiding tight-fitting, narrow shoes that place uncomfortable pressure on the feet and toes.

Herniated Disk

A **herniated disk**, or **ruptured disk**, occurs when the gel inside the vertebral disks of the spine is forced outside the disk `FIGURE 12.14`. This gel can place pressure on spinal nerves or impinge the spinal cord itself.

Herniated disks result from trauma or strain, or from degeneration of the vertebral joints due to disease. Herniated disks most often occur in the lumbosacral region of the spine, or the lower back. The condition usually occurs in adult males under 45 years of age. However, herniated disks may occur in elderly people with degenerative joint disease after minor trauma. Excessive weight, injury, and smoking are also factors for herniated disks at any age.

Signs and Symptoms of a Herniated Disk

Low back pain is the hallmark of a herniated disk. The pain usually radiates through the buttocks and the back of the leg. It is usually one-sided pain. Sensory loss, numbness, motor difficulty, weakness, and muscle atrophy can occur from nerve compression.

Treatment of a Herniated Disk

The goals of treatment of a herniated disk are to relieve pain and prevent future disability. Avoiding painful activities, resting, and taking anti-inflammatory medications are beneficial for relieving the pain associated with herniated disks. If symptoms do not resolve or if there is nerve damage, surgery to remove the offending material and stabilize the vertebrae may be performed.

Kyphosis, Lordosis, and Scoliosis

An abnormal curvature of the spine is classified as kyphosis, lordosis, or scoliosis `FIGURE 12.15`. **Kyphosis** is the abnormal bowing or rounding of the upper back. Kyphosis has two distinct etiologies:

- Adolescent kyphosis occurs in children and is caused by poor posture, growth retardation, or excessive sports activity.

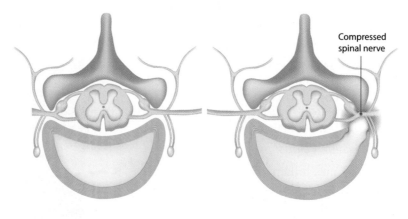

Normal disk   Herniated disk

FIGURE 12.14 A herniated disk, as viewed from above, occurs when the gel inside the vertebral disks of the spine is forced outside the disk.
© Alila Sao Mai/ShutterStock, Inc.

- Adult kyphosis is caused by aging and the degeneration of vertebrae due to bone loss.

Lordosis is the abnormal convex curvature of the low back, commonly called swayback. The spine naturally curves inward at the low back, but lordosis is an excessive or exaggerated curvature. Lordosis is usually caused by poor posture or wearing high-heeled shoes. **Scoliosis** is a sideways or lateral curvature of the spine, usually in the thoracic or upper-back region. Scoliosis is also associated with a rotation of the spine. Scoliosis can be caused by genetic defects of the vertebrae, muscular dystrophy, or paralysis, but most cases have no identifiable cause. Scoliosis is usually diagnosed in adolescent girls; it affects girls 10 times more frequently than boys.

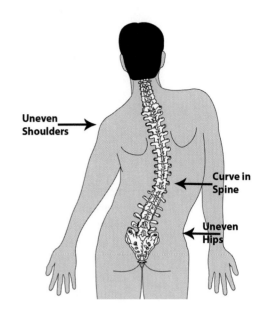

FIGURE 12.15 Kyphosis is the abnormal bowing or rounding of the upper back; scoliosis—shown here—is a sideways or lateral curvature of the spine.
© Blamb/ShutterStock, Inc.

Signs and Symptoms of Kyphosis, Lordosis, and Scoliosis

Any abnormal curvature of the spine results in improper vertebral alignment, which can lead to damaging effects in the entire musculoskeletal system. Most symptoms of spinal curvature develop slowly over time. Patients with kyphosis experience pain, fatigue, localized tenderness, stiffness in the back, and tightening of the hamstring muscles due to poor posture. Respiratory difficulty can present with kyphosis if the curvature of the back is extreme enough to obstruct the normal function of the lungs.

Lordosis and scoliosis do not frequently cause pain, neurologic dysfunction, or respiratory problems. However, cosmetic concerns can cause significant psychological stress, especially for children and adolescents. In cases of scoliosis, hips or shoulders may be visibly uneven or the gait may be awkward.

Treatment of Kyphosis, Lordosis, and Scoliosis

Braces, proper footwear, improved posture, and back-strengthening exercises are appropriate treatment for abnormal curvatures of the spine. In severe, debilitating cases, surgical straightening of the spine with metal rods is indicated to prevent further disability.

Osteoarthritis

Osteoarthritis (OA) is the most common type of joint inflammation and leads to a progressive deterioration of the cartilage within a joint. The hips and knees are common sites of OA. Age is a contributing factor to OA, and it is believed to occur after years of normal wear and tear of joints. Local injury or joint deformity can contribute to OA. A mild inflammatory or metabolic disorder may also play a role in the development of OA. It is believed that OA results from an imbalance in the destruction and regeneration of cartilage. This loss of cartilage leads to inflammation, bone destruction, and further cartilage damage. A family history of OA is also a risk factor for OA.

OA is not a systemic disease. It does not affect life expectancy, but it does impact quality of life. OA carries with it high personal, economic, and societal costs due to its enormous disability and loss of productivity. Nearly 50 million people in the United States suffer from OA.

Signs and Symptoms of Osteoarthritis

OA causes the destruction of cartilage in the joints and the bones themselves, which leads to joint pain, stiffness, and aching. Patients may also complain of a grinding sensation, or **crepitus**, of the joints. Mobility is often limited and function is decreased. Symptoms of OA often appear first in the large, weight-bearing joints.

Treatment of Systemic Osteoarthritis

There is no cure for OA, and the disease is progressive. Its symptoms are most effectively treated with anti-inflammatory drugs and pain relievers, including aspirin and other NSAIDs, steroids, and acetaminophen. The long-term use of NSAIDs should be monitored carefully because they can increase the risk for cardiovascular events, cause gastrointestinal distress, and increase the risk of bleeding. Topical pain-relieving creams can be used for localized symptom relief. Rest also relieves the symptoms of OA, as does the local application of heat or cold. Severe and debilitating pain associated with OA can be treated surgically by removing bone fragments from affected joints and replacing them with artificial joints.

Osteopenia and Osteoporosis

The bone-remodeling process is affected by age. After the age of 30, bone deteriorates more quickly than it regenerates, especially in women. The loss of calcium and phosphate from the bone causes the bone to become porous and fragile **FIGURE 12.16**, a condition called **osteoporosis**, making it prone to fractures. Osteoporosis affects women disproportionately to men. **Osteopenia**, or low bone mass, is the precursor to osteoporosis. With osteopenia, bone loss has begun, but it is not as severe as osteoporosis.

Primary or postmenopausal osteoporosis usually occurs in elderly, postmenopausal women. This type of osteoporosis is due to long-term inadequate calcium intake, estrogen deficiency, and a sedentary lifestyle. Smoking, a family history of osteoporosis, a small body frame, and a low body weight are also risk factors for developing osteoporosis. Men with low levels of testosterone are also at risk for osteoporosis. Secondary osteoporosis occurs with prolonged steroid therapy, bone immobilization or paralysis, malnutrition, excessive alcohol intake, vitamin deficiencies, and hyperthyroidism.

Signs and Symptoms of Osteopenia and Osteoporosis

In general, osteopenia and osteoporosis are silent diseases, with their onset occurring gradually with no outward signs or symptoms. By the time symptoms appear, irreversible damage may have already occurred. Gradually developing kyphosis with loss of height is a hallmark sign of primary osteoporosis. Fractures in the hips or forearms after minor falls or trauma can indicate loss of bone strength and often prompt a diagnosis of osteopenia or osteoporosis. Pain from the collapse of vertebrae or other osteoporotic fractures is sudden and severe. Bone pain may occur with progressive disease. Simple, in-

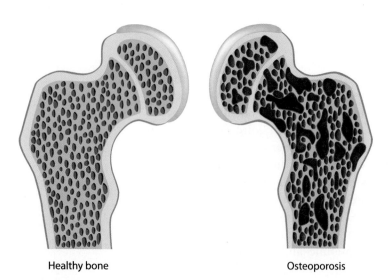

Healthy bone   Osteoporosis

FIGURE 12.16 In osteoporosis, the bone becomes porous and fragile.
© Alila Sao Mai/ShutterStock, Inc.

expensive screening and diagnostic tools can estimate bone loss and aid in setting strategies to maintain bone health.

Treatment of Osteopenia and Osteoporosis

The goals of treatment of osteopenia and osteoporosis are to restore bone strength and prevent bone loss. Osteoporosis is highly preventable. All patients, regardless of age or risk factors, should be advised to participate in regular physical activity and obtain adequate calcium and vitamin D in their diet to support bone remodeling. Postmenopausal women may be candidates for hormone therapy to maintain levels of estrogen that support bone health. Several other classes of drugs are available that slow or prevent bone loss, including bisphosphonates (Boniva [ibandronate] and Reclast [zoledronic acid]), selective estrogen receptor modulators (Evista [raloxifene]), and calcitonin and parathyroid hormone.

> **What Would You Do?**
>
> A 53-year-old postmenopausal woman visits the physician's office where you are a medical assistant for her annual physical. When you obtain her height and weight, you note a slight loss of height over the last several years. The patient responds that she thought this was just a normal part of aging, and that her mother, grandmother, and aunts were all hunched over when they were elderly. She also jokes that, being very petite to begin with, she cannot afford to lose much height. What would you tell the patient?
>
> © NorthGeorgiaMedia/ShutterStock, Inc.

Osteomyelitis

Osteomyelitis is an acute or chronic infection of the bone and bone marrow. It can be caused by bacteria or fungi. Usually, osteomyelitis begins as an infection in another part of the body and travels to nearby bone. Osteomyelitis may also occur from the direct contamination of a wound such as a fracture. Current or past bone injuries make bone more susceptible to osteomyelitis.

Adults should consume 1,000 to 1,200mg of calcium daily.
© auremar/ShutterStock, Inc.

Osteomyelitis affects children more than infants, adolescents, or adults. In children, long bones are usually affected by osteomyelitis. In adults, the bones of the feet, the hips, and the vertebrae are usually affected. Receiving hemodialysis, using injectable drugs, and having a splenectomy are risk factors for osteomyelitis.

Signs and Symptoms of Osteomyelitis

Bone pain, fever, general malaise, and localized swelling, redness, or warmth accompany osteomyelitis. Blood cultures, bone biopsies, and diagnostic imaging aid in the diagnosis of osteomyelitis.

Although the term arthritis indicates any joint inflammation, osteoarthritis and rheumatoid arthritis have unique pathophysiology and presentation.
© auremar/ShutterStock, Inc.

Treatment of Osteomyelitis

The goals of osteomyelitis treatment are to eradicate the infection and reduce damage to the bone and surrounding tissues. Antibiotics are used to control the infection. Often, more than one antibiotic is used, and will be administered for several weeks. Surgery may be necessary to remove damaged bone.

Rheumatoid Arthritis

Rheumatoid arthritis (RA) is a chronic, inflammatory autoimmune disease, meaning that patients have developed antibodies or allergic reactions to the proteins in their own bodies. It primarily affects the joints and surrounding muscles, tendons, ligaments, and blood vessels FIGURE 12.17 . It affects three times as many women as men, and symptom onset usually occurs between the ages of 20 and 60 years.

The cause of RA is unknown, but the autoimmune component of the disease causes macrophages to gather at the joint and stimulate an immune response. The blood vessels within the joint dilate and fluid accumulates in the joint cavity. The joint membrane thickens in response to the fluid accumulation and causes more swelling, eventually leading to the destruction of the joint. There is likely a genetic component to the development of RA.

Signs and Symptoms of Rheumatoid Arthritis

The symptoms of RA develop slowly, but eventually appear in the joints, usually symmetrically and bilaterally. The affected joints swell and stiffen and begin to show signs of deformity. Joints can be painful, tender, and hot, and deformities limit function. The knees, ankles, hands, and elbows are the most frequently affected joints in RA. Children can also be affected by RA. Juvenile RA (JRA) is characterized by red and painful joints, as well as fevers.

Lab tests usually indicate an elevated erythrocyte sedimentation rate (ESR) in RA patients, as well as anemia. Many test positive for a protein known as rheumatoid factor. Fluid aspirated from a joint affected by RA will appear opaque due to the high number of white blood cells (WBCs) in the synovial fluid. Normal synovial fluid is clear and has fewer than 200 WBCs/mm; there may be as many as 100,000 WBCs/mm in RA.

Exacerbations of RA are often triggered by physical or emotional stress. The symptoms of RA change over the course of the disease. Periods of remission become increasingly shorter as the disease progresses, and exacerbations become more severe and difficult to control. Although considered a disease of joints, RA can affect other body systems and present other symptoms, including eye inflammation, nodules under the skin, vasculitis, neurologic dysfunction, cardiopulmonary disease, lymphadenopathy, and splenomegaly.

Treatment of Rheumatoid Arthritis

There is no cure for RA. The goals of treatment are to relieve symptoms and improve quality of life. Corticosteroids, anti-inflammatory drugs, monoclonal antibodies, and

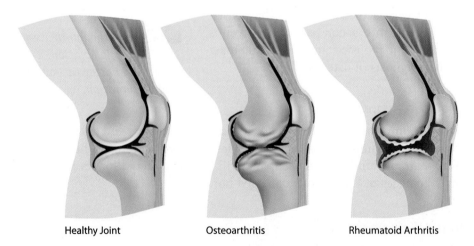

Healthy Joint   Osteoarthritis   Rheumatoid Arthritis

FIGURE 12.17 Types of arthritis: Rheumatoid arthritis affects three times as many women as men.
© Alila Sao Mai/ShutterStock, Inc.

immunosuppressants are mainstays of RA treatment, although each course must be individualized based on a patient's history of remission and exacerbation. Controlling inflammation is the most effective way to prevent or slow disease progression. Disease-modifying anti-rheumatic drugs or biologic agents should be started within three months of an RA diagnosis. Patients with RA should get plenty of rest and maintain an overall healthy lifestyle to manage the symptoms of RA. Range-of-motion exercises, ice, and heat packs can maintain joint integrity.

Strains and Sprains

Strains and sprains are common injuries to the musculoskeletal system. Although they can be painful, neither injury poses significant risks to long-term function. A **strain** is the overstretching of a tendon or overuse of a muscle, such as during lifting or moving heavy objects or repeated sports trauma. A **sprain** is a tear in the supporting ligaments surrounding a joint that is caused by a severe, sudden twisting of the joint. Sprains are slightly more serious injuries than strains.

Signs and Symptoms of Strains and Sprains

An acute strain presents with sudden, sharp, incapacitating pain during an activity. An acute strain may also involve tenderness and swelling of the affected area. Chronic strains present gradually, with pain worsening in the hours after an offending activity. Chronic strains usually do not include swelling or tenderness.

Sprains are characterized by pain, rapid swelling, and black-and-blue discoloration of the joint. The ankle is the most commonly sprained joint. Whiplash is also a type of sprain of the neck. Sprains are often difficult to distinguish from a fracture, due to the overlap of symptoms. An X-ray may be necessary for definitive diagnosis.

Treatment of Strains and Sprains

Treatment of strains and sprains follows the **RICE protocol**: rest, ice, compression, and elevation. The joint should be elevated and rested, and ice should be applied intermittently for 12–24 hours. Immobilization and compression will allow the joint to rest and prevent swelling. Pain control is also appropriate with mild systemic analgesics.

Systemic Lupus Erythematosus

Systemic lupus erythematosus (SLE) is a disease of the connective tissue—specifically, collagen. It is also classified as an autoimmune disorder. Currently, the pathophysiology of SLE is not well understood, and it is very difficult to diagnose and treat.

SLE affects the vascular system and connective tissue found in all areas of the body. More than 85 percent of people who suffer from SLE are women. Symptoms of SLE first appear during childbearing age. SLE is frequently associated with a family history of collagen diseases. Approximately 1,500,000 people in the United States suffer from SLE, and it is more common among African, Asian, and Native Americans.

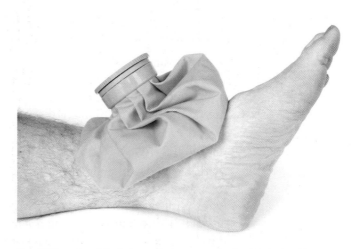

The RICE protocol includes rest, ice, compression, and elevation.

Signs and Symptoms of Systemic Lupus Erythematosus

The first symptoms of SLE are often generalized weakness, fatigue, and fever. Weight loss, headache, depression, loss of appetite, nausea and vomiting, easy bruising, hair loss, and edema also occur. Also, patients frequently present with a butterfly rash—a symmetrical rash over the forehead, cheeks, and bridge of the nose—after exposure to the sun. Patients also experience muscle aches and pains that mimic OA. SLE causes widespread inflammation in the skin, joints, kidneys, lungs, heart, blood vessels, nervous system, and other body systems.

Lab tests indicate an elevated ESR in SLE, as well as anemia. A positive antinuclear antibody test is suggestive of lupus, but does not provide a definitive diagnosis. SLE affects multiple organ systems. It is difficult to differentiate it from other collagen and autoimmune diseases. SLE also mimics the signs and symptoms of syphilis, and SLE almost always yields a false positive result in tests for syphilis.

Treatment of Systemic Lupus Erythematosus

The goals of SLE therapy are to decrease the frequency and severity of symptoms and improve quality of life. Ultimately, inducing remission and maintaining that remission as long as possible are the principle objectives of SLE treatment. The symptoms of SLE vary from person to person and fluctuate over time. Therapy is difficult because it must be tailored to an individual's specific disease activity.

SLE is a long-term, chronic disease. As with all collagen-related and autoimmune diseases, there is no cure for SLE. SLE is characterized by courses of remission and exacerbation over years or decades. Death often results from infarction of vital organs.

Initial treatment for SLE includes large doses of corticosteroids to control inflammation due to the autoimmune response. Muscle and joint pain are treated with analgesics, such as aspirin or NSAIDs. Immunosuppressive agents can be used if patients do not respond to steroids. These drugs place patients at risk for infection because they halt the body's natural immune responses.

During acute exacerbations of SLE, rest is the best treatment. A diet high in vitamins and calories will also combat the fatigue associated with exacerbations. Patients with SLE are advised to stay out of the sun.

Overall, patients with SLE should be advised to maintain a healthy, active lifestyle that includes a balanced diet and regular physical activity. Psychosocial support and adequate rest are essential for preventing SLE exacerbations.

Diagnostic and Treatment-Related Procedures of the Muscular and Skeletal Systems

In diagnosing musculoskeletal conditions, healthcare providers will consider deformities, asymmetry, and restricted motion. Assessments may include simple functional tests such as observation of a patient's gait, or advanced imaging techniques to see inside the bones for signs of disease or trauma.

Arthroscopy

Arthroscopy is an endoscopic procedure that allows for the direct visual inspection of a joint. It can be used to diagnose, treat, or evaluate a joint. Arthroscopy is most often performed on the knee. A surgeon makes a small incision in the skin and inserts a small instrument containing a lens and illuminating and magnifying systems. The images obtained by this **arthroscope** are projected to a screen so the surgeon can see inside the entire joint. Arthroscopy is frequently used to evaluate sports-related injuries and to detect arthritis. Arthroscopy eliminates the need for open surgery, decreasing healing time and reducing the risk of infection.

Cast

A **cast** is used to immobilize a joint or limb as a bone heals from a fracture or surgery. Casts are usually made of plaster or fiberglass. Plaster casts, the mainstay of casting, are formed by wetting bandages that are infused with calcium sulfate and molded to the body part that requires a cast. Plaster casts can be molded very precisely to fit any body part or position required. Fiberglass casts are made by wrapping synthetic tapes around the area that requires casting. Fiberglass casts cannot be molded as precisely as plaster casts but they are lighter, stronger, and more water resistant. The type of casting material used depends on provider preference and the body part to which the cast is being applied.

The type of cast used will depend on the location and severity of the injury. A short arm cast is applied from the fingertips to below the elbow. It is used for fractures or dislocations of the wrist or forearm. A long arm cast is applied from the hand to the upper arm. It is used for fractures of the upper arm. An arm cylinder cast is applied from the wrist to the upper arm. It is used to immobilize the elbow after dislocation or surgery. A short leg cast is applied from below the toes to the knee and a long leg cast is applied from the toes to the upper leg. Both are used for lower leg fractures and severe strains and sprains. They often include a walking heel to aid with ambulation. A leg cylinder cast is applied from the ankle to the upper leg and is used for knee or lower-leg fractures, knee dislocations, and after knee surgery. A Minerva cast is applied around the neck and trunk of the body after surgery to the neck or upper-back area. A spica cast is applied to the trunk and one or more limbs (including the thumb, hand, wrist, and upper arm) and is used to immobilize large joints, including hips and shoulders.

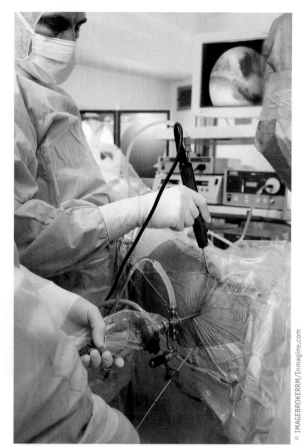

During this arthroscopic surgery of the hip, the surgeon views the inside of the joint on the monitor.

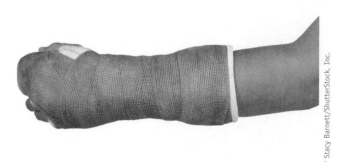

A cast is used to immobilize a joint or limb after an injury.

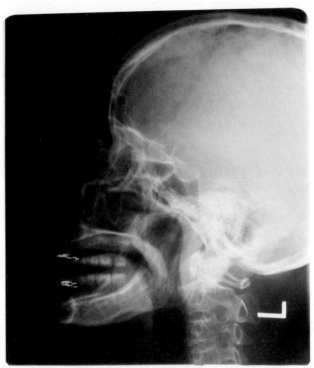

An X-ray of the skull: X-rays allow physicians to see and assess many types of injuries.

X-ray

An **X-ray** is frequently used in the evaluation of skeletal diseases and injuries. An X-ray is often the first imaging test used to assess skeletal integrity. The part of the body being X-rayed is placed between the X-ray camera and film. Electromagnetic waves are passed through the body and the film reflects the internal structure of the body part. Bones, tumors, and dense matter will appear white on the film because they absorb the radiation. Soft tissues and breaks in bones will appear darker because the radiation can pass through the tissue. X-rays do not provide a lot of detail compared with other advanced imaging techniques, but they allow physicians to see and assess many types of injuries. A lead barrier should be used to cover the reproductive organs to protect them from excess radiation during imaging.

Computed Tomography Scan

Computed tomography (CT) scans are specialized X-rays in which the X-ray camera moves around the patient, taking pictures in cross-sectional slices. A computer then compiles the slices into a two-dimensional representation of the patient's anatomy. A CT scan provides much more detail than traditional X-rays and allows visualization of the size, shape, and position of body structures.

Dual Energy X-ray Absorptiometry

Dual energy X-ray absorptiometry (DXA) is the gold standard for evaluating bone density, especially in osteoporosis and osteopenia. Assessments can be made at the heel, finger, or forearm in peripheral DXA, and the hip or spine in central DXA. DXA provides a bone-density score that can be used to diagnose osteoporosis or osteopenia or evaluate response to treatment.

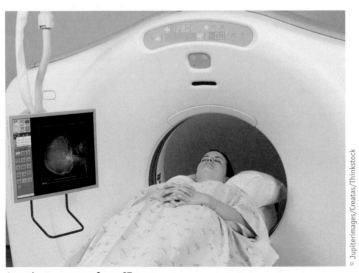

A patient prepares for a CT scan.

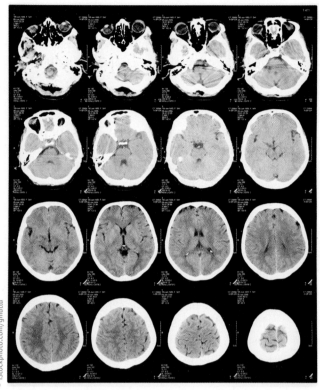

Images created from a CT scan, which provides more detail than traditional X-rays.

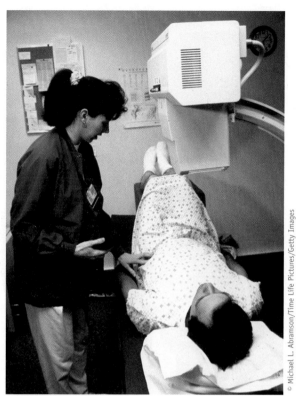

Central DXA is used to assess the bone density of the hip or spine.

Magnetic Resonance Imaging

Magnetic resonance imaging (MRI) uses strong magnets to align protons in a field or body. Radio waves are then passed through a patient, causing the protons to resonate. A computer assesses the vibrational rates of different body structures to create pictures of the proton movement. A computer reconstructs a two-dimensional image in any plane. MRI allows for excellent visualization of soft tissue, but the technology is expensive and time consuming and is not appropriate for patients who are obese or who are claustrophobic. Patients must inform the technician performing the MRI of any metal implants or objects in their body before undergoing an MRI.

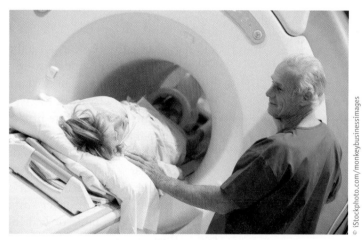

A patient is placed in a large tube for an MRI.

Rehabilitation Medicine

Rehabilitation medicine is a discipline within medicine that uses physical and mechanical agents to diagnose, treat, and prevent disease and bodily injury. It also helps restore or replace body functions that have been lost due to injury or disease. Specialists in rehabilitation medicine include physical therapists, occupational therapists, speech therapists, sports or recreational therapists, massage therapists, acupuncturists, and other professionals who strive to restore patients to the highest level of functioning possible.

Body Mechanics

Body mechanics is the study or use of proper body form and movement to prevent injury and improve performance. Proper body positioning **FIGURE 12.18** reduces physical stress, increases safety, and reduces the risk of injury during any activity that requires moving, lifting, pushing, or pulling. You may be asked to help, lift, or move a patient or equipment, all of which require the use of effective body mechanics.

Correct posture is essential to body mechanics. When standing straight with good posture, the major muscle groups and body parts should be aligned and the body should be balanced. To stand with correct posture, lift your chin and chest, pull your shoulders back and down, tuck your pelvis slightly under your hips, point your toes and knees forward, place your feet shoulder width apart, and distribute your weight evenly between your legs.

Never bend your back when lifting heavy objects. Use the large muscles of your arms

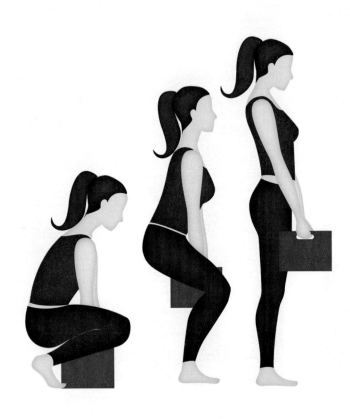

FIGURE 12.18 Illustration of proper lifting technique.
© Hemera/Thinkstock

and legs. Keep the back as straight as possible and your feet shoulder width apart when lifting. This provides a solid base of support and balance for your body. Bend from the hips and knees, not from the waist; squat down and push up with your leg muscles. Do not twist from the waist; instead, pivot the entire body. Get as close as possible to the object you are lifting and hold it close to the body throughout the lift. Ask for help if an object or patient is too large or cumbersome for you to move safely. The safety of you and the patient depend on it.

Always use good body mechanics when transferring a patient. First, however, make sure the area is safe and clear of obstacles and all equipment is secure and stable. If possible, adjust the transfer surfaces to similar heights. For example, if helping a patient on an exam table or bed into a wheelchair, raise or lower the exam table or bed to the same height as the wheelchair. Always use a gait belt when lifting or transferring a patient. A **gait belt** is a device that wraps around the patient's waist to assist in moving him or her from one position or one location to another. Grasp the gait belt to move a patient; never pull on the patient's arms or other body parts or clothes. When lifting, get close to the patient and bend at the hips. Use your leg muscles to straighten and lift the patient. Take small, shuffling steps and avoid crossing your feet. Allow the patient to assist with movement to the best of his or her ability and desire. Be patient and respectful of the patient, but always put safety first.

If a patient begins to fall while you are transferring or lifting him, you must act quickly and responsibly to prevent injury. First, grasp the gait belt; never grab a patient's clothing. Widen your stance to become a stable base of support for the patient. If the patient falls to one side during the transfer, move your foot in the direction of the fall to widen your stance. If the patient falls forward, support his or her waist and step forward with your outer leg. Gently guide the patient to the floor, call for assistance, and check his or her blood pressure and pulse. Have the patient examined by a healthcare provider before attempting to move him again. Document the fall on an incident report and in the patient's chart.

Assistive Devices

Some patients may require **assistive devices** to help with **ambulation** (walking), depending on the extent of their physical disability. Assistive devices are often necessary after surgery or trauma to a lower extremity or after a stroke or other injury that can lead to a loss of balance and coordination.

Some devices simply provide support and stability for the patient, while others require coordination for proper use. Medical assistants are often involved in measuring patients to determine the correct size or type of assistive device required, as well as providing instructions and education for its use. Walkers, crutches, and canes are the most common types of assistive devices. Each has special features and requires certain skills on the part of the patient. Wheelchairs are used for patients who are not able to ambulate, even with assistive devices.

A gait belt helps maintain your safety and the patient's during lifts and transfers.

General guidelines for the safe use of assistive devices should be provided to all patients: Remove all rugs, electrical cords, or other obstacles that can cause a fall; use nonslip bath mats, handles, and shower seats in the bathroom; simplify and tidy the house to keep often-used items within reach and unneeded items out of the way; use a backpack, waist pack, or apron to carry things around; be aware of children and pets, as they can be unpredictable and present obstacles to mobility; and always look forward as you walk, never at your feet.

Walkers

A **walker** provides maximum support and stability for patients when they stand and walk. With a walker, patients may ambulate independently, but a walker requires that a patient possess sufficient upper body strength to hold himself upright. Walkers are available with standard, flat, rubber tips or with wheels for ease of maneuverability.

Most walkers are lightweight and fold easily for storage or transportation. Walkers must be used on level surfaces. They are not useful on stairs or other uneven ground. Walkers are also wide, so patients may have difficulty maneuvering through small spaces or doorways.

Walkers should be adjusted for the patient's height. The handgrips should be positioned just below the patient's waist and the elbow should be bent 30 degrees when grasping the handles. Patients should always be advised to walk slowly when using a walker.

Crutches

Crutches offer more flexibility and mobility than walkers. Crutches provide a solid base of support, but allow for a wider range of gait patterns and speeds. There are five common gaits used for walking with crutches. Patients can advance through the gaits depending on their level of disability, mobility needs, and personal preferences.

Crutch Gaits

The five gaits **FIGURE 12.19** are listed from lowest to highest energy requirement (slowest to fastest):

- **Four-point alternate gait**—This is a slow, stable gait that is appropriate when individuals can bear weight on both legs and can move each leg separately. The sequence is right crutch, left foot, left crutch, right foot.
- **Two-point alternate gait**—This is slightly faster than a four-point gait, but requires more balance. It closely resembles normal walking. The sequence is right crutch and left foot, left crutch and right foot.
- **Three-point alternate gait**—This is a rapid gait that requires arm strength to support weight and maintain balance. The sequence is both crutches and the weaker leg move forward simultaneously, and then the stronger leg is moved forward while the weight is supported by the arms.
- **Swing-to gait**—This is a fast gait that uses parallel movement of the legs. It progresses to a swing-through gait (discussed in the next bullet). The sequence is bear weight on strong leg or legs; move both crutches forward simultaneously; and lean forward while swinging the body into a position even with the crutches.
- **Swing-through gait**—This is the fastest of all crutch gaits. The sequence is bear weight on strong leg or legs; move both crutches forward simultaneously; lean forward while swinging the body into a position ahead of the crutches; and bring crutches forward rapidly.

Axillary crutches are made of wood or aluminum and are used by patients who must not place pressure on a lower extremity while it heals, likely from a fracture. These crutches are appropriate for strong patients and those with minor injuries. Pediatric patients can also use axillary crutches. Axillary crutches require a fair amount of upper-body strength and balance, so they are not recommended for older, frail adults. Crutches can be easily transported and can be used to maneuver through tight spaces.

The height of axillary crutches should be adjusted so the top of the crutch is 1–2 inches below the patient's armpit. The handgrips should be raised or lowered so the patient's elbows are bent at a 30-degree angle when grasping the crutches. When standing, the crutch tips should be placed 6 inches anterior and 2 inches lateral to the foot. The patient's feet and the crutch tips should form a triangle. When walking, allow the hands to support the weight and do not let the tops of the crutches press into the armpits.

Forearm crutches are shorter than axillary crutches. They provide less stability and are usually affixed with a cuff that fits around

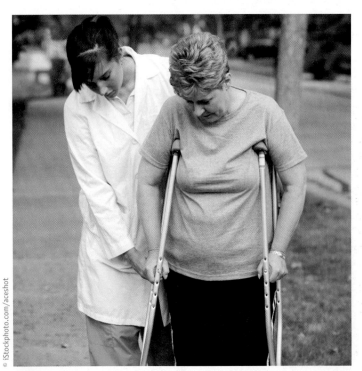

Axillary crutches require upper-body strength for proper use.

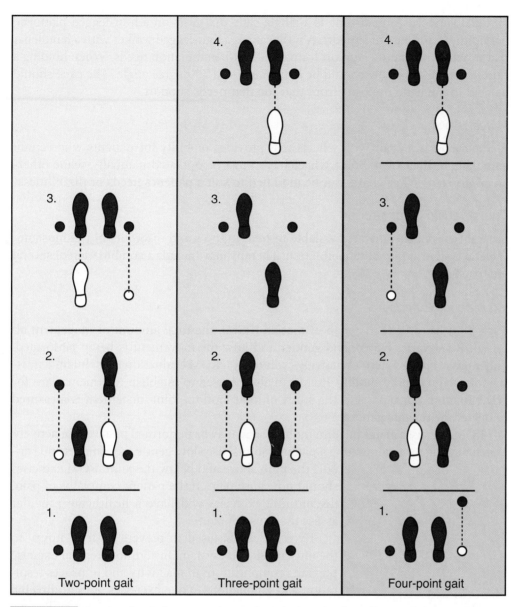

Two-point gait | Three-point gait | Four-point gait

FIGURE 12.19 Crutch gaits: Patients can advance through the gaits depending on their level of disability, mobility needs, and personal preferences.

a patient's forearm. The patient bears almost his entire weight on the handgrip of the crutch. Forearm crutches require significant upper-body strength and balance, and are most appropriate for patients who require long-term or permanent crutches.

Platform crutches are appropriate for patients who should not bear weight on their hands or wrists or who cannot grasp the handgrips of axillary or forearm crutches. A platform at the top of the crutch has a handgrip, but the forearm is maintained at a 90-degree angle and bears nearly all the patient's weight. A platform crutch is an acceptable substitution for a cane.

Canes

A **cane** is appropriate for patients who have weakness on one side of their body or poor balance. Canes are often used for longer periods of time than crutches. A standard cane has a curved handgrip and one tip at the bottom. This type of cane provides minimal support. A quad cane is a single cane that rests on a four-legged platform, providing a wide base of support. A walk cane is a four-legged walker with a handlebar that provides maximum support for patients with ambulation needs. When holding a cane, the patient's elbow should be bent at a 20- to 30-degree angle. The cane should be held in the hand opposite from the side that needs support.

Wheelchairs

A **wheelchair** is a chair with wheels that provides mobility for patients who cannot ambulate on their own. Some wheelchairs must be operated manually, while others are motorized. Wheelchairs can be modified to suit a patient's needs or disabilities.

Therapeutic Approaches

Several types of therapy are available to treat injuries and disorders of the musculoskeletal system as part of rehabilitation. Therapy may include a combination of several approaches.

Therapeutic Exercise

Each joint has a defined **range of motion (ROM)**, the total amount of movement allowed. ROM varies by age and gender and how the movement is being performed, either passively (assisted) or actively (voluntary). ROM evaluation is useful for assessing joint injury and disability. ROM can also be used to establish treatment plans for rehabilitation. **Goniometry** is the study of joint motion. Joint movement is measured in degrees with a **goniometer**.

ROM exercises maintain joint mobility and may be performed passively or actively. When moving or manipulating a patient's joints, use slow, gentle movements and support the limb above and below the joint. ROM exercises should not cause pain. If the patient complains of pain, discontinue exercises and have a healthcare provider assess the cause of pain.

Exercise can be used to prevent or treat injury to the musculoskeletal system. In addition, regular exercise prevents complications of inactivity and improves respiration and circulation. Active exercises are self-directed and performed by a patient without assistance. Passive exercises are performed by another person without participation from the patient. Assisted exercises allow the patient to voluntarily move affected muscles or joints with the assistance of a device, such as a pool. Active resistance exercises are performed by a patient against mechanical or manual pressure to increase muscle strength.

Therapeutic Modalities

If exercise is not suitable for a patient, or if exercise therapy needs to be complemented, several modalities may be employed. Many are easily performed and a combination of modalities may be used.

Thermotherapy, or therapy with heat, causes dilation of the blood vessels, which increases circulation and speeds the repair process of an affected area. Thermotherapy can be used to relax muscles, relieve pain resulting from a strain or sprain, relieve localized swelling,

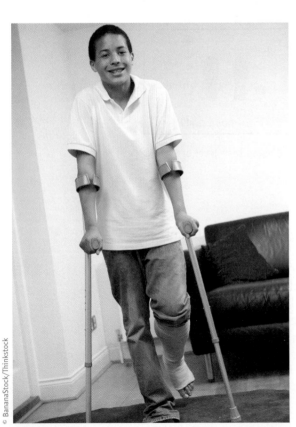

Forearm crutches can be used for pediatric or adult patients.

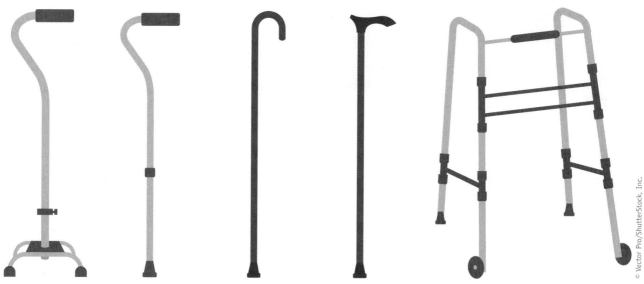

Several styles of canes and walkers are available to assist patients with ambulation.

increase drainage from an infection, increase tissue metabolism and repair, and improve mobility prior to exercise. Be aware that heat also enhances the inflammatory process, which can lead to increased bleeding and swelling, so it should be applied for only short periods of time.

> *All types of hot and cold therapies are inexpensive and simple, and patients can complete these therapies at home with little assistance.*
> © auremar/ShutterStock, Inc.

Moist heat, such as that used in warm soaks, sitz baths, warm wet compresses, and paraffin wax baths, allows heat to penetrate the skin better than dry heat. Moist heat improves circulation, promotes relaxation, and increases mobility. Dry heat applications do not penetrate the skin. Dry heat is used to relax muscles and relieve swelling.

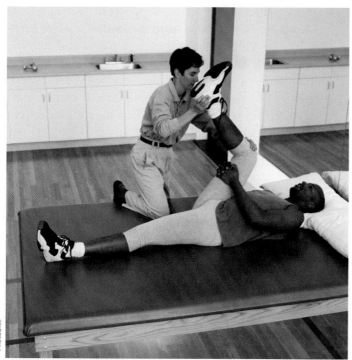

A therapist manipulates a patient's knee.

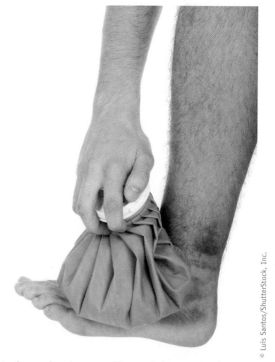

An ice pack reduces swelling and decreases pain.

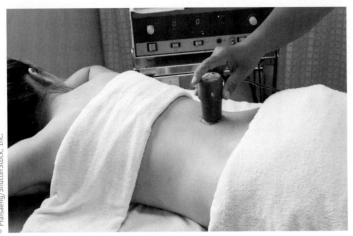

Ultrasound therapy being performed on a back.

Cryotherapy, or applications of cold, constrict blood vessels and restrict blood flow to an area. This slows the inflammatory process and prevents or reduces swelling of inflamed tissues, reduces bleeding, and reduces drainage. Cold also acts as a local anesthetic, relieving pain at the affected area.

As with heat, moist cold therapies penetrate the skin better than dry cold therapies. Moist cold, such as in cold compresses, prevents swelling, relieves pain, and reduces body temperature. Dry cold therapies, such as ice packs, are used for the same purposes as moist cold, but dry cold is better for bleeding and acute injuries.

Ultrasound is a high-frequency acoustic vibration. Ultrasound is part of the electromagnetic spectrum, but it is imperceptible to the human ear. In **ultrasound therapy**, the high-frequency sound waves penetrate deep tissues, where the sound waves are converted to heat. Ultrasound therapy is used for treating chronic and acute injuries including strains, sprains, and chronic pain. Ultrasound waves are conducted through skin and tissue with high water content, such as muscle, with an applicator that uses a gel as a conduit. The duration of treatment is brief—only 5 to 15 minutes—to avoid damage to tissue caused by a high concentration of ultrasound waves. Ultrasound therapy can be administered only by a specially trained assistant or therapist.

Massage therapy is recognized as essential to musculoskeletal rehabilitation. Most states require specialized education and licensure for massage therapists. Many therapists work in conjunction with chiropractors, orthopedists, and physical therapists. Massage therapists are recognized as providers of a complementary and holistic form of medicine.

Massage is used to restore the body's normal function by relieving minor aches and pains and helping patients feels relaxed and refreshed. Massage speeds metabolism, promotes healing, soothes muscles, enhances ROM, and improves circulation. It can be used to manage acute and chronic pain as well as relieve stress and promote relaxation. Massage therapists use their hands to manipulate a patient's soft tissues with various movements and techniques. Massage therapy is not appropriate for patients with open wounds, neuropathies, varicose veins, high blood pressure, or severe osteoporosis.

Skills for the Medical Assistant

As a medical assistant, you will have the opportunity to participate in many procedures relating to musculoskeletal injuries. Most require patience and compassion, as many individuals will be in a great amount of pain or discomfort and others will be facing life with

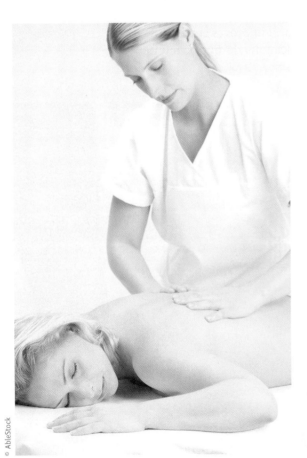

Massage therapy promotes healing and relieves pain.

assistive devices. Your confidence will ease the patient's fears and assist the patient in gaining independence and daily functioning, which will ultimately improve quality of life.

Transferring a Patient to and from an Exam Table

If a patient is unable to stand and walk on his or her own, you may be required to assist him or her to stand and walk when moving to and from an exam table. In this exercise, you will learn how to safely transfer a patient. For this exercise, it is assumed that the patient uses a wheelchair.

Equipment Needed

- Stool with rubber grips and handle
- Gait belt

Steps

1. Wash your hands and assemble the supplies. Identify the patient and introduce yourself. Explain that you will be transferring the patient to the exam table.
2. Position the wheelchair next to the exam table and lock the brakes. The patient's stronger side should be positioned closest to the exam table.
3. Place the gait belt around the patient's waist. Secure the loose end of the belt by tucking it under the belt.
4. Move the footrests of the wheelchair up and have the patient place his or her feet on the floor. Place the stool next to the exam table, as close to the wheelchair as possible.
5. Instruct the patient to slide forward on the seat of the chair, sitting as close to the edge as is safe and comfortable for the patient.
6. Stand in front of the patient, facing him or her, with your feet shoulder width apart. Bend your knees and lean forward at your hips and grasp the gait belt on the patient's sides. Instruct the patient to place his or her hands on the wheelchair's arm rests and push up when you lift him or her FIGURE 12.20 .
7. Straighten your legs and lift the patient. If the patient has adequate lower body strength, he or she should push with his or her legs as you pull up. Maintain hold of the gait belt.
8. Have the patient step up onto the stool with the leg closest to the exam table. Instruct the patient to pivot so his or her back is toward the exam table. The patient's buttocks should be slightly higher than the exam table FIGURE 12.21 .
9. Instruct the patient to grasp the handle of the stool with one hand and place the other hand on the exam table.
10. Gently ease the patient to a seated position on the exam table. Position him or her on the exam table as required. Let go of the gait belt. Remove the gait belt from the patient's waist.

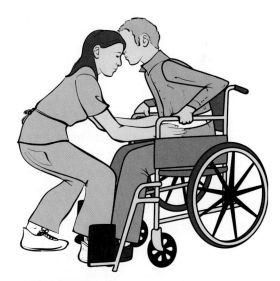

FIGURE 12.20 Grasp the gait belt and use your legs to lift the patient to a standing position.
© Jones & Bartlett Learning

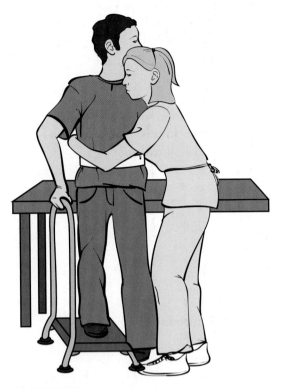

FIGURE 12.21 Help the patient pivot so his or her back is toward the exam table.

© Jones & Bartlett Learning

11. Move the wheelchair and stool away from the exam table.

12. After the exam, return the wheelchair and stool to a position beside the exam table. The wheelchair should be positioned closest to the patient's stronger side. Lock the brakes on the wheelchair and ensure the footrests are lifted out of the way. The stool should be placed as close to the wheelchair as possible.

13. If the patient is not already sitting, assist the patient to a seated position on the exam table. Place the gait belt around the patient's waist, securing the loose ends. With one arm under the patient's arm and around his or her shoulder and the other arm under his or her knees, gently pivot the patient into a position in which his or her legs are dangling off the side of the exam table.

14. Position yourself directly in front of the patient, facing him or her with your feet shoulder width apart. Bend your knees slightly and reach around the patient, grasping the gait belt.

15. Pull the patient toward you so his or her feet come onto the stool. The patient should help push off the exam table with his or her hands, if able, and grasp the stool handle when the feet meet the stool. Have the patient step off the side of the stool with his or her strong leg first, then the weaker leg. Instruct him or her to pivot so the back faces the wheelchair.

16. Instruct the patient to grasp the arms of the wheelchair. Bend at your knees and hips to gently lower the patient into the chair. Make sure the patient is seated comfortably.

17. Lower the footrests and place the patient's feet on the footrests.

Assisting a Patient to Stand and Walk

If a patient is unable to stand and walk on his or her own, you may be required to assist him or her to stand and walk. In this exercise, you will learn how to safely lift a patient to a standing position and help him or her ambulate safely. For this exercise, it is assumed that the patient uses a wheelchair.

Equipment Needed

- Gait belt

Steps

1. Wash your hands and assemble the supplies. Identify the patient and introduce yourself. Explain that you will be assisting him or her to stand and walk.
2. Lock the brakes on the wheelchair.
3. Place the gait belt around the patient's waist. Secure the loose end of the belt by tucking it under the belt.
4. Move the footrests of the wheelchair up and have the patient place his or her feet on the floor.

5. Instruct the patient to slide forward on the seat of the chair, sitting as close to the edge as is safe and comfortable for the patient.

6. Stand in front of the patient, facing him or her, with your feet shoulder width apart. Bend your knees and lean forward at your hips and grasp the gait belt on the patient's sides. Instruct the patient to place his or her hands on the wheelchair's arm rests and push up when you lift him or her.

7. Straighten your legs and lift the patient. If the patient has the lower body strength, he or she should push with his or her legs as you pull up. Maintain hold of the gait belt.

8. Steady the patient and observe him or her for balance, strength, skin color, and signs of distress. If necessary, lower the patient back to the wheelchair before proceeding.

9. When the patient is steady and has achieved balance, stand slightly behind the patient, toward his or her weaker side.

10. Grasp the gait belt with one hand and place the other hand on the patient's arm. Begin walking with the patient, using the same foot as the patient and moving in step with him or her **FIGURE 12.22**.

11. Document the procedure in the patient's chart. For example, write "1430: Assisted patient to walk approximately 20 feet. Patient reports feeling steady and strong. No distress or discomfort noted. J. Jones, CMA."

Applying an Elastic Bandage

An elastic bandage is applied to a strain or sprain to create localized pressure over the injured area. A bandage reduces blood flow to an injury and reduces swelling. In this exercise, you will learn how to apply an elastic bandage.

Equipment Needed

- Elastic bandage and clips

Steps

1. Wash your hands and assemble the supplies. Identify the patient and introduce yourself. Explain that you will be applying an elastic bandage.

2. Position the patient as directed by the physician to allow for access to the injured limb and provide for maximum patient comfort. The injured limb should be supported above and below the injury for patient safety.

3. Hold the bandage with the roll facing up in one hand and the free end of the bandage in the other hand. Place the free end of the bandage close to the injured site and wrap the bandage around the limb twice.

4. Continue wrapping in a circular motion. Maintain even pressure as you wrap around the injured limb. Wrap firmly and securely. As you wrap, ask

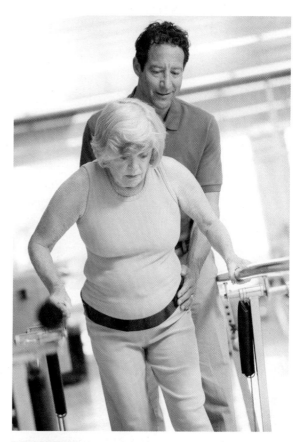

FIGURE 12.22 Maintain a firm hold on the gait belt and walk slowly with the patient.
© iStockphoto/monkeybusinessimages

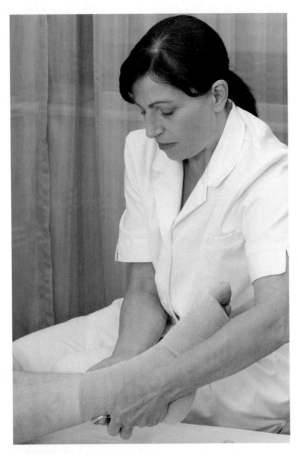

FIGURE 12.23 Wrap the elastic bandage in a circular motion, overlapping each turn.
© iStockphoto.com/Anetta_R

the patient to advise you of any discomfort. Overlap each turn of the bandage by ¹/₂ to ²/₃ of the strip width **FIGURE 12.23**.

5. When the entire length of the bandage is wrapped around the injured limb, secure the ends with clips.

6. Observe the limb and extremity for color changes and ask the patient if he or she is experiencing numbness, tingling, or significant discomfort.

7. Document the procedure in the patient's chart. For example, write "1115: Elastic bandage applied to right wrist and arm, No swelling observed. Patient has no complaints. J. Jones, CMA."

Applying a Splint

A splint is a device used to stabilize an injured part of the body in order to decrease pain and prevent further injury. In this exercise, you will learn how to apply a splint to an injured limb.

Equipment Needed

- Commercially available splint

Steps

1. Wash your hands and assemble the supplies. Identify the patient and introduce yourself. Explain that you will be applying a splint.

2. Position the patient as directed by the physician to allow for access to the injured limb and provide for maximum patient comfort. The injured limb should be supported above and below the injury for patient safety.

3. Gently slide the injured limb or extremity into the splint. Fasten and tighten the splint **FIGURE 12.24**.

4. Observe the injured limb or extremity for color changes and ask the patient if he or she is experiencing numbness, tingling, or significant discomfort.

5. Document the procedure in the patient's chart. For example, write "1350: Splint applied to right wrist. No swelling observed. Patient has no complaints. J. Jones, CMA."

Applying an Arm Sling

A sling is used to provide support for an injured arm or shoulder. In this exercise, you will learn how to apply an arm sling.

Equipment Needed

- Commercially available buckle-type arm sling

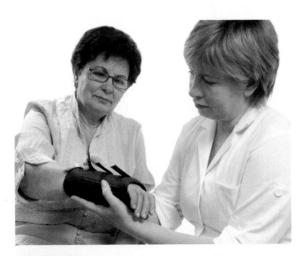

FIGURE 12.24 Fasten the splint so it is tight and secure, but does not cause discomfort.
© Alexander Raths/ShutterStock, Inc.

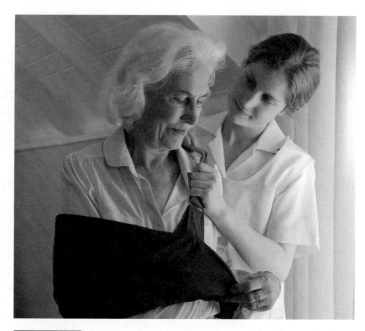

FIGURE 12.25 The injured arm should be snug to the chest and the hand should be positioned above the elbow.

© Clarissa Leahy/Getty Images

Steps

1. Wash your hands and assemble the supplies. Identify the patient and introduce yourself. Explain that you will be applying an arm sling.
2. Position the patient as directed by the physician to allow for access to the injured limb and provide for maximum patient comfort. The injured limb should be supported above and below the injury for patient safety.
3. Gently position the arm at a 90-degree angle and slide it into the sling. The fingers should extend slightly beyond the edge of the sling.
4. Place the adjustable strap around the patient's neck, on the side of the uninjured arm, and slide it into the ring or buckle on the end of the sling. Fasten and tighten the sling. The arm should be fixed snugly to the chest and the hand should be positioned about 4 to 5 inches above the elbow to reduce swelling and relieve discomfort **FIGURE 12.25**.
5. Observe the arm for color changes and ask the patient if he or she is experiencing numbness, tingling, or significant discomfort.
6. Document the procedure in the patient's chart. For example, write "1830: Arm sling applied to left arm. Hand elevated and fingers extend beyond sling. No swelling observed. Patient has no complaints. J. Jones, CMA."

Assisting With Cast Application

A cast is used to immobilize a joint after injury or surgery. Plaster casts are the most common type of casts. In this exercise, you will learn general principles in assisting with the application of any type of cast.

Equipment Needed

- Plaster bandage roll or synthetic tape

- Container of warm water
- Stockinette
- Sheet wadding, webbing material, or cotton padding
- Bandage or casting material
- Scissors
- Disposable gloves
- Sponge rubber for padding

Steps

1. Wash your hands and assemble equipment and supplies. Identify the patient and introduce yourself. Explain that you will be helping to apply a cast.
2. Position the patient as directed by the physician to allow for access to the injured limb and provide for maximum patient comfort.
3. Apply gloves. Clean and dry the area to be cast, as directed by the physician. Note any areas of bruising, redness, or open wounds, and take care to manipulate and touch the area gently, as the patient may be experiencing great amounts of pain.
4. Pad the bony prominences of the limb with a rubber sponge to protect it from pressure from the cast.
5. Apply the stockinette to the limb being cast. Do not use a stockinette that is too large or too small, as either extreme may damage the skin under the cast. Choose a stockinette that fits securely and is not too loose or too tight.
6. Provide the physician with the padding that he or she will use to cover the patient's skin.
7. Place the casting material in the bucket of warm water for five seconds. Gently lift from the bucket and squeeze out extra water. Do not wring. Assist with the application of the cast as requested by the physician. Provide emotional support to the patient during the casting process **FIGURE 12.26** .
8. Review cast care with the patient and provide written instructions for cast care and other exercises ordered by the physician. Reinforce warnings, precautions, and complications provided by the physician.

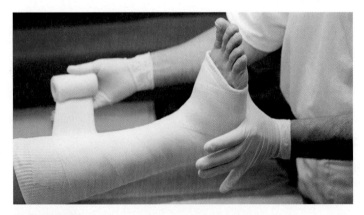

FIGURE 12.26 Assist with the application of the cast, as requested by the physician.
© F1online/Thinkstock

Cast Care

Review the following cast-care points with the patient:

- Keep the cast clean and dry. If a fiberglass cast gets damp, attempt to dry it with a towel or a hairdryer on the cool setting. Call your doctor to find out if it needs to be replaced.
- Cover the cast with a plastic bag or cast cover when bathing.
- Do not lean on the cast or put pressure on it.
- Do not stick objects down the cast.
- Do not put lotions or powders inside the cast.
- Do not trim or cut the cast.
- Call your doctor if:
  - The cast becomes loose because the swelling has gone down.
  - There is an odor, mold, or mildew inside the cast.
  - An edge of the cast is irritating the skin.
  - You experience pain, numbness, or tingling under the cast.
  - You experience loss of feeling or movement in the extremities of the cast limb.
  - You notice increased redness, swelling, or other signs of infection.

---

9. Discard the used water and dispose of casting materials.
10. Clean the work area. Remove gloves and wash your hands.
11. Document the cast application in the patient's chart, including date, time, patient response, and instruction provided.

Assisting With Cast Removal

Casts can remain in place for weeks or months, depending on the severity and location of injury. Patients may be nervous about having a cast removed due to fear of the cutter or saw used for removal, as well as the atrophy of the limb that has been cast. With rehabilitation, however, the patient will likely regain use of the limb. In this exercise, you will learn how to assist with the removal of a cast.

Equipment Needed

- Cast cutter
- Cast spreader
- Bandage scissors
- Bag for disposing of cast materials
- Disposable gloves

Steps

1. Wash your hands and assemble equipment and supplies. Identify the patient and introduce yourself. Explain that you will be helping to remove his or her cast. Reassure the patient that the cast cutter is not sharp and does not spin; it vibrates. The patient may feel slight pressure and warmth from the cast cutter, but the skin cannot be cut or injured by it.

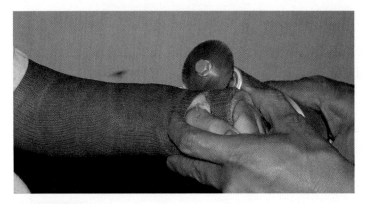

FIGURE 12.27 Assist with cast removal, as requested by the physician.
© Lenice Harms/ShutterStock, Inc.

2. Position the patient as directed by the physician to allow for access to the injured limb and provide for maximum patient comfort.

3. Assist with the removal of the cast, as requested by the physician **FIGURE 12.27** .

4. Review post-cast care with the patient and provide written instruction for care and other exercises ordered by the physician. Reinforce warnings, precautions, and complications provided by the physician.

Care After Cast Removal

Review the following post-cast care points with the patient:

- Wash the skin gently with mild soap and water.
- Do not shave the area for at least three days.
- Use fragrance- and alcohol-free lotion to moisturize the skin.
- Perform rehabilitation exercises as directed by the physician or therapist.

---

5. Dispose of the cast. Clean the work area. Wash your hands.

6. Document the cast removal in the patient's chart, including date, time, patient response, appearance of skin under cast, and instruction provided.

Teaching a Patient to Use Axillary Crutches

Crutches are used to eliminate the need to bear weight on a lower limb to allow the limb time to heal after a fracture or surgery. Crutches can be cumbersome and uncomfortable for patients who are unfamiliar with their use, but with proper instruction, patients can maneuver and ambulate confidently and safely. In this exercise, you will learn how to teach a patient to use crutches.

Equipment Needed

- Axillary crutches
- Gait belt

Steps

1. Wash your hands. Identify the patient and introduce yourself. Explain that you will teach him or her to use crutches. Make sure the patient is wearing appropriate shoes with good support and flat, rubber soles.

2. Apply the gait belt around the patient's waist.

3. Check the crutches to ensure the rubber suction tips are secure. Check the handgrips and bar for damage or rough edges that could cause discomfort or injury.

4. Adjust the height of the crutches. The bar at the top of the crutches should be situated 1–2 inches below the patient's armpit and the patient's elbows should be bent at a 30-degree angle when holding the handgrips. Once adjusted, tighten all screws or wing nuts.

5. Help the patient stand with the crutches under his or her arms and instruct the patient to hold the handgrips. Position yourself behind and slightly to one side of the patient **FIGURE 12.28**.

6. Instruct the patient to transfer his or her weight to the handles while using the crutches; the patient should not bear weight on his or her armpits. Then instruct the patient to step first with the stronger leg, then the weaker leg, using the appropriate gait for the patient's level of disability and need for maneuverability.

7. Have the patient repeat a few steps until he or she feels comfortable with the process. Monitor the patient for signs of fatigue or discomfort. Be alert and ready to aid a patient at risk of a fall.

8. Document the instruction in the patient's chart, including date, time, duration, patient response, and instruction provided.

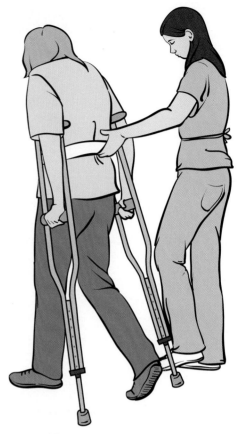

FIGURE 12.28 Position yourself behind and slightly to one side of the patient using crutches.
© Jones & Bartlett Learning

Teaching a Patient to Use a Walker

When a patient requires the use of a walker, he or she may be apprehensive or intimidated at first. As the medical assistant, be patient and allow the patient to express reservations about a new piece of equipment. Although it takes time to learn to use a walker efficiently, the patient will soon find that he or she can gain independence and move freely with a walker. In this exercise, you will teach a patient how to use a walker.

Equipment Needed

- Walker
- Gait belt

Steps

1. Wash your hands. Identify the patient and introduce yourself. Explain that you will teach the patient to use a walker. Make sure the patient is wearing appropriate shoes with good support and flat, rubber soles.

2. Apply the gait belt around the patient's waist.

3. Check the walker to ensure the rubber suction tips are secure on all four legs. Check the handgrips for damage or rough edges that could cause discomfort or injury.

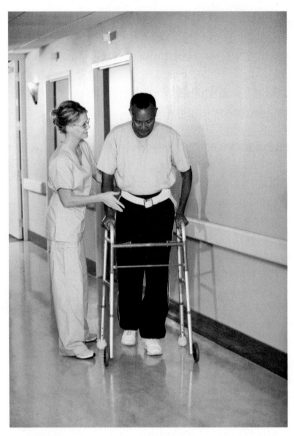

FIGURE 12.29 Position yourself behind and slightly to one side of the patient using a walker.
© iStockphoto.com/kali9

4. Adjust the height of the walker. The handgrips should be level with the top of the patient's thigh and the patient's elbows should be bent at a 30-degree angle when holding the handgrips. Once adjusted, tighten all screws or knobs.

5. Help the patient step inside the walker and instruct the patient to hold the handgrips. Position yourself behind and slightly to one side of the patient **FIGURE 12.29**.

6. Have the patient lift the walker and place all four legs back down on the ground so that the back legs are even with his or her toes.

7. Instruct the patient to lean forward and transfer his or her weight to the handles while stepping into the walker. Instruct the patient to step first with the stronger leg, then the weaker leg. Then instruct the patient to lift the walker and place all four legs on the floor a comfortable distance ahead of him or her. Again instruct the patient to walk into the walker, leading with the strong leg and following with the weak leg.

8. If the walker has wheels, instruct the patient to roll the walker forward a comfortable distance, then step into the walker, leading with the strong leg. Alternatively, the patient may walk normally with a rolling walker, gently pushing it and slightly leaning into it as he or she walks.

9. Have the patient repeat a few steps until he or she feels comfortable with the process. Monitor the patient for signs of fatigue or discomfort. Be alert and ready to aid a patient at risk of a fall.

10. Document the instruction in the patient's chart, including date, time, duration, patient response, and instruction provided.

Teaching a Patient to Use a Cane

Canes are assistive devices that are appropriate for patients who need only a minimal to moderate amount of support or balance. Several types of canes are available, depending on the patient's specific needs, but each is used in the same way. As with other assistive devices, patients may be resistant to using a cane due to the stigma and psychological stress it carries, but patients will soon realize increased independence and renewed functioning. In this exercise, you will learn how to teach a patient to use a cane.

Equipment Needed

- Cane
- Gait belt

Steps

1. Wash your hands. Identify the patient and introduce yourself. Explain that you will teach the patient to use a cane. Make sure the patient is wearing appropriate shoes with good support and flat, rubber soles.
2. Apply the gait belt around the patient's waist.
3. Check the cane to ensure the rubber suction tip (or tips) is secure. Check the handgrips for damage or rough edges that could cause discomfort or injury.
4. Adjust the height of the cane. The handle should reach the top of the patient's hip and his elbow should be bent at a 20- to 30-degree angle when holding the handgrip. Once adjusted, tighten all screws or wing nuts.
5. Help the patient stand with the cane in the hand on the side of the strongest leg. Position yourself behind and slightly to the weaker side of the patient **FIGURE 12.30** .
6. Instruct the patient to transfer his or her weight to the handle while using the cane. Then instruct the patient to step first with the stronger leg and bring the cane forward simultaneously. Next, instruct the patient to bring the weaker leg forward.
7. Have the patient repeat a few steps until he or she feels comfortable with the process. Monitor the patient for signs of fatigue or discomfort. Be alert to aid a patient at risk of a fall.
8. Document the instruction in the patient's chart, including date, time, duration, patient response, and instruction provided.

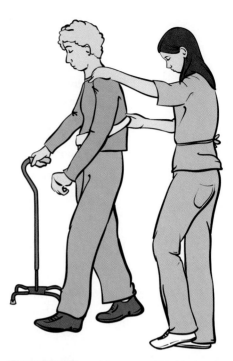

FIGURE 12.30 Position yourself behind and slightly to the weaker side of the patient using a cane.
© Jones & Bartlett Learning

Math Practice

Question: A 56-year-old man who weighs 247 pounds has been diagnosed with bursitis in his shoulder. His orthopedist prescribed the combination analgesic Vicodin to relieve his pain. Each tablet contains 5mg of hydrocodone and 500mg of acetaminophen. The patient is allowed to take 1–2 tablets every 4–6 hours as needed for pain. If he took the maximum allowed dose, how much hydrocodone would he receive in 24 hours? How much acetaminophen would he receive in the same time period?

Answer: Maximum dose: 2 tablets every 4 hours

24 hours × 1 dose/4 hours = 6 doses in 24 hours

2 tablets/dose × 6 doses/24 hours = 12 tablets in 24 hours

12 tablets × 5mg hydrocodone/tablet = 60mg hydrocodone in 24 hours

12 tablets × 500mg acetaminophen/tablet = 6,000mg acetaminophen in 24 hours

Note: This amount of acetaminophen is higher than the maximum daily recommended dose of acetaminophen, which is 4,000mg. Patients should be advised not to consume more than 4,000mg of acetaminophen from any source in a 24-hour period.

Question: A 63-year-old woman visits a health fair to receive a peripheral DXA scan to evaluate her risk for osteoporosis. During her assessment, she reports that her daily diet consists of the following calcium-containing foods:

2 cups skim milk

1 cup low-fat yogurt

1 cup calcium-fortified orange juice

$1/2$ cup broccoli

2 oz cheddar cheese

Given the following calcium contents of the foods, what is her total daily intake of calcium?

Milk: 300mg/8 fluid ounces

Yogurt: 450mg/1 cup

Orange juice: 300mg/8 fluid ounces

Broccoli: 180mg/1 cup

Cheddar cheese: 200mg/1 oz

Answer: Skim milk: 2 cups × 300mg/8 fl oz × 8 fl oz/1 cup = 600mg

Yogurt: 1 cup × 450mg/1 cup = 450mg

Orange juice: 1 cup × 300mg/8 fl oz × 8 fl oz/1 cup = 300mg

Broccoli: $1/2$ cup × 180mg/1 cup = 90mg

Cheddar cheese: 2 oz × 200mg/1 oz = 400mg

Total: 600mg + 450mg + 300mg + 90mg + 400mg = 1,840mg

Question: A 14-year-old female who weighs 105 pounds is prescribed prednisolone (Orapred) 0.25mg/kg/day divided into two doses to reduce swelling and inflammation. What is the total daily dose of prednisolone? How much will the patient receive at each dose?

Answer: 105 lb × 1kg ÷ 2.2 lb = 47.7kg

47.7kg × 0.25mg/kg/day = 11.93mg/day

11.93mg/day × 1 day ÷ 2 doses = 5.97mg

Question: **If prednisolone is available as an oral solution in a concentration of 15mg/5mL, what volume of solution is needed to administer 6mg of prednisolone?**

Answer: $\frac{6mg}{x mL} = \frac{15mg}{5mL}$

15x = 30

x = 2mL

Question: **A 34-year-old female patient is prescribed methylprednisolone 4mg to treat an exacerbation of lupus erythematous. Her instructions are to take six tablets on the first day, five tablets on the second day, four tablets on the third day, three tablets on the fourth day, two tablets on the fifth day, and one tablet on the sixth day. What is the total dose of methylprednisolone she will receive over the course of treatment?**

Answer: Total tablets = 6 + 5 + 4 + 3 + 2 + 1 = 21 tablets

21 tablets × 4mg/tablet = 84mg methylprednisolone

WRAP UP

Chapter Summary

- The musculoskeletal system supports and protects the body, gives it shape, and allows for movement. The bones, muscles, and joints work together to coordinate motion.

- Bones are made of two types of tissue: cancellous (spongy) bone and compact (dense) bone. Each bone has its own supply of blood, nerves, and lymph vessels. Bones are constantly eroded and rebuilt to maintain strength. Bones are classified according to their size, structure, and function.

- A joint is the point at which two bones meet. There are several types of joints, and each allows for different levels of flexibility and freedom of movement, depending on their location and the function of the bones involved.

- Muscles determine physical function. The body contains three distinct types of muscle. Skeletal muscle is the most abundant type of muscle in the human body and it allows for voluntary movement. Skeletal muscles work in pairs, on opposite sides of a joint, to permit extension and flexion of limbs.

- Bursitis and tendonitis are inflammations of bursa or tendons, respectively. Both can occur after repeated joint trauma, infection, or stress. Pain relievers and anti-inflammatory medication are the mainstay of treatment, along with stretching and strengthening of the affected body area.

- Carpal tunnel syndrome is a painful set of symptoms caused by inflammation of the tendons in the wrist. Immobilization of the hand and wrist relieve the swelling, but injections of corticosteroids or surgery may be necessary to relieve the inflammation.

- A dislocation is the displacement of a bone at a joint, usually after an injury, trauma, or disease. A subluxation is a partial dislocation. Both conditions can lead to joint damage as well as damage to the nerves, blood vessels, ligaments, and soft tissues surrounding the joint. Reduction of the joint and rest are the only treatments available for dislocation and subluxation.

- Epicondylitis is the inflammation of the tendons of the forearm, caused by gripping and twisting motions of the forearm. It is more commonly known as tennis elbow. Rest and systemic pain relievers or anti-inflammatory drugs are effective treatments for this condition.

- Fibromyalgia is a syndrome characterized by diffuse, widespread pain. Its cause is unknown, and treatment is highly individualized. Lifestyle changes, muscle relaxants, pain relievers, antidepressants, and anti-epileptic drugs are often used for treating fibromyalgia.

- A fracture is a broken bone. Pain and limb deformity usually accompany a fracture, and prompt realignment and immobilization of the bone facilitates healing and prevents future damage to the bone.

- Gout is an inflammatory disease of the joints caused by the buildup of uric acid. Gout is linked to obesity and metabolic syndrome, as well as the dietary intake of alcohol, meat, and fish. Colchicine is the treatment of choice for gout.

- Hallux valgus is the lateral deviation of the big toe and enlargement of the first metatarsal head. It is often caused by wearing tight or poor-fitting shoes.

- A herniated or ruptured disk is a condition in which the gel between the vertebral disks of the spine is forced to the outside of the disk. This is a painful condition, but symptoms may resolve with avoidance of painful activities, rest, and pain-relieving medications.

- Kyphosis, lordosis, and scoliosis are abnormal curvatures of the spine. In some cases, the conditions may be caused by poor posture, injury, trauma, vitamin deficiencies, or genetic defects. Other cases have no identifiable cause. Treatment varies according to the degree of disability or discomfort caused by the abnormal curvature. Treatment can range from exercises to improve posture to back braces to surgical straightening of the spine.

- Osteoarthritis is the most common type of joint inflammation. It is a chronic condition that leads to the degeneration of the joint. Although it can be painful and costly, osteoarthritis does not decrease life span.

- Osteopenia and osteoporosis are the loss of bone strength. Each condition can be caused by age, disease, altered hormone levels, medications, or poor diet. Every person should be advised to obtain the recommended daily intake of calcium and vitamin D and to participate in regular exercise to maintain strong, healthy bones.

- Osteomyelitis is an infection of the bone and bone marrow. Systemic, long-term antibiotics are usually needed to eradicate a bone infection.

- Rheumatoid arthritis is a chronic, inflammatory autoimmune disease that affects joints and the surrounding muscles, tendons, ligaments, and blood vessels. Joints are affected bilaterally and symmetrically. Treatment includes corticosteroids, monoclonal antibodies, and immunosuppressant drugs.

- Strains and sprains occur after overuse or overstretching of a muscle, ligament, or tendon. Both conditions can be painful, but neither present serious or long-term threats to function. The RICE protocol is the mainstay of strain and sprain treatment.

- Systemic lupus erythematosus is an autoimmune disease of collagen. The symptoms vary from person to person and across the progression of the disease. Treatment is, therefore, highly individualized and changes with periods of remission and exacerbation.

- Arthroscopy is an endoscopic procedure that allows for direct visualization of a joint. It is most often used to examine knees.

- A cast is used to immobilize a joint or limb as a bone heals from a fracture or surgery. Casts are made of a variety of different materials, and in different shapes and sizes, depending on the location and severity of the injury.

- X-rays are used to visualize the skeleton. They are often the first diagnostic imaging technique performed when assessing injuries of the skeletal system.

- Computed tomography scans use X-rays collected in a tube around a patient. A computer captures images as slices and recompiles them into a two-dimensional image that can be used to assess the size, shape, and position of body structures.

- Dual energy X-ray absorptiometry uses X-ray technology and various body positions to evaluate bone strength. It is useful in diagnosing osteoporosis and evaluating response to treatment.

- Magnetic resonance imaging uses magnets and radio waves to create images of a body. It allows for excellent visualization of soft tissues, but it is expensive and time-consuming technology.

- Rehabilitative medicine uses physical or mechanical agents to diagnose, treat, and prevent bodily disease and injury. Therapists in this field work with patients to regain function after an injury. Rehabilitative medicine focuses on the proper use of body mechanics, and may involve assistive devices such as walkers, crutches, and canes to help people ambulate, along with wheelchairs. Therapeutic exercise, as well as thermotherapy, cryotherapy, ultrasound therapy, and massage therapy, are treatment approaches that can be used during rehabilitation.

- As a medical assistant, you will have the opportunity to assist with diagnostic and treatment-related procedures relating to the musculoskeletal system. You may also be called upon to educate patients about their assistive devices. Be mindful that patients with musculoskeletal disease or complaints may be experiencing pain or facing life with new challenges. Be patient and respectful of patients' concerns, and assure patients that, with time and rehabilitation, they should be able to gain function and independence once feared lost.

Learning Assessment Questions

1. How many bones are in the human skeleton?
   A. 80
   B. 126
   C. 206
   D. 600

2. Which of the following divisions of the human skeleton is correctly matched with the bones it contains?
   A. Axial: skull, thoracic cage, and vertebral column
   B. Appendicular: upper limbs, pelvic girdle, and lower limbs
   C. Vertebral: spinal cord and skull
   D. Thoracic: ribs and pectoral girdle

3. What are the two types of bone tissue called?
   A. Visceral and striated
   B. Flexors and extensors
   C. Short and long
   D. Compact and cancellous

4. Which of the following terms is correctly matched with its definition?
   A. Periosteum: the rounded portion at the end of a long bone
   B. Osteoclast: a cell that deposits new bone in the process of bone remodeling
   C. Articulation: the point at which two bones connect
   D. Sesamoid bones: small, irregular bones that are shaped for a specific purpose

5. Which of the following pairs of bone type and example is *not* correctly matched?
   A. Long bones: bones of the feet
   B. Short bones: bones of the hand
   C. Sesamoid bones: patella
   D. Flat bones: plates of the skull

6. Which of the following is an example of a cartilaginous joint?
   A. Ball and socket joint
   B. Pivot joint
   C. Pubic symphysis
   D. Suture lines of the skull

7. Where does bursitis occur?
   A. Between the epiphysis and diaphysis
   B. In the fluid-filled disk within a synovial joint
   C. In the bone and bone marrow
   D. In the forearm flexor tendon

8. Which of the following are *not* symptoms of fibromyalgia?
   A. Localized tenderness
   B. Generalized pain
   C. Increased heart rate
   D. Decreased concentration

9. Which of the following foods or nutrients should be avoided by people with gout?
   A. Liver, beans, spinach, and yeast
   B. Calcium and vitamin D
   C. Protein, iron, and phosphorous
   D. Grapefruit juice and caffeine

10. Which term does *not* signify an inflammation of a joint or joints?
    A. Osteoarthritis
    B. Rheumatoid arthritis
    C. Osteomyelitis
    D. Gout

11. Which of the following is true of osteoporosis?
    A. Smoking, family history, and a small body frame are risk factors for the disease.
    B. It is most prevalent among males with low testosterone.
    C. Hypothyroidism can cause secondary osteoporosis.
    D. Adults should consume at least 1,500mg of calcium daily to prevent bone loss.

12. Which age or demographic group is most often affected by osteomyelitis?
    A. Men under the age of 45 years
    B. Postmenopausal women
    C. Children
    D. Girls aged 10 to 12 years

13. Which of the following lists correctly includes signs and/or symptoms of rheumatoid arthritis?

   A. Decreased ESR and positive syphilis test

   B. Bilateral and symmetrical joint swelling, stiffening, and deformity

   C. Unilateral joint pain with crepitus

   D. General malaise, fever, and bone pain

14. Which of the following is true of casts?

   A. A leg cylinder cast often includes a walking heel.

   B. A Minerva cast is applied to the trunk and at least one of the limbs.

   C. Fiberglass casts are less water resistant and heavier than plaster casts.

   D. Plaster casts can be molded more precisely than fiberglass casts.

15. Which of the following structures appears white on an X-ray film?

   A. Skin

   B. A fracture

   C. A tumor

   D. Water

16. Which of the following correctly describes the proper technique for lifting and/or transferring a patient?

   A. Always use a gait belt. Stand as close to the patient as possible and use the muscles of your legs to lift the patient.

   B. Bend at the waist and stand an arm's length away from the patient as you lift the patient to a standing position.

   C. When walking, stand behind the patient, slightly to his or her stronger side. Advise the patient to take large steps so it will require fewer steps to reach the destination.

   D. Hold the patient's hand for reassurance and allow as much time as necessary for the patient to lift himself or herself into position and walk without assistance.

17. Which of the following is the fastest crutch gait?

   A. Two-point gait

   B. Three-point gait

   C. Four-point gait

   D. Swing-through gait

18. What is the correct technique for performing range-of-motion exercises?

   A. Press against the affected limb as the patient moves through the exercises to help the patient improve strength in the affected limb.

   B. Manipulate the patient's soft tissues to promote healing and increase circulation.

   C. Use slow, gentle movements, and support the limb above and below the joint.

   D. Use quick, controlled movements to loosen the joint; mild discomfort should be expected.

19. Which of the following pairs correctly matches the therapeutic modality with one of its advantages or uses?

   A. Thermotherapy: increases circulation and speeds the healing process

   B. Cryotherapy: increases drainage from a wound

   C. Ultrasound therapy: used to evaluate the size, shape, and position of body structures

   D. Massage therapy: decreases metabolism and reduces blood pressure

20. Which of the following is true of a cast cutter?

   A. The cast cutter may generate a cooling sensation on the patient's skin.

   B. The blade vibrates, but does not rotate.

   C. The patient may experience superficial abrasions during the cast-removal process.

   D. If the patient is uncomfortable with a cast cutter, he or she can use regular scissors to remove the cast at home.

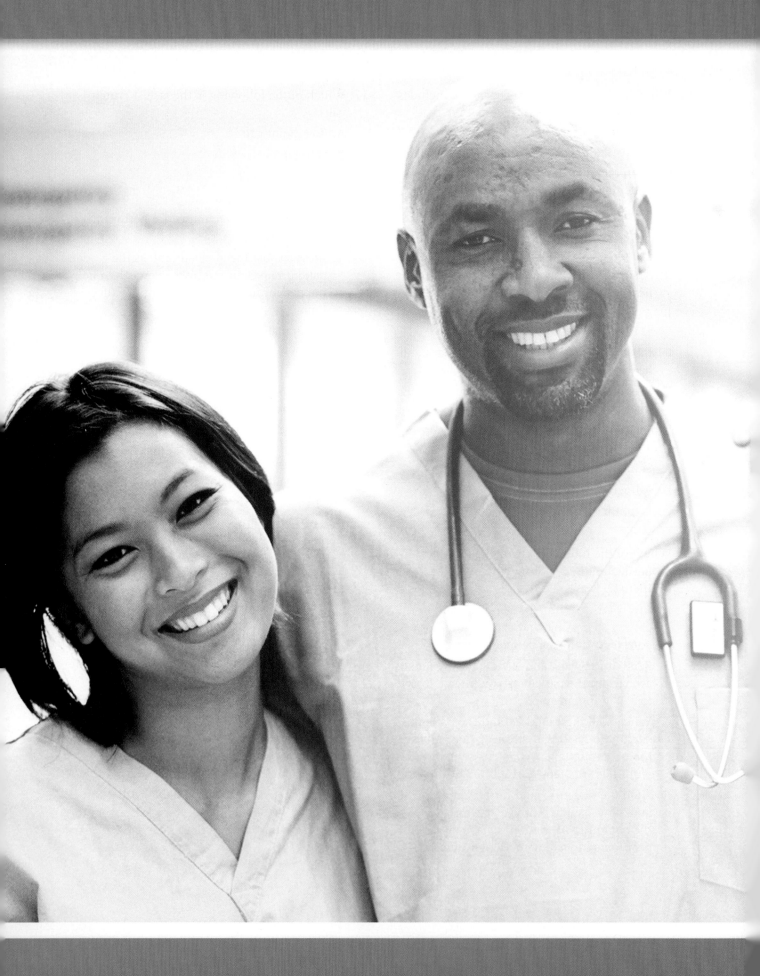

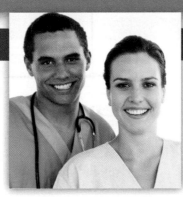

CHAPTER

13

Circulatory System

OBJECTIVES

After reading this chapter, you will be able to:

- Identify combining word forms of the cardiovascular system and their role for the formation of medical terms.
- Define the structures and functions of the circulatory system.
- Identify common diseases, diagnostic procedures, and treatments related to the circulatory system.
- List abbreviations related to the circulatory system.
- Explain the principle of the vacuum tube system.
- State the manner in which anticoagulants prevent coagulation.
- Explain the three skill sets used in collecting blood specimens.
- Explain the importance of correct patient identification; complete specimen labeling; and proper handling, storage, and delivery of the specimen.
- Explain how to handle the various reactions a patient might have to venipuncture.
- Follow the circulation of blood through the heart starting at the vena cava.
- Describe the electrical conduction system of the heart.
- State three reasons why patients may need an electrocardiogram (ECG).
- Explain the purpose of standardization of the ECG.
- Identify the 12 leads of an ECG and describe what area of the heart each lead represents.
- Explain each type of artifact and how each can be eliminated.
- Name and describe the purposes of the various cardiac diagnostic tests and procedures as outlined in this chapter.
- Explain how to calculate heart rates from an ECG tracing.
- Describe the procedure for mounting an ECG tracing.
- Describe the signs and symptoms of a heart attack.

KEY TERMS

Action potential
Angina pectoris
Antecubital space
Aorta
Aortic valve
Arrhythmia
Arteries
Arterioles
Artifact
Atherosclerosis
Atrioventricular (AV) node
Atrioventricular (AV) valves
Augmented leads
Bicuspid valve
Bipolar leads
Capillaries
Capillary puncture
Cardiac catheterization
Cardiac output
Cardiologist
Cerebrovascular accident
Cholesterol
Chordae tendineae
Claudication
Coronary artery disease (CAD)
Deep vein thrombosis (DVT)
Depolarization
Diastolic dysfunction

Echocardiogram (ECHO)
Electrocardiogram (ECG or EKG)
Embolus
Heart
Heart failure (HF)
Hemorrhage
High-density lipoprotein (HDL)
Holter monitoring
Hyperlipidemia
Hypertension
Hypoglycemia
Infarction
Inferior vena cava
Ischemia
Ischemic heart disease
Left atrium
Left ventricle
Lipoproteins
Low-density lipoprotein (LDL)
Mediastinum
Mitral valve
Mounting
Myocardial infarction (MI)
Peripheral artery disease (PAD)
Phlebotomy
Precordial leads
Prehypertension

Pulmonary circulation
Pulmonary embolism (PE)
Pulmonary valve
Right atrium
Right ventricle
Sinoatrial (SA) node
Stress test
Stroke
Superior vena cava
Syncope
Systemic circulation
Systolic dysfunction
Tachycardia
Thoracic surgeon
Thrombus
Total peripheral resistance
Tourniquet
Transient ischemic attack (TIA)
Tricuspid valve
Triglycerides
Vascular surgeon
Vasoconstriction
Veins
Vena cava
Venipuncture
Venous thromboembolism (VTE)
Venules

Chapter Overview

The circulatory system FIGURE 13.1, also called the cardiovascular system, is composed of the heart and blood vessels. Circulation consists of two separate cycles FIGURE 13.2: **pulmonary circulation**, which transports blood between the lungs and the heart so gas exchange can occur, and **systemic circulation**, which transports blood between the heart and the rest of the body so the exchange of nutrients, metabolites, and hormones can occur. Throughout the process of circulation, blood delivers oxygen and nutrients to the body and collects waste products from metabolism to be transported to the lungs and kidneys for elimination from the body.

Diseases and disorders of the circulatory system are common and often affect other organ systems. Several medical specialists are involved in the study of the circulatory system, including cardiologists, thoracic surgeons, and vascular surgeons. A **cardiologist** is an internal medicine specialist who studies diseases and disorders of the human heart. A **thoracic surgeon** performs surgical procedures on the heart, lungs,

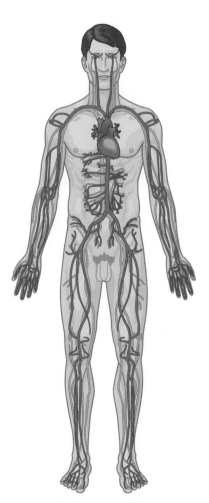

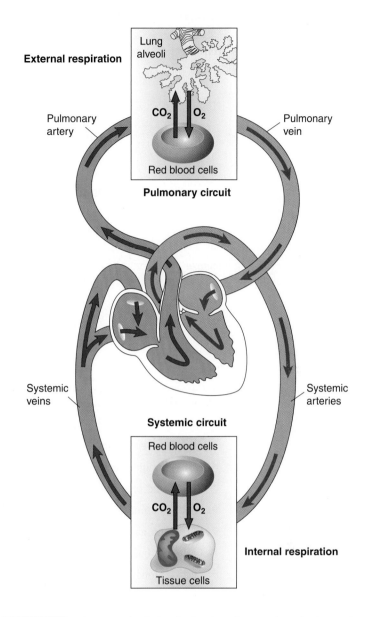

FIGURE 13.1 The circulatory system includes the heart and an intricate web of vessels that transport blood throughout the body.
© Jones & Bartlett Learning

FIGURE 13.2 Pulmonary circulation is the site of external respiration and systemic circulation is the site of internal respiration.
© Blamb/ShutterStock, Inc.

esophagus, and other organs in the chest. A **vascular surgeon** performs surgical procedures involving the blood vessels of the circulatory system. As a medical assistant, you will have the opportunity to interact with patients with a variety of acute and chronic disorders of the circulatory system, as well as participate in diagnostic and treatment-related procedures.

Terminology

TABLE 13.1 lists word roots and terms used in the study of the circulatory system.

Table 13.1 Word Roots of the Circulatory System		
Word Root or Term	**Meaning**	**Example**
Angi/o	Blood vessel	Angiogram (an imaging technique to visualize the inside of blood vessels)
Arteri/o	Artery	Arteriosclerosis (a condition characterized by hardening of the arteries)
Ather/o	Fatty substance	Atherosclerosis (a condition characterized by fatty deposits within the arteries)
Cardi/o	Heart	Cardiomegaly (enlargement of the heart)
Hemangi/o	Blood vessel	Hemangioma (tumor of the blood vessel)
Phleb/o	Vein	Phlebitis (inflammation of the vein)
Sphygm/o	Pulse	Sphygmomanometer (instrument to measure blood pressure)
Steth/o	Chest	Stethoscope (instrument for auscultation and listening to the internal sounds of the chest)
Thromb/o	Clot	Thrombolysis (destruction of a blood clot)
Vas/o	Vessel	Vasospasm (involuntary contraction of a blood vessel)

Abbreviations Related to the Circulatory System

- AF or AFib—Atrial fibrillation
- AV—Atrioventricular
- BBB—Bundle branch block
- BP—Blood pressure
- CABG—Coronary artery bypass graft
- CAD—Coronary artery disease
- Cath—Catheterization
- CCU—Coronary care unit
- CHF—Congestive heart failure
- CPR—Cardiopulmonary resuscitation
- DVT—Deep vein thrombosis
- ECG or EKG—Electrocardiogram
- HDL—High-density lipoproteins
- HTN—Hypertension
- LDL—Low-density lipoproteins
- MI—Myocardial infarction
- mmHg—Millimeters of mercury
- P—Pulse
- PAP—Pulmonary arterial pressure
- PTCA—Percutaneous transluminal coronary angioplasty
- S1—First heart sound
- S2—Second heart sound
- SA—Sinoatrial
- SVT—Supraventricular tachycardia

Structure and Function of the Circulatory System

The primary function of the circulatory system is to propel blood through the body, supplying oxygen and nutrients to and removing waste products from all cells of the body. The heart, along with large and small vessels throughout the body, facilitates this transport of blood. The circulating blood provides a rapid means of transport for cells and molecules from one part of the body to another.

Heart

The **heart** is a muscle and is about the size of a fist FIGURE 13.3 . It maintains uninterrupted blood flow through the arteries, veins, and capillaries. The heart is essentially

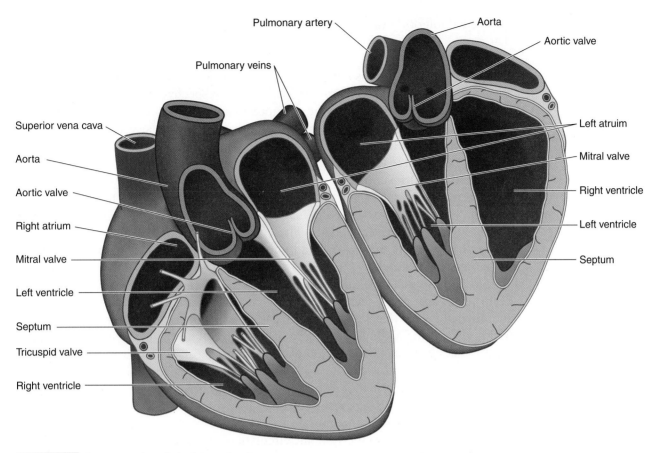

Pulmonary artery

Aorta

Aortic valve

Pulmonary veins

Superior vena cava

Aorta

Aortic valve

Right atrium

Mitral valve

Left ventricle

Septum

Tricuspid valve

Right ventricle

Left atruim

Mitral valve

Right ventricle

Left ventricle

Septum

FIGURE 13.3 A cross section of the human heart.
© Jones & Bartlett Learning

two separate pumps, with the right side and the left side of the heart acting as separate pumps with separate functions. The septum is the muscular wall that divides the two sides of the heart.

The heart is located in the center of the thoracic cavity, in an area of the body called the **mediastinum**. The heart sits below the sternum, between the lungs, and is located slightly to the left side of the body. The heart is composed of three layers of tissue:

- **Endocardium**—The endocardium is the innermost layer of tissue and forms the heart's valves and a smooth layer of epithelial cells.
- **Myocardium**—The myocardium is a thick, muscular layer that is composed of specialized cardiac muscle cells.
- **Pericardium**—The pericardium is a thin membrane that covers the myocardium. The pericardium contains coronary blood vessels, which supply the heart muscle with its blood supply containing oxygen and nutrients. The heart does not receive its blood supply from blood pumped into its interior chambers.

The human heart is composed of four chambers: the **right atrium**, the **left atrium**, the **right ventricle**, and the **left ventricle**. The atria (plural of atrium) are located superiorly (at the top of the heart) and the ventricles

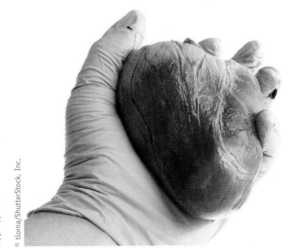

© tlorna/ShutterStock, Inc.

A normal adult heart is slightly larger than a clenched fist.

are located inferiorly (at the bottom of the heart). The atria are collecting chambers that receive blood and the ventricles are distributing chambers that pump blood out of the heart.

The heart also contains four valves: right and left **atrioventricular (AV) valves** (the **tricuspid valve** and **bicuspid valve** or **mitral valve**, respectively), the **pulmonary valve**, and the **aortic valve**. The valves are designed to maintain blood flow in one direction and prevent blood from flowing backward. The atrioventricular valves are composed of squamous epithelial cells that line the heart and make up the endocardium. The valves are attached to the chambers of the heart with special ligaments called **chordae tendineae**. The atrioventricular valves are composed of thinner tissue than the pulmonary and aortic valves and are, therefore, not as strong and are more susceptible to damage and disease. The pulmonary and aortic valves are also called semilunar valves due to their crescent shape. These valves are composed of three very strong cusps (that look like the crown of a tooth) and can withstand the strong contractile pressure of the ventricles.

Blood flows in a continuous loop around the body, beginning before birth until death. Each beat of the heart, or cardiac cycle, is a series of highly integrated and coordinated events that lead to the relaxation and contraction of the atria and ventricles, the closing and opening of the heart's valves, and the filling and emptying of the atria and ventricles. The period of contraction is called systole and the period of relaxation is called diastole. During systole, the pressure exerted by the heart on the blood is at its maximum. Systole can be felt as the pulse in an artery. Blood pressure is at its lowest during diastole, when the heart is at rest. A normal adult heart contracts or beats 60 to 80 times in one minute.

First, the blood from the systemic circulation enters the right atrium through the **vena cava**, the largest vein in the body. The right atrium contracts and pushes blood through the tricuspid valve into the right ventricle. The right ventricle contracts and passes blood through the pulmonary valve into the pulmonary artery. Blood proceeds to the lungs, where it obtains oxygen. After gas exchange in the lungs, blood travels through the pulmonary vein to return to the heart, emptying into the left atrium. The left atrium contracts and blood passes through the bicuspid valve into the left ventricle. After the left ventricle contracts, blood passes through the aortic valve into the aorta and away from the heart into systemic circulation. After blood has traveled through the body and delivered its oxygen, nutrients, and metabolites, it returns to the heart to complete another cycle.

The heart contracts as a result of an electrical impulse. At rest, the cardiac muscle cells are permeable to sodium ions. This influx of sodium causes the myocardium to propagate electrical signals throughout the heart, causing the efficient and coordinated contraction of the atria and ventricles. The nerves that innervate the cardiac muscle are under complete control of the autonomic nervous system **FIGURE 13.4**.

The pathway of electrical activity in the heart is illustrated in **FIGURE 13.5**. Specifically, the **sinoatrial (SA) node** generates an electrical impulse that initiates the wave of contraction around the heart. The SA node is located near the point where the vena cava enters the right atrium and is especially sensitive to the transport of positive sodium ions. The activation of the SA node causes **depolarization**, or the process of becoming more positive, of the cells of the myocardium, initiating an **action potential**, a change in the electrical membrane potential of a cell that leads to contraction. Normally, the SA node generates spontaneous electrical activity, functioning as the physiological pacemaker for the heart. Shortly after depolarization, repolarization occurs as sodium ions travel out of the

Arteries carry oxygenated blood away from the heart; veins carry deoxygenated blood back to the heart. The pulmonary artery and pulmonary vein are the only exceptions.

© auremar/ShutterStock, Inc.

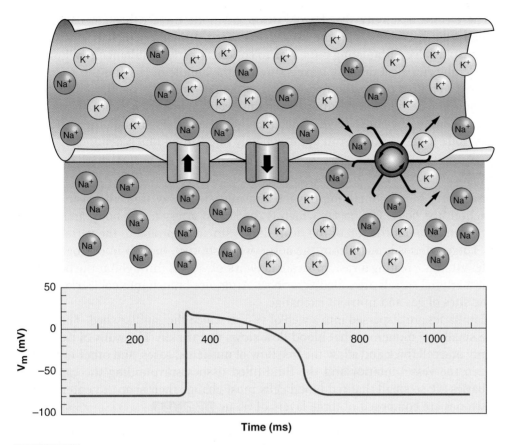

FIGURE 13.4 Electrophysiology of the cardiac muscle.

Adapted from Malmivuo, Jaakko and Plonsey, Robert (1995). Bioelectromagnetism: Principles and Applications of Bioelectric and Biomagnetic Fields. New York, New York: Oxford University Press.

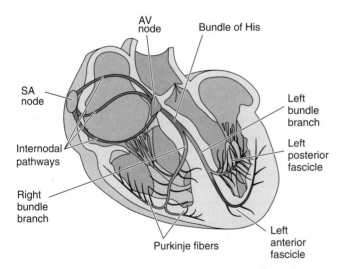

FIGURE 13.5 The electrical system of the heart.

Adapted from *12-Lead ECG: The Art of Interpretation*, courtesy of Tomas B. Garcia, MD

cells of the myocardium. Depolarization causes voltage-gated calcium channels in the cardiac muscle cells to open and potassium channels to close. The influx of positive calcium ions into the cells, along with the release of calcium from the sarcoplasmic reticulum within each cell, causes muscle contraction. After a short delay, potassium channels reopen and the resulting efflux of potassium leads to a repolarization of the cardiac cells and a return to a resting state.

The electrical activity that begins in the SA node travels through Bachmann's bundle to the left atrium and the **atrioventricular (AV) node**, which is located near the tricuspid valve, stimulating both atria to contract nearly simultaneously. From the AV node, the electrical impulse travels through the bundle of His and the AV bundle to the right and left bundle branches, then to the Purkinje fibers and the ventricular myocardium. The ventricles contract when the electrical impulse reaches the ventricular myocardium. The entire wave of electrical impulse travels through the heart, from the SA node to the ventricles, in approximately one-fifth of one second.

Arteries

Arteries carry blood containing oxygen and nutrients away from the heart to cells throughout the body. The **aorta**, which is the largest artery in the body, arches from the left ventricle out the top of the heart and is situated parallel to the vertebral column. Large arteries branch from the aorta, which in turn branch into progressively smaller arteries, creating a vast, intricate network of vessels throughout the body. The smallest arterial vessels are called **arterioles**. Arterioles branch into **capillaries**, which are the sites of gas and nutrient exchange.

Capillaries are dispersed into a web of vessels called the capillary bed. The vessels are so small and numerous that blood flow slows to a trickle. The walls of capillaries are only one cell thick and allow the free flow of nutrients, gases, and other molecules between the vessel interior and the fluid-filled tissues surrounding the capillaries. Capillaries are so small that red blood cells must change their shape to enter them.

Arteries are composed of three layers of tissue **FIGURE 13.6**:

- **Adventitia**—The adventitia is the outermost layer of tissue and is made of connective tissue.
- **Media**—The media is the middle layer of tissue and is composed of smooth muscle.
- **Intima**—The intima is the innermost layer and is made of epithelial tissue and elastic tissue.

Arteries can change their diameter in response to input from hormones or the nervous system **FIGURE 13.7**. The sympathetic nervous system causes **vasoconstriction**, a decrease in the internal diameter of blood vessels. The hormones epinephrine and angiotensin also cause vasoconstriction, as does trauma to a blood vessel. Heat causes arteries to dilate or increase their diameter.

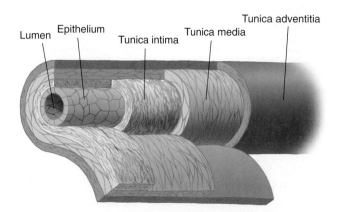

FIGURE 13.6 Arteries are composed of three layers of tissue. *Tunica* is the Latin word for tunic or coat. The *lumen* is the artery's cavity; the *epithelium* is the cavity's lining.

Veins

Veins carry blood that lacks oxygen back to the heart. Capillaries join together to become **venules**, the smallest vessels of the venous system, which, in turn, flow into progressively larger veins. Blood from the trunk and lower extremities flows into the **inferior vena cava** and blood from the head and arms flows into the **superior vena cava**. The vena cava is the largest vein in the body and empties blood into the right atrium of the heart.

Veins are composed of thinner and less elastic tissue than arteries. Veins also contain valves, unlike arteries, which maintain unidirectional blood flow through the venous system. Blood continuously moves from the area of highest pressure (the aorta) to the area of lowest pressure (the veins). Because blood in the venous system flows back to the heart, moving from a low-pressure vessel to a high-pressure one, valves are necessary to prevent the blood from flowing backward. Muscles surrounding the veins also participate in pumping blood in the right direction.

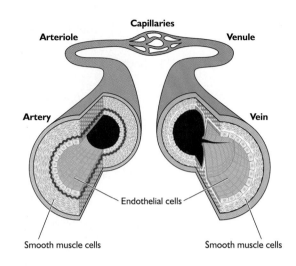

FIGURE 13.7 The anatomy of the circulatory system.
© Blamb/ShutterStock, Inc.

Decreased blood flow to the tissues of the body will result in a lack of oxygen, known as hypoxia, and a lack of nutrients. Dehydration, **atherosclerosis** (the buildup of fatty deposits in the arteries), arterial spasms, and decreased pumping of the muscles surrounding the veins lead to decreased blood flow.

The aorta has an average pressure of 100mmHg, and veins have an average pressure of 6mmHg.

Diseases and Disorders of the Circulatory System

Disorders of the circulatory system are a leading cause of disability and death each year, affecting more than 70 million Americans. Any condition that disrupts the normal, integrated function of the circulatory system impedes an individual's ability to complete activities of daily living and maintain an acceptable quality of life. Often, several disorders that affect the circulatory system occur simultaneously. Many cardiovascular diseases occur without symptoms, especially in early stages of the diseases, so patient education and disease prevention are of utmost importance, perhaps in diseases of the circulatory system more than any other body system.

Cardiovascular changes occur with age, and advanced age is a risk factor for many impairments of the circulatory system. Many circulatory disorders are chronic conditions and patients will require long-term care and follow-up. Further, many disorders are challenging to treat effectively and require multiple treatment modalities and significant changes in lifestyle habits. A medical assistant who deals with cardiovascular patients must be compassionate, understanding, and patient and must stress the importance of compliance with therapeutic regimens.

Arrhythmias

An **arrhythmia** is a variation in the normal heart rate or rhythm. The heart may beat too fast or too slow, or the contractions of the atria and ventricles may not be synchronized. Any disruption in the normal electrical rhythm of the heart can cause an arrhythmia. Arrhythmias occur when an area of the heart other than the SA node generates an electrical impulse that stimulates the myocardium to contract. Arrhythmias can result from **ischemia** (a decreased blood supply to tissues), **infarction** (the death of tissues due to a sudden decrease in blood supply), or alterations or abnormalities in body chemicals.

Signs and Symptoms of Arrhythmias

Abnormal contraction and electrical conduction of the heart lead to conditions such as **tachycardia** (increased heart rate), atrial flutter, and atrial fibrillation. Each of these types of arrhythmias can lead to palpitations, **syncope** (loss of consciousness), light-headedness, visual disturbances, pale complexion, weakness, sweating, chest pain, and decreased blood pressure.

Treatment of Arrhythmias

The goal of arrhythmia treatment is to restore the normal rate or rhythm of the heart. Several classes of antiarrhythmic agents are available, each with a different site or mechanism of action:

- Class I antiarrhythmic agents are termed membrane-stabilizing agents. They reduce the movement of sodium ions into the cardiac cells and decrease the heart's ability to initiate an abnormal action potential.
- Class II antiarrhythmics are traditional beta-blockers, which decrease sympathetic activity in the heart and decrease conduction to the AV node.
- Class III agents are potassium channel blockers and prolong the period of repolarization of the cardiac muscle cells.
- Class IV antiarrhythmics are the calcium channel blockers verapamil and diltiazem, which decrease conduction through the AV node and reduce the contractility of the heart.

Miscellaneous agents, including atropine, digoxin, magnesium sulfate, and isoproterenol, are also effective at treating various arrhythmias, but their mechanisms of action do not fit into one of the other four categories of antiarrhythmic agents. Common antiarrhythmic agents are presented in TABLE 13.2 .

Table 13.2   Drugs Commonly Used to Treat Arrhythmias

Class	Drug (Brand Name)
Class I antiarrhythmics	Disopyramide (Norpace) Flecainide (Tambocor) Lidocaine (Xylocaine) Procainamide (Pronestyl)
Class II antiarrhythmics (beta-blockers)	Acebutolol (Sectral) Atenolol (Tenormin) Bisoprolol (Zebeta) Carvedilol (Coreg) Labetolol (Trandate) Metoprolol (Lopressor, Toprol-XL) Propranolol (Inderal)
Class III antiarrhythmics	Amiodarone (Cordarone) Dofetlide (Tikosyn)
Class IV antiarrhythmics	Verapamil (Covera HS, Calan, Verelan) Diltiazem (Cardizem, Cartia, Dilacor XR,Tiazac)

Congestive Heart Failure

Heart failure (HF), also known as congestive heart failure (CHF), is a condition in which the heart is unable to pump enough blood to meet the body's needs. Most simply, the heart pumps out less blood than it collects. HF is a chronic condition that develops gradually over time. Any condition that reduces the filling of the ventricles (**diastolic dysfunction**) or reduces the contraction of the heart muscle (**systolic dysfunction**) requires the heart to work harder than normal, leading to this failure to meet the body's needs. Conditions may be physical or environmental, including hypertension, atherosclerosis, coronary artery disease, temperature extremes, stress, high salt intake, kidney failure, infection and inflammation, cigarette smoking, obesity, and pregnancy.

HF can occur unilaterally on either the right or left side of the heart, but most cases of HF occur on both sides of the heart. Left-sided heart failure usually occurs first and leads to right-sided failure. Left-sided heart failure often occurs as a result of aortic valve disease or a disorder of the left ventricle. In any case, the left ventricle begins to work harder to compensate for the decreased blood flow and the muscle begins to enlarge. When the heart can no longer compensate for the extra blood-flow requirements, failure occurs, in which case a sufficient supply of blood, and therefore oxygen, does not reach the body's peripheral tissues.

Signs and Symptoms of Congestive Heart Failure

HF develops slowly without symptoms, at first. The first symptom that a patient may notice is often increased shortness of breath during formerly comfortable activities. A patient may also experience discomfort while breathing lying down; he or she may begin using extra pillows at night and prefer sleeping in a semi-upright position. A cough can occur with left-sided heart failure, which is often worse when a patient lies down.

As HF progresses, shortness of breath worsens, even with mild to moderate activities. Hypoxia in the brain and nervous system leads to irritability, restlessness, confusion, and disorientation. When the right side of the heart begins to fail, symptoms worsen and the blood supply to the liver and kidneys decreases. Increased pressure and decreased circulation in these areas leads to fluid and sodium retention. This, in turn, leads to edema in the lower extremities—particularly the feet, ankles, and legs.

Treatment of Congestive Heart Failure

The goal of HF treatment is to improve symptoms, prevent disease progression, prolong survival, and improve quality of life for the patient. Angiotensin-converting enzyme (ACE) inhibitors and beta-blockers are first-line agents for HF. A diuretic, digoxin, and antiplatelet or anticoagulant agents are added as second-line agents to slow disease progression and improve morbidity and mortality rates associated with HF. Vasodilators can also be effective for HF treatment because they expand the internal diameter of the blood vessels and decrease the amount of work required of the heart. Drugs commonly used to treat HF are presented in **TABLE 13.3**. Beta-blockers were presented in Table 13.2.

In addition to pharmacologic therapy, HF patients are advised to alter dietary and lifestyle habits to decrease symptoms and reduce the heart's workload. Primarily, decreased salt intake improves edema. Salt substitutes may be used in place of salt, but many patients find these unpalatable. Improving physical fitness and maintaining a healthy weight are also advisable to combat HF.

Hyperlipidemia

Cholesterol is a component of cell membranes of animals and occurs naturally in foods from animal sources. It is not found in foods from plants. Cholesterol is nec-

Table 13.3 Drugs Commonly Used to Treat CHF	
Class	**Drug (Brand Name)**
ACE inhibitors	Benazepril (Lotensin) Captopril (Capoten) Enalapril (Vasotec) Lisinopril (Prinivil, Zestril) Quinapril (Accupril) Ramipril (Altace)
Vasodilators	Milrinone Nitroprusside (Nitropress) Isosorbide-hydralazine (Bi-Dil)
Cardiac glycosides	Digoxin (Lanoxin)

essary for the proper functioning of several body functions and systems, including producing hormones and digesting food, and the liver is responsible for processing cholesterol consumed from food and manufacturing cholesterol needed by the body. The liver packages molecules of cholesterol together with lipids bound to proteins (**lipoproteins**). Most of the cholesterol in the body travels with **low-density lipoproteins (LDL)** or **high-density lipoproteins (HDL)**. HDL is referred to as good cholesterol and is attached to 20–30 percent of the body's total cholesterol. LDL is referred to as bad cholesterol and is attached to 60–70 percent of the body's cholesterol.

Triglycerides, another type of lipid or fat found in the body, are synthesized from carbohydrates and release free fatty acids into the body. Triglycerides also circulate with cholesterol.

LDL and HDL circulate through the body and deliver cholesterol to parts of the body that need it. LDL is not used by cells, so it is instead deposited in the walls of arteries and forms plaque, which causes the interior space of the artery to narrow; eventually, the blood vessel may become completely blocked. This narrowing of the artery is called atherosclerosis **FIGURE 13.8** and can cause poor circulation or a heart attack or stroke. After circulating, HDL returns to the liver; its presence helps decrease the risk of atherosclerosis.

Signs and Symptoms of Hyperlipidemia

Elevated levels of lipoproteins, triglycerides, and cholesterol, known collectively as **hyperlipidemia**, are influenced by genetics, alcohol consumption, hypothyroidism, liver disease, kidney disease, and age. Diagnosis of hyperlipidemia requires a blood test, as there are no outward symptoms of hyperlipidemia. Ideally, total cholesterol levels (including all types of lipoproteins and triglycerides) should be below 200mg per deciliter of blood. LDL should be less than 100mg and HDL should be greater than 60mg. Triglycerides should be less than 150mg.

Treatment of Hyperlipidemia

As with many cardiovascular diseases, prevention is essential for avoiding complications of hyperlipid-

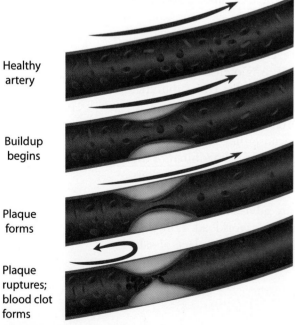

Healthy artery

Buildup begins

Plaque forms

Plaque ruptures; blood clot forms

FIGURE 13.8 The progression of atherosclerosis.
© Alila Sao Mai/ShutterStock, Inc.

emia. A low-fat diet and a healthy, active lifestyle are often effective in maintaining optimum cholesterol levels.

Once diagnosed, the treatment goals for hyperlipidemia include reduction in lipid levels and prevention of cardiovascular complications. Lifestyle modifications are first-line therapy for hyperlipidemia, but drug therapy can be added if diet and exercise habits fail to achieve goal lipid levels. Several classes of cholesterol-lowering agents are available and each has varying effects on LDL, HDL, and triglyceride levels. A combination of drugs from multiple classes may be required for effective cholesterol reduction.

HMG-CoA reductase inhibitors are arguably the most well known of cholesterol-lowering drugs. They are more commonly called statins. These agents inhibit cholesterol formation in the liver. Fibric acid derivatives increase the breakdown of very low-density lipoproteins and promote the excretion of triglycerides. Bile acid sequestrants prevent the absorption of bile acids into the bloodstream; the body must use cholesterol to make more bile acid, thereby reducing stores of cholesterol. Niacin, psyllium, and omega-3 fatty acids are available without a prescription and are effective at reducing cholesterol levels. Common agents for reducing cholesterol levels are presented in TABLE 13.4.

Hypertension

Blood pressure is the product of cardiac output and total peripheral resistance. **Cardiac output** is the amount of blood pumped by the heart each minute, and **total peripheral resistance** is the sum of the entire resistance in the blood vessels of the systemic circulation. Each parameter that affects blood pressure is influenced by a variety of factors, including blood viscosity, blood volume, and nervous system controls.

A blood-pressure measurement is expressed as the systolic blood pressure (the pressure when the heart contracts and ejects blood, or the heart at work) over the diastolic blood pressure (the pressure when the heart relaxes and fills with blood, or the heart at rest). An ideal blood pressure for an adult without diabetes is a systolic blood pressure of 120mmHg or less over a diastolic blood pressure of 80mmHg or less (expressed as 120/80mmHg). Diabetic patients are advised to maintain a blood pressure of less than 130/80mmHg.

Signs and Symptoms of Hypertension

Elevated blood pressure can lead to devastating and disabling consequences, including kidney dysfunction, whole-body edema, and fluid accumulation in the lungs. Most complications are associated with a systolic blood pressure of greater than 140mmHg or a diastolic blood pressure of greater than 90mmHg, defined as **hypertension**. Patients

Table 13.4 Drugs Commonly Used to Treat Hyperlipidemia	
Class	**Drug (Brand Name)**
HMG-CoA reductase inhibitors	Atorvastatin (Lipitor) Fluvastatin (Lescol) Lovastatin (Mevacor) Pravastatin (Pravachol) Rosuvastatin (Crestor) Simvastatin (Zocor)
Fibric acid derivatives	Fenofibrate (TriCor) Gemfibrozil (Lopid)
Bile acid sequestrants	Colesevelam (WelChol) Colestipol (Colestid)

should be advised to maintain healthy blood pressures below this level. **Prehypertension** is defined as a systolic blood pressure of between 120 and 139mmHg or a diastolic blood pressure between 80 and 89mmHg. Patients with prehypertension or hypertension are at risk for cardiovascular disease and complications, and the risk of cardiovascular morbidity and mortality is directly related to elevated blood pressure.

Hypertension is called the silent killer because it presents with few or no symptoms.

Treatment of Hypertension

The goal of hypertension treatment is to reduce blood pressure to healthy levels and decrease the risk of complications associated with hypertension. Lifestyle modifications are the cornerstone of hypertension management and include decreased sodium intake, weight loss for overweight individuals, increased physical activity, decreased alcohol consumption, controlling stress, and smoking cessation.

Pharmacologic therapy can be initiated for hypertension if lifestyle modifications do not result in a substantial decrease in blood pressure. Several classes of antihypertensive agents are available, with different mechanisms and sites of action. Often, drug therapy for advanced hypertension requires combinations of agents from several classes. Diuretics, ACE inhibitors, beta-blockers, and calcium channel blockers are first-line agents for hypertension. Angiotensin receptor blockers (ARBs), central nervous system agents, alpha-blockers, vasodilators, and direct renin inhibitors are used as second-line agents for hypertension. Several classes of antihypertensives are presented in TABLE 13.5. Beta-blockers were presented in Table 13.2, and ACE inhibitors were presented in Table 13.3.

Table 13.5 Drugs Commonly Used to Treat Hypertension	
Class	**Drug (Brand Name)**
Diuretics	Hydrochlorothiazide Chlorthalidone Furosemide (Lasix) Torsemide (Demadex) Eplerenone (Inspra) Spironolactone (Aldactone) Triamterene (Dyrenium) Acetazolamide (Diamox) Mannitol (Osmitrol)
Angiotensin receptor blockers	Candesartan (Atacand) Irbesartan (Avapro) Losartan (Cozaar) Olmesartan (Benicar) Telmisartan (Micardis) Valsartan (Diovan)
Central nervous system agents	Clonidine (Catapres, Catapres-TTS, Duraclon) Guanfacine (Tenex)
Alpha-blockers	Alfuzosin (Uroxatrol) Doxazosin (Cardura) Prazosin (Minipress) Terazosin (Hytrin)
Vasodilators	Epoprostenol (Flolan) Fenoldopam (Corlopram)
Direct renin inhibitors	Aliskiren (Tekturna)

Ischemic Heart Disease

Ischemic heart disease is a condition in which the heart muscles receive a decreased supply of blood. Ischemic heart disease is often a manifestation of atherosclerosis (a buildup of fatty deposits) of the coronary blood vessels.

Signs and Symptoms of Ischemic Heart Disease

Angina pectoris, or angina, is the hallmark symptom of ischemic heart disease. Angina is chest pain caused by the decreased oxygen supply to the heart. Angina causes significant pain and discomfort, but it does not cause irreversible damage to the heart or blood vessels.

Stable angina occurs in response to exertion or exercise. The pain is usually predictable and it is relieved with rest. Unstable angina is pain that occurs with increased frequency and decreased response to treatment. It is not predictable and it may signal an oncoming heart attack. Variant angina is pain that is caused by a coronary artery spasm. This pain is not predictable and is not induced by stress.

Episodes of angina typically involve severe chest pain or discomfort **FIGURE 13.9**. Angina may be accompanied by sweating, dizziness, and shortness of breath. Most episodes of angina are brief.

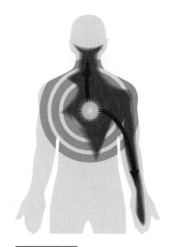

FIGURE 13.9 Angina pain usually radiates up to the neck and jaw or through the left shoulder and arm.

© Jones & Bartlett Learning

Treatment of Ischemic Heart Disease

The goals of treatment of ischemic heart disease are to reduce symptoms and prevent the occurrence of a heart attack. Nitrates, beta-blockers, and calcium channel blockers are the mainstays of ischemic heart disease treatment. Nitrates are the most commonly used agents for angina. These drugs relax vascular smooth muscle and dilate coronary blood vessels, allowing blood to flow to the areas of the heart that require oxygen. Nitroglycerin, a fast-acting nitrate, can be taken at the onset of angina pain to relieve symptoms of an angina episode. Beta-blockers slow the heart rate and lower blood pressure, which, when taken regularly, reduce the frequency and severity of angina attacks. Calcium channel blockers reduce the heart's demand for oxygen, relax coronary smooth muscle, and dilate coronary blood vessels, which together result in increased oxygen delivery to the heart.

Myocardial Infarction

A **myocardial infarction (MI)** is commonly known as a heart attack. An MI occurs after a prolonged period of decreased oxygen delivery to the muscle of the heart, which causes the cells to die. The risk of an MI increases if the coronary blood vessels are occluded.

Signs and Symptoms of Myocardial Infarction

Chest pain is the hallmark symptom of an acute MI and is often described as a tightness, pressure, or squeezing sensation, shortness of breath, nausea, vomiting, palpitations, sweating, and anxiety (often described as a sense of impending doom). Pain may radiate from the chest to the left arm, neck, lower jaw, or back. It may also mimic heartburn by causing pain or discomfort in the upper central portion of the abdomen.

Treatment of Myocardial Infarction

Prevention of an MI by treating underlying cardiovascular disease is paramount. Drug therapy may be needed to reduce hypertension, control diabetes, or reduce cholesterol levels. Stopping smoking, increasing physical activity, following a low-salt and low-fat diet, and maintaining an ideal body weight are also important lifestyle modifications to prevent an MI as well as other cardiovascular complications.

Once an MI occurs, treatment goals include promoting healing of the heart and preventing death or recurrent MI. Beta-blockers and daily aspirin therapy are often initiated after an MI to decrease the heart's workload and prevent clot formation.

Stroke

A **stroke**, also known as a **cerebrovascular accident**, occurs when oxygen supply to an area of the brain is interrupted. This decreased oxygen delivery may be the result of a **hemorrhage** (a release of blood from a blood vessel) or obstructed blood flow. Hemorrhagic strokes occur when a blood vessel ruptures and blood spills into the space surrounding the brain.

Hemorrhagic strokes account for 10 percent of strokes and are most often caused by hypertension. The remaining 90 percent of strokes, termed ischemic strokes, are due to obstructed blood flow, often from a thrombus or atherosclerosis. A **transient ischemic attack (TIA)** is similar to an ischemic stroke, but is brief, often lasting less than 30 minutes. Prompt treatment of a TIA is necessary to prevent the occurrence of a stroke.

Ischemia in the heart causes a heart attack. Ischemia in the brain can cause a stroke, sometimes referred to as a brain attack.

Signs and Symptoms of Stroke

Stroke symptoms usually develop suddenly and include a headache (which may be severe); changes in alertness; changes in hearing, taste, or touch; confusion; dizziness; one-sided muscle weakness; blurred vision; and difficulty speaking. Emergency medical treatment should be obtained if these symptoms occur.

Treatment of Stroke

If an ischemic stroke is diagnosed promptly, fibrinolytic agents can be administered within three hours of symptom onset. Signs and symptoms of stroke can be reversed in many cases. In the case of a hemorrhagic stroke, treatment is supportive, including fluids to maintain hydration status, oxygen to improve oxygenation of the blood to the brain, and blood pressure–lowering medications if blood pressure is elevated. Vital signs are stabilized and pain is relieved while patients experience the acute phase of a hemorrhagic stroke. Once the patient is stable, the cause of the hemorrhagic stroke can be determined and treated. Early rehabilitation following a stroke can lead to a remarkable recovery for many patients, some with no permanent disability.

Modification of risk factors, including weight reduction, smoking cessation, cholesterol reduction, reducing blood pressure, increasing physical activity, and controlling diabetes can prevent the occurrence of a stroke. Anticoagulant and antiplatelet medications can be administered to patients at risk for ischemic strokes. Anticoagulant agents prevent the cascade of clotting steps in the blood, and antiplatelet agents prevent platelets—the component of blood responsible for clotting—from sticking together.

After a stroke, treatment goals include preventing future stroke and restoring levels of pre-stroke functioning and quality of life. If the cause of the stroke is an identifiable blood clot or occlusion, fibrinolytic therapy is useful to break up the clot, as is surgical intervention to remove the occlusion. The cause of a stroke (hemorrhagic versus ischemic) should be unequivocally confirmed before therapy is initiated. Administering antiplatelet, anticoagulant, or fibrinolytic agents after a hemorrhagic stroke could be fatal. **TABLE 13.6** outlines drugs commonly used to prevent and treat stroke.

Table 13.6 Drugs Commonly Used to Prevent and Treat Stroke	
Class	**Drug (Brand Name)**
Anticoagulant agents	Bivalirudin (Angiomax)
	Fondaparinux (Arixtra)
	Heparin
	Lepirudin (Refludan)
	Warfarin (Coumadin)
	Dalteparin (Fragmin)
	Enoxaparin (Lovenox)
	Tinzaparin (Innohep)
Antiplatelet agents	Aspirin
	Clopidogrel (Plavix)
	Abciximab (ReoPro)
	Eptifibatide (Integrilin)
	Tirofiban (Aggrastat)
Fibrinolytic agents	Alteplase (Activase)
	Reteplase (Retevase)
	Tenecteplase (TNKase)

Peripheral Artery Disease

Peripheral artery disease (PAD) is a manifestation of the narrowing of the blood vessels in the extremities due to atherosclerosis. PAD can exist with or without **coronary artery disease (CAD)** (narrowing of the blood vessels supplying the heart itself) due to atherosclerosis. If CAD has not been diagnosed, PAD should serve as an indicator of early CAD, which can lead to MI or stroke.

Signs and Symptoms of Peripheral Artery Disease

Early in the course of PAD, patients often experience no symptoms. The first symptoms to appear are usually pain or discomfort in the legs, which may occur at rest or with exertion. Intermittent claudication and leg pain at rest are classic symptoms of PAD. **Claudication** includes fatigue, discomfort, pain, or numbness in the extremities upon exertion. Resting leg pain occurs due to the decreased circulation and perfusion in the extremity.

Treatment of Peripheral Artery Disease

The goals of PAD treatment are to reduce symptom frequency and severity and to correct the underlying pathology to decrease future cardiovascular complications. Smoking cessation, weight reduction, diabetes control, and healthy lifestyle modifications reduce the risk of future events associated with PAD. Surgical procedures are also available to restore blood flow to affected limbs. Drug therapy may be prescribed to correct hypertension, hyperlipidemia, or clot-forming abnormalities that can increase the occurrence of PAD. PAD-specific drug treatments include the use of cilostazol and pentoxifylline, which can increase walking distance in patients with severe intermittent claudication.

Venous Thromboembolism

A **thrombus** is a blood clot. A thrombus may result from abnormal coagulation, altered blood flow, increased platelet adhesion, or damaged blood vessels. A thrombus is potentially life threatening. An **embolus** is a blood clot that becomes detached and travels through the bloodstream. **Venous thromboembolism (VTE)** results from abnormal clot formation in the venous circulation and is manifested by **deep vein thrombosis (DVT)** and **pulmonary embolism (PE)**.

Blood clots can be silent conditions, presenting no signs or symptoms to prompt diagnosis prior to an acute event **FIGURE 13.10**. A PE occurs when a piece of a blood clot breaks free and travels to the lungs. A PE can lead to a blockage of the pulmonary artery. Death can occur within minutes of a PE, allowing no time for effective treatment.

A DVT is a thrombus that occurs within a vein deep inside the body, most often the legs. A DVT located at or above the knee is at high risk for traveling to blood vessels supplying the brain, heart, or lungs. Risk factors for DVT include age over 40 years, extended periods of immobility, high-dose estrogen therapy, estrogen therapy combined with nicotine exposure, major illness, obesity, pregnancy, previous DVT, surgery, trauma, and varicose veins.

Signs and Symptoms of Venous Thromboembolism

Many blood clots exist without symptoms. A thrombus may go undetected until it becomes an embolus and results in blood vessel occlusion. However, some symptoms of a DVT include changes in the color of skin covering a thrombus and increased warmth, pain, tenderness, or edema in the area of the thrombus. When the thrombus becomes a PE, symptoms can include chest pain, shortness of breath, cough, increased respiratory rate, tachycardia, anxiety, dizziness, lightheadedness, sweating, and wheezing.

Treatment of Venous Thromboembolism

Anticoagulants and antiplatelet agents are the drugs of choice to prevent clot formation in patients at risk for thrombus development. Anticoagulant therapy is often initiated in hospitalized patients with IV heparin, a naturally occurring anticoagulant. Anticoagulant therapy with heparin requires frequent monitoring and individualized dose adjustment. Low molecular weight heparins (LMWHs) are alternatives to heparin and require less monitoring and more standardized dosing. LMWHs include enoxaparin, dalteparin, and tinzaparin. Warfarin is an oral anticoagulant that requires frequent monitoring initially; monitoring requirements decrease as the duration of administration increases. All patients receiving any type of anticoagulant therapy should be educated about the increased risk of bleeding associated with these agents.

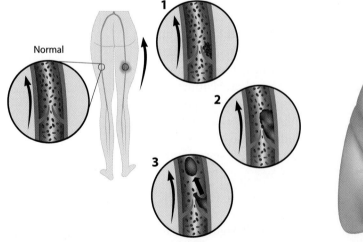
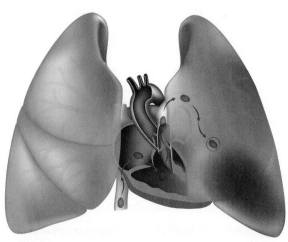

FIGURE 13.10 DVT and PE are manifestations of VTE.
© Alila Sao Mai/ShutterStock, Inc.

Antiplatelet agents, including aspirin and clopidogrel, prevent platelets from forming a clot. Glycoprotein agonists, including abciximab, eptifibatide, and tirofiban, also prevent platelet aggregation and are used in invasive surgical procedures to prevent artery closure.

Once a thrombus has formed, the goal of treatment is to remove or dissolve the clot. Anticoagulant and antiplatelet agents cannot accomplish this, so fibrinolytic agents must be used such as alteplase, reteplase, or tenecteplase. These agents dissolve the clot by binding to the proteins in the thrombus.

Diagnostic and Treatment-Related Procedures of the Circulatory System

More than 60 percent of cardiac deaths occur with no prior history of heart disease and, often, few or no symptoms. The prevalence of cardiovascular disease is increasing around the world due to an aging population and the increasing incidence of overweight and obese people and the health consequences of those conditions. More than ever before, patients must be educated about healthy lifestyle habits that decrease the risks of cardiovascular disease, even in the absence of defined risk factors or related conditions.

A thorough medical history and physical examination, as well as visualization techniques and diagnostic tests, are important in prevention and early identification of diseases that affect the circulatory system. Comprehensive cardiovascular testing also aids in evaluating patient compliance with health regimens. Although patients may be hesitant to incorporate drastic lifestyle changes, healthy diet and exercise alone can significantly reduce the risk of future cardiovascular events.

Cardiovascular History

A detailed medical history is the cornerstone of cardiovascular evaluation. Family history is particularly important. Patients should be questioned about MI, stroke, diabetes, hypertension, hypercholesterolemia, and other cardiovascular disease in their relatives.

If patients offer specific complaints related to cardiovascular health, an in-depth description of the symptoms will help identify the cause of the condition. For example, solicit a patient for specifics about chest pain: Where does it begin? How long does it last? What does it feel like? What were you doing when it started? What relieved the pain?

Symptoms of cardiovascular diseases overlap with each other, as well as disorders of other body systems. Specific qualities or characteristics of the symptoms can differentiate among various conditions.

Physical Examination

A component of a global patient evaluation includes a physical assessment of all body systems. For the cardiovascular system, the blood pressure and pulse are two important physical findings that a medical assistant will often obtain. Refer to Chapter 6 for more detailed information on collecting patients' vital signs.

Heart rate can be described by both rate and rhythm. In healthy adults, the pulse is usually taken at the radial artery and is counted for 15 seconds. This result is multiplied by 4 to obtain the total number of beats per minute. In patients with an irregular pulse, the apical pulse should be measured over one to two minutes to determine an average rate and rhythm. Also note whether the beats are strong or weak.

Always describe heart rate by the number of beats per minute, the rhythm, and quality of the pulsations.

© auremar/ShutterStock, Inc.

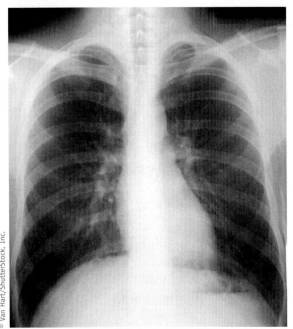

A chest X-ray.

© Van Hart/ShutterStock, Inc.

Measuring blood pressure requires careful listening and correct technique. It is measured with a stethoscope and a sphygmomanometer. Blood-pressure cuffs are available in multiple sizes. It is imperative to use the correct size cuff on each patient; a cuff that is too small will lead to a false high reading, and a large cuff will lead to a false low reading.

Testing Modalities

Visualization techniques and diagnostic tools can supplement the medical history and physical examination to determine risk factors for cardiovascular disease, diagnose disorders of the circulatory system, and evaluate disease progression.

Radiography

Chest radiography is often the first cardiovascular test performed after the initial history and physical. It cannot provide details about internal cardiac structures, but a radiograph can provide global information about the position of the heart, its size, and the surrounding anatomy.

Electrocardiogram

The **electrocardiogram (ECG or EKG)** measures the heart's electrical activity through electrodes placed on the surface of the body. It measures the electrical activity that results from the depolarization and repolarization of the heart. An ECG is simple to perform, inexpensive, and noninvasive. It is the first-choice test to evaluate chest pain, syncope, and dizziness.

The ECG characterizes heart rhythm or rate abnormalities and provides information on the anatomy and structure of the heart and any physiological changes in the heart. ECGs are interpreted for several characteristics: heart rate, rhythm, intervals, voltage, axis, waveforms, and abnormal features.

A standard ECG involves 12 leads or recordings. In this test, 10 electrodes are placed at distinct places on the body. The voltage between two electrodes is referred to as a lead. The standard placement of electrodes is described in TABLE 13.7 and FIGURE 13.11. Four electrodes are placed on the limbs and six electrodes are placed on the chest.

The first three leads are standard or **bipolar leads**, because they connect two electrodes. Lead I records the voltage difference between the left and right arm electrodes. Lead II records the voltage difference between the left leg and right arm electrodes, and lead III records the voltage difference between the left leg and left arm. Limb leads I, II, and III form a triangle known as Einthoven's triangle, which has the heart at its center.

The second three leads are **augmented leads** and also measure the voltage difference between two points. The first of the augmented leads, aVR, records the voltage difference between the right arm electrode and a point midway between the left arm and left leg electrodes, termed the augmented voltage of the right arm. The augmented voltage of the left arm is recorded by lead aVL, which records the voltage difference between the left arm and a point midway between the right arm and left leg. The

When describing ECG leads, augmented means to become larger. Leads aVR, aVL, and aVF record such small electrical impulses that the ECG machine must amplify the voltage to record it on the graph paper.

© auremar/ShutterStock, Inc.

Table 13.7	Electrode Placement for a 12-Lead ECG
Electrode Label	**Placement**
RA	Right arm
LA	Left arm
RL	Right lateral calf muscle
LL	Left lateral calf muscle
V_1	In the fourth intercostal space (between the fourth and fifth ribs) to the right of the sternum
V_2	In the fourth intercostal space (between the fourth and fifth ribs) to the left of the sternum
V_3	Midway between leads V_2 and V_4
V_4	In the fifth intercostal space (between the fifth and sixth ribs) in the midclavicular line
V_5	Horizontal to V_4 at the left anterior axillary line
V_6	Horizontal to V_4 and V_5 at the midaxillary line

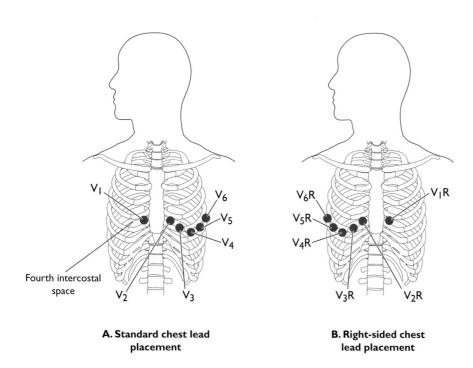

A. Standard chest lead placement

B. Right-sided chest lead placement

FIGURE 13.11 Placement of chest electrodes for a standard ECG.
© Blamb/ShutterStock, Inc.

augmented voltage of the left foot or leg, recorded by aVF, is the voltage difference between the left leg electrode and a point midway between the right arm and left arm.

The remaining six leads are chest or **precordial leads**. They are unipolar leads and monitor only one electrode and a point within the heart. The precordial leads are named for the anatomical placement of the electrodes they monitor. The precordial leads assess the activity of the heart in the horizontal plane, which is referred to as the z-axis. Leads of a standard 12-lead ECG are presented in TABLE 13.8 .

Table 13.8 Leads for a 12-Lead ECG	
Label	**Electrodes Connected**
I	LA and RA
II	LL and RA
III	LL and LA
aVR	RA and (LA-LL)
aVL	LA and (RA-LL)
aVF	LL and (RA-LA)
V_1	V_1 and LA-RA-LL
V_2	V_2 and LA-RA-LL
V_3	V_3 and LA-RA-LL
V_4	V_4 and LA-RA-LL
V_5	V_5 and LA-RA-LL
V_6	V_6 and LA-RA-LL

ECG results are recorded on graph paper **FIGURE 13.12**. The vertical axis of the paper represents voltage and the horizontal axis measures time. The paper moves through the machine at 25mm per second. Each small square of ECG paper measures 1mm by 1mm and represents 0.04 second. Each larger square measure 5mm by 5mm and represents 0.2 second. Together, five large squares represent one second. Therefore, 300 large squares represent one minute.

The recording provided by an ECG is read from left to right as a series of waves, named alphabetically **FIGURE 13.13**:

- The P wave results from the depolarization, or electrical activation, of the right and left atria.
- The PR interval corresponds to the electrical impulse traveling through the AV node and bundle of His and right and left bundle branches.

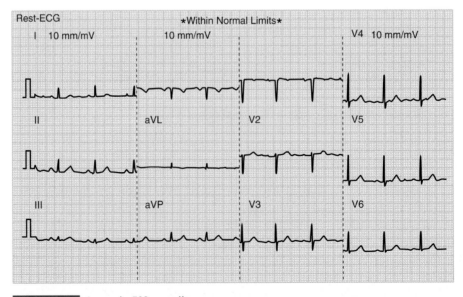

FIGURE 13.12 A sample ECG recording.

- The QRS complex records the depolarization of the ventricles. The complex begins with a negative deflection (the Q wave), followed by a positive deflection (the R wave). It concludes with another negative deflection (the S wave).

- The ST segment follows the QRS complex and appears as a plateau on the ECG at or slightly above the baseline. Repolarization of the ventricle appears as the T wave.

- The entire QT interval denotes the duration of ventricular depolarization and repolarization, and varies with heart rate. The U wave is a small wave that follows the T wave. It is not seen on all ECGs. The U wave likely arises from the repolarization of the Purkinje fibers, but its origin is not entirely clear.

- The RR interval (from one R wave to the next R wave) is an indicator of ventricular rate.

- The PP interval is an indicator of atrial rate. The duration, magnitude, and configuration of the waves and segments are reported on an ECG.

The heart rate can be calculated by examining the ECG tracing. If the heart rhythm is regular, calculate the distance, in large boxes, from one QRS interval to the next, or the RR interval. Divide 300 by the number of large boxes to achieve the heart rate. For example, if the RR interval spans four boxes, 300 ÷ 4 = 75 beats per minute. If the RR interval spans three boxes, 300 ÷ 3 = 100 beats per minute. Alternatively, count the number of small boxes spanned by the RR interval and divide 1,500 by this number to calculate the heart rate.

Any abnormal appearance or interference in ECG recordings is known as an artifact. An **artifact** is a recording of an electrical impulse that is not generated by the heart. Artifacts occur as a result of outside electrical interference, electrical activity in other areas of the body, poor electrode contact, or machine malfunction. They are common and easy to recognize. If an artifact is detected on an ECG tracing, it should be corrected and the test should be run again. Causes of artifacts include the following:

- A somatic tremor due to shivering from cold, nervousness, or neurological impairment can produce artifacts. To correct for an artifact caused by a somatic

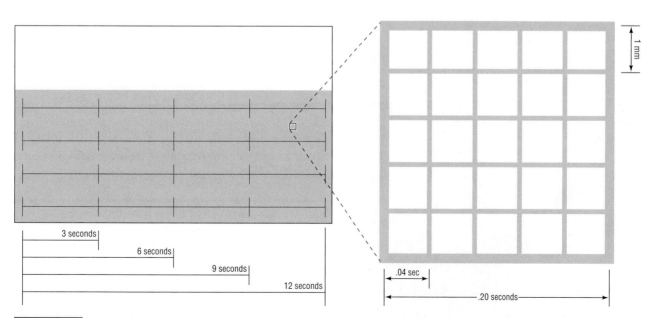

FIGURE 13.13 On an ECG tracing, five large squares represent one second, and 300 large squares represent one minute.

From *Arrhythmia Recognition: The Art of Interpretation*, courtesy of Tomas B. Garcia, MD

tremor, place the arm electrodes close to the shoulders to decrease the interference of a tremor.

- Alternating current (AC) interference is due to outside electrical activity, often from the ECG's power cord or other equipment. To prevent the occurrence of an artifact from this type of interference, the power cord should not come close to the patient or the lead wires during the ECG. Also, the patient should be seated away from other equipment that may have its own electrical activity. Finally, electrodes must be properly placed and in good contact with the skin to reduce AC interference.

A wandering baseline can be caused by improperly applied electrodes or poor skin contact with the electrode. Oils, creams, and lotions on the skin, as well as excess hair, should be removed before applying electrodes. Patient movement during the test can also cause a wandering baseline.

An interrupted baseline is caused by an electrode becoming separated from the lead wire or by a broken wire. Prior to performing an ECG, ensure that the equipment is in good working order. Follow the manufacturer's instructions for replacing or repairing damaged equipment or supplies.

Some patients do not allow for accurate electrode placement, such as obese patients, patients with thick chest muscles, and those with limb amputations. In each case, place the electrode as close to the preferred site as possible. Never place electrodes on wounds, open sores, sutures, or staples. If a patient is unable to lie down to complete the test, an ECG may be recorded with the patient placed in semi-Fowler's position. Document any changes in electrode placement or patient position in the patient's chart.

After a provider has reviewed the ECG tracing, the medical assistant is likely responsible for mounting the tracing, because it is often printed on thin, fragile paper. The process of **mounting**, or preparing the tracing for placement in the patient's medical record, preserves the integrity of the tracing and allows it to be readily accessible for review. You may need to trim the edges of the tracing and adhere it to a study card or paper. Some ECG machines already provide durable tracings, and these can be placed directly in the patient's record.

Ambulatory ECG monitoring, or **Holter monitoring**, documents and evaluates arrhythmias and other abnormalities over an extended period of time. The device used to perform this type of monitoring, called a Holter monitor, is worn by a patient for 24–48 hours and assesses electrical activity of the heart during daily activities. Holter monitoring is useful for patients with unexplained syncope or episodes of dizziness, recurrent palpitations, suspected arrhythmias, or atypical symptoms.

The Holter monitor is named for its inventor, American biophysicist Norman Holter.

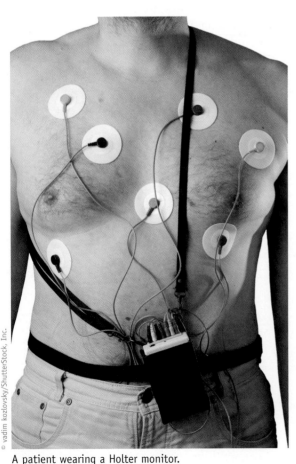

© vadim kozlovsky/ShutterStock, Inc.

A patient wearing a Holter monitor.

Stress Test

A **stress test**, also known as exercise electrocardiography, is used to assess cardiovascular disease by evaluating the circulatory system's ability to respond to physiologic

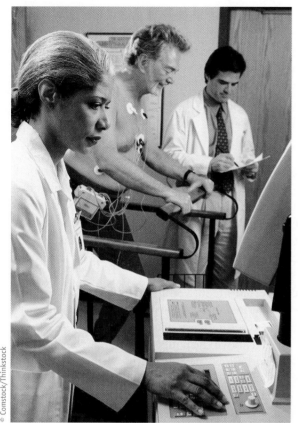

An exercise stress test.

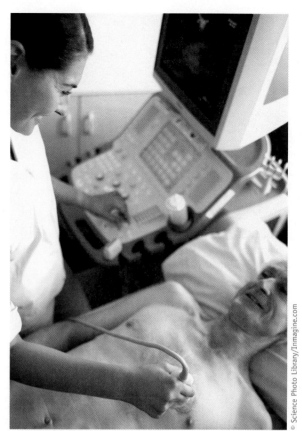

An echocardiogram uses sound waves to create a picture of the heart.

changes. Stress tests identify indicators of ischemia and abnormalities of coronary blood supply or demand.

Exercise stress tests are performed on a treadmill or stationary bicycle while the patient undergoes an ECG. The patient exercises, which increases the workload on the heart. During the test, the patient's physical and physiological parameters are measured, including changes in heart rate and blood pressure, shortness of breath, chest pain, and arrhythmias.

If a patient is unable to exercise, a pharmacologic stress test can be performed. In this case, the patient is administered a medication that mimics stress on the heart without requiring physical activity. Currently, dipyridamole, adenosine, and dobutamine are used for pharmacologic stress testing. The same parameters are measured as in an exercise stress test.

Echocardiogram

An **echocardiogram (ECHO)** uses sound waves to create a moving picture of the heart. An ECHO can be used in conjunction with a stress test or independently. An ECHO can provide details of the size and shape of the heart, as well as how well it is working. An ECHO can detect abnormalities or dysfunction in the muscles of the heart, identify heart defects, display blood clots, and evaluate fluid accumulation around the heart.

Cardiac Catheterization

Cardiac catheterization is the process of passing a thin tube (catheter) through the blood vessels leading to the heart. It is performed to detect cardiac abnormalities, collect blood samples, and determine the pressure in the area surrounding the heart.

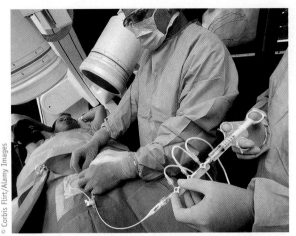

During a cardiac catheterization, a catheter is inserted through a peripheral blood vessel and threaded to the heart.

The catheter is usually inserted into a blood vessel in the arm, groin, or neck and threaded to the heart. Once a cardiac catheter is inserted in the blood vessels surrounding the heart, a physician can perform diagnostic tests or treatment-related interventions through the catheter. Cardiac catheterization is usually performed in a hospital setting.

Blood Tests

Laboratory blood tests are performed on whole blood, serum, or plasma. **Phlebotomy** is the process of collecting blood samples. The practice of collecting blood samples from veins is called **venipuncture**. Often, a trained and certified phlebotomist will collect blood samples, but the role of the medical assistant in phlebotomy varies greatly among practice sites.

The preferred site for venipuncture is the **antecubital space**, located anterior to the elbow on the inside of the arm. The veins in this area are large and close to the skin's surface, providing easy access for blood collection. Before venipuncture, a tourniquet is applied above the collection area. A **tourniquet** is a device that is used to slow blood flow and allow the vein to fill with excess blood. This allows for easier palpation and visualization. In phlebotomy, most tourniquets are disposable and made of rubber or latex. The tourniquet should be tied tightly enough to compress the limb, but should still allow enough room for one finger to be inserted between the limb and the tourniquet.

Three primary mechanisms of blood collection are commonly used: a vacuum tube, a butterfly assembly, and a syringe. Vacuum tubes are the preferred means of blood collection and are used whenever possible for routine collection. Vacuum tubes are fast, safe, allow for large volumes to be collected, and maintain the quality of blood. Vacuum tubes do not work well with small or fragile veins or small children. Butterfly assemblies are preferred for small or fragile veins. They may be used for children.

Vacuum tubes are vacuum-packed test tubes with rubber stoppers. They come in a variety of sizes for various uses. They also contain chemicals or substances specific to the test that will be run. Each colored rubber cap denotes the contents inside the tube. Although the colors are nearly universal among manufacturers, when in doubt, read the label to determine what additive is in the tube. Colors and uses for common phlebotomy tubes are provided in TABLE 13.9. The order of blood draw is important. Sterile collections must be obtained first to prevent contamination. After sterile tubes, blood is drawn according to the additives in the tubes. The standard order of draw is yellow top or culture bottles, light blue top (sodium citrate), red top and red-gray mottled top (serum tubes), light and dark green tubes (heparin), lavender, then pink, white, or royal blue top (EDTA), gray top (glycolytic inhibitor), and, finally, dark blue top (FDP).

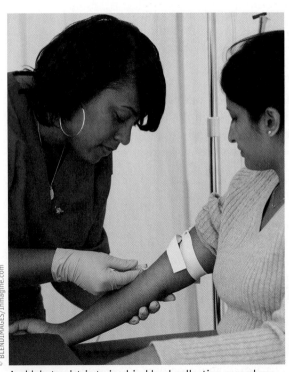

A phlebotomist is trained in blood-collection procedures.

Table 13.9	Characteristics of Phlebotomy Collection Tubes, in Order of Collection	
Color	Contents	Uses
Light blue top	Sodium citrate	Coagulation tests
Red top	None	Chemistries, immunology and serology, blood bank (crossmatch)
Red-gray mottled top	Serum separating tube (SST) with clot activator	Blood type screening and chemistries
Gold top	Separating gel and clot activator	Serology, endocrinology, immunology
Light green top	Plasma separating tube (sodium heparin)	Chemistries
Dark green top	Sodium heparin or lithium heparin	Ammonia, lactate, lithium levels
Tan/brown top	Sodium heparin	Serum lead
Lavender/purple top	Liquid EDTA	Hematology, blood bank (crossmatch)
Royal blue top	Sodium heparin or sodium EDTA	Toxicology, trace elements, drug levels
Light gray top	Sodium fluoride and potassium oxalate	Lithium level, glucose
Black top	Sodium citrate (buffered)	Westergren sedimentation rate
Orange top	Thrombin	STAT serum chemistries
Yellow top	Acid-citrate-dextrose (ACD)	Paternity testing, DNA studies

Butterfly assemblies are not likely to collapse a vein and are the least painful means of blood collection. A syringe or tube adapter can be attached to the assembly. Syringes can be used on any patient, including children and infants, obese patients, and critically ill patients. Syringes can also be used to collect blood from fragile or inaccessible veins. Blood collection with a syringe is easy to perform and allows for small collection volumes, but it is not a preferred technique for dehydrated patients or those with poor circulation. Blood collection by syringe cannot be used for blood cultures or to measure the erythrocyte sedimentation rate.

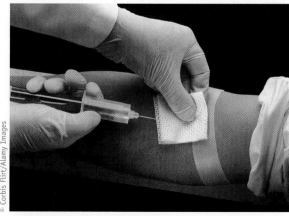

Venipuncture using a vacuum tube.

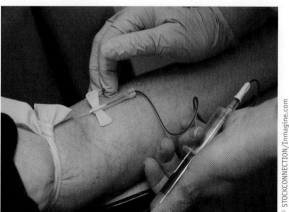

Venipuncture using a butterfly assembly.

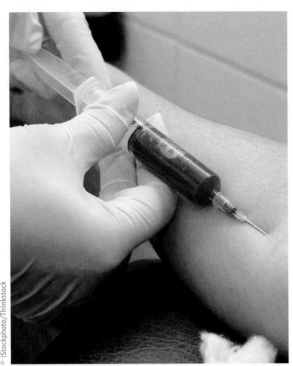

© iStockphoto/Thinkstock

Venipuncture using a syringe.

Patient reaction to venipuncture can vary widely. A medical assistant must be able to anticipate and respond to a patient's needs. Commonly, patients experience pain during venipuncture. Proper technique will prevent pain, but if pain does occur, reposition the needle and loosen the tourniquet to relieve the discomfort. Discontinue the venipuncture if pain persists.

Patients may also experience syncope, or fainting, in response to a venipuncture. If this happens, immediately remove the tourniquet; then remove the needle from the patient's arm. Stop the patient from falling, if necessary. Wipe the patient's forehead and back of the neck with a cold compress. Obtain help from another medical professional or care provider if the patient does not respond. Help the patient to remain comfortable and safe until he or she is completely alert and oriented.

Patients may experience nausea in response to a venipuncture. It is advisable to maintain an emesis basin in close reach. If a patient complains of nausea, apply a cold compress to his or her forehead and provide an emesis basin. Advise deep, slow breaths until the nausea subsides.

With venipuncture, **hypoglycemia**, or low blood sugar, can occur, especially among patients undergoing a fasting blood sugar test. A patient may experience a cold sweat and pale complexion, as well as become weak, shaky, and disoriented. Confusion and altered mental status can accompany hypoglycemia. Obtain assistance from the provider if the patient loses consciousness.

If a patient loses consciousness and experiences convulsions during a venipuncture, do not try to restrain the patient. Move objects or furniture from the area to prevent injury to the patient. Help the patient to the floor and allow him or her to rest until fully recovered. Notify the provider about the patient's reaction and follow the provider's orders for how to proceed with the blood collection and when to release the patient.

Capillary blood collection is useful when only a small amount of blood is required. **Capillary puncture** is also referred to as finger sticks. Capillaries are located just under the surface of the skin, so a small puncture is a practical, safe, and nearly pain-free method of obtaining small amounts of blood.

When concluding a blood-collection procedure, proper documentation is imperative. Patient and specimen identification is essential to accurate testing. Each specimen tube should be labeled with the patient's name, date of birth, medical record or other identifying number, and the date and time of collection. Label the tubes immediately after collection is complete, while still in the patient's presence. Complete laboratory paperwork, in its entirety, as required by your employer or the laboratory. Ensure proper storage and handling of the sample after collection, before delivery to the laboratory. Under improper storage conditions, specimens will not maintain their integrity, and the test results will be useless.

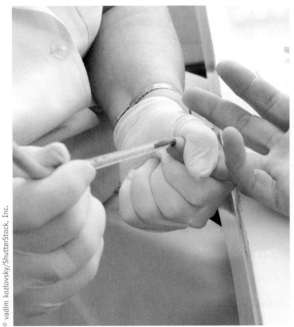

© vadim kozlovsky/ShutterStock, Inc.

Capillary puncture.

What Would You Do?

A patient presents to your medical office and requires a blood specimen to be collected. She appears nervous and pale. She starts breathing rapidly and complaining that she is afraid of needles. What do you do?

© NorthGeorgiaMedia/ShutterStock, Inc.

Skills for the Medical Assistant

As a medical assistant, you will have the opportunity to participate in several procedures relating to the circulatory system. Patients may be nervous or uncomfortable when undergoing an ECG or a blood collection. Your confidence will ease the patient's fears and allow for safe and accurate testing.

Performing Venipuncture by Syringe

When a blood sample is needed from a small or fragile vein, blood can be collected using a needle and syringe. Generally, a 21- or 23-gauge needle, 1 to 1½ inches in length, is used for blood collection, and a 10 to 20mL syringe is used. In this exercise, you will learn how to perform venipuncture and collect blood using a needle and syringe.

Equipment Needed

- Sterile needle, 21- or 23-gauge
- Syringe, 10 to 20mL
- Specimen tubes
- Laboratory packaging materials and forms, as required
- Alcohol wipes or cotton balls and isopropyl alcohol
- Disposable gloves
- Tourniquet
- Gauze pads
- Tape
- Sterile adhesive bandage
- Biohazard waste container
- Sharps container

Steps

1. Introduce yourself and identify the patient. Explain the procedure that you will be performing. Answer the patient's questions and ensure he or she is calm and comfortable before proceeding with the venipuncture.
2. Select an appropriate puncture site. This is most often the antecubital area, just below the patient's elbow. Instruct the patient to sit comfortably with the puncture site exposed and accessible and supported by the arm of a chair or table. Select a vein that can be easily palpated.
3. Gather the required equipment. Wash your hands and apply gloves.

4. Secure the needle to the syringe using sterile technique. Pull the plunger back approximately halfway; then depress the plunger completely to remove all air from the barrel of the syringe.

5. Apply a tourniquet to the patient's upper arm, approximately 3 inches above the elbow. Once a tourniquet is applied, proceed quickly, as it is uncomfortable for a patient and should not be left in place for more than one minute **FIGURE 13.14** .

A tourniquet decreases blood flow to the area below the tourniquet, which increases volume in the vein and aids in palpation and visualization of the vein.

6. Clean the puncture site by making a smooth circular pass over the site with the alcohol pad, moving in an outward spiral from the zone of penetration. Allow the skin to dry before proceeding. Do not touch the puncture site after cleaning.

7. Ask the patient to make a fist if a vein is still not easily visible. Tap the antecubital area gently with two fingers to help the vein stand out.

8. Remove the needle guard or cap and pull the skin taut by placing one or two fingers 1 to 2 inches below the venipuncture site. Insert the needle into the vein with the bevel facing up. Use a quick, steady motion and follow the path of the vein. Maintain the needle at approximately a 10- to 15-degree angle to the arm. Do not insert the needle more than ¼ to ½ inch. Let go of the skin.

A vein can collapse if blood is withdrawn too quickly. If this occurs, stop withdrawing blood and allow the vein to refill before continuing with the blood collection.

9. Hold the barrel of the syringe with your nondominant hand. With your dominant hand, pull back the plunger slowly and steadily until the barrel is filled with the required amount of blood. While the syringe is filling with blood, ask the patient to release his or her fist. Remove the tourniquet **FIGURE 13.15** .

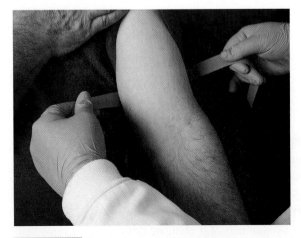

FIGURE 13.14 A tourniquet should be placed approximately three inches above the venipuncture site.
© Jones & Bartlett Learning. Photographed by Sarah Cebulski.

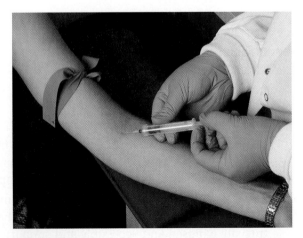

FIGURE 13.15 Pull the plunger of the syringe back with a slow, steady motion.
© Jones & Bartlett Learning. Photographed by Sarah Cebulski.

10. Gently pull the needle out of the vein, following the same path as it was inserted. Place a dry cotton ball or gauze pad at the site of needle insertion. Apply tape over the cotton ball or gauze pad. Ask the patient to hold the gauze or cotton in place for several minutes. Instruct him or her to apply gentle pressure to the puncture site and elevate the arm slightly to slow the bleeding.

11. Attach a blood-transfer device to the syringe and allow the blood to flow into the collection tube. Do not depress the plunger of the syringe. Do not shake the blood during the transfer process to avoid damaging the blood sample.

12. Place the syringe, needle, and blood-transfer device into the sharps container. Dispose of other used equipment and supplies in appropriate receptacles.

13. Apply an adhesive bandage to the puncture site.

14. Remove the gloves and wash your hands.

15. Document the procedure in the patient's chart. For example, write "1340. Performed venipuncture with needle and syringe at left antecubital area; collected 15mL of blood. Sent to AB lab for analysis. Patient tolerated procedure well. J. Jones, CMA."

Performing Venipuncture by Vacuum Tube System

The vacuum tube system for blood collection is the preferred method for blood collection because it is simple and requires the fewest steps. In this system, blood flows directly into the collection tube, so no transfer of blood is necessary. In this exercise, you will learn how to perform a venipuncture and collect blood using a vacuum tube collection system.

Equipment Needed

- Sterile needle, 21- or 23-gauge
- Plastic needle adapter
- Vacuum collection tubes
- Laboratory packaging materials and forms, as required
- Alcohol wipes or cotton balls and isopropyl alcohol
- Disposable gloves
- Tourniquet
- Gauze pads
- Sterile adhesive bandage
- Biohazard waste container
- Sharps container

Steps

1. Introduce yourself and identify the patient. Explain the procedure that you will be performing. Answer the patient's questions and ensure he or she is calm and comfortable before proceeding with the venipuncture.

2. Select an appropriate puncture site. This is most often the antecubital area, just below the patient's elbow. Instruct the patient to sit comfortably with the puncture site exposed and accessible and supported by the arm of a chair or table. Select a vein that can be easily palpated.

3. Gather the required equipment. Wash your hands and apply gloves.

4. Apply the plastic adapter to the needle.

5. Apply a tourniquet to the patient's upper arm, approximately 3 inches above the elbow. Once a tourniquet is applied, proceed quickly, as it is uncomfortable for a patient and should not be left in place for more than one minute.

6. Clean the puncture site by making a smooth circular pass over the site with the alcohol pad, moving in an outward spiral from the zone of penetration. Allow the skin to dry before proceeding. Do not touch the puncture site after cleaning.

7. Ask the patient to make a fist if a vein is still not easily visible. Tap the antecubital area gently with two fingers to help the vein stand out.

8. Remove the needle guard or cap and pull the skin taut by placing one or two fingers 1 to 2 inches below the venipuncture site. Insert the needle into the vein with the bevel facing up. Use a quick, steady motion and follow the path of the vein. Maintain the needle at approximately a 10- to 15-degree angle to the arm. Do not insert the needle more than ¼ to ½ inch. Let go of the skin **FIGURE 13.16** .

9. Hold the needle adapter with your nondominant hand. With your dominant hand, insert the vacuum tube into the adapter, pressing down on the tube with your thumb and holding the protruding wings of the adapter with the index and middle fingers of your dominant hand, allowing the needle to puncture the rubber stopper of the tube **FIGURE 13.17** . While the tube is filling with blood, ask the patient to release his or her fist. Remove the tourniquet. Repeat this procedure until the required number of tubes is filled with blood.

10. Gently pull the needle out of the vein, following the same path as it was inserted. Place a dry cotton ball or gauze pad at the site of needle insertion. Ask the patient to hold the cotton in place for several minutes. Instruct the patient to apply gentle pressure to the puncture site and elevate the arm slightly to slow the bleeding.

11. Place the needle in the sharps container. Dispose of other used equipment and supplies in the appropriate receptacles.

12. Apply an adhesive bandage to the puncture site.

13. Remove the gloves and wash your hands.

14. Document the procedure in the patient's chart. For example, write "1055. Performed venipuncture with vacuum tubes at left antecubital area; collected 3 tubes of blood. Sent to AB lab for analysis. Patient tolerated procedure well. J. Jones, CMA."

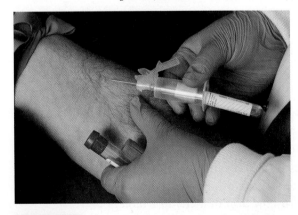

FIGURE 13.16 Insert the needle into the vein with the bevel facing up.
© Jones & Bartlett Learning. Photographed by Sarah Cebulski.

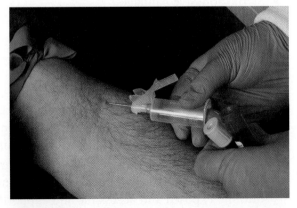

FIGURE 13.17 Insert the vacuum tube into the adapter with your dominant hand.
© Jones & Bartlett Learning. Photographed by Sarah Cebulski.

Performing Venipuncture by Butterfly Needle System

A butterfly needle system is used to perform a venipuncture in small, fragile veins or those that are difficult to see or access. Often, the butterfly system is used for infants and children. In this exercise, you will learn how to perform a venipuncture using the butterfly needle system.

Equipment Needed

- Sterile butterfly needle
- Syringe or plastic needle adapter and vacuum collection tubes
- Laboratory packaging materials and forms, as required
- Alcohol wipes or cotton balls and isopropyl alcohol
- Disposable gloves
- Tourniquet
- Gauze pads
- Sterile adhesive bandage
- Biohazard waste container
- Sharps container

Steps

1. Introduce yourself and identify the patient. Explain the procedure that you will be performing. Answer the patient's questions and ensure he or she is calm and comfortable before proceeding with the venipuncture.
2. Select an appropriate puncture site. Acceptable venipuncture sites include the antecubital area or the back of the hand. Instruct the patient to sit comfortably with the puncture site exposed and accessible and supported by the arm of a chair or table. Select a vein that can be easily palpated.
3. Gather the required equipment. Wash your hands and apply gloves.
4. Apply a tourniquet approximately 3 inches above the venipuncture site. Once a tourniquet is applied, proceed quickly, as it is uncomfortable for a patient and should not be left in place for more than one minute.
5. Clean the puncture site by making a smooth circular pass over the site with the 70 percent alcohol pad, moving in an outward spiral from the zone of penetration. Allow the skin to dry before proceeding. Do not touch the puncture site after cleaning.
6. Ask the patient to make a fist and hold it tightly.
7. Remove the needle guard or cap and pull the skin taut by placing one or two fingers 1 to 2 inches below the venipuncture site. Insert the needle into the vein with the bevel facing up. Use a quick, steady motion and follow the path of the vein. Maintain the needle at approximately a 10- to 15-degree angle to the arm. Do not insert the needle more than $\frac{1}{4}$ to $\frac{1}{2}$ inch. Let go of the skin.
8. Collect blood using vacuum collection tubes or a syringe. After collection, ask the patient to release his or her fist. Remove the tourniquet.
9. Gently pull the needle out of the vein, following the same path as it was inserted. Place a dry cotton ball or gauze pad at the site of needle insertion. Ask the patient to hold the cotton in place for several minutes. Instruct the patient to apply gentle pressure to the puncture site and elevate the arm slightly to slow the bleeding.

10. Place the needle in the sharps container. Dispose of other used equipment and supplies in the appropriate receptacles.
11. Apply an adhesive bandage to the puncture site.
12. Remove the gloves and wash your hands.
13. Document the procedure in the patient's chart. For example, write "1425. Performed venipuncture with butterfly needle and vacuum tubes at left antecubital area; collected 1 tube of blood. Sent to AB lab for analysis. Patient tolerated procedure well. J. Jones, CMA."

Performing Capillary Puncture

A skin puncture using a sterile lancet is used to collect a small amount of capillary blood. This procedure is widely used for many types of blood tests, including blood glucose tests. Patients who are required to test their blood glucose levels on a regular basis will need to learn to perform a capillary puncture at home. In this exercise, you will learn how to perform a skin puncture using a sterile lancet to collect capillary blood.

Equipment Needed

- Disposable gloves
- Sterile lancet
- Isopropyl alcohol and cotton balls or alcohol wipes
- Collection tube
- Biohazard waste container
- Sharps container
- Dry gauze pad
- Sterile adhesive bandage

Steps

1. Introduce yourself and identify the patient. Explain the procedure that you will be performing. Answer the patient's questions and ensure he or she is calm and comfortable before proceeding with the capillary puncture.
2. Select an appropriate puncture site. This is most often the tip of the ring or middle finger, but an adult's earlobe or the lateral areas of an infant's heel can also be used for a capillary puncture. Some patients have a preference for a particular puncture site. Do not use a site that is bruised, calloused, or injured.
3. Gather the required equipment. Wash your hands and apply gloves.
4. Clean the puncture site by making a smooth circular pass over the site with the alcohol pad, moving in an outward spiral from the zone of penetration. Allow the skin to dry before proceeding. Do not touch the puncture site after cleaning.

Do not blow on the skin to speed up drying after cleansing with alcohol. Doing so can spread microorganisms from expired air to the skin and contaminate the collection area.

5. Remove the sterile lancet from its package. Do not touch the tip of the lancet.
6. Hold the patient's finger (or other site of puncture) firmly with two fingers of your nondominant hand. Hold the lancet in your dominant hand. Place the lancet on the puncture site, with the tip of the lancet oriented perpendicular

to the fingerprints. A correct puncture should not be in the direction of the fingerprints. Press down on the lancet using either your thumb or index finger and a quick, firm, and steady motion **FIGURE 13.18**.

7. Discard the lancet in the sharps container.

8. Wipe away the first drop of blood from the puncture site by blotting it with a cotton ball or dry gauze pad.

9. Apply gentle pressure to either side of the puncture to release the blood and collect it in the collection tube appropriate for the test being performed. Continue this process until the required amount of blood has been collected.

10. Wipe the puncture site with a cotton ball and instruct the patient to hold the cotton in place for several minutes. Inspect the puncture to ensure bleeding has stopped. If bleeding continues, instruct the patient to hold the cotton in place for a few more minutes. When the bleeding has stopped, apply an adhesive bandage to the puncture site.

11. Discard used items in the appropriate receptacles. Remove the gloves and wash your hands.

12. Document the procedure in the patient's chart. For example, write "0950. Performed capillary puncture on right ring finger; filled one microcapillary tube. Patient tolerated procedure well. J. Jones, CMA."

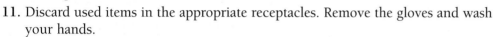

FIGURE 13.18 Puncture the fingertip with a firm, steady motion.
© Jones & Bartlett Learning. Photographed by Sarah Cebulski.

Performing a 12-Lead ECG

An ECG is performed to obtain a graphical representation of the electrical activity of the heart. Every detail of the ECG procedure must be performed correctly to ensure accurate results. The test should be performed in a quiet, private area. In this exercise, you will learn how to prepare a patient for an ECG and place the electrodes correctly for a 12-lead ECG.

Equipment Needed

- ECG and graph paper
- Disposable, pre-gelled adhesive electrodes
- Cables and lead wires with clips to attach to electrodes
- Drape or gown for patient
- Gauze pads
- Alcohol wipes
- Disposable razor

Steps

1. Introduce yourself and identify the patient. Explain the procedure that you will be performing. Answer the patient's questions and ensure he or she is calm and comfortable before proceeding with the ECG.

2. Wash your hands. Gather supplies and prepare the equipment.

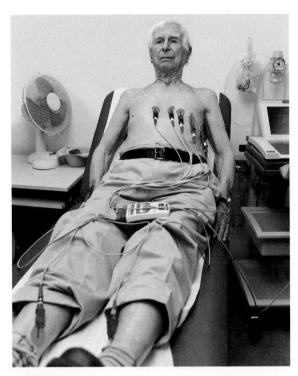

FIGURE 13.19 Limb electrode placement for a 12-lead ECG.

© Antonia Reeve/Photo Researchers

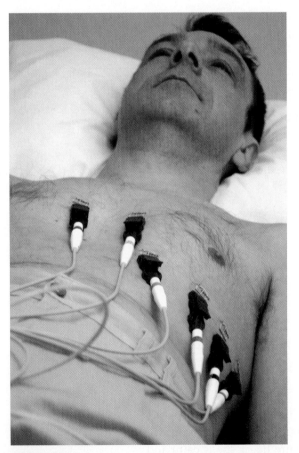

FIGURE 13.20 Chest electrode placement for a 12-lead ECG.

© AJPhoto/Photo Researchers

3. Ask the patient to disrobe from the waist up and remove clothing from the lower legs. Ask the patient to lie down on the examination table.

4. Place electrodes on the fleshy outer area of the upper arms, with the connectors pointing down. Place leg electrodes on the fleshy inner area of the lower leg, with the connectors pointing up. Limb lead placement is described in Table 13.7. Connect the lead wires to the appropriate electrodes **FIGURE 13.19**.

5. Place the six chest electrodes in the correct anatomical positions **FIGURE 13.20**, as described in Table 13.7 and Figure 13.11.

If the area for electrode placement is covered with lotion or oil, use a gauze pad to wipe it clean to promote adhesion of the electrode. If the area contains excess hair, obtain the patient's permission to shave the area. If a patient's breast covers the placement area for a chest electrode, gently lift the breast tissue with the back of your hand to expose the area under the breast.

6. Cover the patient with a drape or gown to provide warmth and privacy during the exam.

7. Follow the manufacturer's instructions on the ECG equipment, as well as the healthcare provider's preferences for what information is recorded.

8. Remind the patient to remain still during the test. Begin the test by pressing the appropriate button on the ECG machine.

9. When the test is completed, review the tracing to confirm that there are no artifacts present. If artifacts are present, repeat the test, correcting for the interference. Alert the provider to the results and remove the lead wires and the electrodes. Clean the electrode sites with an alcohol pad, if necessary.

10. Assist the patient to a sitting position and instruct him or her to dress. Assist the patient with dressing, if necessary.

11. Wash your hands.

12. Place the ECG tracing in the patient's chart and document the procedure. For example, write "1115. 12-lead ECG obtained. Patient experienced shortness of breath while lying flat. J. Jones, CMA."

Performing an Ambulatory ECG

Patients who experience irregular or intermittent chest pain or unusual symptoms, but who still have normal standard ECG results, may require ambulatory ECG monitoring. In this case, an ECG is obtained over an extended period of time while patients perform their normal activities of daily living. Monitors are digital; in most cases, the information is recorded on a portable memory card or flash drive. The patient is also instructed to maintain a log of activities and symptoms of chest pain during the time the monitor is worn. In this exercise, you will learn how to apply an ambulatory ECG monitor.

Equipment Needed

- Holter monitor
- Disposable, pre-gelled adhesive electrodes
- Gauze pads
- Alcohol wipes
- Disposable razor

Steps

1. Introduce yourself and identify the patient. Explain the procedure that you will be performing. Answer the patient's questions and ensure he or she is calm and comfortable before proceeding with applying the Holter monitor.
2. Wash your hands. Gather supplies and prepare the equipment.
3. Ask the patient to disrobe from the waist up. Ask the patient to sit at the end of the examination table.
4. Place the six chest electrodes in the correct anatomical positions, according to the manufacturer's instructions.
5. Place the belt supplied with the monitor around the patient's waist or drape it around his or her shoulders. Assist the patient in dressing without disturbing the placement of the electrodes.
6. Instruct the patient to maintain his or her normal daily routine, but note activities and symptoms of chest pain, including time of onset, characteristics, and duration of discomfort, in a diary.
7. Wash your hands.
8. Document the procedure in the patient's chart. For example, write "1445. Holter monitor applied. Provided patient with instructions regarding activity diary and care of monitor and electrodes. J. Jones, CMA."
9. When the patient returns to have the Holter monitor removed, disconnect the wires and remove the electrode pads, washing the site of application with an alcohol wipe, if necessary.
10. Remove the recording device from the monitor and give it to the provider for computer analysis. Document the procedure in the patient's chart. For example, write "1445. Holter monitor removed. Memory card given to Dr. Henry. Patient diary placed in chart for review. J. Jones, CMA."

Math Practice

Question: A 67-year-old man is prescribed warfarin as an anticoagulant to prevent thromboembolic disorders. He takes a nonuniform dose of 7.5mg Coumadin on Mondays and Fridays and 5mg daily the remaining days of the week. What is his total weekly dose of warfarin?

Answer: 7.5mg/day × 2 days/week = 15mg

5mg/day × 5 days/week = 25mg

15mg + 25mg = 40mg warfarin weekly

Question: **A 36-year-old 176-pound male is prescribed dalteparin for DVT treatment. The physician orders 200 units/kg/day divided into two doses. What is the total daily dose of dalteparin? What is the dose of dalteparin that the patient will receive with each administration?**

Answer: 176 lb × 1kg ÷ 2.2 lb = 80kg

80kg × 200 units/kg = 16,000 units per day

16,000 units/day × 1 day ÷ 2 doses = 8,000 units/dose

Question: **A 135-pound female is prescribed subcutaneous heparin for DVT treatment. The physician orders an initial dose of 333 units/kg followed by a maintenance dose of 250 units/kg every 12 hours. What is the initial dose of heparin? What is the maintenance dose of heparin?**

Answer: 135 lb × 1kg ÷ 2.2 lb = 61.36kg

61.36kg × 333 units/kg = 20,433 units in initial dose

61.36kg × 250 units/kg = 15,340 units in maintenance dose

Question: **A 175-pound 16-year-old male is prescribed digoxin for the treatment of an arrhythmia. The initial dose is 12mcg/kg by mouth followed by a maintenance dose of 3.75mcg/kg once daily by mouth. What is the initial dose of digoxin? What is the maintenance dose?**

Answer: 175 lb × 1kg/2.2 lb = 79.55kg

79.55kg × 12mcg/kg = 954.6mcg digoxin in initial dose

79.55kg × 3.75mcg/kg = 298.3mcg digoxin in maintenance dose

WRAP UP

Chapter Summary

- The circulatory system is composed of the heart and the blood vessels (arteries, veins, and capillaries) that circulate blood through the body. Pulmonary circulation transports blood from the heart to the lungs so gas exchange can occur, and systemic circulation transports blood from the heart to the rest of the body so the exchange of nutrients, metabolites, and hormones can occur.

- The heart is a double pump. It contains two collecting vessels (atria) and two distributing chambers (ventricles). Four valves in the heart direct the unidirectional flow of blood through its chambers.

- Blood flows in a continuous loop around the body. Each beat of the heart is a series of integrated, coordinated events that lead to the contraction and relaxation of the heart's atria and ventricles that propel the blood through the body. The heart contracts as a result of an electrical impulse initiated in the sinoatrial node, known as the heart's pacemaker.

- Arteries carry oxygenated blood away from the heart to the rest of the body. The only exception is the pulmonary artery, which carries deoxygenated blood from the heart to the lungs. The aorta is the largest artery in the body and is situated at the top of the heart. The aorta branches into progressively smaller vessels, the smallest of which are called arterioles. The arterioles branch into an intricate web of capillaries, where gas exchange occurs.

- Veins carry deoxygenated blood back to the heart. The only exception is the pulmonary vein, which carries oxygenated blood from the lungs to the heart. Capillaries join to form venules, which join to make larger and larger veins. The vena cava is the largest vein in the body and empties directly into the right atrium of the heart.

- An arrhythmia is any abnormal variation in heart rate or rhythm. Arrhythmias can result from ischemia, infarction, or alterations in body chemicals. Signs and symptoms of arrhythmias include palpitations, syncope, light-headedness, visual changes, pale complexion, weakness, sweating, chest pain, and decreased blood pressure. Arrhythmias can be treated with a variety of antiarrhythmic agents.

- In heart failure (HF), the heart is not able to pump enough blood to meet the body's needs. HF develops slowly over time, often without symptoms early in the disease. Later, patients may experience labored breathing, irritability, disorientation, and fluid and sodium retention. HF treatment includes blood pressure–lowering agents, diuretics, and antiplatelet or anticoagulant agents.

- Hyperlipidemia, or elevated cholesterol levels, is influenced by genetic and lifestyle factors. Fatty deposits in the arteries caused by excess circulating cholesterol leads to atherosclerosis, which can eventually cause poor circulation and other cardiovascular complications, including stroke and heart attack. Lifestyle modifications, including a low-fat diet and physical activity, are first-line options for the prevention and treatment of hyperlipidemia. When lifestyle modifications do not control cholesterol levels, several types of drug therapy are available to manage hyperlipidemia.

- Hypertension, or elevated blood pressure, can lead to kidney failure, edema, and fluid accumulation in the lungs. Adults without diabetes should maintain a blood pressure of less than or equal to 120/80mmHg. Goal blood pressure for diabetic adults is 130/80mmHg. Lifestyle modifications are critical in hypertension, but several classes of medications are available to control blood pressure through a variety of medications. Drugs from multiple classes can be used together to achieve optimum control.

- Ischemic heart disease is a condition in which the heart muscle does not receive an adequate supply of oxygen, usually due to atherosclerosis of the coronary blood vessels. Angina, or chest pain, is the hallmark symptom of ischemic heart disease. Angina may be predictable and occur in response to exertion, or it may be unpredictable. Nitrates are the most commonly used agents to treat symptoms of angina. Untreated ischemic heart disease can lead to a heart attack.

- A myocardial infarction (MI), more commonly known as a heart attack, occurs after a prolonged period of decreased oxygen supply to the muscle of the heart. Chest pain is the classic presentation of a heart attack. Lifestyle modification and control of comorbid (simultaneously occurring) conditions is essential to prevention of a heart attack. Once a heart attack occurs, beta-blockers and daily aspirin promote healing of the heart and prevent future cardiovascular complications.

- A stroke occurs as a result of a decreased oxygen supply to the brain. A stroke may be hemorrhagic or ischemic. Stroke prevention can be accomplished through lifestyle modification and risk factor reduction by treating comorbid conditions. Anticoagulant and antiplatelet therapy can also help prevent an ischemic stroke from occurring. Fibrinolytic agents dissolve clots once an ischemic stroke has occurred.

- Peripheral artery disease (PAD) is atherosclerosis of the arteries of the lower extremities. PAD is an indicator of coronary artery disease. Intermittent claudication and leg pain at rest are hallmark symptoms of PAD. Cilostazol and pentoxifylline are drugs of choice for managing symptoms of PAD.

- Pulmonary embolism (PE) and deep vein thrombosis (DVT) are manifestations of venous thromboembolism (VTE). In VTE, blood clots form and travel through veins, eventually occluding blood vessels. VTE can result in significant disability or death and often occurs without warning or prior symptoms. Anticoagulant or antiplatelet agents are administered to patients at risk for DVT or PE.

- An accurate diagnosis of diseases and disorders of the circulatory system begins with a thorough medical history and physical examination. Proper technique and accurate measurement are critical to ensuring precise diagnoses and evaluating therapeutic outcomes. Testing modalities, including chest radiography, electrocardiogram (ECG), stress test, echocardiogram, cardiac catheterization, and blood tests, also help provide a complete picture of cardiovascular disorders.

- As a medical assistant, you will have the opportunity to assist in procedures related to the diagnosis and evaluation of disorders of the circulatory system, including venipuncture by a variety of methods, capillary puncture, and performing an ECG. You should be calm, confident, and professional throughout the procedures to maintain the safety and comfort of the patient. You also have the opportunity to promote healthy lifestyle choices to patients and encourage lifestyle modifications to manage risk factors for cardiovascular diseases and complications.

Learning Assessment Questions

1. What are the components of the circulatory system?

   A. The right atrium, right ventricle, left atrium, and left ventricle

   B. The heart, arteries, veins, and capillaries

   C. Pulmonary circulation and systemic circulation

   D. Systole and diastole

2. Which of the following layers of tissue is correctly matched with its function?

   A. Pericardium: the thin membrane covering the myocardium

   B. Mediastinum: the thick, muscular layer of heart muscle

   C. Endocardium: the outer layer of the heart that contains coronary blood vessels

   D. Myocardium: the thin layer of epithelial cells that forms the valves of the heart

3. Which of the following statements is true regarding the heart's valves?

   A. The valves are made of cardiac muscle cells.

   B. The valves are attached to the heart's chambers by specialized ligaments called chordae tendineae.

   C. The aortic and pulmonary valves allow blood to flow in two directions.

   D. The atrioventricular valves separate the right side of the heart from the left side.

4. Which of the following represents the correct flow of blood through the body?

   A. Right atrium, left atrium, pulmonary vein, left ventricle, right ventricle, pulmonary artery, systemic circulation

   B. Left atrium, left ventricle, lungs, right atrium, right ventricle, systemic circulation

   C. Left atrium, left ventricle, lungs, pulmonary vein, right atrium, right ventricle, pulmonary artery, systemic circulation

   D. Right atrium, right ventricle, pulmonary artery, lungs, left atrium, left ventricle, aorta, systemic circulation

5. What area of the heart is known as the pacemaker?

   A. Bundle of His

   B. Atrioventricular node

   C. Sinoatrial node

   D. Purkinje fibers

6. Which of the following does *not* cause vasoconstriction?

   A. Heat

   B. Angiotensin

   C. Epinephrine

   D. Trauma to a blood vessel

7. Which of the following can cause hypoxia?

   A. Infarction

   B. Increased blood flow

   C. Vasospasms

   D. Atherosclerosis

8. Which of the following can cause an arrhythmia?

   A. Tachycardia

   B. Ischemia

   C. Syncope

   D. Hyperlipidemia

9. What is usually the first apparent symptom of congestive heart failure?

   A. Shortness of breath during formerly comfortable activities

   B. Kidney dysfunction

   C. Disorientation

   D. Lower limb edema

10. What is also known as good cholesterol?

    A. VLDL

    B. Triglycerides

    C. LDL

    D. HDL

11. Which of the following represents an ideal level of lipids in the blood?

    A. LDL ≥ 100mg/dL

    B. Triglycerides ≤ 150mg/dL

    C. HDL ≤ 40mg/dL

    D. Total cholesterol between 120 and 139mg/dL

12. What is goal blood pressure for adults without diabetes?

    A. 80–89mmHg

    B. < 140mmHg

    C. 120/80mmHg

    D. 130/90mmHg

13. Which of the following is characteristic of angina?

    A. Angina usually lasts for several hours before relief.

    B. Angina usually involves severe chest pain or discomfort.

    C. Angina causes irreversible damage to the muscle of the heart.

    D. Stable angina is not precipitated by a predictable event.

14. Which of the following are symptoms of a stroke?

    A. Headache, changes in alertness, confusion, dizziness, one-sided weakness, and trouble speaking

    B. Pain radiating from the chest to the jaw, left arm, or neck

    C. Leg pain at rest, edema, tachycardia, and disorientation

    D. Warmth, pain, and tenderness in the lower leg

15. All but which of the following are risk factors for deep vein thrombosis?

    A. Extended periods of immobility

    B. Major illness

    C. Age under 40 years

    D. Obesity

16. What is the consequence of a blood pressure cuff that is too large?

    A. A false low blood pressure reading

    B. A false high blood pressure reading

    C. A false high heart rate

    D. A false low heart rate

17. Which of the following waves or intervals seen on an ECG is correctly matched with its origin?

    A. P wave: the activation of the atrioventricular node

    B. QRS complex: the depolarization of the ventricles

    C. ST segment: the repolarization of the atria

    D. U wave: the depolarization of the bundle of His

18. If the RR interval on an ECG spans three large boxes, what is the patient's heart rate?

    A. 100 beats per minute

    B. 500 beats per minute

    C. 15 beats per minute

    D. 60 beats per minute

19. All but which of the following can produce artifacts on an ECG?

    A. The patient shivering during the test

    B. Excess hair on a patient's chest

    C. A broken electrode

    D. The power cord being too far away from the lead wires during the test

20. What is a benefit of the vacuum tube blood collection system?

    A. It is appropriate for fragile veins.

    B. It is the least painful method of blood collection.

    C. It allows for the collection of large samples of blood.

    D. It is appropriate for both children and adults.

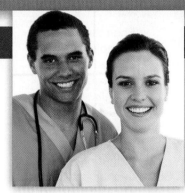

Nervous and Sensory Systems

After reading this chapter, you will be able to:

- Identify combining word forms of the nervous system and their role for the formation of medical terms.
- Define the structures and functions of the nervous system.
- Identify common diseases, diagnostic procedures, and their treatment.
- Identify combining word forms of the special senses and their role for the formation of medical terms.
- Define the structures and functions of the special senses.
- List abbreviations related to the systems.
- Differentiate between instillation and irrigation.
- Discuss the different types of visual acuity charts and how to use them appropriately.
- Explain the medical assistant's role when assisting with audiometry.
- List items required by a provider for a neurological examination and explain the medical assistant's role in the examination.
- Define a cerebral vascular accident (CVA).

KEY TERMS

Afferent system	Amyotrophic lateral	Autonomic nervous
Age-related macular	sclerosis (ALS)	system
degeneration (AMD)	Arachnoid	Axons
Alzheimer's disease (AD)	Audiometer	Bell's palsy

Biopsy	Encephalitis	Otitis media
Blepharitis	Epilepsy	Parasympathetic
Brain scan	Evoked potentials	nervous system
Brain stem	Frontal lobe	Parietal lobe
Cataract	Ganglia	Parkinson's disease (PD)
Cerebellum	Glaucoma	Pia mater
Cerebral angiogram	Hyperopia	Plexuses
Cerebral vascular	Instillation	Pons
accident (CVA)	Irrigation	Positron emission
Cerebrospinal fluid (CSF)	Jaeger chart	tomography (PET)
Cerebrospinal fluid	Keratoconjunctivitis	Retinal detachment
analysis	Medulla oblongata	Schwann cells
Cerebrum	Meningitis	Seizures
Conjunctivitis	Midbrain	Snellen chart
Corneal ulcers	Mixed nerve	Somatic nervous system
Cranium	Myelin sheath	Strabismus
Dendrites	Myelography	Stye
Diabetic retinopathy	Myopia	Subarachnoid space
Dura mater	Nerve	Subdural space
Efferent system	Neurological examination	Sympathetic nervous
Electroencephalography	Neuron	system
(EEG)	Neurosonography	Temporal lobe
Electromyography (EMG)	Neurotransmitters	Thalamus
Electronystagmography	Nissl bodies	Vertigo
(ENG)	Occipital lobe	Videonystagmograph

Chapter Overview

This chapter covers the basics of medical terminology related to the nervous system and the special senses. It includes a description of the nervous system and coverage of the special senses along with common diseases, diagnostic procedures, and treatment.

Terminology

As a medical assistant, you must have a strong working knowledge of medical terminology. You must be able to define and apply these terms when working with patients and other healthcare professionals. These terms serve as a universal language that all medical doctors, nurses, pharmacists, medical assistants, and other medical personnel can understand. TABLE 14.1 lists common combining forms related to the nervous system, while TABLE 14.2 lists common combining forms pertaining to the senses.

A combining form is a word root that has a vowel added to the end to help connect suffixes or other word roots or combining forms. Most often, the combining form ends in the vowel a, o, or i.
© auremar/ShutterStock, Inc.

The Nervous System

The nervous system has two main divisions: the central nervous system (CNS) and the peripheral nervous system (PNS). The peripheral nervous system is divided into the somatic nervous system and the autonomic nervous system. The central nervous

Table 14.1 Common Combining Forms Related to the Nervous System

Combining Form	Meaning	Example
Cerebell/o	Cerebellum	Cerebellar
Cerebr/o	Cerebrum	Cerebral
Electr/o	Electricity	Electromyography
Encephal/o	Brain	Encephalitis
Mening/o	Membranes covering brain and spinal cord	Meningitis
Myel/o	Spinal cord	Myelogram
Neur/o	Nerve	Neurology
Phas/o	Speech	Aphasia

Table 14.2 Common Combining Forms Related to the Senses

Combining Form	Meaning	Example
Acous/o, ot/o	Ears or hearing	Acoustic
Blephar/o	Eyelid	Blepharitis
Conjunctiv/o	Conjuctiva	Conjunctivitis
Kerat/o	Cornea	Keratoconus
Ir/i, ir/o, irid/o	Iris	Irides
Labyrinth/o	Inner ear	Labyrinthitis
Macul/o	Spot	Macular degeneration
Myring/o	Middle ear	Myringotomy
Ocul/o	Eye	Ocular
Opt/i, opthalm/o	Eye	Opthalmologist
Phac/o, phak/o	Lens	Phacoemulsification
Scler/o	White of the eye	Scleritis
Tympan/o	Membrane of middle ear	Tympanostomy

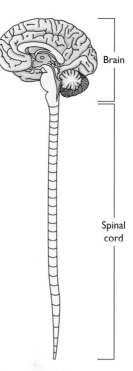

FIGURE 14.1 The central nervous system, composed of the brain and spinal cord.

© Jones & Bartlett Learning

system includes the brain and spinal cord **FIGURE 14.1**. The brain and spinal cord serve as the main processing center that controls all the functions of the body. Both the brain and the spinal cord are covered by meninges. The spinal cord and parts of the brain are filled with cerebrospinal fluid, which helps the brain maintain its normal pressure.

The central nervous system includes the brain and spinal cord. It is the body's control center.

© auremar/ShutterStock, Inc.

The brain is divided into right and left hemispheres. Each hemisphere has different functions. The left hemisphere controls language, math, and logic. The right hemisphere controls spatial abilities, facial recognition, visual imagery, and music **FIGURE 14.2**. Each hemisphere is essential to the other. The spinal cord contains nerve pathways called tracts that send signals from sensors in the body to the brain. The brain interprets these signals and sends signals to the body organs telling them what to do.

The signals that are sent to and from the brain are electrical signals. These electrical signals stimulate the release of **neurotransmitters**, or chemicals, at many nerve endings. These neurotransmitters allow the electrical signal to continue to the next nerve.

The central nervous system is the body's control center.

© auremar/ShutterStock, Inc.

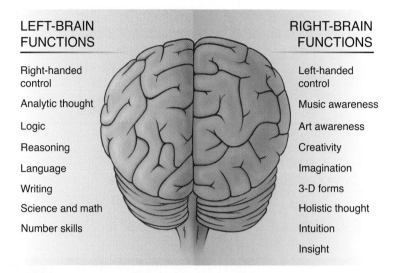

LEFT-BRAIN FUNCTIONS	RIGHT-BRAIN FUNCTIONS
Right-handed control	Left-handed control
Analytic thought	Music awareness
Logic	Art awareness
Reasoning	Creativity
Language	Imagination
Writing	3-D forms
Science and math	Holistic thought
Number skills	Intuition
	Insight

FIGURE 14.2 Human right-brain and left-brain functions.
© Jones & Bartlett Learning

Neurotransmitters can either stimulate or inhibit these signals. Lack or incorrect amounts of these neurotransmitters can cause many different physical, emotional, and mental disorders.

The basic functioning unit of the nervous system is a nerve cell, or **neuron**. There are three types of neurons in nerve tissue: sensory, connecting, and motor. Neurons receive stimuli or impulses, transmit impulses to other neurons, and deliver messages to muscles and glands. **FIGURE 14.3** shows the structure of a motor neuron.

Like all cells, nerve cells have a nucleus, cytoplasm, and cell membrane. Throughout the cytoplasm are microscopic **Nissl bodies**, which are involved in protein synthesis and metabolism. The cell body of a neuron has processes that are extensions of the cytoplasm called **dendrites** and **axons**. The neuron sends electrical impulses from its cell body through the axon to target cells. Each nerve cell has one axon. Around the long, thin axons of peripheral nerves are **Schwann cells**. These cells form a protective covering called the **myelin sheath** and also play a part in the transmission of messages. Dendrites are threadlike extensions of a neuron that conduct impulses from adjacent cells inward toward the cell body.

A **nerve** is composed of bundles of nerve fibers that are bound together by connective tissue. If a nerve is composed of fibers sending information from the sensory organs to the spinal cord or brain, it is a sensory or afferent nerve. If the nerve is carrying impulses from the brain or spinal cord to a gland, muscle, or organ, it is an efferent or motor nerve. Some nerves are both afferent and efferent in nature and are called **mixed nerves**. **FIGURE 14.4** shows the anatomy of a nerve.

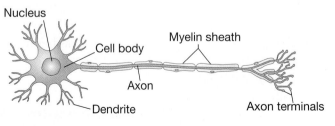

The neuron is the basic functioning unit of the nervous system.
© auremar/ShutterStock, Inc.

Nucleus
Cell body
Myelin sheath
Axon
Dendrite
Axon terminals

FIGURE 14.3 The structure of a motor neuron.
© Jones & Bartlett Learning

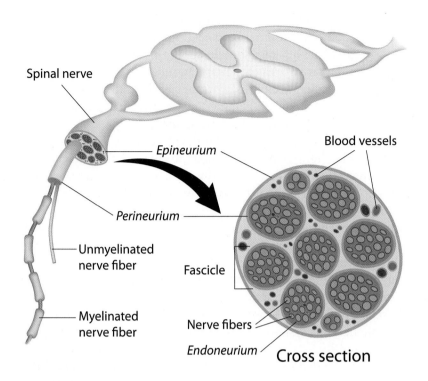

FIGURE 14.4 Anatomy of a nerve.
© Alila Sao Mai/ShutterStock, Inc.

Sensory neurons transmit messages from receptor cells to the spinal cord and then to the brain for interpretation and action. If a reaction is needed, impulses are then transmitted from the brain and spinal cord to the muscle or organ via the motor neurons. Connecting interneurons throughout the body enable one nerve to communicate with another nerve.

The peripheral nervous system (PNS) includes all the nerves that connect the CNS to every organ and area of the body. It includes 12 pairs of cranial nerves that connect the brain directly to the sense organs, the heart, the lungs, and other internal organs **FIGURE 14.5**. It also includes 31 pairs of spinal nerves.

The PNS is divided into the afferent system and the efferent system. The **afferent system** includes all the nerves and sense organs. These nerves and organs take in information and send it to the CNS. The **efferent system** includes all the nerves and pathways that send information from the CNS to other organs and body systems. The efferent system is further divided into the autonomic nervous system, parasympathetic nervous system, and somatic nervous system. The **autonomic nervous system** controls internal organs and other self-regulating body functions. The parasympathetic nervous system returns the body to a normal state. The **somatic nervous system** controls all the skeletal muscles in the body.

The autonomic nervous system is the part of the nervous system that controls involuntary functions,

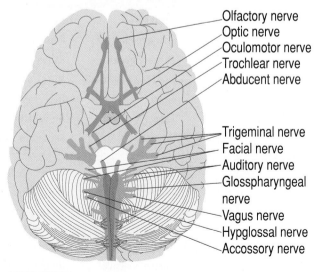

Olfactory nerve
Optic nerve
Oculomotor nerve
Trochlear nerve
Abducent nerve

Trigeminal nerve
Facial nerve
Auditory nerve
Glosspharyngeal nerve
Vagus nerve
Hypglossal nerve
Accessory nerve

FIGURE 14.5 Cranial nerves. These connect the brain to various organs.
© illustrator/ShutterStock, Inc.

The peripheral nervous system includes all the nerves in the body except those in the central nervous system.
© auremar/ShutterStock, Inc.

such as breathing, digestion, widening or narrowing of the arteries, and beating of the heart. It consists of nerves, **ganglia** (clusters of neurons), and **plexuses** (networks of nerves). In most situations, people are unaware of the workings of the autonomic nervous system in their bodies because it functions in an involuntary, reflexive manner.

The autonomic system is important in two situations: emergencies that cause stress and require us to "fight" or take flight, frequently called the "flight-fight mechanism," and in nonemergencies that allow us to rest and digest. The autonomic system is always working. It acts to maintain normal internal functions and works with the somatic nervous system.

There are two primary neurotransmitters in the peripheral nervous system: acetylcholine, a neurotransmitter that plays a role in skeletal muscle movement and regulation of smooth and cardiac muscle; and norepinephrine, a neurotransmitter secreted by the adrenal medulla and nerve endings of the sympathetic nervous system that increases heart rate and increases the actions of the peripheral nervous system by constricting blood vessels. Epinephrine, a hormone secreted by the adrenal medulla, stimulates the sympathetic nervous system, increasing blood pressure, heart rate, and cardiac output.

The autonomic system is divided into the sympathetic nervous system and parasympathetic nervous system. The **sympathetic nervous system** accelerates activity in the smooth, involuntary muscles of the body's organs. The **parasympathetic nervous system** reverses the action and slows down activity. These activities continuously balance each other to maintain homeostasis. Some organs do not have a dual supply of parasympathetic nerves and sympathetic nerves, so these opposing mechanisms do not apply to all organs. **TABLE 14.3** outlines various aspects of the autonomic nervous system. **FIGURE 14.6** shows the sympathetic nervous system, while **FIGURE 14.7** shows the parasympathetic nervous system.

The autonomic nervous system is important in flight-fight responses.
© auremar/ShutterStock, Inc.

Table 14.3   Autonomic Nervous System

Structure	Sympathetic Stimulation	Parasympathetic Stimulation
Iris (eye muscle)	Pupil dilation	Pupil constriction
Salivary glands	Saliva production reduced	Saliva production increased
Oral/nasal mucosa	Mucus production reduced	Mucus production increased
Heart	Heart rate and force increased	Heart rate and force decreased
Lung	Bronchial muscle relaxed	Bronchial muscle contracted
Stomach	Peristalsis reduced	Gastric juice secreted; motility increased
Small intestine	Motility reduced	Digestion increased
Large intestine	Motility reduced	Secretions and motility increased
Liver	Increased conversion of glycogen to glucose	Stimulates release of bile
Kidney	Decreased urine secretion	Increased urine secretion
Adrenal medulla	Norepinephrine and epinephrine secreted	
Bladder	Wall relaxed, sphincter closed	Wall contracted, sphincter relaxed

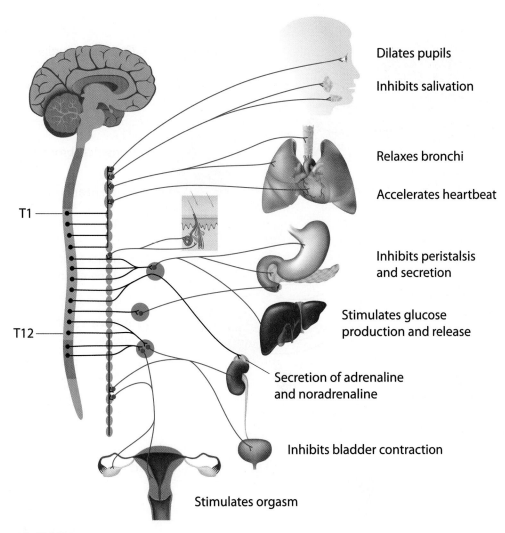

Dilates pupils

Inhibits salivation

Relaxes bronchi

Accelerates heartbeat

Inhibits peristalsis
and secretion

Stimulates glucose
production and release

Secretion of adrenaline
and noradrenaline

Inhibits bladder contraction

Stimulates orgasm

T1

T12

FIGURE 14.6 The sympathetic nervous system accelerates activity in the smooth, involuntary muscles of the body's organs.
© Alila Sao Mai/ShutterStock, Inc.

The Central Nervous System

The central nervous system includes the brain and spinal cord. The brain controls all bodily functions. The spinal cord is a bundle of nerve fibers that connects the brain to the rest of the body. It extends from the neck to the lower back and transmits information from body organs to the brain and information from the brain to other areas of the body.

The Brain

The brain is the control center of the body. It controls thoughts, speech, memory, and movement. It also regulates the function of many organs.

The brain and spinal cord are protected by three connective tissue layers collectively called the meninges. The meninges support blood vessels and contain cerebrospinal fluid. The brain is also protected by the **cranium** (skull).

The brain is divided into five parts **FIGURE 14.8** :

■ **Cerebrum**—The **cerebrum** is the largest part of the brain. It controls sensory and motor activities. The cerebrum is divided into the frontal lobe, occipital

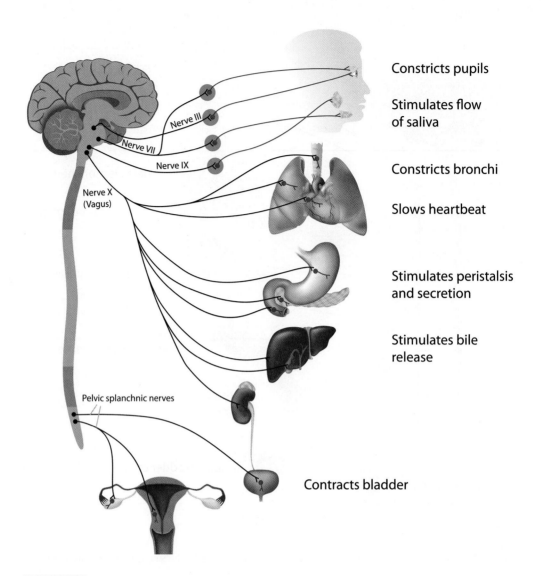

Constricts pupils

Stimulates flow of saliva

Constricts bronchi

Slows heartbeat

Stimulates peristalsis and secretion

Stimulates bile release

Contracts bladder

Nerve III

Nerve VII

Nerve IX

Nerve X (Vagus)

Pelvic splanchnic nerves

FIGURE 14.7 The parasympathetic nervous system reverses the action and slows down activity.
© Alila Sao Mai/ShutterStock, Inc.

lobe, parietal lobe, and temporal lobe. The **frontal lobe** seems to be related to motor functions, planning, reasoning, judgment, impulse control, and memory. The **occipital lobe** is associated with vision. The **parietal lobe** is associated with cognition, information processing, pain and touch sensation, spatial orientation, speech, and visual perception. The **temporal lobe** plays an important role in organizing sensory input, auditory perception, and language and speech production.

■ **Cerebellum**—The **cerebellum** lies just beneath the cerebrum. It is responsible for motor-movement coordination, balance, equilibrium, and muscle tone.

■ **Brain stem**—The **brain stem** connects the brain to the spinal cord. It is composed of three sections: the medulla oblongata, the pons, and the midbrain. The **medulla oblongata** controls autonomic functions such as breathing, digestion, heart and blood-vessel function, and sneezing. It helps transfer messages between the spinal cord and various parts of the brain. Above the medulla oblongata is the pons. The **pons** serves as the communication center between the two hemispheres of the brain. It is the reflex center for secreting saliva, chewing,

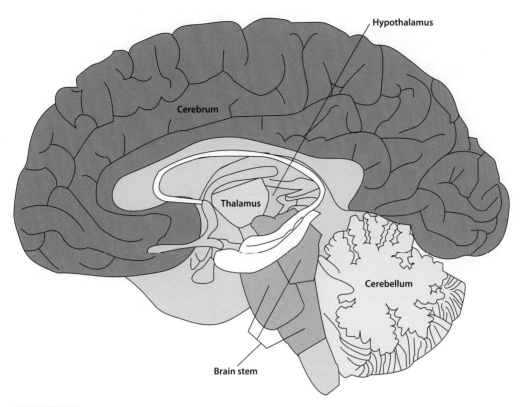

FIGURE 14.8 The five parts of the brain.
© Anita Potter/ShutterStock, Inc.

and tasting, and plays a role in generating dreams. The **midbrain** is superior to the pons and is the control center for visual reflexes, such as moving the head and eyes, sleep/wake control, arousal, and temperature control. It also conducts impulses between the brain parts above and below it.

■ **Thalamus**—The **thalamus** lies between the cerebrum and the midbrain. It is involved in sensory perception and regulation of motor functions. The thalamus controls sleep and awake states of consciousness. It acts as a relay station for impulses going to and from the brain and those impulses from the cerebellum and other parts of the brain.

■ **Hypothalamus**—The hypothalamus lies below the thalamus and between the cerebrum and the midbrain. It is connected to the pituitary gland, midbrain, and thalamus by a bundle of nerve fibers. It is the control center for many autonomic functions of the PNS. It is involved in many functions, including autonomic function control, endocrine function control, homeostasis, motor function control, regulation of food and water intake, and sleep-wake cycle regulation.

Meninges

The brain and spinal cord are protected by three connective tissue layers collectively called the meninges **FIGURE 14.9**. These three layers consist of the **pia mater** (the innermost layer, closest to the CNS structures), the **arachnoid** (the middle layer), and the **dura mater** (farthest from the CNS). The pia mater contains blood vessels to nourish the nerve tissue, and the dura mater is a tough, fibrous tissue that protects the CNS. The space between the dura mater and the arachnoid is called the **subdural space**. The space between the arachnoid and the pia mater is the **subarachnoid space**.

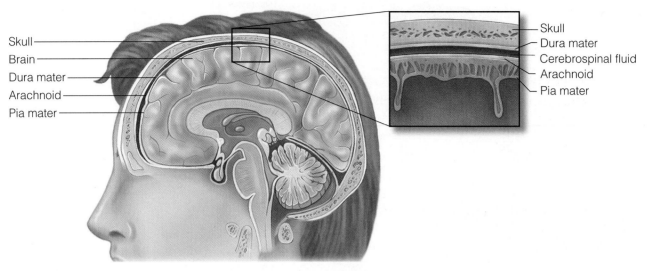

Skull
Brain
Dura mater
Arachnoid
Pia mater

Skull
Dura mater
Cerebrospinal fluid
Arachnoid
Pia mater

FIGURE 14.9 The meninges, with the pia mater, arachnoid, and dura mater.
© Jones & Bartlett Learning

The brain is protected by three layers of connective tissue called the meninges.

Cerebrospinal Fluid

Cerebrospinal fluid (CSF) acts as a cushion, protecting the brain and spinal cord from injury. It provides a mechanical barrier to protect the brain and spine from shock. The fluid also transports nutrients to the brain and spinal cord.

Diagnostic Tests

Diagnostic tests and procedures are vital tools that help doctors confirm or rule out the presence of a neurological disorder or other medical condition. Based on the result of a neurological examination, physical examination, patient history, and X-rays of the patient's chest and skull, physicians may order diagnostic tests to determine the nature of a neurological disorder or injury. These tests generally involve either nuclear medicine imaging, in which very small amounts of radioactive materials are used to study organ function and structure, or diagnostic imaging, which uses magnets and electrical charges to study human anatomy.

Making sure that patients have a good understanding of what they can expect during these tests is the first step in preparing them for any examination. The medical assistant will probably be the main person with whom the patient interacts before the examination or diagnostic test.

The medical assistant plays an important role in making sure the patient is comfortable and understands what to expect during testing.

Neurological Examination

A **neurological examination** assesses motor and sensory skills, hearing, speech, vision, coordination, balance, mental status, changes in mood or behavior, and the functioning of cranial nerves. It can be used to help diagnose brain tumors, encephalitis, meningitis,

Parkinson's disease, Huntington's disease, amyotrophic lateral sclerosis (ALS), and epilepsy.

X-rays

X-rays of the patient's skull are often taken as part of the neurological workup. X-rays are often used to view vertebral misalignment or fractures.

Cerebral Angiogram

A **cerebral angiogram** can detect the degree of narrowing of an artery or blood vessel in the brain, head, or neck. It is used to diagnose stroke and to determine the location and size of a brain tumor, aneurysm, or vascular malformation. It is usually performed in a hospital outpatient setting and takes up to three hours, followed by a six- to eight-hour resting period. While the patient is awake, a physician anesthetizes a small area of the leg near the groin and then inserts a catheter into a major artery located there. The catheter is threaded up to the carotid artery in the neck. Radiopaque dye is injected into the catheter and travels through the bloodstream into the head and neck. A series of X-rays are taken. Patients may feel a warm or hot sensation or slight discomfort as the dye is released.

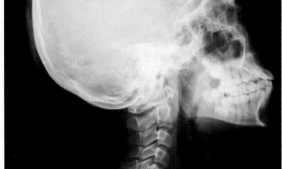
A doctor administers a neurological examination.

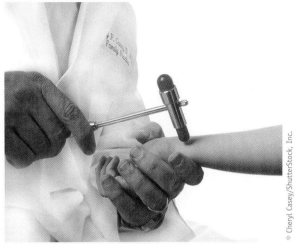

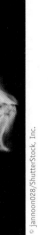

Brain Biopsy

Biopsy involves the removal and examination of a small piece of tissue. A biopsy of the brain is the removal and examination of tissue from the brain. It is used to determine the type of brain tumor.

Brain Scan

Brain scans are imaging techniques used to study organ function, injury, and disease, and to diagnose tumors, blood-vessel malformations, and hemorrhage in the brain. Types of brain scans include computed tomography (CT or CAT scans), magnetic resonance imaging (MRI), and positron emission tomography (PET).

An X-ray of the head and neck.

Cerebrospinal Fluid Analysis

Cerebrospinal fluid analysis involves the removal of a small amount of the CSF by lumbar puncture **FIGURE 14.10** or spinal tap. The doctor inserts a special needle into the subarachnoid space between the vertebrae of the lower back and removes a small amount of fluid for testing. The fluid is tested to detect bleeding or brain hemorrhage, diagnose infection to the brain and/or spinal cord, identify some cases of multiple sclerosis and other neurological conditions, and measure intracranial pressure.

Computed Axial Tomography

Computed tomography (CT or CAT scan) is used to produce rapid, clear images of organs, bones, and tissues. Neurological CT scans are used to view the brain and spine. They can detect bone and vascular irregularities, certain brain tumors and cysts,

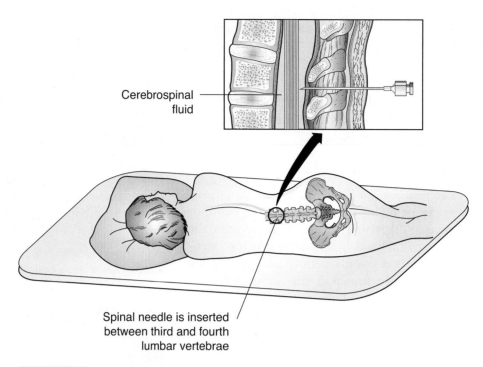

Cerebrospinal fluid

Spinal needle is inserted
between third and fourth
lumbar vertebrae

FIGURE 14.10 Cerebrospinal fluid analysis involves a lumbar puncture.
© Jones & Bartlett Learning

herniated disks, epilepsy, encephalitis, spinal stenosis (narrowing of the spinal canal), a blood clot or intracranial bleeding in patients with stroke, brain damage from head injury, and other disorders. Many neurological disorders share certain characteristics; a CT scan can aid in proper diagnosis by differentiating the area of the brain affected by the disorder.

During a CT scan, the patient lies on a special table that slides into a narrow chamber. As the patient lies still, X-rays are passed through the body at various angles and are detected by a computerized scanner. The data is processed and displayed as cross-sectioned images, or slices, of the brain. Occasionally, a contrast dye is injected into the bloodstream to highlight the different tissues in the brain. Although very little radiation is used in CT, pregnant women should avoid the test because of potential harm to the fetus from ionizing radiation.

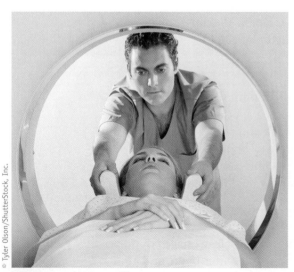

© Tyler Olson/ShutterStock, Inc.

A patient undergoes a CT scan.

Intrathecal Contrast-Enhanced CT Scan

An intrathecal contrast-enhanced CT scan is used to detect problems with the spine and spinal nerve roots. During this procedure, the physician removes a small amount of CSF via lumbar puncture. The CSF is mixed with a contrast dye and injected into the spinal sac located at the base of the lower back. The patient is then asked to move to a position that will allow the contrast fluid to travel to the area to be studied. The dye allows the spinal canal and nerve roots to be seen more clearly on a CT scan.

Electroencephalography

Electroencephalography (EEG) monitors brain activity through the skull. EEG is used to help diagnose certain seizure disorders, brain tumors, brain damage from head injuries, inflammation of the brain and/or spinal cord, alcoholism, certain psychiatric disorders, and metabolic and degenerative disorders that affect the brain. It is also used to evaluate sleep disorders, monitor brain activity when a patient has been fully anesthetized or loses consciousness, and confirm brain death.

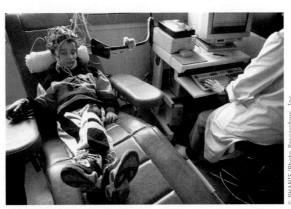

A patient receives an EEG.

During an EEG, a series of electrodes is attached to the patient's scalp, either with a special conducting paste or with extremely fine needles. The electrodes (also called leads) are small devices that are attached to wires and carry the electrical energy of the brain to a machine for reading. A very low electrical current is sent through the electrodes and the baseline brain energy is recorded. Patients are then exposed to a variety of external stimuli—including bright or flashing light, noise, or certain drugs—or asked to open and close the eyes or to change breathing patterns. The electrodes transmit the resulting changes in brain wave patterns.

Electromyography

Electromyography (EMG) records the electrical activity from the brain and/or spinal cord to a peripheral nerve root found in the arms and legs that controls muscles during contraction and at rest. It is used to diagnose nerve and muscle dysfunction and spinal cord disease.

During an EMG, very fine wire electrodes are inserted into a muscle to assess changes in electrical voltage that occur during movement and when the muscle is at rest. The electrodes are attached through a series of wires to a recording instrument. An EMG is usually done in conjunction with a nerve conduction velocity (NCV) test, which measures electrical energy by assessing the nerve's ability to send a signal.

Electronystagmography

Electronystagmography (ENG) is used to diagnose involuntary eye movement, dizziness, and balance disorders, and to evaluate some brain functions. Small electrodes are taped around the eyes or infrared photography is used to record eye movements.

Evoked Potentials

Evoked potentials (also called evoked response) measure the electrical signals to the brain generated by hearing, touch, or sight. These tests are used to assess sensory nerve problems and confirm neurological conditions, including multiple sclerosis, brain tumor, and spinal cord injury. Evoked potentials are also used to test sight and hearing (especially in infants and young children), monitor brain activity among coma patients, and confirm brain death.

Two sets of needle electrodes are used to test for nerve damage. One set of electrodes is used to measure the electrophysiological response to stimuli. The second set of electrodes is attached to the part of the body to be tested. The physician then records the amount of time it takes for the impulse generated by stimuli to reach the brain. Under normal circumstances, the process of signal transmission is instantaneous.

Auditory evoked potentials are used to assess high-frequency hearing loss and diagnose damage to the acoustic nerve and auditory pathways in the brain stem. The patient sits in a soundproof room and wears headphones. Clicking sounds are delivered one at a time to one ear while a masking sound is sent to the other ear.

Visual evoked potentials detect loss of vision from optic-nerve damage (in particular, damage caused by multiple sclerosis). The patient sits close to a screen and is asked to focus on the center of a shifting checkerboard pattern. Only one eye is tested at a time; the other eye is either kept closed or covered with a patch.

Somatosensory evoked potentials measure response from stimuli to the peripheral nerves and can detect nerve or spinal-cord damage or nerve degeneration from multiple sclerosis and other degenerating diseases. Tiny electrical shocks are delivered by electrode to a nerve in an arm or leg. Responses to the shocks are recorded.

Magnetic Resonance Imaging

Magnetic resonance imaging (MRI) uses computer-generated radio waves and a magnetic field to produce detailed images of body structures, including tissues, organs, bones, and nerves. Neurological uses include the diagnosis of brain and spinal cord tumors, eye disease, inflammation, infection, and vascular irregularities that may lead to stroke. MRI can also detect and monitor degenerative disorders such as multiple sclerosis and can document brain injury from trauma.

The equipment houses a hollow tube that is surrounded by a very large cylindrical magnet. The patient lies on a special table that slides into the tube. A computer creates either a three-dimensional picture or a two-dimensional slice of the tissue being scanned, differentiating between bone, soft tissues, and fluid-filled spaces by their water content and structural properties. A contrast dye may be used to enhance visibility of certain areas or tissues.

Myelography

Myelography is an X-ray examination of the spinal canal. A contrast agent is injected through a needle into the space around the spinal cord to display the spinal cord, spinal canal, and nerve roots on an X-ray. It is used to diagnose spinal nerve injury, herniated disks, fractures, back or leg pain, and spinal tumors.

A small amount of CSF is removed by spinal tap and the contrast dye is injected into the spinal canal. After a series of X-rays is taken, most or all of the contrast dye is removed by aspiration.

Positron Emission Tomography

Positron emission tomography (PET) scans provide two- and three-dimensional pictures of brain activity by measuring radioactive isotopes that are injected into the bloodstream. PET scans of the brain are used to detect tumors and diseased tissue, measure cellular and/or tissue metabolism, show blood flow, evaluate patients who have seizure disorders who do not respond to medical therapy and patients with certain memory disorders, and determine brain changes following injury or drug abuse. A low-level radioactive isotope, which binds to chemicals that flow to the brain, is injected into the bloodstream and can be traced as the brain performs different functions. The patient lies still while overhead sensors detect gamma rays in the body's tissues. A computer processes the information and displays it on a video monitor or on film.

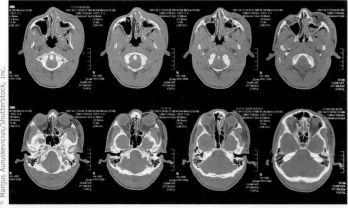

© Marijus Auruskevicius/ShutterStock, Inc.

An MRI of the human body.

Neurosonography

Neurosonography (ultrasound of the brain and spinal column) analyzes blood flow in the brain and can diagnose stroke, brain tumors, hydrocephalus (excess cerebrospinal fluid in the brain), and vascular problems.

During the procedure, the patient lies on an imaging table after removing clothing around the area of the body to be scanned. A jellylike lubricant is applied and a transducer, which both sends and receives high-frequency sound waves, is passed over the body. The sound wave echoes are recorded and displayed as a computer-generated real-time visual image of the structure or tissue being examined.

Videonystagmograph

A **videonystagmograph** is a special examination that measures eye movements and is used to evaluate balance. The test uses special goggles that record eye movement. Patients are asked to identify locations of objects when shown.

Diseases and Disorders

A disease of the nervous system can affect the brain or spinal cord. The nervous system is vulnerable to many disorders. These disorders can be caused by trauma, infections, structural defects, degeneration, tumors, autoimmune diseases, or disruption of blood flow.

Alzheimer's Disease

Alzheimer's disease (AD) is a degenerative disorder of the brain that leads to loss of brain function. It results in memory impairment and in loss of judgment, decision-making ability, and speech. It also results in changes in personality and behavior.

Alzheimer's disease is a degenerative disorder of the brain that results in loss of brain function.
© auremar/ShutterStock, Inc.

The exact cause of AD is unknown. Patients with AD often have amyloid plaques and neurofibrillary tangles. Cognitive loss in AD is associated with depletion of acetylcholine, which is involved in learning and memory. In the early stages of the disease, the patient may experience language problems, the misplacing of items, personality changes, loss of social skills, and difficulty performing tasks that require some thought. As the disease progresses, the symptoms become worse and can interfere with normal functioning. As the disease becomes even more severe, patients with AD can no longer understand language, recognize family members, or perform basic tasks.

None of the treatments currently available for AD cure, reverse, or stop the progression of AD. Unlike other cells, nerve cells cannot reproduce themselves. The primary goal of therapy is to preserve patient function, lessen agitation, improve sleeping, and treat depression. Drugs that increase the concentrations of acetylcholine may have beneficial effects on the symptoms of dementia, but can also cause adverse cholinergic effects, such as nausea, vomiting, and diarrhea.

Amyotrophic Lateral Sclerosis

Amyotrophic lateral sclerosis (ALS), also known as Lou Gehrig's disease, is a progressive neurological disease that attacks the neurons that control voluntary muscles. In ALS, the upper and lower motor neurons (nerve cells that send messages from the brain to the voluntary muscles in the body) die and stop sending messages to the muscles. This causes the muscles to weaken, waste away, and twitch. Eventually, all

Lou Gehrig's disease is a progressive neurological disease that results in the inability to control voluntary muscles.
© auremar/ShutterStock, Inc.

the voluntary muscles of the body are affected and patients lose the ability to move their arms and legs and control their body.

There is no cure for ALS. Treatment is aimed at controlling symptoms and providing emotional and physical support. Physical therapy and speech therapy can enhance the patient's quality of life. The FDA has approved the use of the drug riluzole (Rilutek) to treat ALS patients. Riluzole is believed to reduce damage to motor neurons by decreasing the release of glutamate. It does not reverse the damage already done to motor neurons.

Bell's Palsy

Bell's palsy is a disorder of the nerve that controls movement of the facial muscles. Damage to the seventh cranial nerve (facial nerve), the nerve that controls the movement of the muscles of the face, causes muscle weakness or paralysis of facial muscles. Symptoms often start suddenly and are almost always on one side of the face. It causes the mouth to droop on the affected side, resulting in excess drooling. It may also cause drooping of the face, difficulty eating and swallowing, and difficulty closing the eye of the affected side. The cause is thought to be an infection, which causes swelling of the facial nerve.

Often, no treatment is needed because symptoms begin to improve right away. Corticosteroids can be used to reduce inflammation around the facial nerve. Antiviral medications can also be used to treat the infective process that may be causing the inflammation.

Encephalitis

Encephalitis is a severe inflammation of the brain that can destroy nerve cells, cause bleeding in the brain, and result in brain damage. It is most often caused by a viral infection. The virus causes inflammation of the brain tissue. Symptoms include fever, headache, poor appetite, confusion, drowsiness, irritability, loss of consciousness, muscle weakness, and seizures.

The goals of therapy are to provide supportive care and relieve symptoms. Antibiotics or antivirals may be given to treat the cause of the infection, antiepileptics to prevent seizures, steroids to reduce brain swelling, and sedatives to treat irritability or restlessness.

Epilepsy

Epilepsy is a neurological condition that is also known as a seizure disorder. It is characterized by sudden and recurring seizures. It is usually diagnosed after a person has two seizures that are unrelated to another medical disorder. **Seizures** result from an abnormal, sudden, excessive firing of a small number of neurons, which interferes with normal brain functioning. This abnormal electrical activity can occur in a specific area of the brain or can spread more extensively throughout the brain.

All patients with epilepsy have seizures, but not all patients with seizures have epilepsy. Seizures can also be attributed to other conditions. Seizures can vary in severity, appearance, consequence, and management, and can affect different people in different ways.

Anticonvulsants, also known as antiepileptic drugs, are the drugs of choice for seizure control. Goals of therapy are to control or reduce the frequency of seizures and to prevent behavioral and psychological changes that result from seizures.

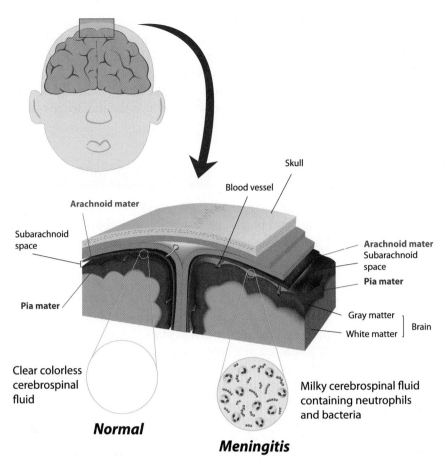

Meningitis

Meningitis is an inflammation of the membranes that cover the brain and spinal cord. It can be caused by viral or bacterial infection. Symptoms may include fever, chills, altered mental status, nausea, vomiting, light sensitivity, severe headache, stiff neck, and fast heart rate FIGURE 14.11.

Treatment consists of antibiotics if the cause is bacterial or antivirals if the cause is viral. Medications to reduce cerebral edema and relieve pain may also be given.

Parkinson's Disease

Parkinson's disease (PD) is a motor-system disorder caused primarily by progressive degeneration of dopamine-containing neurons in the substantia nigra, which is the layer of gray substance in the brain FIGURE 14.12.

Nerve impulses travel from the cerebral cortex to the basal nuclei and back to the cerebral cortex by electrical impulses and neurotransmitters. Normal movement requires a balance of two neurotransmitters: dopamine and acetylcholine. In healthy persons, dopaminergic neurons in the substantia nigra release enough dopamine to counterbalance the stimulating effects of acetylcholine. In patients with PD, not enough dopamine is produced

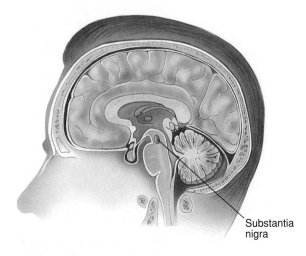

FIGURE 14.12 A cross section of the brain.

to counteract the production of acetylcholine, resulting in trembling in the hands, arms, legs, jaw, and face, rigidity, slowness of movement, and postural instability.

There is no known cure for PD. The goal of drug therapy is to provide symptomatic relief, minimize disability, and help patients maintain their quality of life. Dopamine itself cannot be used to treat PD because it does not cross the blood-brain barrier. All drugs for the treatment of PD are administered orally to reduce the incidence of side effects outside the CNS.

Sensory Systems

There are five major senses: sight, hearing, smell, taste, and touch. Equilibrium is associated with the sense of hearing and plays a major role in our ability to maintain balance. The organs associated with these senses include the eyes, ears, nose, tongue, and skin.

The Eyes

As one of the five sensors of the body, the eyes perceive images and translate them into impulses. Each area of the eye has a specific function that works to protect it, maintain it, and enhance vision. Each eye is housed in a bony socket called the orbit. Covering the eyes are the eyelids. The eyelids are composed of four individual layers: the outer skin, the muscles, the connective tissue, and the conjunctiva. The conjunctiva is a thin mucous membrane that covers the inner surface of the eyelid and the sclera. The sclera is the white fibrous tissue that covers the outside of the eye. It helps maintain the shape of the eyeball. The cornea is the clear, dome-shaped surface that covers the front of the eye and allows light into the eye for visual acuity. The iris filters light and is responsible for the color of the eye. The retina is the light-sensitive layer of tissue at the back of the eye that contains the nerve endings that transmit electrical impulses to the brain. FIGURE 14.13 shows the anatomy of the eye.

The Ears

The ears are responsible for hearing and maintaining balance. Each ear is composed of three sections: the external ear, middle ear, and inner ear. The external ear is composed of cartilage and skin. It transmits sound waves to the middle ear and protects the middle ear from foreign objects. The middle ear transmits sound waves that enter this cavity to the inner ear. As sound waves enter the inner ear, the inner ear transmits impulses to the brain. The inner ear also provides information to the brain about the orientation of the body at rest and when in motion, thus helping maintain balance and equilibrium FIGURE 14.14.

The Nose

The olfactory organ at the top of the nasal cavity is responsible for the sense of smell. The nerve fibers connect the mucous membranes of the olfactory organ to the olfactory center in the brain and are responsible for responding to stimuli from molecules dissolved in the moisture from the mucous membranes. It detects smells once it is dissolved in the mucous secretions FIGURE 14.15.

The Tongue

Receptors on the tongue give us the ability to taste different flavors. Taste buds are located on the tip, sides, and back of the tongue. In order to taste something, it must be dissolved by saliva FIGURE 14.16.

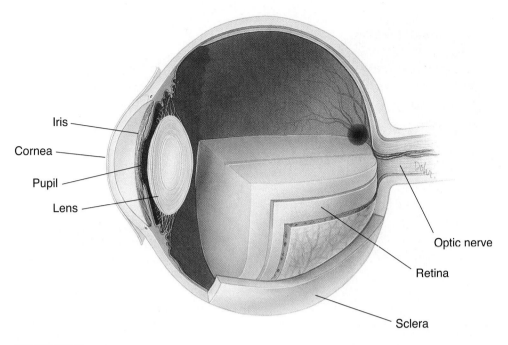

FIGURE 14.13 Anatomy of the eye.
© Jones & Bartlett Learning

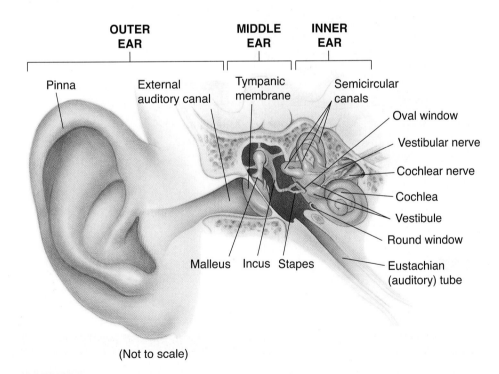

FIGURE 14.14 Anatomy of the ear.
© Jones & Bartlett Learning

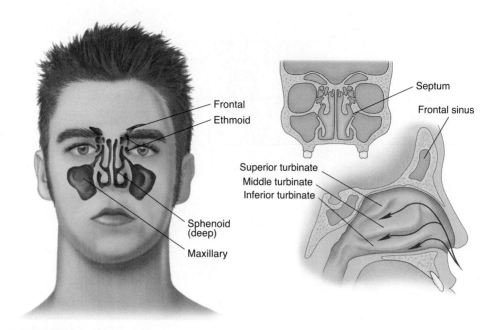

FIGURE 14.15 Anatomy of the nose.
© Jones & Bartlett Learning

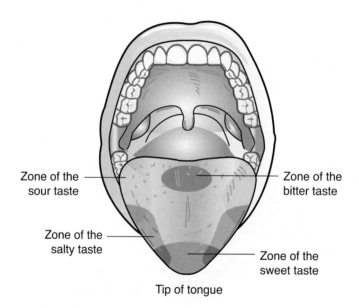

FIGURE 14.16 Basic tastes.
© Jones & Bartlett Learning

Diseases and Disorders of the Eye

The location and exposure of the eye make it susceptible to contamination and infection. However, the eye has protective mechanisms to prevent the entry of foreign bodies into the eye and to maintain the health and comfort of the eye.

Age-Related Macular Degeneration

Age-related macular degeneration (AMD) is a disease that affects the macula and causes loss of central vision. There are two types of AMD: dry AMD and wet AMD. In wet AMD, abnormal blood vessels behind the retina start to grow under the macula and leak blood and fluid. In dry AMD, the light-sensitive cells in the macula slowly break down. Both can cause blurred and distorted vision in the center of the image being viewed.

AMD results from damage to the blood vessels that supply the retina, which eventually causes thinning of the macula. There is no cure for AMD. Treatment includes nonsurgical interventions such as the use of various optical devices, including magnifying glasses and injections of medications. Surgical intervention has been used for wet AMD to stop progression of the leaky blood vessels.

Blepharitis

Blepharitis is an inflammation of the edges of the eyelids. It can cause a burning sensation, excessive tearing, light sensitivity, redness, and crusting of the eyelashes. It can be caused by bacteria and scalp dandruff or by pediculosis of the brows and lashes.

Treatment depends on the cause. Frequent hair washing and daily cleansing of the eyelids with a mild baby shampoo can keep eyelids clean. Warm wet washcloths over the eyelids can help soften scales and loosen debris. Artificial tears to relieve dryness and antibiotic or steroid eye drops can also be used.

Cataract

A **cataract** is a condition in which the normally clear lens of the eye becomes cloudy **FIGURE 14.17**. It frequently occurs as part of the aging process. People with cataracts complain of seeing halos around lights.

Causes of cataracts include use of steroids, diseases such as diabetes, prolonged exposure to ultraviolet light, trauma, and aging. The goal of therapy is to slow progression. New eyeglasses, antiglare sunglasses, and brighter lighting may help ease symptoms. If these measures do not help, surgical removal of the clouded lens and replacement with an artificial lens is the only effective treatment.

Chronic Dry Eye

Chronic dry eye (**keratoconjunctivitis**) is one of the most common disorders affecting the eye. With this condition, the eye is not able to produce enough tears to lubricate and nourish the eye. It is characterized by a sandy or gritty sensation in the eye, and may be accompanied by redness.

Chronic dry eye may be caused by environmental factors, medications, or chronic medical conditions. OTC lubricating or rewetting drops can be instilled in the eye

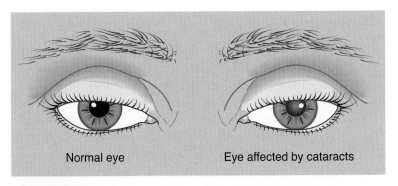

Normal eye   Eye affected by cataracts

FIGURE 14.17 A normal eye and an eye affected by cataracts.

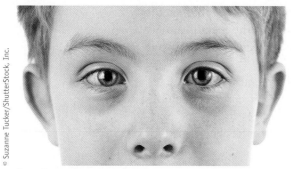

The effects of conjunctivitis.

to relieve the symptoms associated with dry eye. Recent evidence has proved the role of an immune-mediated inflammatory process in chronic dry eye. Dry eye can be successfully treated with an immunomodulatory agent, which is a drug that alters the response of the immune system.

Conjunctivitis

Conjunctivitis is an inflammation of the outer membrane of the eye. It usually begins in one eye and spreads to the other from contamination by hands or by a washcloth. It is more commonly known as pink eye. Conjunctivitis appears as redness, increased tear production, itching, and swelling. It may be caused by infections or allergies. Several topical therapies are available for reducing the signs and symptoms of conjunctivitis. Antibiotics or antiviral medications can be administered if the cause is infection.

Corneal Ulcer

Corneal ulcers are caused by infections of the cornea. Symptoms include red eyes, light sensitivity, blurry vision, swollen eyelids, pain, or a white or gray round spot on the cornea.

Treatment can include pain medications and antibiotics to prevent corneal scarring.

Diabetic Retinopathy

Diabetic retinopathy is a complication of diabetes. It affects the blood vessels in the retina and, if left untreated, can lead to blindness. There are two types of diabetic retinopathy: nonproliferative retinopathy and proliferative retinopathy. Nonproliferative retinopathy is less severe and consists of vascular abnormalities called microaneurysms. Proliferative retinopathy is more severe and consists of new growth of abnormal blood vessels on the surface of the retina that frequently bleed into the vitreous. (This is called neovascularization.) In diabetes, the excess glucose in the blood is metabolized through an alternate pathway that results in sorbitol deposits in the walls of the blood vessels in the retina. This causes the retinal vessels to become leaky or to compensate by making new blood vessels to get enough oxygen to the retina.

Treatment is by laser surgery or surgery on the vitreous. Diabetic retinopathy can often be prevented by lifestyle modification and strict control of high blood sugar. Intraocular injections of drugs into the vitreous cavity are used to treat microaneurysms and macular edema.

Glaucoma

Glaucoma is a common disorder of the eye characterized by increased ocular pressure. The increased pressure is a result of an imbalance of the production and drainage of fluid within the eye. The pressure damages the optic nerve and causes partial vision loss. Glaucoma may occur as a result of a genetic predisposition or eye injury or disease **FIGURE 14.18**.

The goals of glaucoma treatment are to reduce the pressure in the eye and to prevent further damage to the optic nerve. In certain cases, corrective surgery may be appropriate for treatment of glaucoma.

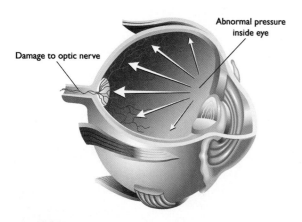

Damage to optic nerve

Abnormal pressure inside eye

FIGURE 14.18 The effects of glaucoma.

Hyperopia

Hyperopia, also known as farsightedness, is a disorder in which people have difficulty focusing on close objects. It occurs because the light entering the eye focuses behind the retina instead of directly on it.

Eyeglasses, contact lenses, or surgery can change the way the light rays bend when entering your eye and can all be used to correct hyperopia.

Myopia

Myopia is also known as nearsightedness. People with myopia have difficulty seeing distant objects and can only see objects when those objects are close to the eyes. In myopia, the eyeball is larger or longer or the cornea has too much curvature.

This eye disorder is easily corrected with eyeglasses, contact lenses, or surgery. Radial keratotomy (RK) is a procedure in which radial incisions are cut into the cornea to induce a flattening of the cornea. In LASIK surgery, excimer lasers are used to remove thin layers of the cornea to correct myopia.

Retinal Detachment

Retinal detachment is a disorder in which the retina is separated from its underlying tissue. It is usually the result of a retinal break, hole, or tear. This can be caused by the normal aging process, diseases that cause buildup of fluids underneath the retina, or trauma to the eye. After the retina has torn, liquid from the vitreous humor accumulates behind the retina. The buildup of fluid behind the retina causes the retina to separate from the back of the eye. Symptoms include flashing lights, floaters, and gradual vision loss.

Treatment will depend on the cause of the hole or tear. Surgery, limiting eye movements, and heat and cold therapies to create a sterile inflammatory reaction that causes the retina to re-adhere can be used to reattach the retina.

Strabismus

Strabismus, also known as crossed eyes, is a condition in which one eye deviates from the other. One of the eyes may look in or out or turn up or down. An abnormally inward gaze is called esotropia and an abnormally outward gaze is known as exotropia.

The absence of coordinated eye movement can cause double vision or the inability to see objects clearly. It results from an imbalance in eye muscles or as a result of extreme farsightedness. If the affected eye is not treated, a condition known as amblyopia (lazy eye) can occur. This results when the eyes are misaligned.

Treatment for mild to moderate strabismus focuses on use of an eye patch to cover the stronger eye, forcing the weaker eye to work. Eye exercises and eyeglasses can also help strengthen the affected eye. In more severe cases, surgery to adjust the muscles is often indicated.

Stye

A **stye** is a painful red bump inside the eyelid or at the base of an eyelash. It results from an infection of the glands of the eyelids that occurs after the glands have become clogged or from an infected hair follicle at the base of an eyelash. Symptoms include tenderness, redness, light sensitivity, and pain in the affected area.

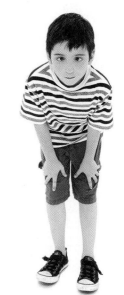

Strabismus is also known as crossed eyes.

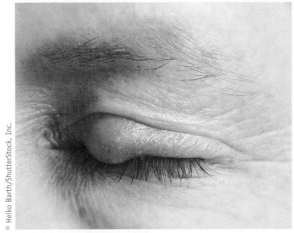

A stye is a painful bump inside the eyelid or at the base of an eyelash.

Applying a warm compress to the affected area can relieve symptoms and facilitate rupture of the stye.

Diseases and Disorders of the Ear

Disorders of the ear are common, and range from pain (otalagia), to excess wax in the ear canal, to complicated infections. In contrast to other medical conditions, 87 percent of patients with ear complaints seek medical care.

Auditory Canal Obstruction

This occurs when something blocks the opening of the ear canal. Excess cerumen (earwax) in the ear canal is one of the most common complaints seen in general practice. It can lead to pain, ringing in the ears, **vertigo** (a type of dizziness in which an individual feels a sense of motion even when still), hearing loss, and damage to the ear canal. It can also be caused by a foreign body, such as a bean, pea, or pebble.

Treatment consists of removal of the foreign object or the excess wax from the ear. Earwax solvents soften, loosen, and remove excess wax that builds up in the ear canal. Earwax can also be removed by gentle scraping with a cerumen spoon or irrigation by syringe.

Otitis Media

Otitis media is an infection of the middle ear. It is often caused by an infection. It is characterized by ear pain, fever, and hearing loss. Excessive pressure can cause the tympanic membrane to rupture, resulting in drainage into the canal.

Treatment may require antibiotics and pain medication. Some children may require a tympanostomy, which involves the insertion of a tiny polyethylene tube through the tympanic membrane to equalize the pressure. Solutions should not be administered to people with tubes in their ears or a ruptured eardrum. Suspensions, however, may be safely used in these patients.

Eye and Ear Care

Good eye health and eye care can prevent eye injuries, prevent common eye disorders, and protect your sight. As a medical assistant, you can encourage patients to have their eyes and ears checked routinely. You can also advise patients not to put anything into their ears to avoid damaging the tympanic membrane. Instruct patients that ear and eye medications must only be used with the consent of their healthcare provider.

Medical Abbreviations

In most cases, directions for use are written in shorthand, or an abbreviated form that allows for the easy writing of directions. Directions generally include how and when to take the medication ordered.

The medical assistant must have knowledge of commonly used abbreviations found in prescription orders or directions. These directions must be spelled out as simply as possible for the patient to ensure that the patient uses the medication properly. TABLE 14.4 lists common medical abbreviations related to the sensory organs. Because of concerns about drug errors that have occurred from misinterpretation of prescription orders, the Institute for Safe Medication Practices (ISMP) has compiled a list of common misread abbreviations. These are listed in TABLE 14.5.

Table 14.4 Common Medical Abbreviations Related to the Sensory Organs	
Abbreviation	**Translation**
AD	Right ear
AS	Left ear
AU	Both ears
IN	Intranasal
INH	Inhalation
OD	Right eye
OS	Left eye
OU	Both eyes
top	Topically
ud	As directed

Table 14.5 Common Problematic Abbreviations Related to the Sensory Organs			
Abbreviation	**Intended Meaning**	**Misinterpretation**	**Correction**
AD	Right ear	OD (right eye)	Write out right ear
AS	Left ear	OS (left eye)	Write out left ear
AU	Both ears	OU (both eyes)	Write out both ears
IN	Intranasal	IM or IV (intramuscular or intravenous)	Write out intranasal or NAS
OD	Right eye	AD (right ear)	Write out right eye
OS	Left eye	AS (left ear)	Write out left eye
OU	Both eyes	AU (both ears)	Write out both eyes
ud	As directed	Unit dose	Write out as directed

Instillation and Irrigation

Instillation refers to the dispensation of a sterile ophthalmic medication into a patient's eye or ear. **Irrigation** is the introduction of flushing fluid into the inner corner of the eye that is next to the nose and letting the fluid run across the eye to the outer edge or the introduction of flushing fluid to the ear canal. Irrigation is used to remove foreign objects from the eye or ear.

Steps for Instilling Eye Drops or Ointments

The purpose of instilling eye drops or ointments is to treat eye infections, dilate pupils, soothe irritation, and anesthetize.

Equipment Needed

- Sterile eyedropper
- Sterile ophthalmic medication drops or ophthalmic ointment
- Disposable gloves
- Sterile cotton balls
- Tissues

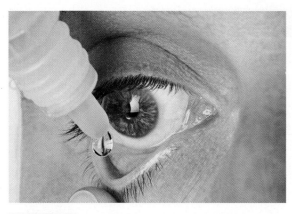

FIGURE 14.19 Instilling eye drops.
© zoompix/Alamy Images

Steps

1. Wash your hands thoroughly.
2. Gather all supplies using sterile technique.
3. Check the medication ordered, including the expiration date, and verify that the medication ordered is for this patient.
4. Identify the patient.
5. Position the patient in a sitting or lying-down position.
6. Explain the procedure to the patient.
7. Apply disposable gloves.
8. Tilt the patient's head back. Tell the patient to stare at a fixed spot during instillation of the drops or application of ointment.
9. Place the eyedropper directly over the eye. Be careful not to touch the surface of the eye with the eyedropper. If applying ointment, place tube of ointment directly over the eye. Be careful not to touch the surface of the eye with the tube.
10. Using your fingers, pull down on the lower lid of the affected eye to expose the conjunctival sac.
11. Instill a drop into the pocket of the eyelid or squeeze a ribbon of ointment from the tube and let it fall into the pocket of the eyelid **FIGURE 14.19**.
12. Slowly release the lower eyelid and close the eye. Instruct the patient to gently roll the eye around to distribute the ointment or drops. Tell the patient to minimize blinking or squeezing the eyelid for several minutes.
13. You or the patient should then gently press on the tear duct and blot excess medication from the eyelids with a cotton ball or tissue. Always wipe from the inner to outer eye.
14. If more than one drop is required, wait five minutes between drops to ensure that the first drop is not washed away by subsequent drops.
15. Dispose of all supplies.
16. Remove your gloves and wash your hands thoroughly.
17. Record the procedure in the patient's chart or medical record. Include the following information in the patient's chart or medical record: the name of the eyedrops or ophthalmic ointment, the quantity administered, the frequency of administration, and the eye in which it was administered.

Steps for Irrigating the Eye

The purpose of irrigating the eye is to remove foreign objects or discharge, soothe eyes, or relieve inflammation.

Equipment Needed

- Sterile eye irrigation solution
- Sterile irrigation syringe
- Disposable gloves
- Sterile cotton balls

- Small basin
- Towel
- Biohazard waste container

Steps

1. Wash your hands thoroughly.
2. Gather all supplies using sterile technique. If both eyes are to be irrigated, use separate equipment for each eye to prevent cross-contamination.
3. Check the medication ordered, including the expiration date, and verify that the medication ordered is for this patient.
4. Position the patient in a sitting or lying-down position.
5. Apply disposable gloves.
6. Warm the irrigation solution to body temperature.
7. Place a towel on the patient to protect his or her clothing.
8. Tilt the patient's head toward the affected eye and place the small basin beside the affected eye. Ask the patient to hold the basin in place. It is important to prevent any solution from entering the other eye.
9. Gently wipe the eye from the inner to outer eye to remove any particles.
10. Hold the affected eye open with the index finger and thumb and slowly release the solution over the eye from the inside canthus to the outer corner of the eye. Ask the patient to stare at a fixed spot **FIGURE 14.20**.
11. Using sterile cotton balls or tissue, wipe the eyelid and eyelashes.
12. Dispose of all supplies.
13. Remove your gloves and wash your hands thoroughly.
14. Record the procedure in the patient's chart or medical record. Include the following information in the patient's chart or medical record: the name of the irrigation fluid, the quantity administered, the frequency of administration, and the eye in which it was administered.

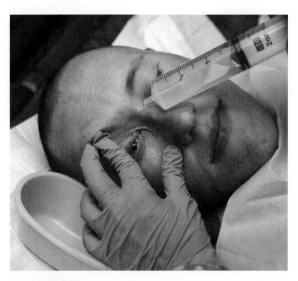

FIGURE 14.20 Performing eye irrigation.
© Jones & Bartlett Learning. Courtesy of MIEMSS.

Steps for Instilling Ear Drops

The purpose of instilling ear drops is to treat ear infections, soothe irritation, soften cerumen, or relieve pain.

Equipment Needed

- Sterile ear dropper
- Otic medication drops
- Disposable gloves
- Sterile cotton balls

Steps

1. Wash your hands thoroughly.
2. Gather all supplies using sterile technique.

3. Check the medication ordered, including the expiration date, and verify that the medication ordered is for this patient.

4. Position the patient in a sitting or lying-down position with his or her head tilted toward the unaffected ear.

5. Apply disposable gloves.

6. Gently pull the top of the ear upward and backward (adult) or pull the earlobe downward and backward (child).

7. Instill a drop into the affected ear.

8. Ask the patient to lie still for five minutes to retain medication in the ear.

9. Place a moistened cotton ball in the external ear canal to help the medication stay in the ear (if instructed by the physician).

10. Dispose of all supplies.

11. Remove your gloves and wash your hands thoroughly.

12. Record the procedure in the patient's chart or medical record. Include the following information in the patient's chart or medical record: the name of the ear drops, the quantity administered, the frequency of administration, and the affected ear in which it was administered.

Steps for Irrigating the Ear

The purpose of irrigating the ear is to remove foreign objects or discharge or impacted cerumen.

Equipment Needed

- Ear irrigation solution
- Irrigation syringe
- Disposable gloves
- Cotton balls
- Small basin or ear basin
- Towel
- Biohazard waste container
- Otoscope

Steps

1. Wash your hands thoroughly.

2. Gather all supplies using sterile technique.

3. Check the medication ordered, including the expiration date, and verify that the medication ordered is for this patient.

4. Position the patient in a sitting position.

5. Warm the irrigation solution to body temperature.

6. Place a towel on the patient to protect his or her clothing.

7. Apply disposable gloves.

8. View the affected ear with an otoscope.

9. Tilt the patient's head toward the affected ear and place the small basin beside the affected ear. Ask the patient to hold the basin in place.

10. Gently wipe the outer ear with a wet cotton ball to remove any particles.

11. With one hand, gently pull the top of the ear upward and backward (adult) or pull the earlobe downward and backward (child).

12. With the other hand, place the tip of the syringe into the canal and direct the flow of the solution upward toward the roof of the canal.

13. Allow the solution to drain from the ear by instructing the patient to tilt his or her head to the side.

14. Using an otoscope, inspect the ear canal. Repeat the irrigation as needed.

15. Using cotton balls or tissue, wipe the ear.

16. Dispose of all supplies.

17. Remove your gloves and wash your hands thoroughly.

18. Record the procedure in the patient's chart or medical record. Include the following information in the patient's chart or medical record: name of the irrigation fluid, the quantity administered, the frequency of administration, and the ear in which it was administered.

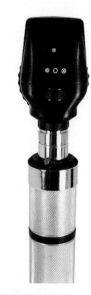

FIGURE 14.21 An ophthalmoscope.
© bsites/ShutterStock, Inc.

Eye Examination

The medical assistant may be expected to assist the provider with eye examinations. Assembling the instruments in the correct order of use and making sure that the instruments are clean and in working order is an essential role of the medical assistant.

Most often, the instrument needed for visualization of the inner part of the eye (ophthalmoscope) is mounted to the wall of the examination room **FIGURE 14.21**. The ophthalmoscope should be checked to make sure that the lightbulb is strong enough to provide adequate light for examination. The lightbulb should be changed periodically. In some cases, the ophthalmoscope may be battery operated; you may be responsible for changing the batteries.

Visual examinations may need to be performed if a patient has an eye injury or an infection, or as a screening to check visual acuity. The doctor or healthcare provider may ask you to perform the vision screenings.

Visual acuity is measured as part of the physical examination. It is most often performed by the medical assistant as a diagnostic screening procedure. The test should be performed in a well-lit area, free from distractions. The medical assistant should note signs or behaviors that may indicate visual disturbances, such as tilting of the head to one side or forward, blinking of the eyes, straining to see, squinting or closing of one eye when testing both eyes, or puckering of the face.

The most common screening for distance vision is the **Snellen chart** **FIGURE 14.22**. This is a visual screening test used to determine a patient's distance visual acuity. There are many variations of the Snellen chart, but it usually contains 11 rows of capital letters. Small children or those who don't know the alphabet can use a modified version of the Snellen chart called the tumbling E chart **FIGURE 14.23**. This

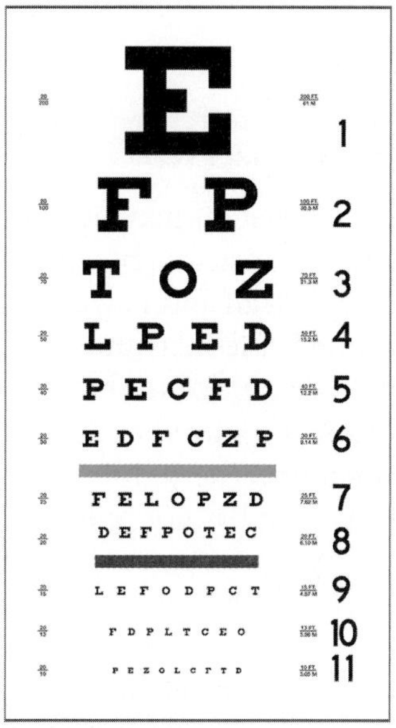

FIGURE 14.22 The Snellen chart is used to determine a patient's distance visual acuity.
© Germán Ariel Berra/ShutterStock, Inc.

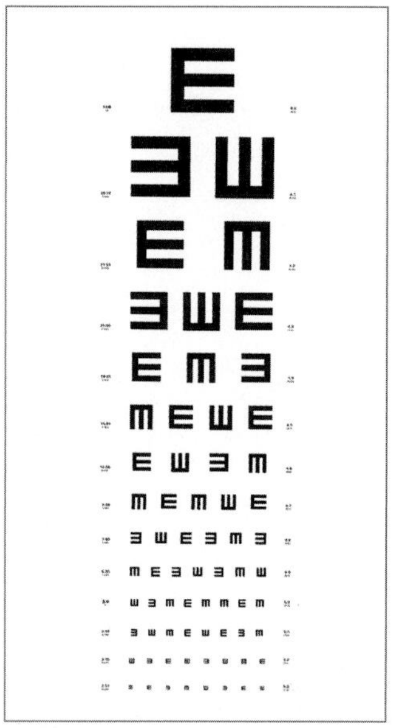

FIGURE 14.23 The tumbling E chart is used for small children or those who don't know the alphabet.
© anaken2012/ShutterStock, Inc.

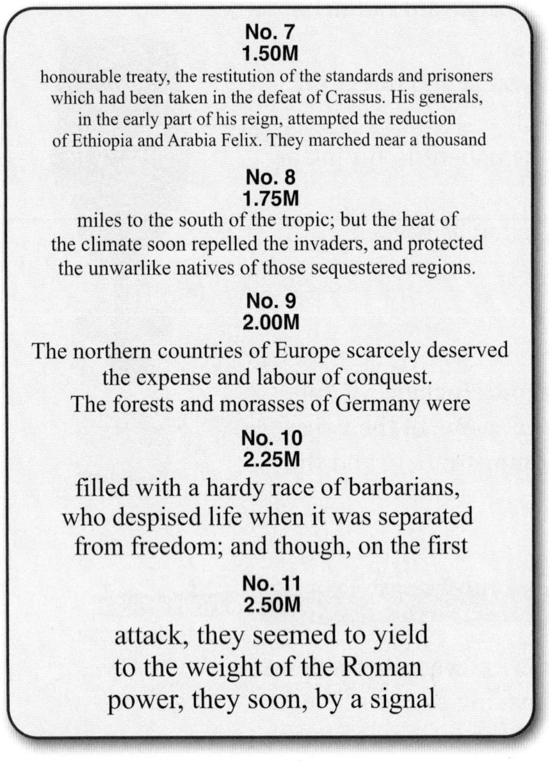

No. 7
1.50M

honourable treaty, the restitution of the standards and prisoners
which had been taken in the defeat of Crassus. His generals,
in the early part of his reign, attempted the reduction
of Ethiopia and Arabia Felix. They marched near a thousand

No. 8
1.75M

miles to the south of the tropic; but the heat of
the climate soon repelled the invaders, and protected
the unwarlike natives of those sequestered regions.

No. 9
2.00M

The northern countries of Europe scarcely deserved
the expense and labour of conquest.
The forests and morasses of Germany were

No. 10
2.25M

filled with a hardy race of barbarians,
who despised life when it was separated
from freedom; and though, on the first

No. 11
2.50M

attack, they seemed to yield
to the weight of the Roman
power, they soon, by a signal

FIGURE 14.24 The Jaeger chart is used to screen for near vision acuity.

© Jones & Bartlett Learning

chart has the same scale as the standard Snellen chart, but all the letters on the chart are different spatial orientations of the capital E. The chart is hung on a wall and the patient is instructed to stand 20 feet away. The patient covers one eye with an occluder so that each eye can be tested individually. The patient is asked to read the smallest line possible without making a mistake. If that line cannot be read, the patient should be instructed to read the line above it. The results are then recorded.

Distance visual acuity is expressed as a fraction. Scoring for the Snellen chart is based on a distance of 20 feet and is represented as a fraction. The patient must stand 20 feet away from the chart in order for the test results to be accurate. The denominator is the number listed to the right of each row on the eye chart. It represents the normal distance at which people with "normal" vision can read a letter of that row's size. The patient must be able to read the whole line to receive that score. The numerator is the distance from the chart. A 20/20 reading is average and means that the patient can see at 20 feet what should be able to be seen at a distance of 20 feet. A 20/60 reading means that the patient can see at 60 feet what should be able to be seen at a distance of 20 feet.

The **Jaeger chart** is used to screen for near vision acuity **FIGURE 14.24**. The patient should be tested with and without eyeglasses or contact lenses. This chart is a handheld chart that is held 14–16 inches away (the distance a person with normal vision can read printed material) from the eye. The chart contains excerpts of short paragraphs with type of various sizes. The patient is asked to read the smallest type possible without making a mistake. The results are then recorded.

Ear Examination

The medical assistant may be expected to assist the provider with ear examinations. Assembling the instruments in the correct order of use and making sure that the instruments are clean and in working order is an essential role of the medical assistant.

Most often, the instrument needed for visualization of the inner part of the ear (otoscope) is mounted to the wall of the examination room. The otoscope should be checked to make sure that the lightbulb is strong enough to provide adequate light for examination. The lightbulb should be changed periodically. In some cases, the otoscope may be battery operated; you may be responsible for changing the batteries. Most physicians use a disposable plastic ear speculum to prevent transmission of disease. If nondisposable specula are used, the specula should be sterilized after each use.

Auditory acuity may also be measured as part of the physical examination. The medical assistant should note signs or behaviors that may indicate auditory disturbances such as frequently asking to repeat what was said, talking in a loud voice, not responding when spoken to, turning the best ear toward the sound source, standing close during conversation, and not communicating well. Symptoms that can indicate hearing loss include ringing in the ears and bleeding from the ear.

During a physical examination, the doctor may use a tuning fork to test hearing. This test can be used to assess nerve or conduction deafness. An **audiometer** measures the frequency of sound waves and the ability of the patient to hear various frequencies of sound waves. The patient is instructed to wear earphones. The machine provides a series of tones and tests one ear at a time. The patient signals each time a sound is heard **FIGURE 14.25**.

Neurological Examination

A neurological examination assesses motor and sensory skills, hearing, speech, vision, coordination, mental status, mood, behavior, memory, and cognition. One example of a test performed during a neurological examination is the knee-jerk reflex test **FIGURE 14.26**. To test the knee-jerk reflex, also called the patellar reflex, a small hammer is used to tap the tendon below the kneecap. This test is used to assess for nerve damage.

The mental status examination can be performed by the medical assistant when taking the patient's medical history. The medical assistant must pay careful attention to the level of awareness, memory, coordination, balance, cognition, and mood of a patient. The medical assistant will also assist the doctor and patient as needed before, during, and after the examination.

Items required by a provider for a neurological examination include the following **FIGURE 14.27**:

- Tuning fork
- Reflex hammer
- Ophthalmoscope
- Safety pin or sensory wheel
- Cotton ball
- Flashlight
- Tongue blade
- Material for odor identification (examples include coffee grounds or soap)

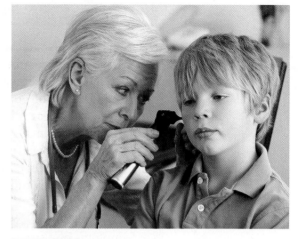

FIGURE 14.25 A patient receiving an ear examination.
© Monkey Business Images/ShutterStock, Inc.

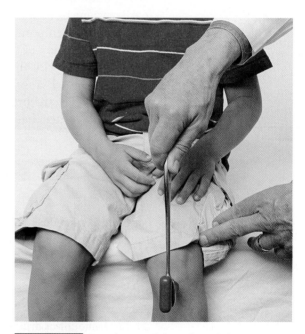

FIGURE 14.26 A patient receiving a knee-jerk test.
© AISPIX by Image Source/ShutterStock, Inc.

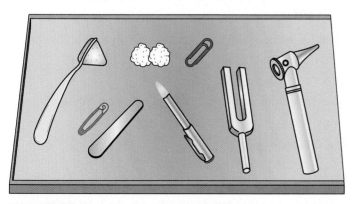

FIGURE 14.27 Tools used in a neurological exam.
© Jones & Bartlett Learning

Cerebral Vascular Accident

A **cerebral vascular accident (CVA)** is more commonly known as a stroke or brain attack. It is a medical emergency that is caused when blood flow to part of the brain stops. Immediate emergency medical attention (call 911) should be sought in the event of a stroke. The goal is to get the patient to the hospital as quickly as possible. If the blood flow ceases for more than a few seconds, it can cause the brain cells to die, resulting in permanent damage.

There are two main types of stroke: ischemic stroke and hemorrhagic stroke. Ischemic stroke occurs when a clot forms in a narrow artery (thrombotic stroke) or when a clot breaks off from another part of the body and travels to the brain (embolic stroke), causing the blood vessel that supplies the brain to be blocked. A hemorrhagic stroke occurs when a blood vessel in the brain bursts, causing blood to leak into the brain.

Symptoms of a stroke will vary depending on what part of the brain is damaged. They can include headache, altered mental status, loss of balance, changes in taste and hearing, numbness or tingling on one side of the body, and mood changes.

A transient ischemic attack (TIA) is a short-lived stroke that resolves within 24 hours. It causes temporary loss of brain function in the area of the body that is controlled by the portion of the brain that was affected. The loss of brain function is usually the result of a clot that causes loss of blood supply to the brain. The clot usually forms in the blood vessels of the brain, but it can also occur in another part of the body and travel to the brain. A TIA should also be considered an emergency because there is no guarantee that the situation will resolve and brain function will be restored.

Math Practice

Question: **If each dose is 7.5mL, and the total amount of drug to be administered is 150mL, what is the total number of doses available?**

Answer: The total number of doses available is 150mL ÷ 7.5mL = 20

Question: **If the dose is 25mg daily, and the duration of therapy is 14 days, what is the total amount of drug needed to complete the course of therapy?**

Answer: The total amount of drug needed to complete therapy is 25mg × 14 days = 350mg

Question: **What is the total amount of drug to be administered if each dose is 25mg and the total number of doses is 40?**

Answer: Multiply the number of doses by the quantity of each dose: 25mg/dose × 40 doses = 1,000mg

Question: **What is the total dose for a child weighing 15kg and requiring a dose of 0.25mg/kg?**

Answer: The total dose is 15kg × 0.25mg/kg = 3.75mg

Question: **A 36-year-old 145-pound female is prescribed a drug to treat her seizures. The physician orders 50mg/kg/day divided into two doses. What is the total daily**

dose of the drug? What is the dose of the drug that the patient will receive with each administration?

Answer: First, convert the woman's weight from pounds to kilograms: 145 lb × 1kg ÷ 2.2 lb = 66kg

Then, determine the number of milligrams per day: 66kg × 50mg/kg = 3,300mg/day

Finally, determine the milligrams per dose: 3,300mg/day × 1 day ÷ 2 doses = 1,650mg/dose

Question: **A pediatric patient with attention deficit disorder is prescribed methylphenidate 6mg/kg/day divided into two doses each day. If the patient weighs 32 pounds, what is the total daily dose that he will receive? What is the dose of the drug that the patient will receive with each administration?**

Answer: First, convert the child's weight to kilograms: 32 lb × 1kg ÷ 2.2 lb = 15kg

Next, determine the number of milligrams per day: 15kg × 6mg/kg/day = 90mg/day (rounded up)

Finally, determine the milligrams per dose: 90 ÷ 2 doses = 45mg/dose

WRAP UP

Chapter Summary

- Medical assistants must have a good working knowledge of medical terminology.

- The central nervous system (CNS) is the body's control center and includes the brain and spinal cord.

- The peripheral nervous system (PNS) includes all the nerves that connect the CNS to every organ and area of the body. It includes 12 pairs of cranial nerves that connect the brain directly to the sense organs, the heart, the lungs, and other internal organs. It also includes 31 pairs of spinal nerves.

- The PNS is divided into the afferent system and the efferent system. The afferent system includes all the nerves and sense organs. These nerves and organs take in information and send it to the CNS. The efferent system includes all the nerves and pathways that send information from the CNS to other organs and body systems.

- The autonomic nervous system controls internal organs and other self-regulating body functions. The parasympathetic nervous system returns the body to a normal state. The somatic nervous system controls all the skeletal muscles in the body.

- The brain and spinal cord are protected by three connective tissue layers collectively called the meninges. The meninges support blood vessels and contain cerebrospinal fluid.

- The brain is divided into five parts. The cerebrum is the largest part of the brain. It controls sensory and motor activities. The cerebellum lies just beneath the cerebrum. It is responsible for motor movement coordination, balance, equilibrium, and muscle tone. The brain stem connects the brain to the spinal cord. The thalamus lies between the cerebrum and the midbrain. It is involved in sensory perception and regulation of motor functions. The hypothalamus lies below the thalamus and between the cerebrum and the midbrain. It is connected to the pituitary gland, midbrain, and thalamus by a bundle of nerve fibers. It is the control center for many autonomic functions of the PNS. It is involved in many functions, including autonomic function control, endocrine function control, homeostasis, motor function control, food and water intake regulation, and sleep-wake cycle regulation.

- The brain stem is divided into three parts. The medulla oblongata controls autonomic functions, such as breathing, digestion, heart and blood-vessel function, and sneezing. It helps transfer messages between the spinal cord and various parts of the brain. The pons serves as the communication center between the two hemispheres of the brain. It is the reflex center for secreting saliva, chewing, and tasting. The midbrain is superior to the pons and is the control center for visual reflexes such as moving the head and eyes. It also conducts impulses between the brain parts above and below it.

- Diagnostic tests and procedures are vital tools that help doctors confirm or rule out the presence of a neurological disorder or other medical condition.

- A neurological examination assesses motor and sensory skills, hearing, speech, vision, coordination, balance, mental status, changes in mood or behavior, and the functioning of cranial nerves.

- A cerebral angiogram can detect the degree of narrowing of an artery or blood vessel in the brain, head, or neck.

- Brain scans are imaging techniques used to study organ function, injury, and disease, and to diagnose tumors, blood-vessel malformations, and hemorrhage in the brain.

- Cerebrospinal fluid analysis involves the removal of a small amount of the CSF by lumbar puncture or spinal tap.

- Computed tomography, also known as a CT or CAT scan, is used to produce rapid, clear images of organs, bones, and tissues. Neurological CT scans are used to view the brain and spine.

- Electroencephalography (EEG) monitors brain activity through the skull.

- Electromyography (EMG) records the electrical activity from the brain and/or spinal cord to a peripheral nerve root found in the arms and legs that controls muscles during contraction and at rest.

- Electronystagmography (ENG) is used to diagnose involuntary eye movement, dizziness, and balance disorders, and to evaluate some brain functions.

- Evoked potentials (also called evoked response) measure the electrical signals to the brain generated by hearing, touch, or sight.

- Magnetic resonance imaging (MRI) uses computer-generated radio waves and a magnetic field to produce detailed images of body structures, including tissues, organs, bones, and nerves.

- Myelography is an X-ray examination of the spinal canal. A contrast agent is injected through a needle into the space around the spinal cord to display the spinal cord, spinal canal, and nerve roots on an X-ray.

- Positron emission tomography (PET) scans provide two- and three-dimensional pictures of brain activity by measuring radioactive isotopes that are injected into the bloodstream.

- Neurosonography (ultrasound of the brain and spinal column) analyzes blood flow in the brain and can diagnose stroke, brain tumors, hydrocephalus (excess cerebrospinal fluid in the brain), and vascular problems.

- A videonystagmograph is a special examination that measures eye movements and is used to evaluate balance.

- Alzheimer's disease (AD) is a degenerative disorder of the brain that leads to loss of brain function. It results in memory impairment and in loss of judgment, decision-making ability, and speech. It also results in changes in personality and behavior.

- Amyotrophic lateral sclerosis (Lou Gehrig's disease) is a progressive neurological disease that attacks the neurons that control voluntary muscles.

- Bell's palsy is a disorder of the nerve that controls movement of the facial muscles. Damage to the seventh cranial nerve (facial nerve), the nerve that controls the movement of the muscles of the face, causes muscle weakness or paralysis of facial muscles.

- Encephalitis is a severe inflammation of the brain that can destroy nerve cells, cause bleeding in the brain, and cause brain damage.

- Epilepsy is a neurological condition that is also known as a seizure disorder. It is characterized by sudden and recurring seizures.

- Meningitis is an inflammation of the membranes that cover the brain and spinal cord.

- Parkinson's disease is a motor-system disorder caused primarily by progressive degeneration of dopamine-containing neurons in the substantia nigra, which is the layer of gray substance in the brain.

- There are five major senses: sight, hearing, smell, taste, and touch. Equilibrium is associated with the sense of hearing and plays a major role in our ability to maintain balance. The organs associated with these senses include the eyes, ears, nose, tongue, and skin.

- Age-related macular degeneration (AMD) is a disease that affects the macula and causes loss of central vision. There are two types of AMD: dry AMD and wet AMD.

- Blepharitis is an inflammation of the edges of the eyelids. It can cause a burning sensation, excessive tearing, light sensitivity, redness, and crusting of the eyelashes.

- A cataract is a condition in which the normally clear lens of the eye becomes cloudy. It frequently occurs as part of the aging process. People with cataracts complain of seeing halos around lights.

- Chronic dry eye (keratoconjunctivitis) is one of the most common disorders affecting the eye. With this condition, the eye is not able to produce enough tears to lubricate and nourish the eye.

- Conjunctivitis is an inflammation of the outer membrane of the eye. It usually begins in one eye and spreads to the other from contamination by hands or by a washcloth. It is more commonly known as pink eye.

- Corneal ulcers are caused by infections of the cornea.

■ Diabetic retinopathy is a complication of diabetes. It affects the blood vessels in the retina and, if left untreated, can lead to blindness. There are two types of diabetic retinopathy: nonproliferative retinopathy and proliferative retinopathy.

■ Glaucoma is a common disorder of the eye characterized by increased ocular pressure. The increased pressure is a result of an imbalance of the production and drainage of fluid within the eye. The pressure damages the optic nerve and causes partial vision loss.

■ Hyperopia, also known as farsightedness, is a disorder in which people have difficulty focusing on close objects. It occurs because the light entering the eye focuses behind the retina instead of directly on it.

■ Myopia is also known as nearsightedness. People with myopia have difficulty seeing distant objects and can only see objects when the objects are close to the eyes. In myopia, the eyeball is larger or longer or the cornea has too much curvature.

■ Retinal detachment is a disorder in which the retina is separated from its underlying tissue. It is usually the result of a retinal break, hole, or tear. This can be caused by the normal aging process, diseases that cause buildup of fluids underneath the retina, or trauma to the eye. Once the retina has torn, liquid from the vitreous humor accumulates behind the retina. The buildup of fluid behind the retina causes the retina to separate from the back of the eye.

■ Strabismus, also known as crossed eyes, is a condition in which one eye deviates from the other. One of the eyes may look in or out or turn up or down.

■ A stye is a painful red bump inside the eyelid or at the base of an eyelash. It results from an infection of the glands of the eyelids that occurs after the glands have become clogged or from an infected hair follicle at the base of an eyelash.

■ Otitis media is an infection of the middle ear. It is commonly caused by a bacterial infection but may also be viral. Instillation refers to the dispensation of a sterile ophthalmic medication into a patient's eye or ear. Irrigation is the introduction of flushing fluid into the inner corner of the eye that is next to the nose and letting the fluid run across the eye to the outer edge or introduction of flushing fluid upward toward the roof of the ear canal and allowing the solution to drain from the ear.

■ Irrigation is used to remove foreign objects from the eye or ear.

■ The most common screening for distance vision is the Snellen chart. This is a visual screening test used to determine a patient's distance visual acuity.

■ The Jaeger chart is used to screen for near vision acuity.

■ A neurological examination assesses motor and sensory skills, hearing, speech, vision, coordination, mental status, mood, behavior, memory, and cognition.

■ A cerebral vascular accident is more commonly known as a stroke or brain attack. It is a medical emergency that is caused when blood flow to part of the brain stops. If the blood flow ceases for more than a few seconds, it can cause the brain cells to die, resulting in permanent damage.

Learning Assessment Questions

1. What is the basic functioning unit of the nervous system?
   A. Axon
   B. Dendrite
   C. Neuron
   D. Meninges

2. What function(s) does the autonomic nervous system control?
   A. Breathing
   B. Digestion
   C. Heartbeat
   D. All of the above

3. What is the name of the condition in which the normally clear lens of the eye becomes cloudy?

   A. Myopia

   B. Glaucoma

   C. Cataract

   D. Retinal detachment

4. Which disorder is also known as nearsightedness?

   A. Myopia

   B. Presbyopia

   C. Glaucoma

   D. Cataract

5. Which disorder is also known as farsightedness?

   A. Myopia

   B. Presbyopia

   C. Hyperopia

   D. Cataract

6. Which of the following is a motor-system disorder caused primarily by progressive degeneration of dopamine-containing neurons in the substantia nigra?

   A. Alzheimer's disease

   B. Parkinson's disease

   C. Lou Gehrig's disease

   D. Encephalitis

7. Which of the following is more commonly known as a stroke?

   A. Cerebral vascular accident

   B. Epilepsy

   C. Parkinson's disease

   D. Meningitis

8. What part of the brain is involved in sensory perception and regulation of motor functions?

   A. Thalamus

   B. Hypothalamus

   C. Midbrain

   D. Pons

9. Which of the following examinations assesses motor and sensory skills, hearing, speech, vision, coordination, balance, mental status, changes in mood or behavior, and the functioning of cranial nerves?

   A. Snellen chart

   B. Neurological examination

   C. CT scan

   D. PET scan

10. What test would you use to detect the degree of narrowing of an artery or blood vessel in the brain, head, or neck?

    A. CT scan

    B. PET scan

    C. MRI

    D. Cerebral angiogram

11. Which of the following diagnostic tests uses computer-generated radio waves and a magnetic field to produce detailed images of body structures, including tissues, organs, bones, and nerves?

    A. CT scan

    B. PET scan

    C. MRI

    D. Cerebral angiogram

12. Which of the following disorders is the result of damage to the seventh cranial nerve?

    A. Bell's palsy

    B. Parkinson's disease

    C. Amyotrophic lateral sclerosis

    D. Epilepsy

13. Which of the following is characterized by increased ocular pressure?

    A. Glaucoma

    B. Myopia

    C. Conjunctivitis

    D. Blepharitis

14. Which of the following is characterized by an inflammation of the membranes that cover the brain and spinal cord?
    A. Parkinson's disease
    B. Amyotrophic lateral sclerosis
    C. Epilepsy
    D. Meningitis

15. Which of the following is the thin mucous membrane that covers the inner surface of the eyelid and the sclera?
    A. Retina
    B. Iris
    C. Conjunctiva
    D. Strabismus

16. Which test is used to screen for near vision acuity?
    A. Snellen chart
    B. Jaeger chart
    C. Reflex chart
    D. Sasson chart

17. Which of the following would be needed for a neurological examination?
    A. Tuning fork
    B. Reflex hammer
    C. Sensory wheel
    D. All of the above

18. What procedure is used to remove foreign objects from the eye or ear?
    A. Irrigation
    B. Instillation
    C. Application
    D. Fumigation

19. Which of the following is a type of dizziness in which an individual feels a sense of motion even when still?
    A. Myopia
    B. Epilepsy
    C. Vertigo
    D. Seizure

20. Which of the following is the clear, dome-shaped surface that covers the front of the eye and allows light into the eye for visual acuity?
    A. Retina
    B. Iris
    C. Cornea
    D. Pons

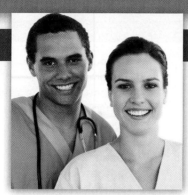

Endocrine System

KEY TERMS

Acromegaly
Addison's disease
Adenohypophysis
Adrenal cortex
Adrenal medulla
Adrenocorticotropic
    hormone (ACTH)
Androgens
Antidiuretic hormone
    (ADH)
Corticosteroids
Cushing's syndrome
Diabetes insipidus
Diabetes mellitus (DM)
Diabetic nephropathy
Diabetic neuropathy
Endocrine glands
Endocrinologist
Exocrine glands
Exophthalmos
Fasting blood glucose
    (FBG) test
Follicle-stimulating
    hormone (FSH)
Giantism
Glucagon

Glucocorticoid
Glucometer
Glucose tolerance test
    (GTT)
Glycosuria
Goiter
Gonads
Graves' disease
Hemoglobin A1c (HbA1c)
Hyperglycemia
Hypergonadism
Hyperparathyroidism
Hyperpituitarism
Hyperthyroidism
Hypogonadism
Hypoparathyroidism
Hypopituitarism
Hypothyroidism
Insulin
Islets of Langerhans
Isthmus
Luteinizing hormone (LH)
Melanocyte-stimulating
    hormone (MSH)
Melatonin
Mineralocorticoids

Myxedema
Neurohypophysis
Oxytocin
Parathormone
Parathyroid hormone
    (PTH)
Pineal gland
Precocious puberty
Prolactin
Tetany
Thymus
Thyroglobulin
Thyroid-stimulating
    hormone (TSH)
Thyrotoxicosis
Thyrotropin
Thyroxine (T4)
Triiodothyronine (T3)
Type 1 diabetes mellitus
    (DM)
Type 2 diabetes mellitus
    (DM)

Chapter Overview

The endocrine system is a network of glands that secrete hormones into the bloodstream FIGURE 15.1. Hormones are chemical messengers used by the body to communicate between cells. Hormones are diverse, ranging in structure and function. Some hormones directly affect a target cell and some hormones alter gene expression in target cells, changing the production of regulatory proteins.

Diseases and disorders of the endocrine system are common and often affect other organ systems, including the integumentary, digestive, reproductive, urinary, nervous, and circulatory systems. A medical specialist who studies the endocrine system is called an **endocrinologist**. As a medical assistant, you will have the opportunity to interact with patients with a variety of disorders of the endocrine system, as well as participate in diagnostic and treatment-related procedures. Most endocrine disorders are chronic, long-term conditions. You will also have the opportunity to educate patients about their endocrine disease and teach them to monitor their conditions with blood tests performed at home. Developing a strong rapport with your patients will promote compliance and improve health outcomes.

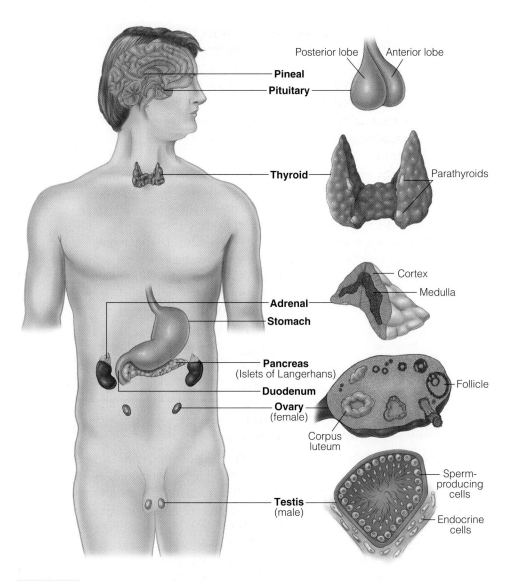

FIGURE 15.1 The endocrine system is a network of glands.

© Jones & Bartlett Learning

Terminology

TABLE 15.1 lists word roots and terms used in the study of the endocrine system.

Table 15.1 Word Roots of the Endocrine System		
Word Root or Term	**Meaning**	**Example**
Acr/o	Extremities	Acromegaly (enlargement of the extremities)
Aden/o	Glands	Adenoma (a benign tumor of the glands)
Andr/o	Male	Androgen (hormones that produce characteristics of maleness)
Cortic/o	Cortex, outer layer	Adrenocortical carcinoma (cancer of the outer layer of the adrenal gland)
Crin/o	Secrete	Endocrine (to secrete inside)
Dips/o	Thirst	Polydipsia (increased thirst)
Gluc/o	Sugar	Gluconeogenesis (producing sugar)

(Continues)

Table 15.1   Word Roots of the Endocrine System *(Continued)*

Word Root or Term	Meaning	Example
Glyc/o	Sugar	Hyperglycemia (increased levels of sugar in the blood)
Myx/o	Mucus	Myxocystoma (a mucus-filled tumor produced by ovarian epithelial cells)
Natr/o	Sodium	Natriuresis (the excretion of large amounts of sodium in the urine)
Phag/o	Hunger	Polyphagia (increased hunger)

Abbreviations Related to the Endocrine System

The following are abbreviations related to the endocrine system:

- ACTH—Adrenocorticotropic hormone
- ADH—Antidiuretic hormone
- Ca—Calcium
- DI—Diabetes insipidus
- DM—Diabetes mellitus
- FBS—Fasting blood sugar
- FSH—Follicle-stimulating hormone
- GH—Growth hormone
- GTT—Glucose tolerance test
- HbA1c—Hemoglobin A1c
- K—Potassium
- LH—Luteinizing hormone
- Na—Sodium
- PTH—Parathyroid hormone
- RIA—Radioimmunoassay
- T3—Triiodothyronine
- T4—Thyroxine
- T7—Free thyroxine index
- TFT—Thyroid function test
- TSH—Thyroid-stimulating hormone

Components of the Endocrine System

The body contains distinct types of glands: exocrine glands and endocrine glands. **Exocrine glands** secrete substances, including liquids, digestive enzymes, and hormones, through a duct or an organ. Sweat glands, mammary glands, and salivary glands are examples of exocrine glands. **Endocrine glands** secrete hormones directly into the bloodstream. Endocrine glands can also be called ductless glands because there are no ducts connecting the glands to another organ.

Endocrine glands comprise the endocrine system: the adrenal glands, gonads, parathyroid glands, pituitary gland, thymus gland, and thyroid gland. The glands of the endocrine system affect the functions of the entire body, including regulating fluid volume and electrolyte levels, managing digestion, stimulating sex-hormone production, and promoting growth. The entire endocrine system is interrelated through feedback mechanisms, a process in which the presence or absence of one hormone affects the secretion of another.

Adrenal Glands

A small, triangular adrenal gland is located above each kidney **FIGURE 15.2**. The adrenal gland is composed of two sections: the cortex (the outer portion) and the medulla (the inner portion). The **adrenal cortex** manufactures hormones called **corticosteroids**, which can be divided into mineralocorticoids, glucocorticoids, and androgens. **Mineralocorticoids** such as aldosterone control the concentration of salt and potassium in the body's fluids. **Glucocorticoids** control the formation of glycogen (stored sugar) in the liver. Glucocorticoids also promote the metabolism of fats and proteins and release fats stored in adipose tissue to be used as energy. Cortisol, or hydrocortisone, is the most active glucocorticoid. **Androgens** are similar to hormones produced in the testes that are responsible for male sex characteristics. Overproduction of androgens leads to exaggerated male characteristics. Low levels of the female sex hormones estrogen and progesterone are also produced by the adrenal cortex.

The **adrenal medulla** produces the catecholamines epinephrine (also called adrenaline) and norepinephrine, which are hormones of the sympathetic nervous system that are responsible for the fight-or-flight response to stressful situations. Epinephrine releases glycogen from the liver to provide energy for the body and increases the heart rate, which in turn increases cardiac output. Norepinephrine causes vasoconstriction but has similar effects to epinephrine.

Pituitary Gland

The pituitary gland (also known as the master gland) is located behind the optic nerve, below the cerebrum, in the brain. The pituitary gland controls the function of many other endocrine glands. It is divided into anterior and posterior lobes. The anterior portion, also known as the **adenohypophysis**, produces hormones that control growth and development through the production of growth hormone, **adrenocorticotropic hormone (ACTH)**, **thyrotropin** or **thyroid-stimulating hormone (TSH)**, **melanocyte-stimulating hormone (MSH)**, **prolactin**, and gonadotropic hormones that induce the maturation of sperm and eggs in the reproductive system, including **follicle-stimulating hormone (FSH)** and **luteinizing hormone (LH)**.

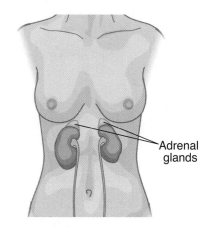

FIGURE 15.2 The adrenal glands sit on top of the kidneys.

© Jones & Bartlett Learning

Adrenal glands

The posterior portion of the pituitary gland, also known as the **neurohypophysis**, produces **antidiuretic hormone (ADH)**, also known as vasopressin, which facilitates water reabsorption in the kidneys. The posterior pituitary also produces **oxytocin**, the hormone responsible for stimulating the uterus to contract during childbirth and expelling milk from mammary glands.

The pituitary gland is known as the master gland in the body because it affects the function, growth, and development of many other glands and body systems.

© auremar/ShutterStock, Inc.

Pituitary Hormones

- **Growth hormone**—Directs the growth of body tissues, including bone length
- **Thyrotropin**—Increases the production of thyroid hormones in the thyroid
- **ACTH**—Stimulates the adrenal cortex to produce hormones
- **MSH**—Increases skin pigmentation
- **Prolactin**—Promotes breast development and the production of milk in the mammary glands
- **FSH**—Stimulates the ovarian follicle to produce estrogen in females and stimulates the production of sperm in males
- **LH**—Stimulates the ruptured ovarian follicle to become a corpus luteum and secrete progesterone in females and stimulates the testes to produce testosterone in males
- **Oxytocin**—Stimulates uterine contractions and milk secretion from the breast
- **ADH**—Concentrates and conserves water in the body

Thyroid Gland

The thyroid gland resembles the shape of a butterfly, with two lobes located on either side of the trachea and larynx **FIGURE 15.3**. The **isthmus** connects the two lobes of the thyroid. The thyroid is composed of large, cystlike units called follicles. Thyroid cartilage, more commonly called the Adam's apple, sits just below the thyroid gland and is visible in the neck. The thyroid produces the thyroid hormones **thyroxine (T4)** and **triiodothyronine (T3)** from the mineral iodine. The thyroid stores thyroxine in

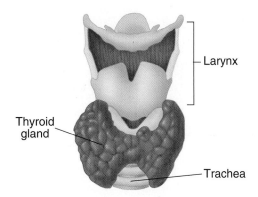

FIGURE 15.3 The thyroid glands sit on either side of the trachea and larynx.
© Jones & Bartlett Learning

the form of **thyroglobulin**. The thyroid also produces calcitonin, which reduces the level of calcium in the blood.

Thyroxine is released directly from the thyroid into the bloodstream and accounts for 95 percent of all thyroid hormone in the blood. Triiodothyronine accounts for the rest. Together, T3 and T4 increase the metabolic rate of almost all tissues. Thyroid hormones increase growth, speed mental processes, and stimulate digestion. Hormone production and release in the thyroid is controlled by a negative feedback loop between the thyroid and the pituitary gland.

Parathyroid Glands

Four parathyroid glands are located on the back of the thyroid **FIGURE 15.4**. They help regulate the amount of calcium in the blood by producing **parathyroid hormone (PTH)**, also called **parathormone**, which, in the presence of vitamin D, promotes the absorption of calcium in the gastrointestinal mucosa. If low levels of calcium are detected in the body, feedback mechanisms stimulate the parathyroid to produce more PTH, which decreases the absorption of calcium from the intestines and increases the release of stored calcium from bone. Alternatively, if high levels of calcium are detected, the PTH works to decrease calcium absorption in the intestines and increase the excretion of calcium from the kidneys.

Hypothalamus

The hypothalamus is located in the midbrain **FIGURE 15.5** and coordinates and monitors the body's state of homeostasis. The hypothalamus controls the function of the pituitary gland through neurosecretory cells that act both as electrochemical nerve cells and pituitary-stimulating hormones.

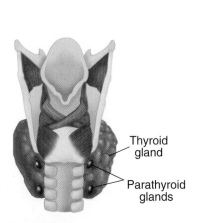

FIGURE 15.4 The parathyroid glands (represented in pink ovals) sit on the back of the thyroid gland.
© Jones & Bartlett Learning

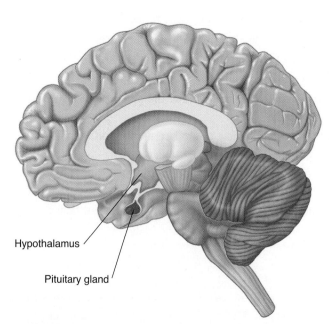

FIGURE 15.5 The pituitary gland and the hypothalamus are located inside the brain.
© Jones & Bartlett Learning

Pineal Gland

The **pineal gland** is located in the third ventricle of the brain. It produces melatonin. **Melatonin** regulates circadian rhythms, which promotes cycles of sleep and wakefulness. Melatonin also influences the timing of the onset of puberty.

Gonads

Collectively, the ovaries and testes are known as **gonads**, or sex glands. Gonads produce hormones responsible for reproduction and sexual characteristics. Females have two ovaries located in the lower abdominal region on either side of the uterus. Males have two testes located in the scrotal sac.

The ovaries secrete estrogen, which promotes the development and maintenance of female sexual organs, and progesterone, which promotes the proliferation of the uterine lining and maintains pregnancy. The testes produce testosterone, which promotes the development of male sex characteristics such as a deep voice, muscle development, and the growth of body hair.

Thymus

The **thymus** is a very small, two-lobed organ located in the mediastinum, under the sternum and in front of the heart **FIGURE 15.6**. The thymus is present in newborns and grows until puberty. After puberty, the thymus atrophies and is replaced by connective and adipose tissue. The primary function of the thymus is the development of the immune system. It stimulates the growth of T cells, a critical component of the immune system.

Pancreas

The pancreas is located behind the stomach, in front of the second and third lumbar vertebrae **FIGURE 15.7** . The top of the pancreas is attached to the duodenum of the bowel. The group of cells in the pancreas that produce the hormones insulin and glucagon are called the **islets of Langerhans**. Alpha cells in the islets produce glucagon and beta cells produce insulin.

Insulin decreases the amount of circulating glucose in the blood by facilitating the transport of glucose through cell membranes. Insulin also governs the storage of glycogen and the metabolism of carbohydrates. **Glucagon** increases the amount of

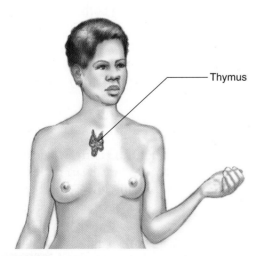

Thymus

FIGURE 15.6 The thymus sits between the lungs, near the heart.
© Jones & Bartlett Learning

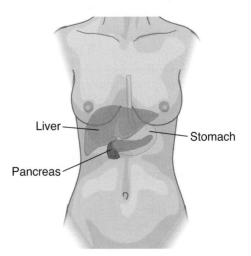

Liver

Stomach

Pancreas

FIGURE 15.7 The pancreas sits behind the stomach, under the liver.
© Jones & Bartlett Learning

Approximately half of the body's insulin is produced as a constant, basal dose, and half is produced in response to eating.

© auremar/ShutterStock, Inc.

glucose in the blood by increasing the excretion of glycogen from the liver and increasing the rate at which glucose is produced. The islets of Langerhans also contain delta cells, which contain somatostatin (also known as growth hormone–inhibiting hormone, it regulates the endocrine system) and pancreatic polypeptide-containing cells, which influence intestinal function.

The pancreas also produces pancreatic juices, which flow into the duodenum through a duct and participate in digestion.

The pancreas is an endocrine gland *and* an exocrine gland.

Diseases and Disorders of the Endocrine System

The endocrine system is integrated with several other body systems to coordinate all body functions. Essentially, the endocrine system is responsible for maintaining homeostasis and regulating growth and maturation. Many diseases and disorders of the endocrine system result from an over- or underproduction of hormones. Overt signs and symptoms of such conditions may not appear until after several years of abnormal hormonal secretions. Additionally, because disorders of the endocrine system affect several body systems and offer diffuse, nonspecific symptoms, diagnosis can be challenging.

Fortunately, many conditions can be successfully treated by correcting the over- or underproduction of hormones. The goal of treatment of all endocrine disorders is to normalize the levels of hormone in the body and reduce symptoms associated with the abnormality, as well as prevent future complications. Treatment of all endocrine disorders is highly individualized and varies with the appearance of signs and symptoms and response to treatment.

Thyroid Disorders

Thyroid activity that is below normal is called **hypothyroidism** or **myxedema**. Thyroid activity that is above normal is called **hyperthyroidism**. Thyroid hormones are necessary for the control of normal growth and metabolism, so both hypothyroidism and hyperthyroidism result in altered metabolic rates. The most common form of hyperthyroidism is **Graves' disease**, which is caused by a genetic susceptibility to an autoimmune disease. Hyperthyroidism occurs more frequently in women than men, and symptoms usually appear between the ages of 20 and 40. Hyperthyroidism is also called **thyrotoxicosis**.

Signs and Symptoms of Thyroid Disorders

Hypothyroidism decreases metabolic processes throughout the body. A person with hypothyroidism often feels cold and experiences fatigue. Also, the heart rate and body temperature of a person with hypothyroidism are abnormally low. Hypothyroidism often causes a person to be overweight due to decreased metabolism. Dry, brittle skin and hair are also symptoms of hypothyroidism.

In an overactive state, as seen in Graves' disease, the thyroid enlarges and increases metabolic processes in the body. A **goiter** is an enlarged thyroid gland **FIGURE 15.8**. Goiters can become so large that they interfere with respiration and swallowing. A person with hyperthyroidism will experience anxiety, nervousness, restlessness, and

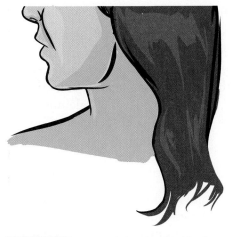 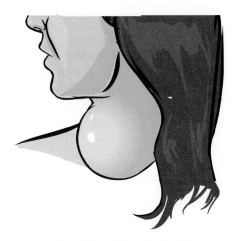

FIGURE 15.8 A normal thyroid gland is shown on the left and an enlarged thyroid gland, or goiter, is shown on the right.
© hkannn/ShutterStock, Inc.

irritability. The heart rate and blood pressure will also be elevated. The patient will likely lose weight despite a normal diet. **Exophthalmos** is a hallmark symptom of hyperthyroidism and is a condition in which the eyes protrude dramatically **FIGURE 15.9**. Generally, exophthalmos is experienced bilaterally, but it can occasionally be seen in only one eye. Mood swings and emotional instability may also occur with Graves' disease. The skin is usually warm and moist.

A severe form of hyperthyroidism, often precipitated by stress or infection, is a thyrotoxic crisis or thyroid storm. This condition produces an extremely accelerated metabolism, severe nervous-system malfunction, overheating, and heart failure. A thyroid storm can be fatal.

Treatment of Thyroid Disorders

Hypothyroidism is treated by supplementing thyroid hormones, the most common of which is levothyroxine (Synthroid). Patients diagnosed with hypothyroidism will take thyroid hormones orally for the remainder of their lives.

Treatment of hyperthyroidism involves removing or destroying part of the thyroid. Surgical procedures can remove all or part of the thyroid to decrease its function. Radioactive iodine or antithyroid drugs such as propylthiouracil also limit the function of the thyroid.

Parathyroid Disorders

Similar to thyroid disorders, overactivity of parathyroid glands is called **hyperparathyroidism** and underactivity of glands is called **hypoparathyroidism**. Hyperparathyroidism is usually caused by a tumor in one of the glands. Hypoparathyroidism can be caused by damage to or the accidental removal of the parathyroid glands during the surgical removal of the thyroid. Inherited forms of hypoparathyroidism are rare.

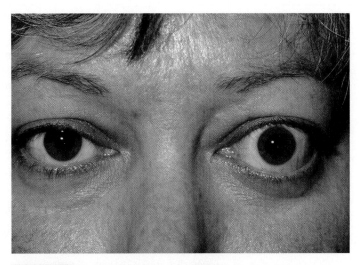

FIGURE 15.9 Exophthalmos is a symptom of hyperthyroidism.
© Dr. P. Marazzi/Photo Researchers, Inc.

Signs and Symptoms of Parathyroid Disorders

If parathyroid glands are overactive, there will be a very high level of calcium in the body. Excess calcium causes lethargy. Kidney stones are also common because the body tries to rid itself of calcium by eliminating it through the urine. Hyperparathyroidism also leads to the progressive decalcification of the bones, which leads to fractures.

If parathyroid glands are underactive, there will be a low level of calcium in the body. **Tetany**, or muscle excitability and tremors, can result from such a calcium deficiency.

Treatment of Parathyroid Disorders

If the calcium levels in hyperparathyroidism are only slightly elevated and are not causing symptoms, no treatment is necessary. Continued monitoring to evaluate progression of the condition is appropriate. If calcium levels or symptoms are extreme, removal of the parathyroid gland is indicated. Hypoparathyroidism is treated with calcium supplementation.

Sex Hormone Disorders

In both males and females, decreased function of the gonads, or **hypogonadism**, inhibits the maturation of sex organs and prevents the appearance of secondary sex characteristics. **Hypergonadism** is the overproduction of sex hormones and also affects sexual maturity. The cause of hypergonadism is not always identifiable, but may be associated with disorders or tumors of the gonads, adrenal glands, or hypothalamus.

Primary hypogonadism, a dysfunction in the gonads themselves, may be caused by an autoimmune disorder, a genetic or developmental disorder, an infection, liver or kidney disease, radiation therapy, or surgery. Turner syndrome and Klinefelter syndrome are the most common genetic causes of hypogonadism in women and men, respectively.

Central hypogonadism is caused by an abnormality in the glands that control the function of the gonads, namely the hypothalamus and the pituitary gland. Central hypogonadism can be caused by steroid administration, long-term opiate use, genetic abnormalities, infection, nutritional deficiencies, radiation therapy, rapid weight loss, trauma, and tumors.

Signs and Symptoms of Sex Hormone Disorders

Hypogonadism in childhood prevents the onset of puberty. With hypogonadism, girls will not begin menstruating and breast development will not occur normally. Hypogonadism that occurs in adult women, including during menopause, is associated with hot flashes, hair loss, decreased libido, and an end to menstruation. Hypogonadism in boys prevents muscle development and facial-hair growth. In men, symptoms include breast enlargement, decreased facial and body hair, muscle loss, and sexual problems. Hypogonadism in both genders may lead to infertility.

Hypergonadism is the overactive production of sex hormones. Most often, this leads to **precocious puberty** (puberty that occurs at a young age) in children, an overactive sex drive, excess body hair, rapid growth, and acne.

Treatment of Sex Hormone Disorders

Levels of sex hormones decline naturally with age, but when the symptoms impair quality of life, hormone replacement therapy can be considered. Replacement therapy with the deficient sex hormones resolves the signs and symptoms associated with hypogonadism. In children, replacement therapy is usually initiated around the age of the normal onset of puberty. In adult women, estrogen can be administered in the form of an oral pill or a transdermal patch. Progesterone should be administered for women whose uterus has not been removed. Testosterone is available in injectable, oral, transdermal, and topical formulations.

Hypergonadism is treated with hormones that inhibit the production or function of sex hormones.

Adrenal Gland Disorders

Addison's disease results from the decreased production of hormones in the adrenal cortex. This decreased function of the adrenal gland is often due to an autoimmune destruction of the cells of the adrenal cortex. Infections, malignancies, and hemorrhages in or around the adrenal gland can also alter its function.

Cushing's syndrome results from an excessive production of glucocorticoids from the adrenal cortex. Cushing's syndrome may be caused by an adrenal tumor or a pituitary tumor.

Signs and Symptoms of Adrenal Gland Disorders

The lack of corticosteroids in Addison's disease impairs normal metabolism and causes electrolyte disturbances, particularly high levels of potassium. Also, patients develop increased pigmentation in their skin due to the excess ACTH and MSH production by the pituitary gland. Weakness, low blood pressure, fatigue, chronic diarrhea, and salt cravings are common symptoms associated with Addison's disease.

Excess glucocorticoids in Cushing's syndrome result in the rapid storage of body fat, eventually resulting in obesity. Hypertension, muscle weakness, and easy bruising are also symptoms of Cushing's disease. A rounded face, known as moon face, also results from excess glucocorticoids. Excess glucocorticoids also stimulate the metabolism of amino acids and the production of glucose. In turn, excess glucose leads to hyperglycemia, which either worsens existing diabetes mellitus (DM) or provokes the onset of DM.

Treatment of Adrenal Gland Disorders

Treatment of Addison's disease requires supplementation of the deficient hormones. Administration of glucocorticoids and mineralocorticoids, including hydrocortisone, prednisone, and fludrocortisone, normalizes the body's hormone levels and feedback mechanisms. Lifelong treatment is required for patients with Addison's disease.

Cushing's syndrome is managed by treating the underlying cause of excess glucocorticoid production. If the cause is a tumor, removal of the tumor corrects the hormone production and removes the symptoms.

Pituitary Gland Disorders

Hyperpituitarism is the abnormal increase in hormones produced by the pituitary gland. Giantism results from the excess production of growth hormone in children. Acromegaly results from the excess production of growth hormone in adulthood. This pituitary-gland dysfunction is almost always due to the presence of a benign tumor in the pituitary gland. **Hypopituitarism**, the decreased production of hormones in the pituitary gland, is also caused by a benign tumor of the pituitary gland.

Signs and Symptoms of Pituitary Gland Disorders

Giantism results in abnormally tall children due to the excessive growth of the long bones before puberty. **Acromegaly** leads to an overgrowth of connective tissue and enlargement of the hands, feet, jaw, brow, nose, and lips.

Hypopituitarism in childhood results in dwarfism, a condition in which children grow in normal proportions but are simply smaller than average. Intelligence is not affected. In adults, hypopituitarism often appears as a deficiency in the presence of sex hormones due to altered feedback mechanisms. Women may fail to ovulate or menstruate, while men may fail to produce sperm.

Hypopituitarism can also lead to a decreased production of ADH, which results in a condition caused **diabetes insipidus**. This form of hypopituitarism may be genetic, be idiopathic (meaning that it arises from a spontaneous or unknown cause), or result from a hypothalamic tumor. ADH promotes the reabsorption of water by the kidneys, so a lack of ADH results in patients producing large quantities of very dilute urine. This, in turn, creates excessive thirst.

Treatment of Pituitary Gland Disorders

Giantism and acromegaly are treated by removing the pituitary tumor or the entire gland, if necessary. This is usually accomplished by surgery and radiation therapy. Drugs such as sandostatin and bromocriptine reduce the secretion of growth hormone from the pituitary gland, which can decrease the symptoms associated with acromegaly.

Hypopituitarism is, likewise, treated by removing an offending tumor. Dwarfism in children can be treated with regular injections of human growth hormone throughout childhood and adolescence. In both hyperpituitarism and hypopituitarism, hormone replacement therapy may be necessary to maintain levels of hormones influenced by the pituitary gland. In the case of diabetes insipidus, vasopressin can be administered to correct levels of ADH.

Pancreas Disorders

The most common disorder associated with the dysfunction of the pancreas is **diabetes mellitus (DM)**, a condition in which individuals do not produce or cannot use insulin. There are several types of DM, but all result from a deficiency of or resistance to insulin. **Type 1 diabetes mellitus (DM)** is an autoimmune disorder in which the beta cells of the islets of Langerhans do not produce insulin **FIGURE 15.10**. **Type 2 diabetes mellitus (DM)** is a condition in which the body's cells are resistant to insulin. In type 2 DM, the beta cells produce insulin, but the body is unable to use it. Approximately 10 percent of diabetic patients have type 1 DM, while the remaining 90 percent have type 2.

Signs and Symptoms of Pancreas Disorders

In both type 1 and type 2 DM, the body's cells are unable to metabolize glucose, which leads to abnormally high levels of glucose circulating in the bloodstream. This excess glucose in the blood is called **hyperglycemia**. The excess glucose in the blood is excreted by the body in the urine, resulting in **glycosuria**.

The symptoms of type 1 DM usually appear in childhood and include increased thirst, increased urination, and weight loss. Children are usually dehydrated. The symptoms of type 2 DM usually appear in adulthood and include fatigue, increased thirst, increased urination, and increased hunger. Type 2 DM is the result of insulin resistance due to genetic factors, aging, and being overweight or obese. A poor diet and lack of physical activity are the main factors contributing to the onset of type 2 DM. Left untreated, type 2 DM leads to a buildup of glucose in the blood, which causes damage to nerves, blood vessels, and other tissues. Poor circulation in type 2 DM disrupts the normal healing process, and diabetic patients often suffer permanent injury or amputations due to wounds in the extremities that do not heal and lead to aggressive infections.

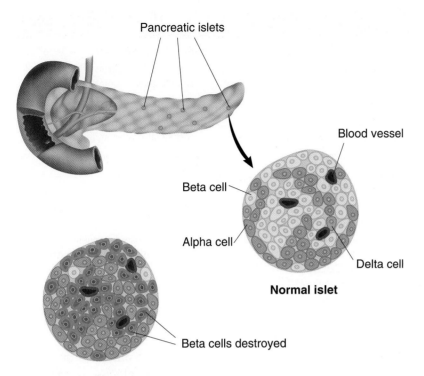

Normal islet

Type 1 diabetes mellitus

FIGURE 15.10 In type 1 DM, the beta cells of the islets of Langerhans do not produce insulin.
© Alila Sao Mai/ShutterStock, Inc.

If left untreated, both types of DM cause damage to the retina (diabetic retinopathy), which leads to blindness; damage to the kidneys (**diabetic nephropathy**); atherosclerosis, which leads to an increased risk of stroke and MI; damage to the nerves (**diabetic neuropathy**); and a decreased ability to fight infections. Diabetes management should include regular ophthalmology visits and assessments of lipid levels, including total cholesterol, LDL, HDL, and triglycerides to identify patients at high risk for coronary heart disase.

The Three Ps of Diabetes

Symptoms of diabetes include polydipsia (excessive thirst), polyuria (excessive urination), and polyphagia (excessive hunger).

Treatment of Pancreas Disorders

Type 1 DM can be treated only with insulin. Because the body does not produce insulin, injections of insulin are required to control glucose levels for the duration of the patient's life. Short-, intermediate-, and long-acting forms of insulin are available to be used in combination to mimic basal levels of insulin production as well as after-meal insulin production.

Type 2 DM is treated by correcting insulin resistance. Diet and lifestyle modifications are the first step to controlling the symptoms of type 2 DM. Weight loss through exercise and a low-fat, high-fiber diet can reduce blood glucose levels enough

By the year 2050, the prevalence of type 2 DM in the United States is expected to be as high as 1 in 3 adults.
© auremar/ShutterStock, Inc.

Table 15.2   Oral Antidiabetic Agents

Category	Drug Name (Brand Name)	Mechanism of Action
α-glucosidase inhibitors	Acarbose (Precose) Miglitol (Glyset)	Prevent the breakdown of sucrose and complex carbohydrates
Biguanides	Metformin (Glucophage)	Reduce hepatic glucose production
Thiazolidinediones	Rosiglitazone (Avandia) Pioglitazone (Actos)	Reduce insulin resistance in peripheral tissues and in the liver
Sulfonylureas	Glipizide (Glucotrol) Glyburide (Diabeta) Glimepiride (Amaryl)	Stimulate the secretion of insulin from the pancreas
Short-acting secretagogues	Repaglinide (Prandin) Nateglinide (Starlix)	Stimulate the secretion of insulin from the pancreas
Peptide analogues	Exenatide (Byetta) Liraglutide (Victoza) Sitagliptin (Januvia) Saxagliptin (Onglyza) Linagliptin (Tradjenta)	Increase glucose-dependent secretion of insulin from pancreas

to control symptoms in early stages of type 2 DM. Exercise not only aids in weight loss, which facilitates efficient use of glucose, but also increases glucose metabolism and insulin sensitivity, which enables the body's cells to use the insulin that the body produces. Unfortunately, type 2 DM is a progressive disease and symptoms gradually worsen over time, despite most diet and lifestyle interventions. Oral hypoglycemic drugs can be added to a healthy lifestyle to facilitate the body's use of glucose by altering sensitivity to insulin or increasing its secretion from the pancreas. These agents can delay the progression of diabetes and prevent complications of chronic hyperglycemia. The drugs are often used in combination as the disease worsens.

Common oral medications for type 2 DM are presented in **TABLE 15.2**. Eventually, most type 2 diabetic patients will require insulin injections. Short-, intermediate-, and long-acting insulins are summarized in **TABLE 15.3**. The most significant side effect associated with antidiabetic agents, including insulin, is the risk of abnormally low blood sugar, or hypoglycemia. Hypoglycemia can cause fainting, lightheadedness, anxiety, visual disturbances, sweating, and heart palpitations.

Table 15.3   Types of Insulin

Insulin	Time to Onset of Action	Time to Peak Activity	Duration of Activity
Rapid-acting (insulin aspart, insulin lispro, insulin glulisine)	15–30 minutes	1–2 hours	3–6 hours
Short-acting (regular insulin)	30–60 minutes	2–3 hours	5–7 hours
Intermediate-acting (NPH insulin, insulin zinc)	2–4 hours	6–10 hours	10–18 hours
Long-acting (insulin glargine, insulin detemir)	4 hours	No peak	24 hours

Insulin Safety

Insulin is available in a variety of brands and formulations that can be easily confused. Verify that the prescribed insulin is the one being administered. Double-check the dose, which is always reported in units. Doses are individualized and vary in response to activity levels and eating habits. Insulin is available in a concentration of 100 units/mL (U-100). Regular insulin is also available in a concentration of 500 units/mL (U-500) for patients who require a large dose of insulin.

© auremar/ShutterStock, Inc.

Diagnostic Procedures of the Endocrine System

Many diagnostic tests of the endocrine system can be performed with blood or urine samples. These tests measure hormone levels or assess their function. Blood and urine tests can be used to diagnose diseases or disorders of the endocrine system or to monitor therapeutic responses. In addition to the tests listed here, nearly every hormone can be measured, often with a blood test, if abnormalities are suspected.

Blood Glucose Monitoring

Blood glucose concentrations rise after a meal, and the levels are regulated by insulin and glucagon. Blood glucose tests are used to measure the level of glucose in the blood. Tests can be conducted after fasting or after meals. Each test provides different information about the function of the pancreas and the effects of insulin in the body. Blood glucose tests measure short-term glucose control.

A **fasting blood glucose (FBG) test** measures the amount of glucose in the bloodstream after a 12-hour fast. An FBG is a diagnostic tool for DM. In adults, a normal fasting glucose level is between 70 and 100mg/dL. A fasting glucose level between 100–125mg/dL is now considered impaired fasting glucose and a sign of prediabetes. A result greater than 126mg/dL on two or more samples is diagnostic of DM.

A two-hour postprandial glucose test measures the amount of glucose in the bloodstream after a meal. This test screens for DM and assesses how the body uses insulin. Two hours after eating a high carbohydrate meal, blood sugar levels should return to near-fasting levels (below 100mg/dL) in healthy individuals.

Many types of meters and systems are available for measuring blood glucose levels. Most are small and designed to be used by the patient or at the point of care. As a medical assistant, you should familiarize yourself with a variety of blood glucose testing meters (**glucometers**) to aid patients who use them on a daily basis.

It is important for diabetic patients to maintain logs of their daily blood sugars and insulin doses. They should also record physical activity, meals, snacks, and other medications they take. Maintaining a log will help establish long-term patterns of glucose control and enable patients and healthcare providers to identify variations in insulin requirements.

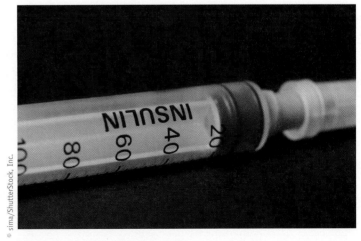

© sima/ShutterStock, Inc.

Insulin syringes are marked in units.

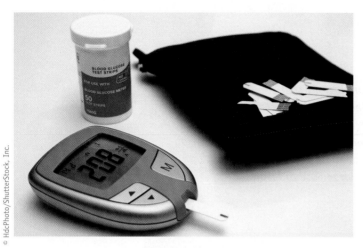

Many types of glucometers and test strips are available.

Glucose Tolerance Testing

A **glucose tolerance test (GTT)** measures the body's ability to process a large amount of glucose in a short amount of time. GTTs are often conducted during pregnancy to assess the mother's risk for gestational diabetes.

A GTT is conducted after a 10-hour fast. A concentrated glucose solution containing 75–100mg of glucose is then administered to the patient, usually in the form of a solution called Glucola. The patient must consume the entire solution in five minutes. Blood and urine specimens are collected at specified time intervals after the ingestion of the solution: 30 minutes, one hour, two hours, and three hours. The blood and urine samples are used to measure the amount of glucose at each time point, which indicates how well the body responds to increased glucose loads. In healthy patients, blood glucose levels reach a maximum of 160–180mg/dL 30 to 60 minutes after ingestion. FBG levels return within two to three hours.

What Would You Do?

A newly diagnosed type 1 DM patient presents for a follow-up to review her first month on insulin therapy. She has her blood glucose logs with her for the physician to review. While you are obtaining her vital signs, she notes that her blood sugars fluctuated markedly throughout the day and she cannot identify any patterns to her blood glucose readings or insulin requirements. You ask her what meter and test strips she has been using to test her blood sugar, and she offers that she has an old meter that used to belong to her grandmother and she uses whatever strips she can find on sale. What would you suggest to the patient?

© NorthGeorgiaMedia/ShutterStock, Inc.

Hemoglobin A1c Testing

Hemoglobin A1c (HbA1c) is assessed with a blood test and measures long-term glucose control. Glycosylated hemoglobin, or HbA1c, is the molecule that is formed when glucose attaches to hemoglobin in a red blood cell. An elevated finding is indicative of excess glucose in the bloodstream. HbA1c results indicate how much glucose has been circulating in the blood for the past two to three months. It does not vary with day-to-day glucose control. Patients do not need to fast for the HbA1c test. An HbA1c result of less than 6 percent is normal and healthy. A result above 6.5 percent is diagnostic for diabetes.

Thyroid Testing

Blood tests assess the levels of T3, T4, and TSH, which describe the function of the thyroid. Also, thyroid scans help providers visualize the activity of the thyroid. Radioactive iodine uptake tests involve administering an oral dose of radioactive iodine to a patient with suspected thyroid dysfunction. At intervals of 6 and 24 hours, a scintillator assesses the amount of iodine taken up by the thyroid. Thyroid function is determined by the thyroid's ability to use iodine.

After a dose of radioactive iodine, the thyroid can also be scanned with a camera that is capable of viewing radioactive isotopes. This type of scan identifies areas of increased or decreased function within the thyroid. A thyroid ultrasound can assess thyroid size and the presence of thyroid nodules.

Skills for the Medical Assistant

As a medical assistant, you will have the opportunity to participate in several procedures relating to the endocrine system. You will also have the opportunity to teach patients about self-monitoring of blood glucose levels and insulin administration. Your confidence will ease the patient's fears and allow for safe and accurate testing.

Blood Glucose Testing

Blood glucose testing using a glucometer or other automated testing device is common, both for screening for diabetes and for evaluating therapeutic regimens. In addition to performing this procedure in office or clinic settings, you may be called upon to teach a patient how to perform this test himself or herself. Patients with diabetes must check their blood glucose level frequently during the day, so proper technique will help minimize discomfort and promote accurate test results. In this exercise, you will learn the proper technique for obtaining a blood sample for blood glucose testing so you are able to perform it yourself and teach patients how to perform the procedure.

Equipment Needed

- Sterile lancet
- Reagent strips
- Glucometer
- Disposable gloves
- Cotton balls
- Alcohol wipes or isopropyl alcohol
- Sterile adhesive bandage

Steps

1. Introduce yourself and identify the patient. Explain the procedure that you will be performing. Answer the patient's questions and ensure he or she is calm and comfortable before proceeding with the procedure.

> If the glucose test is meant to be a fasting test, confirm that the patient has had nothing to eat or drink for 8 to 12 hours.

2. Wash your hands and apply disposable gloves.
3. Perform a capillary puncture. (See Chapter 13.)
4. Remove one of the reagent strips from its container, taking care not to touch the testing end of the strip.
5. Apply a large drop of blood from the patient's finger to the test strip so that the blood completely covers the testing portion of the strip FIGURE 15.11.
6. Time the test, according to the manufacturer's instructions.
7. Give the patient a cotton ball to place over the puncture site. Provide a sterile bandage.
8. Read the results displayed by the glucometer. The number is the patient's blood glucose level.
9. Record the results in the patient's chart. For example, write "1345: Finger stick of middle

When using a glucometer, ensure that the proper test strips are used for the selected meter. Also, check the expiration date of the strips.

© auremar/ShutterStock, Inc.

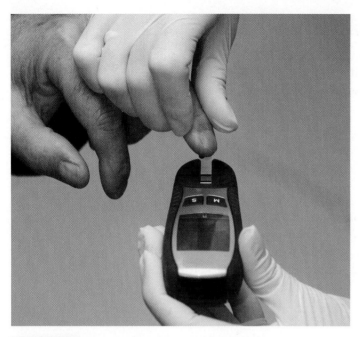

FIGURE 15.11 Apply a large drop of blood to the test strip.

finger performed for capillary FBG. Result: 98mg/dL. J. Jones, CMA."

10. Record the lot number, control ranges, and expiration date of reagent strips used.

11. Discard all used items in the proper receptacles. Remove the gloves and wash your hands.

HbA1c Testing

HbA1c measures long-term glucose control, which should be done one to two times each year for diabetic patients. In this exercise, you will learn the proper technique for obtaining a blood sample for HbA1c testing.

Equipment Needed

- Sterile lancet
- Disposable gloves
- Testing instrument and reagents
- Cotton balls
- Alcohol wipes or isopropyl alcohol
- Sterile adhesive bandage

Steps

1. Introduce yourself and identify the patient. Explain the procedure that you will be performing. Answer the patient's questions and ensure he or she is calm and comfortable before proceeding with the procedure.
2. Wash your hands and apply disposable gloves.
3. Perform a capillary puncture. Collect a capillary blood sample according to the manufacturer's instructions for the testing equipment.
4. Give the patient a cotton ball to place over the puncture site. Provide a sterile bandage.
5. Complete the test, according to the manufacturer's instructions.
6. Read the results displayed by the testing equipment. The number is the patient's glycosylated hemoglobin level.
7. Record the results in the patient's chart. For example, write "0925: Performed capillary puncture for HbA1c test. Result: 6.2%. J. Jones, CMA."
8. Discard all used items in the proper receptacles. Remove the gloves and wash your hands.

Insulin Administration

Patients with type 1 DM and some with type 2 DM require frequent injections of insulin. Some types of insulin are available in prefilled pens for ease of administration, but most are available in vials that must be administered with a syringe. In this exercise, you will learn the proper technique for administering insulin so you are able to perform it yourself and teach patients how to perform the procedure.

Equipment Needed

- Vial of insulin
- Insulin syringe with needle
- Disposable gloves
- Cotton balls
- Alcohol wipes or isopropyl alcohol
- Sterile adhesive bandage

> *Rotate the site of insulin injection frequently to prevent tissue damage. To maintain consistency in insulin absorption, try to inject insulin in the same general area at the same time of the day, but rotate within each injection site.*
>
> © auremar/ShutterStock, Inc.

Steps

1. Introduce yourself and identify the patient. Explain the procedure that you will be performing. Answer the patient's questions and ensure he or she is calm and comfortable before proceeding with the procedure.
2. Wash your hands and apply disposable gloves.
3. Check the expiration date of the insulin. Roll the vial between your palms to warm it slightly and allow the suspension to mix uniformly. Do not shake the vial of insulin.
4. Select an injection site **FIGURE 15.12**. Pull the skin taut and, using a circular motion, wipe it clean with an alcohol wipe. Appropriate injection sites include the

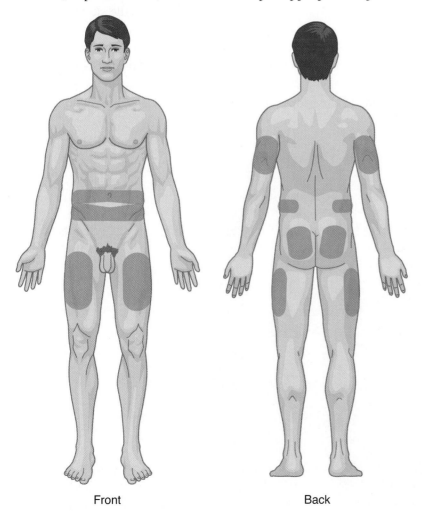

Front   Back

FIGURE 15.12 Sites for insulin injection.

© Jones & Bartlett Learning

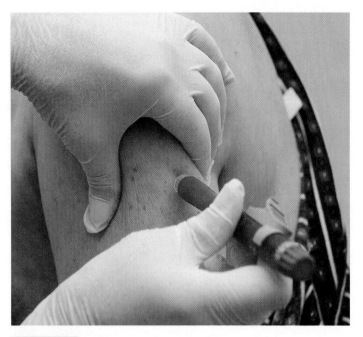

FIGURE 15.13 Insert the needle at a 90-degree angle when administering insulin.
© iStockphoto.com/art-4-art

abdomen, upper arms, thighs, and hips or buttocks. Insulin is absorbed most rapidly from the abdomen. Do not inject close to the belly button, scars, moles, or damaged skin.

5. Use proper technique for withdrawing medication from a vial. (See Chapter 11.)

6. Use your thumb and index finger to pinch the skin at the injection site, pulling up at least $\frac{1}{2}$ inch of fat and skin. Quickly insert the needle at a 90-degree angle into the folded skin **FIGURE 15.13**. Insert the needle all the way to the hub. Depress the plunger slowly, injecting the full amount of insulin from the syringe.

Pinch the skin to avoid administering insulin intramuscularly.

7. Place a cotton ball over the injection site and withdraw the needle slowly.

8. Record the procedure in the patient's chart. For example, write "1400: Administered 50 units of regular insulin to left side of lower abdomen, per Dr. Parker's order. J. Jones, CMA." Many patients with diabetes will learn to self-administer insulin **FIGURE 15.14**.

9. Discard all used items in the proper receptacles. Remove the gloves and wash your hands.

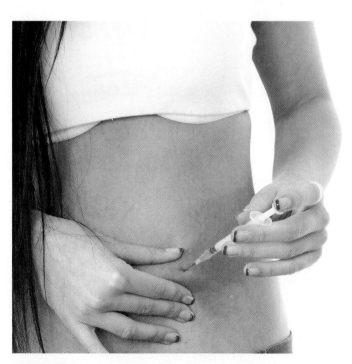

FIGURE 15.14 Many patients with diabetes will learn to self-administer insulin.
© photomak/ShutterStock, Inc.

Math Practice

Question: **A physician orders 20 units of regular insulin for a patient with diabetes. If the insulin is available in a concentration of 100 units/mL, what is the total volume of insulin that will be injected?**

Answer: Step 1: Multiply the number of units ordered by the number of units in one milliliter. To do this, first convert the number of units to a fraction: $20 = {}^{20}/_1$

   Therefore, 20 units × 1mL/100 units = 20 units/1 × 1mL/100 units

   Now, multiply the two numerators: 20 units × 1mL = 20 units × mL

   Then, multiply the denominators: 1 × 100 units = 100 units

   The result is 20 units × mL/100 units

   Cancel the units and divide the fraction: ${}^{20}/_{100}$ mL

Step 2: Finally, convert the fraction to a decimal: ${}^{20}/_{100}$ mL = 0.2mL

Question: **A physician orders 35 units of U-100 insulin for a patient with diabetes. If a 10mL vial is available, what is the total volume of insulin that will be administered?**

Answer: Step 1: Multiply the number of units ordered by the number of units in one milliliter. To do this, first convert the number of units to a fraction: $35 = {}^{35}/_1$

   Therefore, 35 units × 1mL/100 units = 35 units/1 × 1mL/100 units

   Now, multiply the two numerators: 35 units × 1mL = 35 units × mL

   Then, multiply the denominators: 1 × 100 units = 100 units

   The result is 35 units × mL/100 units

   Cancel the units and divide the fraction: 35 units × mL/100 units = ${}^{35}/_{100}$mL

Step 2: Finally, convert the fraction to a decimal: ${}^{35}/_{100}$mL = 0.35mL

Question: **A pediatric patient with diabetes weighs 167 lb. Her physician orders regular insulin four units/kg/day. What is the total dose of insulin? To decrease the volume of insulin that needs to be administered, the physician prescribes U-500 insulin. What is the total volume of insulin for the daily dose?**

Answer: Step 1: Remember that 1kg equals 2.2 lb: 1kg = 2.2 lb
Convert this to a ratio: 1kg:2.2 lb

   Next, convert the number of pounds to a fraction: $167 = {}^{167}/_1$ lb

   Multiply the number of pounds by the number of kilograms per pound: 167 lb/1 × 1kg/2.2 lb

   Now, multiply the numerators: 167 × 1 = 167 lb × kg

   Then, multiply the denominators: 1 × 2.2 lb = 2.2 lb

   The result is 167 lb × kg/2.2 lb

   Cancel the units and divide the fraction: 167kg/2.2 lb = 75.9kg

Step 2: Now, multiply the number of kilograms by the number of units of insulin ordered: 75.9kg × 4 units/kg/day = 303.6 units/day

Step 3: Finally, multiply the number of units by the number of units in a milliliter. To do this, convert the number of units to a fraction: 303.6 units $= {}^{303.6}/_1$ units

   Therefore, 303.6 units × 1mL/500 units = 303.6 units/1 × 1mL/500 units

Now, multiply the two numerators: 303.6 × 1mL = 303.6 units × mL

Then, multiply the denominators: 1 × 500 = 500mL

The result is 303.6 units × mL/500 units. Cancel the units and divide the fraction: $^{303.6}/_{500}$mL

Step 4: Finally, convert the fraction to a decimal: $^{303.6}/_{500}$mL = 0.6mL

Question: **A patient with newly diagnosed type 1 diabetes is beginning an insulin regimen. The physician orders that her total insulin dose be 0.7 units/kg/day. Half the dose will be a basal dose of long-acting insulin and half will be administered as shorter-acting insulin in response to meals. If the patient weighs 118 lb, what will her basal dose of long-acting insulin be?**

Answer: Step 1: Remember that 1kg equals 2.2 lb: 1kg = 2.2 lb
Convert this to a ratio: 1kg: 2.2 lb

Next, convert the number of pounds to a fraction: 118 = $^{118}/_1$ lb

Multiply the number of pounds by the number of kilograms per pound: 118 lb/1 × 1kg/2.2 lb

Now, multiply the numerators: 118 lb × 1kg = 118 lb × kg

Then, multiply the denominators: 1 × 2.2 lb = 2.2 lb

The result is 118 lb × kg/2.2 lb

Cancel the units and divide the fraction: 118 lb × kg/2.2 lb = 53.6kg

Step 2: Now, multiply the number of kilograms by the number of units of insulin ordered: 53.6kg × 0.7 units/kg/day = 37.52 units/day

Step 3: Finally, divide the daily dose in half to find the basal dose: 37.52 units ÷ 2 = 18.76 units

---

Question: **A pediatric patient with growth hormone deficiency is prescribed somatropin 0.16mg/kg/week divided into six doses each week. If the patient weighs 51 lbs, what is the total weekly dose that he will receive? How much drug will be administered at each of the six sessions during the week?**

Answer: Step 1: Remember that 1kg equals 2.2 lb: 1kg = 2.2 lb
Convert this to a ratio: 1kg:2.2 lb

Next, convert the number of pounds to a fraction: 51 = $^{51}/_1$ lb

Multiply the number of pounds by the number of kilograms per pound: 51 lb/1 × 1kg/2.2 lb

Now, multiply the numerators: 51 lb × 1kg = 51 lb × kg

Then, multiply the denominators: 1 × 2.2 lb = 2.2 lb

The result is 51 lb × kg/2.2 lb

Cancel the units and divide the fraction: 51 lb × kg/2.2 lb = 23.2kg

Step 2: Now, multiply the number of kilograms by dose ordered: 23.2kg × 0.16 mg/kg/week = 3.7 mg/week

Step 3: Finally, multiply the weekly dose by the number of sessions per week. To do this, convert the number of sessions in one week to a fraction: 6 sessions per week = 1 week/6 sessions

Therefore, 3.7 mg/week × 1 week/6 session = 0.62 mg/session

WRAP UP

Chapter Summary

- The endocrine system is a network of glands that secrete hormones. Hormones are a diverse group of chemical messengers that communicate between cells.

- Endocrine glands release hormones directly into the bloodstream. Several major glands make up the endocrine system. The adrenal glands are located above the kidneys and produce corticosteroids, as well as epinephrine and norepinephrine. The pituitary gland is located behind the optic nerve and controls the function of many other endocrine glands. The thyroid gland is situated on either side of the larynx and trachea and produces thyroid hormones that control the metabolic rate of nearly all tissues. The parathyroid glands, located on the back of the thyroid glands, produce parathyroid hormone, which controls the amount of calcium in the blood. The hypothalamus controls the function of the pituitary gland. The pineal gland produces melatonin and controls circadian rhythms. The ovaries and testes are gonads, or sex glands, that control sexual characteristics and reproductive functions. The thymus contributes to the development of the immune system and atrophies after puberty.

- The pancreas produces insulin and glucagon to control the amount of glucose in the blood.

- Increased or decreased activity in any of the endocrine glands results in abnormal growth, metabolism, body function, or homeostasis.

- Diabetes mellitus (DM) is one of the most common disorders associated with the endocrine system. DM is the inability of the body to produce or use insulin, resulting in high levels of glucose in the blood. Untreated diabetes can lead to significant long-term consequences, including damage to the retina, kidneys, and nerves.

- Blood tests can help identify disorders of the endocrine system and assess treatment regimens. Diabetic patients require frequent blood glucose testing, and should maintain a log of daily blood glucose results and food and activities to identify patterns in glucose control.

- As a medical assistant, you will have the opportunity to assist with several types of blood tests to evaluate endocrine conditions. Remaining calm and confident will ease patients' fears and apprehensions about a long-term chronic condition that will likely require frequent blood tests.

Learning Assessment Questions

1. Which of the following is *not* a primary function of the endocrine system?
   A. Facilitate metabolism
   B. Promote sexual maturation
   C. Regulate respiration
   D. Maintain electrolyte levels

2. Which two hormones are responsible for the fight-or-flight response?
   A. Cortisol and aldosterone
   B. Epinephrine and norepinephrine
   C. Vasopressin and growth hormone
   D. Insulin and glucagon

3. The adrenal cortex produces which category of hormones?
   A. Corticosteroids
   B. Gonadotropic hormones
   C. Thyroid hormones
   D. Catecholamines

4. Which gland is known as the master gland of the body?
   A. Parathyroid gland
   B. Pineal gland
   C. Hypothalamus
   D. Pituitary gland

5. Which component of the endocrine system is responsible for maintaining homeostasis?
   A. Thyroid
   B. Hypothalamus
   C. Adrenal glands
   D. Thymus

6. Which of the following hormones is produced by the ovaries?
   A. Follicle-stimulating hormone
   B. Luteinizing hormone
   C. Estrogen
   D. Testosterone

7. What gland is inactive after childhood?
   A. Pineal gland
   B. Gonads
   C. Hypothalamus
   D. Thymus

8. Where is insulin produced?
   A. In the beta cells of the islets of Langerhans
   B. In the adrenal medulla
   C. In the neurohypophysis
   D. In the duodenum

9. Which gland has exocrine and endocrine functions?
   A. Thyroid gland
   B. Pancreas
   C. Pituitary glands
   D. Gonads

10. Which of the following is *not* a symptom of hypothyroidism?
    A. Slow heart rate
    B. Fatigue
    C. Dry skin
    D. Exophthalmos

11. Which of the following is a sign or symptom of hyperparathyroidism?
    A. Tetany
    B. Decreased potassium levels
    C. Elevated calcium levels
    D. Increased skin pigmentation

12. Which of the following conditions can cause precocious puberty?
    A. Hypergonadism
    B. Hyperaldosteronism
    C. Cushing's syndrome
    D. Graves' disease

13. Which of the following are signs and symptoms of Addison's disease?
    A. Hypertension, bruising, diarrhea, and moon face
    B. Glucose in the urine and salt cravings
    C. Elevated potassium, low blood pressure, weakness, and fatigue
    D. Increased growth of connective tissue, leading to an enlarged jaw, nose, and brow

14. What type of diabetes is characterized by the body's inability to produce insulin?
    A. Type 1 DM
    B. Type 2 DM
    C. Gestational diabetes
    D. Diabetes insipidus

15. Which term describes sugar in the urine?
    A. Gluconeogenesis
    B. Glycosuria
    C. Hypoglycemia
    D. Natriuresis

16. Which of the following is important to tell patients regarding management of their diabetes?
    A. Intramuscular injection of insulin results in the most rapid onset of action.
    B. Glucose test strips are compatible with any glucometer.
    C. Administer insulin at the same injection site all the time to standardize insulin absorption.
    D. Obtain regular ophthalmology exams and cholesterol tests to monitor for complications of diabetes.

17. What test measures long-term control of blood glucose levels?

    A. Hemoglobin A1c

    B. Fasting blood glucose

    C. Radioactive iodine uptake test

    D. Glucose tolerance test

18. Which of the following HbA1c levels is considered normal or healthy?

    A. 7.6 percent

    B. 126mg/dL

    C. 5.9 percent

    D. 72mg/dL

19. What type of insulin has the fastest onset of action?

    A. Insulin detemir

    B. Regular insulin

    C. NPH insulin

    D. Insulin lispro

20. Which of the following FBG levels indicates a diagnosis of diabetes mellitus?

    A. 85mg/dL

    B. 140mg/dL

    C. 42mg/dL

    D. 115mg/dL

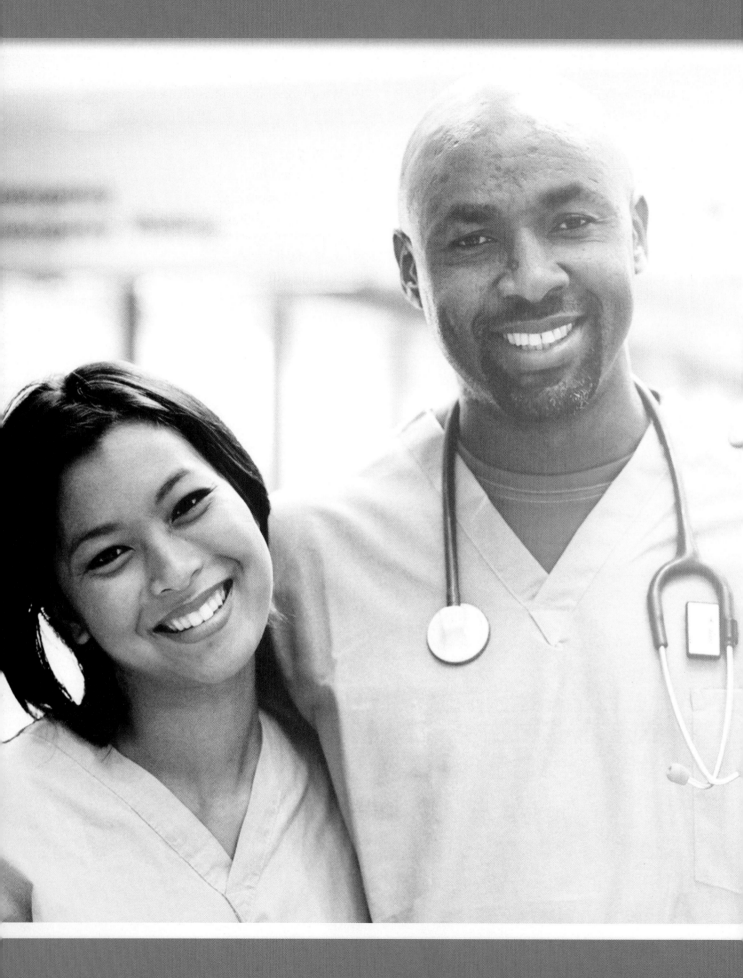

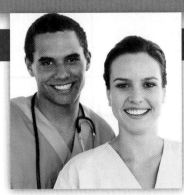

Digestive System

OBJECTIVES

After reading this chapter, you will be able to:

- Identify combining word forms of the digestive system and their role in the formation of medical terms.
- Define the structures and functions of the digestive system.
- Identify common diseases of the digestive system and their treatment, as well as diagnostic procedures relating to the digestive system.
- List abbreviations related to the digestive system.
- Describe the relation of nutrition to the functioning of the digestive system.
- Identify the basic nutrient types.
- Explain the relationship and balance among the three energy-providing nutrients.
- Distinguish between water-soluble and fat-soluble vitamins.
- Discuss herbal supplements.
- Explain the reason for nutrition labels on food packaging.
- Discuss various therapeutic diets and explain how each can help to control a particular disease state or accommodate a change in the life cycle.
- Describe patient preparation for occult blood testing.

KEY TERMS

Acidosis	Anion	Ascites
Alimentary canal	Anus	Basal metabolic rate
Alkalosis	Appendectomy	(BMR)
Amylase enzymes	Appendicitis	Bicuspids
Anal canal	Ascending colon	Bile

Body mass index (BMI)
Bolus
Calorie
Canines
Carbohydrates
Cardiac sphincter
Cation
Cecum
Cholecystectomy
Cholelithiasis
Chyme
Cirrhosis
Colon
Colonoscopy
Colostomy
Common bile duct
Complementary and
    alternative medicine
    (CAM)
Constipation
Crohn's disease
Cuspids
Cystic duct
Deciduous teeth
Defecation
Dehydration
Descending colon
Diarrhea
Digestion
Disaccharides
Duodenum
Electrolyte
Elimination
Enema
Esophagogastroduo-
    denoscopy (EGD)
Esophagus
External anal sphincter
Extreme obesity
Fat-soluble vitamins
Fatty acid
Fecal occult blood test
    (FOBT)

Feces
Fiber
Fundus
Gallbladder
Gallstones
Gastric emptying time
Gastroenteritis
Gastroenterologist
Gastroesophageal reflux
    disease (GERD)
Gastroscopy
GI transit time
Hematemesis
Hematochezia
Hepatic duct
Hepatic flexure
Hydrogenation
Hyponatremia
Ileocecal valve
Ileostomy
Ileum
Incisors
Inflammatory bowel
    disease (IBD)
Ingestion
Internal anal sphincter
Intrinsic factor
Ion
Irritable bowel syndrome
    (IBS)
Jaundice
Jejunum
Large intestine
Laxative
Lipids
Liver
Macronutrients
Malnutrition
Melena
Mesentery
Micronutrients
Mineral
Molars

Monosaccharides
Nutrients
Nutrition
Obesity
Overnutrition
Overweight
Pancreatitis
Pepsin
Peptic ulcer disease
    (PUD)
Peptic ulcers
Peptidases
Peristalsis
Polyps
Polysaccharides
Premolars
Proctologist
Protein
Ptyalin
Pyloric sphincter
Rectum
Rugae
Saliva
Salivary glands
Saturated fatty acid
Sigmoid colon
Small intestine
Splenic flexure
Stomach
Stool
Taste buds
Trace elements
Trans fats
Transverse colon
Ulcerative colitis (UC)
Undernutrition
Unsaturated fatty acid
Vermiform appendix
Villi
Vitamin
Water-soluble vitamins

Chapter Overview

The digestive system is also known as the gastrointestinal (GI) system. It includes several structures and accessory organs located along 30 feet of hollow tubing between the mouth and the anus that work to store and digest food, eliminate waste, and utilize nutrients FIGURE 16.1 . Simply, the digestive system breaks down food into components that can be used as nutrients for all the cells of the body. To function effectively, the di-

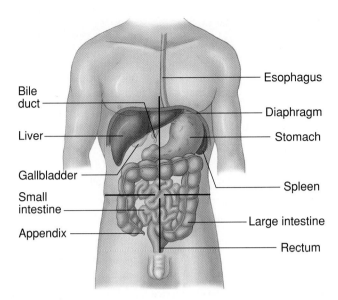

Bile duct
Liver
Gallbladder
Small intestine
Appendix

Esophagus
Diaphragm
Stomach
Spleen
Large intestine
Rectum

FIGURE 16.1 The human digestive system is made up of a series of organs and structures.

© Jones & Bartlett Learning

gestive system requires coordination with and input from other body systems, including the immune system, the muscular system, and the nervous system.

The digestive system, unlike many other body systems, provides clear and often immediate indications of dysfunction, disease, and conditions that require attention. Diseases and disorders of the digestive system are common and often affect other organ systems, including the integumentary, circulatory, respiratory, urinary, and nervous systems. A medical specialist who studies the digestive system is called a **gastroenterologist**. A specialist who specializes in diseases and disorders of the lower digestive tract is called a **proctologist**.

As a medical assistant, you will have the opportunity to interact with patients with a variety of disorders of the digestive system, as well as participate in diagnostic and treatment-related procedures. Patients undergoing procedures relating to the GI system are often required to consume strong laxatives, receive dyes or substances that allow visualization of internal structures, or collect stool samples. It is imperative that the medical assistant provide clear instructions for the preparation of the procedures because the tests may not be able to be performed if the preparation is not completed as ordered.

Terminology

TABLE 16.1 lists word roots and terms used in the study of the digestive system.

Table 16.1 Word Roots of the Digestive System

Word Root or Term	Meaning	Example
Aliment/o	Nourish	Alimentary canal (the tube through which food enters the body, is digested, and waste is eliminated)
Bucc/o	Cheek	Buccal cavity (the area of the mouth surrounded by the cheeks, lips, and gums)
Chol/o or chol/e	Bile, gall	Cholelithiasis (the formation of stones in the gallbladder)
Cholecyst/o	Gallbladder	Cholecystectomy (removal of the gallbladder)
Col/o or colon/o	Colon or large intestine	Colostomy (an artificial opening of the large intestine)
Dent/o	Tooth	Dentist (a medical specialist who studies the oral cavity and teeth)

(Continues)

Table 16.1 Word Roots of the Digestive System *(Continued)*

Word Root or Term	Meaning	Example
Enter/o	Small intestine	Enteroscope (a flexible fiber-optic tube and camera that is used to visualize the small intestine)
Gastr/o	Stomach	Gastroscopy (visual examination of the stomach)
Gingiv/o	Gums	Gingivitis (inflammation of the gums)
Gloss/o	Tongue	Glossitis (inflammation of the tongue)
Hepat/o	Liver	Hepatomegaly (enlargement of the liver)
Lingu/o	Tongue	Sublingual (under the tongue)
Phag/o	To eat/swallow	Dysphagia (difficulty swallowing)
Proct/o	Rectum	Proctologist (a medical specialist who studies the colon, anus, and rectum)
Sial/o	Saliva/salivary gland	Sialorrhea (excessive salivation)
Stomat/o	Mouth	Stomatitis (inflammation of the mouth)

Structure and Function of the Digestive System

The chain of organs that makes up the digestive system is sometimes referred to as the **alimentary canal**, and the organs form a continuous tube from the mouth to the anus. The organs facilitate the processes of ingestion, digestion, absorption, and elimination of food. Various mechanical and chemical processes take place during this entire digestive process and each organ in the digestive system has a critical role in altering the composition of food, absorbing its nutrients, and eliminating the waste products.

Ingestion is the process by which food is consumed and broken down into small pieces. Most often, in humans, food is taken into the body through the mouth. **Digestion** is the process of converting food to a form that can be used by the cells of the body. Absorption is the process by which digested food particles are transported to the cells of the body. **Elimination** is the removal of solid waste products of digestion.

Abbreviations Related to the Digestive System

The following are abbreviations related to the digestive system:

- Ba—Barium
- BM—Bowel movement
- BS—Bowel sounds
- E. coli—*Escherichia coli*
- EGD—Esophagogastroduodenoscopy
- GB—Gallbladder
- GI—Gastrointestinal
- HAV—Hepatitis A virus
- HBV—Hepatitis B virus
- HCV—Hepatitis C virus
- IBD—Inflammatory bowel disease
- IBS—Irritable bowel syndrome
- NG—Nasogastric
- NPO—Nothing by mouth
- N&V—Nausea and vomiting
- PEG—Percutaneous endoscopic gastrostomy
- PP—Postprandial (after meals)
- RDA—Recommended daily/dietary allowance
- TPN—Total parenteral nutrition
- UC—Ulcerative colitis
- UGI—Upper gastrointestinal series

GI transit time is the amount of time it takes for food to pass through the GI tract. Transit time varies depending on the amount of food consumed, the amount of fat consumed, smoking, medications, and various disease states. Gastric emptying time, a component of GI transit time, is the time it takes for food to pass through the stomach. Reduced transit time can lead to decreased absorption of nutrients, and increased transit time can lead to increased absorption. Increased transit time can also lead to abdominal pain and discomfort, nausea, vomiting, lack of appetite, and bloating.

Each day, the adult gastrointestinal tract produces 7–10 liters of fluid to facilitate the digestive process.
© auremar/ShutterStock, Inc.

Mouth

The digestive tract begins at the mouth, the point at which food enters the body. The entire digestive process begins with chewing and swallowing. The teeth break up food into smaller, smoother particles to facilitate swallowing. Teeth first appear at approximately six months of age. The first set of teeth are called deciduous teeth and will gradually fall out and be replaced by permanent teeth beginning around six years of age. Each type of tooth has a specific function related to chewing. Incisors have sharp edges that can bite through food. Canines or cuspids are pointed to puncture or tear food. Bicuspids, premolars, and molars, which are located toward the back of the mouth, are used for crushing and grinding food FIGURE 16.2.

The tongue also aids in chewing by moving food around the mouth to facilitate contact with the teeth. The tongue is a strong muscle that can alter its shape to reach all areas of the mouth. Taste buds, the sensory receptors for taste, are located on the surface of the tongue. There are four types of taste buds: sweet, bitter, sour, and salty.

Saliva is produced by three sets of salivary glands located in the mouth: the parotid, the submandibular, and the sublingual salivary glands. Saliva contains mucus, which moistens the food and the entire oral cavity, and amylase enzymes (also known as ptyalin), which break down polysaccharides (a type of carbohydrate) in food. Saliva also cleanses the teeth and removes food particles that are left in the mouth that may allow bacteria to grow.

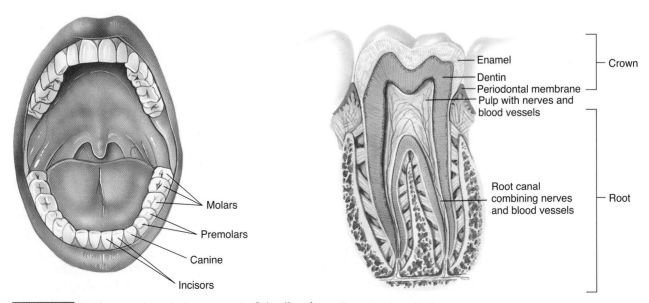

FIGURE 16.2 Teeth are an important component of the digestive system.
© Jones & Bartlett Learning

After food is chewed and moistened and formed into a round mass called a **bolus**, it is swallowed. Swallowing requires coordinated movement of the tongue, the muscles in the cheeks, and the soft palate on the roof of the mouth. Swallowed food is directed into the esophagus.

Esophagus

The **esophagus** is a tube that is approximately 10 inches long and covered in two layers of smooth muscle. The inner layer of muscle forms circles around the esophagus and the outer layer is arranged longitudinally. The esophagus is lined with a mucous membrane that moistens and lubricates food and protects the esophagus from damage.

The esophagus begins the movement of food through the digestive tract through involuntary smooth muscle actions called **peristalsis**. During peristalsis, the two layers of muscles of the esophagus contract and relax, squeezing the bolus of food. This peristaltic action moves food from the esophagus to the stomach.

Stomach

The **stomach** is the saclike structure that stores and digests large particles of food. The stomach is approximately 10 inches in length and slightly curved at the bottom. The opening at the top of the stomach is controlled by the **cardiac sphincter**. The cardiac sphincter is a circular muscle that acts as a one-way gate to assist the unidirectional movement of food from the esophagus to the stomach. The body of the stomach is called the **fundus**.

The stomach is covered in three layers of strong muscles situated in opposite directions. The innermost layer of muscle is an oblique layer, the middle layer is a circular layer, and the outermost layer is a longitudinal layer. The three layers work together to churn the food and continue the process of digestion.

The inner lining of the stomach is composed of a mucous membrane that contains folds, called **rugae**, that can straighten and allow the stomach to expand. The stomach can hold approximately one-half gallon of food and liquid. The mucous membrane also contains glands that secrete mucus and hydrochloric acid, as well as other enzymes to aid in digestion, such as **pepsin**. **Intrinsic factor**, a protein that is necessary for the absorption of vitamin B_{12}, is also secreted by the stomach.

Liquids pass through the stomach within only a few minutes, but food requires several hours to be broken down and prepared for the rest of the digestive tract. Carbohydrates are usually digested first, followed by proteins, then fats. After three to five hours, the partially digested food in the stomach becomes a semiliquid substance called **chyme**. When chyme is the appropriate consistency, the **pyloric sphincter** at the distal end of the stomach opens and the chyme flows into the small intestine **FIGURE 16.3**.

Small Intestine

The **small intestine** is a tube that is one inch in diameter and about 20 feet long. It receives chyme from the stomach and completes the process of digestion. Absorption of nutrients also takes place in the small intestine.

The small intestine is divided into three segments: the **duodenum**, the **jejunum**, and the **ileum**. The first segment, the duodenum, is a C-shaped segment that is approximately nine inches long. The jejunum comprises the next eight feet of small intestine and the ileum is the last 12 feet of small intestine. Both the jejunum and the ileum are suspended in the abdominal cavity by **mesentery**, a fan-shaped fold of tissues attached to the abdominal wall. At the end of the ileum, just prior to joining the large intestine, the diameter of the small intestine reduces to about half an inch.

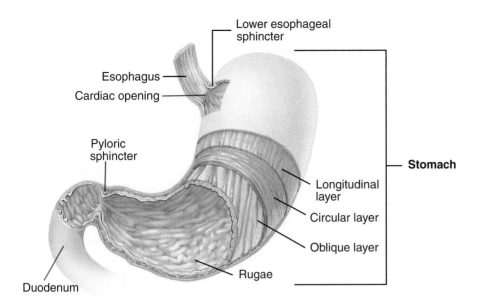

FIGURE 16.3 The stomach stores and digests food.
© Jones & Bartlett Learning

The duodenum secretes **peptidases**, enzymes that digest protein. The small intestine also produces sucrose, maltase, and lactase, which break down complex sugars into simple **monosaccharides** (one-ringed sugars). By the time the chyme reaches the jejunum, it mostly consists of monosaccharides, amino acids, fatty acids, monoglycerides, diglycerides, triglycerides, and water. Mono-, di-, and triglycerides are glycerol molecules attached to one, two, or three fatty acid chains, respectively.

Most absorption takes place in the small intestine, occurring primarily in the jejunum. The lining of the small intestine is covered in thousands of microscopic finger-like projections called **villi** **FIGURE 16.4**. The villi move continuously, which moves and mixes chyme through the digestive tract. The villi also contain capillaries that supply blood and access to the lymphatic system. The villi absorb nutrients and water from the chyme. Carbohydrates, proteins, and some fats are also absorbed by the villi and transported to the portal vein and, ultimately, the liver.

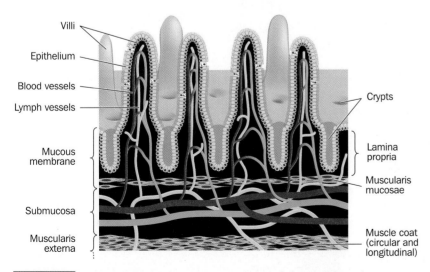

FIGURE 16.4 Villi extend from the mucous membrane of the small intestine.
© Blamb/ShutterStock, Inc.

Large Intestine

The **large intestine** is five feet long and two inches in diameter. It is also called the **colon**. The junction between the large and small intestines is controlled by the **ileocecal valve**, a sphincter that directs the one-way movement of chyme into the large intestine. By the time chyme reaches the large intestine, all of the useful nutrients have been removed and absorbed by the small intestine. The chyme that reaches the large intestine includes waste products, indigestible material, and excess water. The waste products and excess water are excreted from the body as feces or urine. **Feces** is the solid waste that passes through the rectum as a bowel movement; it contains undigested food, bacteria, mucus, and dead cells. Feces is also called **stool**.

The **cecum** is the first segment of the large intestine. It is a small, pouchlike segment from which the **vermiform appendix** extends. The appendix is a small, fingerlike projection that can become filled with chyme. It drains slowly, however, and substances that are irritating to the lining can cause an inflammation of the appendix, known as appendicitis.

After the cecum, the large intestine is divided into three segments: the ascending colon, transverse colon, and descending colon. The **ascending colon** begins after the cecum and ascends up the right side of the abdominal cavity. It bends at the **hepatic flexure**, which is located in front of the right kidney and behind the right lobe of the liver. The **transverse colon** begins at the hepatic flexure and travels across the abdominal cavity to a point near the spleen. At the **splenic flexure**, the **descending colon** begins extending down through the abdominal cavity to the pelvis.

Once the colon enters the pelvic cavity, it bends into an S-shape and is called the **sigmoid colon**. The sigmoid colon joins with the rectum. The **rectum** is six to eight inches long and collects the solid remains from the digestive process. When a large enough amount of material is collected, sensors in the rectum initiate **defecation**, the act of eliminating waste from the body. The **anal canal** extends from the bottom of the rectum to the **anus**, the opening in the body through which waste is expelled from the digestive tract. Sphincters are located at both ends of the one-inch-long anal canal. The **internal anal sphincter**, at the junction of the anal canal and the rectum, is

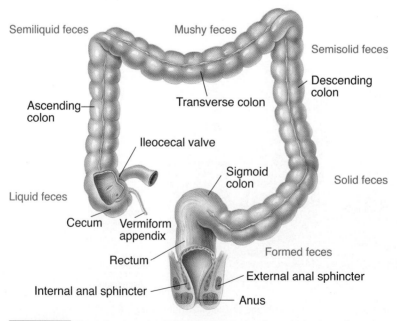

FIGURE 16.5 Feces forms and solidifies as it passes through the large intestine.

an involuntary muscle. The **external anal sphincter**, at the junction of the anal canal and the anus, is a voluntary muscle and can be consciously controlled to encourage or prevent defecation FIGURE 16.5.

Liver

The **liver** is the largest gland in the body. The liver contributes to the functioning of several body systems, and the exocrine functions of the liver are essential to the digestive system and include the production of bile, which is excreted from the liver through the right and left hepatic ducts, which join to form the **hepatic duct**. **Bile** is a bitter liquid that digests fats. Bile is made mostly of water, but its yellow-orange color comes from pigments of destroyed red blood cells that are carried to the liver from the spleen. Iron from the destroyed blood cells is reabsorbed by the body, but the remaining components of bile are excreted in feces.

The liver is also involved in protein and carbohydrate metabolism. It synthesizes nonessential amino acids, builds plasma proteins, and forms and stores glycogen, which the body uses to produce glucose when it needs more fuel. Additionally, the liver manufactures substances that are essential to the clotting process for blood, including fibrinogen and prothrombin. The liver manufactures some antibodies and removes and destroys toxins that have entered the blood. The liver also stores blood and body fluid. The liver receives blood from the hepatic

The liver produces more than one pint of bile every day.
© auremar/ShutterStock, Inc.

artery, which delivers blood to support the liver, and from the portal vein, which brings blood containing absorbed nutrients and waste products from abdominal organs to the liver to be filtered and processed. The liver also stores fat-soluble vitamins, some B vitamins, and iron FIGURE 16.6.

Gallbladder

The **gallbladder** is a small sac underneath the liver that concentrates and stores bile. When the body needs bile to digest fats, the gallbladder releases green-yellow concentrated bile through the **cystic duct** to supplement bile that is released from the liver. The cystic duct and the hepatic duct converge to form the **common bile duct**, which empties bile directly into the duodenum.

The bile ducts can become obstructed by small stones, which are formed from the crystallization of mineral salts present in bile FIGURE 16.7. This condition, known as **gallstones** or **cholelithiasis**, is precipitated by poor drainage of the bile ducts or extended storage of bile. When stones pass into the cystic duct, they can become lodged, which causes pain. Often, surgery is required to remove the stones. If the gallstones become lodged in the common bile duct, neither the gall bladder nor the liver can empty bile into the digestive system. The bile is, instead, absorbed into the bloodstream and produces a yellow discoloration of the skin, mucosa, and sclera (whites of the eyes) known as **jaundice**. The gallbladder may also become infected and can fill with stones. A **cholecystectomy** (surgical removal of the gall-bladder) is usually warranted in this case FIGURE 16.8.

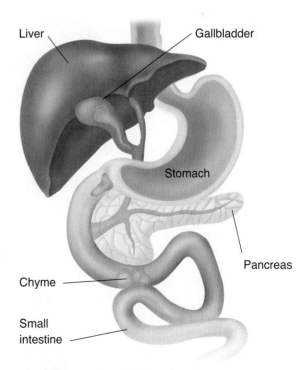

FIGURE 16.6 The liver, gallbladder, and pancreas are accessory organs of the digestive system.
© Jones & Bartlett Learning

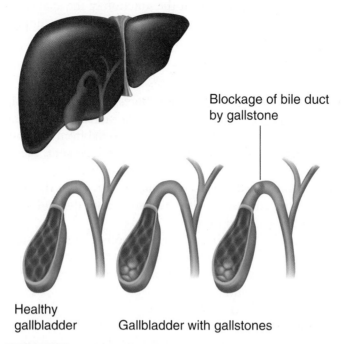

FIGURE 16.7 Gallstones can obstruct bile ducts.
© Alila Sao Mai/ShutterStock, Inc.

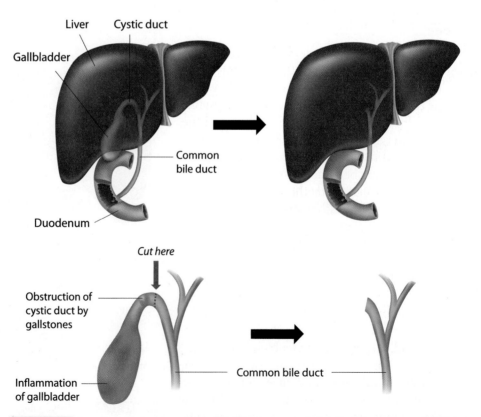

FIGURE 16.8 In a cholecystectomy, the gallbladder is removed, but the bile ducts are left intact.
© Alila Sao Mai/ShutterStock, Inc.

Pancreas

The pancreas is a gland that has both endocrine and exocrine functions. The exocrine functions of the pancreas include secreting pancreatic juice through the pancreatic ducts, which eventually joins the common bile duct, into the duodenum. Pancreatic juice contains powerful enzymes that digest carbohydrates, fat, and protein, and prepare them for the remainder of the digestive process. Trypsin, chymotrypsin, nucleases, and carboxypeptidases break down proteins into amino acids and nucleic acids. Pancreatic lipase digests fats into fatty acids and glycerol. Pancreatic amylase digests carbohydrates. The endocrine functions of the pancreas, which include the production of insulin and glucagon, are described in Chapter 15.

Nutrition

Proper nutrition is essential to the function of the digestive system. **Nutrition** is the process of taking nutrients into the body to replace those that have been used. Healthy individuals consume an amount of nutrients close to that which the body uses. Poor nutrition, including both excess consumption and inadequate consumption of nutrients, contributes to poor outcomes of many disease states. Poor nutrition is also associated with an increased use of healthcare resources. The amount and quality of food consumed contributes to an individual's quality of life, overall health, and longevity.

Malnutrition refers to any nutrition disorder and encompasses a variety of nutrition statuses. **Overnutrition** describes excess nutrient intake and leads to conditions of being overweight and obesity. **Undernutrition** describes inadequate nutrient intake and leads to weight loss and altered organ function. Nutrition disorders, both overnutrition and undernutrition, can result from a variety of conditions, including medical, social, economic, and psychological factors. Substance abuse, fad diets, and eating disorders also contribute to nutritional deficiencies.

Poor nutrition increases the risk for cancer, infections, and complications from surgery or other medical treatments. Wound-healing time and mortality are increased across a range of diseases and conditions due to nutritional deficiencies. Nutritional deficiencies cause inadequate nutrient delivery, synthesis, and absorption, and lead to depletion of the body's nutrient stores, biochemical changes in the functioning of the body, physical manifestations of deficiency, and morbidity and mortality.

Nutrients

Nutrients provide energy for the cells of the body and regulate body processes. Nutrients are the building blocks for proteins and fats that are produced by the body. Nutrients are divided into two groups: **macronutrients** that provide energy and **micronutrients** that do not provide energy. Energy-providing macronutrients include carbohydrates, fats, and protein. Micronutrients, including vitamins, minerals, trace elements, and water, cannot be converted to energy but, instead, regulate body processes.

Carbohydrates

Carbohydrates are the body's main source of energy. All carbohydrates are made of carbon, hydrogen, and oxygen formed into units of sugar called saccharides. Monosaccharides are one-sugar carbohydrates; **disaccharides** are two-sugar carbohydrates. Monosaccharides and disaccharides are known as simple sugars. Glucose, fructose, and galactose are monosaccharides, and lactose, maltose, and sucrose are disaccharides. Glucose is the sugar that the body uses most to produce energy, and most sugar that is ingested is eventually converted to glucose for the body to use. Fructose is the sugar

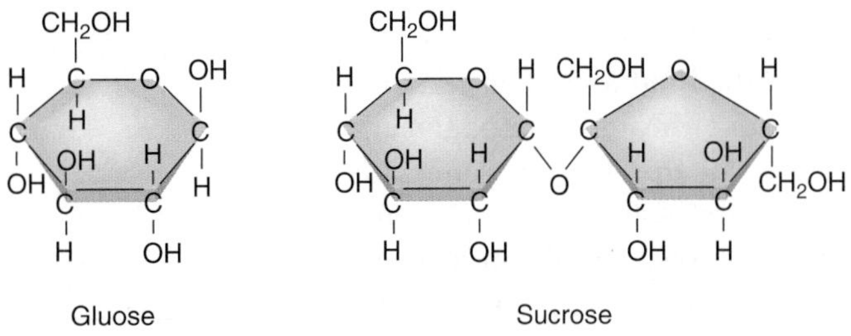

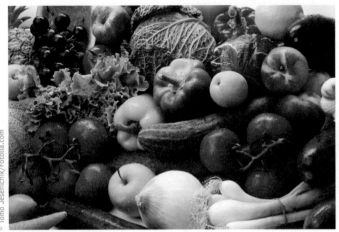

Gluose   Sucrose

FIGURE 16.9 Glucose is a one-sugar carbohydrate and sucrose is a two-sugar carbohydrate.
© Jones & Bartlett Learning

Fruits and vegetables are sources of fiber.

© Tomo Jesenicnik/Fotolia.com

found in many fruits. Galactose is a product of lactose digestion. Lactose is the sugar found in dairy products, and maltose is a product of the digestion of polysaccharides. Sucrose is a sweet sugar that occurs naturally in fruits and vegetables, as well as the sugar cane and the sugar beet, the sources for commercial refined sugar. Because simple sugars are small, their digestion takes little time and absorption occurs rapidly after ingestion **FIGURE 16.9** .

Polysaccharides are called complex carbohydrates. They are made up of three or more sugar units. Starches, glycogen, and fiber are common polysaccharides. These larger compounds require more time for digestion than simple sugars. **Fiber** is a polysaccharide that is derived from plant sources. It is available in the diet in the form of fruits, vegetables, and grains. Fiber cannot be digested by the body, but acts to add bulk to feces. A lack of fiber in the diet is associated with constipation, inflammation of the colon, and colorectal cancer. Excess fiber can lead to diarrhea or flatulence.

Fats

Fats, or **lipids**, are also composed of carbon, hydrogen, and oxygen, but in different ratios and arrangements than carbohydrates. In the body, fats most often exist as triglycerides, or glycerol molecules with three fatty acid chains. A **fatty acid** is a carboxylic acid with a long hydrocarbon chain, usually with an even number of carbon atoms ranging from 4 to 28. The only fatty acid that is essential for the human diet is linoleic acid. All other fatty acids can be derived from linoleic acid **FIGURE 16.10**.

Fatty acids are classified as saturated or unsaturated. In a **saturated fatty acid**, every carbon atom in the chain is attached to as many hydrogen atoms as possible. In chemistry terms, the carbons are all attached with single bonds. In an **unsaturated fatty acid**, some of the carbons are attached by double bonds, meaning that they are not attached to as many hydrogen atoms as possible. Unsaturated fats tend to be liquids at room temperature, and saturated fats are solids at room temperature. Saturated fats are more common from animal sources and tend to increase levels of cholesterol in the blood.

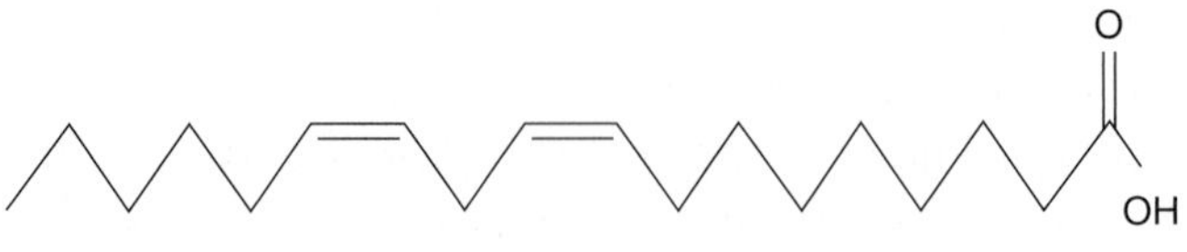

FIGURE 16.10 Linoleic acid has an 18-carbon chain.
© Jones & Bartlett Learning

Trans unsaturated fatty acids, known as **trans fats**, are not naturally occurring fats. They are produced by a process called **hydrogenation**, in which vegetable oil is heated and hydrogen is added to it. This process is used in the commercial food industry to give foods a longer shelf life and better taste. Convenience foods and commercially available snack foods often contain trans fats, although the food industry is working toward eliminating these unhealthy trans fats from many consumer products. The Food and Drug Administration (FDA) recommends that people consume as few trans fats as possible and requires food packaging labels to clearly state the amount of trans fat present in each serving.

Protein

In addition to the carbon, hydrogen, and oxygen found in the other energy-providing nutrients, proteins contain nitrogen. A **protein** is composed of repeating units of amino acids. There are 22 amino acids that form proteins. Eight of them must be included in the diet and the rest can be synthesized by the body. Histidine is essential only during childhood. Animal products such as meat, milk, and eggs are the best dietary sources for protein that contains all eight essential amino acids. Plant products provide some protein, but often do not contain all eight amino acids. Proteins do not provide energy in the same way as carbohydrates and fats, but serve mostly as building blocks for essential body functions, including the production of hormones, enzymes, and structural components of cells. The body can use protein as an energy source when carbohydrates or fats are in short supply. However, this process can have detrimental effects on the body. Protein from organs and muscles will be used for energy, damaging the structure of the body systems.

Vitamins

A **vitamin** is an organic molecule that regulates metabolic processes in the body. These processes support growth, homeostasis, and reproduction. Vitamins, with the exception of vitamins D and K, cannot be produced by the body in sufficient quantities for optimal growth and health, and they must be obtained from food sources or supplementation.

Vitamins are classified as water-soluble or fat-soluble. **Water-soluble vitamins** (vitamin B complexes and vitamin C) are present in extracellular fluids and excreted by the kidneys and are not stored by the body, so they must be supplied by continuous dietary intake. **Fat-soluble vitamins** (vitamins A, D, E, and K) are stored by the body, usually in the liver. High doses of either class of vitamins can cause toxicity, but the risk of toxicity is higher with fat-soluble vitamins because they are stored by the body. Vitamin deficiencies can lead to significant health consequences.

Vitamin C (ascorbic acid) is a water-soluble vitamin found in green, leafy vegetables, tomatoes, strawberries, kiwi, citrus fruits, and potatoes. Vitamin C is an antioxidant, promotes immune-system function, and possesses anti-inflammatory properties. Scurvy, a disorder that causes anemia, hemorrhages, spongy gums, and hardening of leg muscles, is caused by a vitamin C deficiency. Muscle

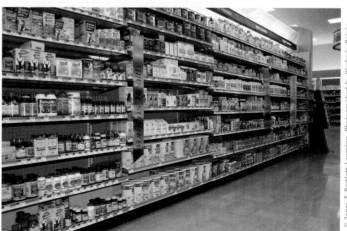

Vitamin supplements are a multibillion dollar industry in the United States.

cramps and ulcers on the gums also result from a vitamin C deficiency. Vitamin C toxicity can cause anemia and kidney stones.

Vitamin B complexes and vitamin C are water-soluble.
Vitamins A, D, E, and K are fat-soluble.

Vitamin B is a group of water-soluble vitamins that contains several members. B-complex vitamins are not associated with signs or symptoms of toxicity. Vitamin B_1 (thiamine) is found in animal products such as liver, kidney, and pork, whole grains, peas, beans, wheat germ, and yeast. It supports carbohydrate metabolism, cardiac function, mental and cognitive proficiency, and energy production. A vitamin B_1 deficiency causes beriberi and leads to edema, cardiac abnormalities, weight loss, muscular dysfunction, and impaired sensory perception. Alcoholics frequently suffer from a thiamine deficiency.

Vitamin B_2 (riboflavin) is found in meats, poultry, fish, dairy products, and green vegetables. It supports hair, skin, and nail growth. It also plays a small role in nerve function and the production of red blood cells.

Vitamin B_3 (nicotinic acid or niacin) is found in lean meats, fish, liver, poultry, grains, eggs, peanuts, and milk. It facilitates fat synthesis and protein metabolism. Niacin is used therapeutically to lower cholesterol levels. A niacin deficiency is known as pellagra and leads to diarrhea, depression, mental confusion, and dermatitis.

Vitamin B_5 (pantothenic acid) is found in most vegetables, meat, fish, eggs, and yeast. Pantothenic acid is found in at least small quantities in almost all foods. It supports growth, energy production, and normal physiological functioning. A pantothenic acid deficiency leads to fatigue, headache, sleepiness, nausea, muscle spasms, and decreased coordination.

Vitamin B_6 (pyridoxine) is found in meats, cereals, lentils, nuts, legumes, milk, and egg yolks. It is found in virtually every food of plant or animal origin. It supports nerve growth and function. Pyridoxine is used therapeutically to treat alcoholics who have nerve damage.

Vitamin B_7 (biotin) is also known as vitamin H. It is found in liver, yeast, eggs, most vegetables, bananas, mushrooms, peanuts, and milk. It supports fatty-acid synthesis and carbohydrate, protein, and fat metabolism for energy production. It promotes healthy hair, skin, and nail growth, as well as nerve-tissue, bone marrow, and sweat-gland formation. Biotin is found in many foods and can be recycled by the body, unlike most water-soluble vitamins. Biotin can also be produced by intestinal flora.

Vitamin B_9 (folic acid or folate) is found in liver, lean beef, wheat, whole grains, eggs, fish, and fresh green vegetables. Folic acid works with vitamin B_{12} to promote the growth of red blood cells and can be used therapeutically to treat anemia. Folic acid is also responsible for fetal development in the first few weeks of pregnancy. Therefore, it is important that women of child-bearing age who might become pregnant receive adequate intake of folic acid. Inadequate folic acid intake during pregnancy is related to neural-tube birth defects. Depression is a symptom of folic acid deficiency.

Vitamin B_{12} (cyanocobalamin) is found in animal tissues and dairy products. It is a cofactor that supports the production of red blood cells. Cyanocobalamin must work with the intrinsic factor in the stomach to exert its effect. A deficiency in either vitamin B_{12} or the intrinsic factor leads to anemia. Cyanocobalamin is poorly absorbed from the GI tract, so intramuscular or intravenous administration is recommended for supplementation. If taken orally, cyanocobalamin supplements must be taken in extremely large quantities.

Many compounds that were once believed to be vitamins have been reclassified as other substances, leaving gaps in the numbering of B-complex vitamins.

Fat-soluble vitamins are absorbed with the fats in the diet and are stored by the body. Deficiencies in fat-soluble vitamins occur after prolonged periods of decreased intake.

Vitamin A (retinol) is found in liver, milk, eggs, and dairy products. The body can produce vitamin A from pigments and carotene present in many fruits and vegetables. Vitamin A supports normal growth, bone formation, reproduction, and repair of epithelial tissue. A vitamin A deficiency leads to keratomalacia, a softening of the cornea. Night blindness, respiratory infections, and cessation of bone growth can also result from vitamin A deficiency. Vitamin A toxicity results in cessation of menstruation in women, joint pain, stunted growth, and enlargement of the liver.

Vitamin D (D_2, ergocalciferol; D_3, cholecalciferol) is found in dairy products, eggs, and fish oils. It is formed in the skin following exposure to ultraviolet radiation; calciferol, the active form of vitamin D, is formed from the precursors vitamins D_2 and D_3 and transported to the bloodstream. A vitamin D deficiency disrupts calcium-phosphate balance and inhibits healthy bone growth and formation. In children, vitamin D deficiency causes rickets, a disorder in which the bones of the legs and the spine become distorted. In adults, vitamin D deficiency causes osteomalacia, a condition in which the skeleton is weakened due to the demineralization of the bones. Vitamin D toxicity can lead to kidney stones and the calcification of soft tissue.

Vitamin E (tocopherol) is a group of compounds found in soybeans, wheat germ, nuts, corn, butter, eggs, liver, and green vegetables. Vitamin E is an antioxidant and prevents cataracts, enhances immune response, prevents cardiovascular disease, and decreases the progression of dementia. Vitamin E deficiency can cause neurological defects and the destruction of red blood cells. An overdose of vitamin E can damage the heart.

Vitamin K (phytonadione) is found in liver, vegetable oils, spinach, kale, broccoli, and cauliflower. Vitamin K promotes blood clotting through the formation of thrombin in the liver, and a vitamin K deficiency leads to prolonged clotting times. Vitamin K is used as an antidote to reverse overdoses of anticoagulants. Hemolytic anemia and jaundice occur as a result of vitamin K toxicity.

Vitamin Deficiencies

Five primary vitamin deficiencies seen in humans are as follows:

- Keratomalacia (vitamin A)
- Rickets (vitamin D)
- Beriberi (vitamin B_1)
- Pellagra (vitamin B_3)
- Scurvy (vitamin C)

The symptoms of vitamin deficiencies can be reversed with supplementation of the deficient vitamin.

Minerals

A **mineral** is an inorganic substance that exists in body fluids and regulates homeostasis or functions as constituents of organic compounds. Like most vitamins, minerals cannot be produced by the body and must be supplied by the diet. However, unlike vitamins, which are complex molecules, minerals are single elements.

An **electrolyte** is a mineral that exists as an ion when dissolved in water. An **ion** is an electrically charged atom or molecule that possesses either a positive charge (**cation**) or negative charge (**anion**). Electrolytes maintain homeostasis and coordinate the electrophysiological processes of the body.

Sodium (Na^+) is the primary cation present in the fluid outside of cells. Sodium retains fluid in the body, generates nerve impulses, and regulates enzymatic activity. The kidneys maintain optimal sodium levels in the body. Sodium supplementation is not usually necessary because the average dietary intake is more than sufficient to meet physiological needs.

Potassium (K^+) is the primary cation present inside the cells. Potassium regulates nerve signaling and muscle function. Potassium is also critical to insulin release from the pancreas and protein synthesis. Excess potassium leads to cardiac abnormalities. Potassium deficiencies may be seen in patients who take diuretics. Potassium supplementation can correct the deficiency.

Calcium (Ca^{2+}) is the mineral present in the highest quantity in the body. It functions in bone and teeth formation, muscle contraction, and blood coagulation. When dietary intake does not provide enough calcium to meet the body's needs, the body removes calcium from bone, which can lead to decreased bone mass and osteoporosis. A complete discussion of osteoporosis is available in Chapter 12.

Hydrogen (H^+) determines the acid-base balance of body fluids. Normal blood pH is slightly alkalinic, with a pH of 7.4. **Acidosis** (a blood pH below 7.35) is a metabolic condition caused by the excessive loss of sodium or bicarbonate due to dehydration or starvation. In the respiratory system, acidosis causes increased carbon dioxide levels. **Alkalosis** (a blood pH above 7.45) is a metabolic condition caused by the excessive loss of potassium or chloride due to vomiting or diarrhea. Alkalosis causes hyperventilation and decreased carbon dioxide levels.

Magnesium (Mg^{2+}) is a cation located inside cells and bones. It regulates enzymatic functions, controls nerve and muscle impulse generation, and coordinates energy metabolism. Magnesium can be lost from the body due to alcohol abuse, stress, or medications that increase magnesium excretion such as digoxin, estrogen, and diuretics.

Chloride (Cl^-) maintains homeostasis and acid-base balance. It is the primary extracellular anion.

Trace elements are minerals that are required in smaller quantities than other minerals, but are no less important. Trace elements include iron, copper, chromium, molybdenum, selenium, manganese, iodine, zinc, cobalt, and fluorine. Iron is essential to the heme molecule, which carries oxygen in the blood and delivers it to the cells of the body. Iron is also part of myoglobin, which is involved in metabolic reactions in muscle cells. Zinc is an important trace element because it promotes tissue growth and immune-system function. Iodine is critical in the formation of thyroid hormone; without iodine, the thyroid would not be able to regulate the functions of other glands. Other trace elements are involved in countless metabolic reactions and tissue functions.

Water

The human body is composed of roughly 50 percent water. Water is the primary component of all living cells, and the fluids that are outside the cells, such as lymph and plasma, are composed of high proportions of water. Water is the major solvent in the human body and removes toxic waste from the body. Water also transports substances, lubricates surfaces, and controls temperatures in the body. Water must be continually ingested and replenished. Water is lost in sweat, urine, feces, and respiration. Food contains some water, but water should also be consumed to supplement the fluid found in food.

The amount of water in the human body varies by age, disease state, gender, and body weight. There is an inverse relationship between fatty tissue and water. Overweight individuals have a smaller percentage of body water than lean, muscular individuals. Newborns have the highest percentage of body water, with 75 percent or more. The body loses water as it ages; the elderly generally have the lowest proportion of body water.

> Water accounts for 50–60 percent of body weight for the average adult male and 45–50 percent of body weight for the average adult female.
> © auremar/ShutterStock, Inc.

Changes in the normal proportion of water in the body can lead to organ dysfunction, electrolyte imbalance, and cardiac and muscle irregularities. The proportion of body water can change due to certain medications, disease states, environmental conditions, exercise, or increased or decreased intake of fluid. **Dehydration**, or the loss of body water, can be caused by vomiting, diarrhea, edema, excessive sweating, significant weight loss, or large urine output. Dehydration can cause dry skin and mucous membranes, decreased blood pressure, increased heart rate, and lowered body temperature. Chronic dehydration causes mental disturbances, headache, depression, and fatigue. A loss of 25 percent of body water can cause death.

The human body can survive several weeks without food, but only three days without water.

Sometimes referred to as water intoxication, drinking too much water in a short amount of time is as dangerous as dehydration. Large volumes of water cannot be quickly filtered by the kidneys, so the blood begins to absorb the water, leading to decreased concentrations of electrolytes in the blood. This sudden and severe drop in electrolyte concentration disrupts the body's normal electrophysiological processes and leads to water entering the brain and other organs. **Hyponatremia**, or a decreased concentration of sodium in the blood, is the most severe consequence of large water intake, and can lead to lethargy, confusion, seizures, coma, and death.

Imbalances in fluid and electrolyte concentrations can lead to a variety of signs and symptoms. Fluid- and electrolyte-replacement therapy can be used to replenish lost fluids and electrolytes or maintain homeostasis.

Signs and Symptoms of Fluid and Electrolyte Imbalances

Signs and symptoms of fluid and electrolyte imbalances include the following:

- Thirst
- Dry mouth
- Hypotension
- Decreased urine output
- Sunken eyes
- Weakness
- Fatigue
- Diminished reflexes
- Muscle cramps
- Tingling in extremities
- Confusion
- Shortness of breath
- Nausea and vomiting

Calories and Energy Balance

The amount of energy supplied by each nutrient is measured in calories. One **calorie** is the amount of energy required to raise the temperature of one gram of water one degree Celsius. When calculating the energy in food, the term *calories* is often used, but food energy is actually measured in kilocalories (1,000 calories.) To distinguish the two terms, the small base unit of calories is sometimes written with a lowercase *c* and the larger kilocalorie is written with a capital *C*—that is, *calorie* and *Calorie*, respectively. Carbohydrates and proteins provide four Calories per gram and fats provide nine Calories per gram.

Nutrition Facts

Serving Size 1 Bar (85g)
Servings Per Container 4

Amount Per Serving

Calories 170	Calories from Fat 50

	% Daily Value *
Total Fat 6g	**9%**
Saturated Fat 4g	**19%**
Trans Fat 0g	
Polyunsaturated Fat 0.5g	
Monounsaturated Fat 1g	
Cholesterol 13mg	**4%**
Sodium 83mg	**3%**
Total Carbohydrate 33g	**11%**
Dietary Fiber 4g	**16%**
Sugar 25g	
Protein 3g	

Vitamin A 110%	•	Vitamin C 2%
Calcium 10%	•	Iron 3%

*Percent Daily Values are based on a 2,000 calorie diet. Your daily values may be higher or lower depending on your calorie needs.

	Calories	2,000	2,500
Total Fat	Less than	65g	80g
Sat Fat	Less than	20g	25g
Cholesterol	Less than	300mg	300mg
Sodium	Less than	2,400mg	2,400mg
Total Carbohydrate		300g	375g
Dietary Fiber		25g	30g

Calories per gram:
Fat 9   •   Carbohydrate 4   •   Protein 4

© Eugene Feygin/Dreamstime.com

Food labels provide nutrition information.

Energy is used continuously by the body for all activities, including voluntary and involuntary activities and restful and active behaviors. The level of energy required for the body's activities while at rest is the **basal metabolic rate (BMR)**. An individual's BMR will vary with age, gender, and disease state. BMR is high during periods of rapid growth, and lean individuals have a higher BMR than those with more body fat. Activities above and beyond the BMR also require energy, and total calorie requirements for an individual vary with physical activity.

To maintain a healthy energy balance, individuals should consume the same number of calories each day that their body uses for energy. When more calories are consumed than used, the body stores the excess calories as fat. When fewer calories are consumed than used, the body will use stored fat to create energy. Optimally, the largest proportion of calories should come from carbohydrates, followed by fats, then proteins. Carbohydrates should account for 50 to 60 percent of total consumption, fats should account for less than 30 percent, and protein should make up the remaining 10 to 20 percent.

To help individuals understand and visualize healthy food choices, the United States Department of Agriculture has introduced MyPlate as a part of a larger communications initiative based on 2010 Dietary Guidelines for Americans to help consumers make better food choices. MyPlate is designed to remind Americans to eat healthfully; it is not intended to change consumer behavior alone. MyPlate illustrates the five food groups using a familiar mealtime visual, a place setting.

Food labels are also available for nutrition information. Each label provides clear representations of the serving size of the food item, and the Calories, fat, protein, vitamins, and minerals present in each serving. It is imperative to read the food label on prepackaged foods to fully understand the ingredients and nutritional content. Many manufacturers place phrasing in their advertising and labeling that promote the healthfulness of the food. Only by reading the food label will a consumer be able to discriminate healthy food from unhealthy food.

Herbal and Dietary Supplements

Complementary and alternative medicine (CAM) encompasses diverse medical and healthcare systems, therapies, and products. CAM includes dietary supplements, such as herbs, minerals, and botanical preparations. CAM therapies are often used concurrently with traditional medications and therapies. They may be used to treat chronic conditions, acute illnesses, pain, sleep disturbances, sexual dysfunction, and mental health, as well as a host of other diseases and conditions. Use of CAM crosses all gender, age, socioeconomic, educational, and racial lines. Many supporters of CAM feel that "natural" preparations, such as those derived from plants or other naturally occurring compounds, are safer than traditional pharmaceutical products. In general, CAM also encourages a philosophy of integrative and holistic treatment.

The use of dietary supplements is increasing due to healthcare costs and patient desire for autonomy. Common dietary supplements and their potential side effects are listed in **TABLE 16.2**.

Safety is a primary concern with the use of CAM supplements. These products are not regulated by the U.S. FDA; therefore, no guarantees of a product's safety or effectiveness can be made. The

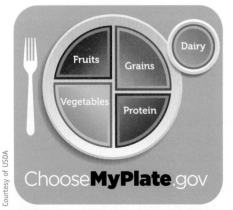

Courtesy of USDA

The U.S. Department of Agriculture's MyPlate illustrates the five food groups using a familiar mealtime visual, a place setting.

Table 16.2 Common Dietary Supplements		
Name	**Intended Use**	**Side Effects/Safety**
Black cohash	Symptoms of PMS and menopause	GI upset, weight gain, headache
Chondroitin	Osteoarthritis	None reported
Coenzyme Q10	Cardiovascular disease	Mild insomnia, elevated liver enzymes
Echinacea	Enhanced immune function	GI upset, tingling of the tongue, headache; may lead to immunosuppression with long-term use; should not be used in patients with autoimmune disorders
Evening primrose oil	Breast pain, symptoms of PMS and menopause	GI upset, headache
Feverfew	Headache	GI upset, allergic reactions, antiplatelet effects, withdrawal symptoms
Garlic	Hyperlipidemia, hypertension, diabetes mellitus	GI upset, bad breath, allergic reactions; caution when used with anticoagulants
Ginger	Antiemetic	Weak antiplatelet effects
Ginkgo biloba	Alzheimer's disease and dementia, vascular disease	GI upset, headache, dizziness, allergic reactions; possible seizures or lowering of seizure threshold
Ginseng	Anemia, diabetes mellitus, insomnia, impotence, fever	Insomnia, headache, blood-pressure changes, anorexia, rash, vaginal bleeding
Glucosamine	Osteoarthritis	GI upset
Kava-kava	Muscle relaxant, anticonvulsant	Rash
Licorice	Peptic ulcer disease	Pseudoaldosteronism, hypokalemia; caution for patients with renal or liver disease
Melatonin	Sleep disorders	Vivid dreams, drowsiness, GI upset, headache, irritability, breast enlargement, decreased sperm count in men
Milk thistle	Liver disease and cirrhosis	Mild diarrhea
Red yeast	Hypercholesterolemia	Should not be used in patients with liver disease
Saw palmetto	Benign prostatic hyperplasia	GI upset
St. John's wort	Depression	Insomnia, vivid dreams, restlessness, GI upset, fatigue, dry mouth, dizziness, headache; caution in patients with bipolar disorder or schizophrenia
Valerian	Sedative/hypnotic	Headache, excitability, insomnia; may induce uterine contractions in pregnant women

FDA simply mandates that dietary supplements cannot claim to treat, prevent, or diagnose any disease or condition. Evidence from randomized, controlled clinical trials is limited for dietary supplements, and patients should be warned of the risks associated with taking dietary supplements. It is possible to have an allergic reaction or toxicity from herbal and dietary supplements.

Dietary Supplement and Health Education Act

As part of the Dietary Supplement and Health Education Act (DSHEA) of 1994, the FDA requires that all dietary supplements that make a disease-specific claim contain the following statement on the label: "This statement has not been evaluated by the Food and Drug Administration. This product is not intended to diagnose, treat, cure, or prevent any disease."

Patients should always be advised to keep a complete list of all the medications and dietary supplements they are taking, and to share the list with their physician and pharmacist. Respecting cultural or ideological differences facilitates trust between patients and the healthcare system. The more open patients are about the drugs and supplements they are taking, the more effective healthcare providers can be at delivering safe, accurate health information.

Recommend that all patients tally a list of all medications, vitamins, and supplements that they are taking. Tell them to keep this list with them at all times and share it with their physicians and pharmacist.
© auremar/ShutterStock, Inc.

Diseases and Disorders of the Digestive System

When any of the steps in the digestive process (ingestion, absorption, digestion, or elimination) is hindered or altered, gastrointestinal complications can occur. Complications range from mild discomfort to dehydration and malnutrition. Common signs and symptoms of diseases and disorders of the digestive tract include nausea, vomiting, diarrhea, epigastric pain, loss of appetite, weight loss, fatigue, **hematemesis** (vomiting blood), **melena** (blood in the feces), and **hematochezia** (bright red blood in the feces).

Appendicitis

Appendicitis is the acute inflammation of the appendix. Appendicitis is often the result of an obstruction in the intestines, which, in turn, leads to an infection.

Signs and Symptoms of Appendicitis

Appendicitis usually begins with generalized abdominal pain that eventually localizes to the lower-right abdomen. Tenderness in the abdomen, loss of appetite, nausea, and vomiting are often present with appendicitis. Fever may also occur. An elevated white blood cell count might be apparent on laboratory evaluations. The sudden cessation of symptoms indicates a rupture of the appendix. A ruptured appendix causes the release of infectious material into the abdominal cavity, which can be fatal if left untreated.

Treatment of Appendicitis

The goals of appendicitis treatment are to relieve symptoms and prevent further infection or complication. Surgical removal of the appendix, called an **appendectomy**, is the only treatment for appendicitis.

Cirrhosis

Cirrhosis of the liver is a progressive and irreversible condition in which the cells of the liver are gradually destroyed due to chronic hepatic inflammation FIGURE 16.11 . This destruction leads to impaired blood and lymph circulation and loss of liver function. Cirrhosis is most frequently caused by malnutrition associated with alcoholism. Hepatitis or diseases of the bile ducts can also cause cirrhosis.

Signs and Symptoms of Cirrhosis

Early signs of cirrhosis are general and diffuse. They include lack of appetite, indigestion, nausea, vomiting, constipation, and diarrhea. Later symptoms of cirrhosis include nosebleeds, anemia, and bleeding gums. With advanced cirrhosis, the liver will enlarge and jaundice is apparent. Fluid also collects in the abdomen, a condition called **ascites**. A liver biopsy is required for a definitive diagnosis of cirrhosis.

Treatment of Cirrhosis

The goals of treatment for cirrhosis are preventing further damage to the liver or other organ systems. Dietary changes and vitamin supplementation to correct malnutrition are indicated. Alcohol must be avoided by patients diagnosed with cirrhosis. Ascites is managed by sodium restriction and removal of fluid from the body by the use of diuretics. Unfortunately, mortality related to cirrhosis is high.

> Cirrhosis is the 12th most common cause of death in the United States.

Constipation

Constipation is the decreased frequency of bowel movements or difficulty defecating. Constipation is not a disease, but can be a symptom of an underlying GI issue. The two most common causes of constipation are a lack of dietary fiber and drug-induced constipation. Common drug-related causes of constipation include ACE inhibitors, antacids, antihistamines, benzodiazepines, beta-blockers, calcium channel blockers, iron preparations, non-potassium-sparing diuretics, NSAIDs, and opioid analgesics. The chronic use of laxatives and routinely ignoring the urge to defecate can also cause constipation.

Signs and Symptoms of Constipation

Constipation is characterized by hard, dry, and infrequent bowel movements. The bowel movements may be painful.

Treatment of Constipation

The goal of constipation treatment is to restore normal bowel function. The most effective treatment of constipation begins by determining and treating the cause. In the case of drug-induced constipation, the offending agent should be discontinued if possible. If it cannot be discontinued, a lower dose may relieve the constipation, but dietary management or pharmacological therapy may be necessary.

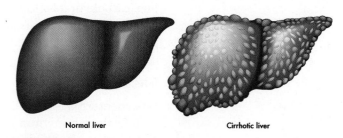

Normal liver   Cirrhotic liver

FIGURE 16.11 Hepatic cirrhosis leads to destruction of the liver and fluid collection in the abdomen.
© Jones & Bartlett Learning

Dietary modification relieves a majority of cases of constipation. Fiber, the indigestible portion of plant-based foods, increases stool bulk, helps retain water in the stool, and increases transit time through the GI tract. According to the American Dietetic Association, adults should consume 25 to 30 grams of fiber in their diets daily to maintain healthy bowel function; most Americans consume only half this amount.

Laxatives are also available to encourage defecation. A **laxative** softens the stool and increases the frequency of bowel movements. Laxatives should not be used for long-term control of bowel movements. They are indicated for short-term use only, unless directed by a physician.

Diarrhea

Diarrhea is defined as an increased frequency and decreased consistency of fecal matter compared with an individual's normal bowel habits. Diarrhea is a gastrointestinal discomfort that affects virtually every person at some point during his or her life.

Diarrhea can be a sign or symptom of a systemic condition.

Diarrhea can be caused by a number of bacterial or viral organisms, but may also be caused by other disease states, conditions, medications, or food intolerances. Most cases of diarrhea, although inconvenient and uncomfortable, are self-limiting and short-lived. Acute diarrhea is defined as diarrhea lasting less than 14 days. Persistent diarrhea lasts more than 14 days, and chronic diarrhea lasts more than 30 days.

Diarrhea accounts for 7 percent of all adverse drug events. Of these, 25 percent are caused by antibiotics.
© auremar/ShutterStock, Inc.

Common drug-related causes of diarrhea include laxatives, magnesium-containing drugs, antibiotics, antihypertensives, NSAIDs, misoprostol, and colchicine.

Signs and Symptoms of Diarrhea

Diarrhea is characterized by frequent, liquid stools. Diarrhea decreases transit time through the GI tract. Therefore, it leads to altered absorption of nutrients. Diarrhea can be dangerous when it occurs as a chronic condition or leads to dehydration.

Treatment of Diarrhea

The goals of diarrhea treatment include maintaining hydration and electrolyte balance, as well as treating the underlying cause of diarrhea, if identifiable. Dietary management of diarrhea is important to maintain fluid and electrolyte balance. A normal diet is recommended for most patients because bowel rest is not necessary after acute episodes of diarrhea that do not result in dehydration. In general, a diet rich in complex carbohydrates (found in rice, potatoes, breads, and cereals), yogurt, lean meats, fruits, and vegetables is appropriate. Patients should avoid foods and drinks high in fat, simple sugars, and caffeine because these ingredients can worsen diarrhea.

Gastroenteritis

Gastroenteritis is an inflammation of the stomach and intestines. It may be caused by an infectious bacterium or virus, diarrhea, food poisoning, allergies, drug reactions, or ingestion of a toxin or poison. In general, cases of gastroenteritis are self-limiting and resolve within a few days. Mild gastroenteritis is not a serious health condition for otherwise healthy adults.

Signs and Symptoms of Gastroenteritis

Gastroenteritis is characterized by fever, nausea, abdominal pain, cramping, diarrhea, and vomiting. General malaise often accompanies gastroenteritis. Loss of appetite is common in gastroenteritis.

Treatment of Gastroenteritis

The goals of gastroenteritis treatment are to relieve symptoms and prevent complications related to dehydration or malnutrition. Rest, increased fluid intake, and a bland diet are indicated for gastroenteritis. If a bacterial cause of gastroenteritis is identified, antibiotic treatment is appropriate.

Gastroesophageal Reflux Disease

Gastroesophageal reflux disease (GERD), often referred to as heartburn, is a common problem. It is most often seen in patients over 40 years of age in Westernized countries.

GERD is caused by a dysfunctional lower esophageal sphincter, which normally prevents stomach contents from flowing back into the esophagus. This dysfunction causes a flow of gastric and, sometimes, duodenal contents into the esophagus **FIGURE 16.12**.

Several behaviors, medications, and foods can precipitate or worsen GERD: eating quickly, eating late at night, overeating, smoking, alcohol, caffeine, citric acid, garlic, gas-producing foods, high-fat foods, onions, peppermint and spearmint, spicy foods, tomato juice, aspirin, estrogen, nitrates, NSAIDs, potassium chloride, progesterone, theophylline, and tetracycline.

Signs and Symptoms of Gastroesophageal Reflux Disease

The most common complaint associated with GERD is a warm or burning sensation rising from the abdomen toward the neck. The symptoms vary in frequency and intensity but often include chest pain, sore throat, nausea, cough, asthma, sinusitis, bad breath, dental erosions, and recurrent ear infections. Symptoms are often worse after a meal and when patients are lying down.

GERD results in damage to the mucosa of the GI tract caused by an abnormal reflux of stomach contents into the esophagus. If this reflux occurs for a prolonged period, the highly acidic contents of the stomach can cause permanent damage to the esophagus and can lead to the development of several forms of cancer. If patients experience difficult or painful swallowing, significant weight loss, bleeding in the GI tract, or anemia, prompt medical attention is warranted, as these could be signs or symptoms of serious complications of GERD, including ulceration or fibrosis of the esophagus and esophageal cancer.

One in five Americans experiences symptoms of GERD on a weekly basis.

Treatment of Gastroesophageal Reflux Disease

The goals of GERD treatment are to relieve the symptoms of heartburn, prevent the return of symptoms, and

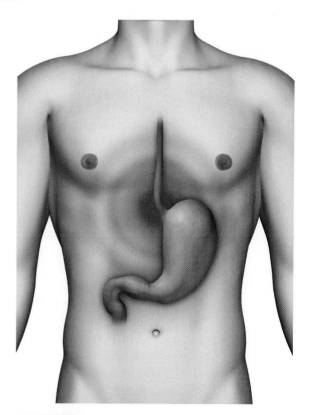

FIGURE 16.12 GERD leads to pain near the location of the lower esophageal sphincter.
© Andrea Danti/ShutterStock, Inc.

promote the healing of the esophageal mucosa. Therapies may include a combination of lifestyle modifications and pharmacological therapy.

There are over-the-counter and prescription drugs available to treat GERD. Persistent GERD, lasting longer than two weeks, should not be treated without supervision from a healthcare provider. Antacids, including aluminum hydroxide and magnesium hydroxide, neutralize the acidic contents of the stomach. Antacids do not prevent reflux, but do help prevent irritation of the esophagus if reflux occurs. Antacids must be dosed frequently and can cause GI disorders of their own, including diarrhea and constipation, depending on the product. Patient compliance is a barrier to effective therapy.

Histamine receptor antagonists (H2RAs), including cimetidine, famotidine, nizatidine, and ranitidine, lower gastric acidity. Histamine stimulates the secretion of gastric acid and pepsin in the stomach, so blocking the histamine receptors prevents the secretion of these acidic agents. Proton pump inhibitors (PPIs), including omeprazole, esomeprazole, and pantoprazole, block the secretion of gastric acid in the stomach. PPIs are more effective than H2RAs at producing long-term relief of GERD symptoms. PPIs must be administered daily to ensure relief.

Hepatitis

Hepatitis is an inflammation caused by a viral infection of the liver. The three most common types of hepatitis are A, B, and C. These infections cause damage to the cells of the liver, and cause the liver to become swollen and tender. Permanent liver damage may occur if not treated properly.

Hepatitis A virus (HAV) is transmitted through blood and body fluids, usually by the fecal-oral route. It is most prevalent among populations with poor sanitation and hygiene. Hepatitis A occurs most commonly in children. Hepatitis B virus (HBV) is transmitted sexually, through infected needles, and from an infected mother to her unborn child. Infants and children are at the highest risk for HBV infections and complications. Hepatitis C virus (HCV) is a blood-borne pathogen. HCV infections may occur in users of illegal injectable drugs, patients who received blood transfusions prior to 1992, patients who received clotting factors prior to 1987, chronic hemodialysis patients, patients infected with HIV or other sexually transmitted diseases, or people who received tattoos with contaminated instruments. Healthcare workers who are routinely in contact with blood or blood products are also at risk for HCV infection.

Signs and Symptoms of Hepatitis

Symptoms of HAV appear suddenly, but some patients, particularly children, have no symptoms of an infection; symptoms of HBV are slower to develop, often 60 to 180 days after exposure to the infectious virus. Acute HCV infections may not cause symptoms, and the infection is often not diagnosed until significant disease progression has occurred.

Signs and symptoms of hepatitis include fatigue, malaise, headache, loss of appetite, sensitivity to light, sore throat, cough, nausea, vomiting, and fever. The lymph nodes and liver may be enlarged.

An HAV infection is always acute and rarely fatal. HBV can cause either acute or chronic infections. Acute infections are usually short-lived and self-limiting, but chronic infections can lead to permanent liver damage and death. HCV infections may be either acute or chronic. Most infections lead to long-term complications.

Prevention and Treatment of Hepatitis

Two inactive HAV vaccines are available in the United States: Havrix and Vaqta. Treatment of HAV infections is supportive, with no specific medication available to treat the infection. Preventing dehydration is the most important component of HAV treatment.

Two HBV vaccines are also available: Recombivax HB and Engerix B. Twinrix is a combination vaccine that protects against both HAV and HBV. Antiviral therapy can be used to treat HBV infections. Interferon products are approved for the long-term treatment of HBV infections, and reverse-transcriptase inhibitors (a class of antiviral agents) are also effective against HBV.

No vaccine is available for HCV. Avoidance of contact with infected blood products is the most effective prevention for HCV. Combination treatment with peginterferon and the antiviral ribavirin is first-line therapy for HCV infections. Side effects of riba-virin limit patient compliance and often require discontinuation of therapy. Extreme fatigue, flulike symptoms, anemia, and psychiatric symptoms, including severe depression and suicidal behaviors, have been associated with ribavirin. In 2011, the antiviral agents boceprevir and telaprevir were approved by the FDA for the treatment of HCV.

Irritable Bowel Syndrome

Irritable bowel syndrome (IBS) is a common GI syndrome characterized by chronic abdominal pain and altered bowel habits. It is not associated with any specific cause, but is among the most commonly diagnosed GI conditions. IBS may affect any age group or gender, but younger female patients are the most likely to be diagnosed with IBS. Although no particular cause has been identified for IBS, new research points toward altered levels of serotonin in IBS sufferers.

Signs and Symptoms of Irritable Bowel Syndrome

IBS is classified as diarrhea-predominant or constipation-predominant. It often includes lower abdominal pain, altered defecation, and bloating. Because the symptoms of IBS present as general indications of GI dysfunction, a thorough physical examination and laboratory evaluations are necessary to exclude other causes of the condition.

Treatment of Irritable Bowel Syndrome

The goal of treatment of IBS is to relieve symptoms and restore normal bowel function. In general, the treatment of IBS depends on the type and severity of symptoms present. Often, common treatments for diarrhea and constipation are sufficient to control IBS symptoms. Diet and behavioral modifications, along with pharmacological interventions for diarrhea or constipation, can be used.

Inflammatory Bowel Disease

Inflammatory bowel disease (IBD) includes **ulcerative colitis (UC)** and **Crohn's disease**. UC is an inflammation of the mucosa and submucosa of the rectum or colon. Crohn's disease causes continuous lesions that extend through all the layers of tissue in the GI tract. Lesions in Crohn's disease are not confined to the colon, but may occur in any part of the GI tract, from the mouth to the anus FIGURE 16.13 .

The exact cause of IBD is not known, although an immune component is suspected to play a role. Genetic susceptibility also contributes to the development of IBD.

Signs and Symptoms of Inflammatory Bowel Disease

UC often presents with abdominal pain, frequent bowel movements, weight loss, fever, increased heart rate, blurred vision or eye pain, arthritis, hemorrhoids, anal fissures, and decreased hemoglobin and hematocrit. The most common symptom of UC is bloody diarrhea. Many patients with UC suffer from dehydration due to chronic diarrhea.

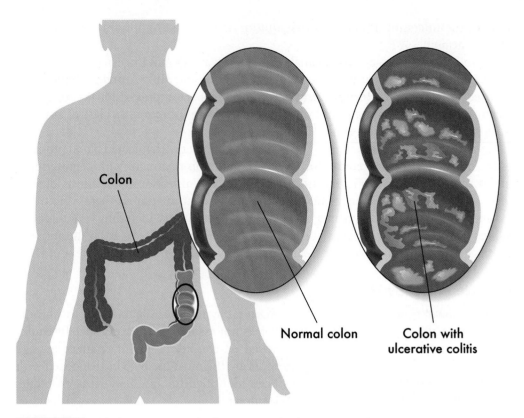

Colon

Normal colon

Colon with
ulcerative colitis

FIGURE 16.13 UC lesions are present in the rectum and colon.
© rob3000/ShutterStock, Inc.

Crohn's disease often presents with fever, fatigue, abdominal pain, frequent bowel movements, weight loss, arthritis, abdominal tenderness, abdominal mass, perianal fissures, and increased white blood cell count. Crohn's disease is not confined to a specific portion of the GI tract and results in discontinuous lesions throughout the tract. Nutritional deficiencies are common with Crohn's disease because nutrient absorption is altered due to inflammation and damage in the small intestine. Crohn's disease is characterized by periods of remission and exacerbation, and some patients may be symptom free for years at a time.

Treatment of Inflammatory Bowel Disease

The goals of IBD treatment depend on the type of disease present and the severity of disease. It may require immunosuppressant agents, antimicrobials, or anti-inflammatory agents. Nutritional support to alleviate symptoms and prevent malnutrition is necessary in IBD. Treatment may be short-term, involving only a few weeks before IBD remits, or long-term, with maintenance of remission possibly requiring years of therapy.

Obesity

Nearly 100 million American adults are overweight or obese, and the proportion of children and adolescents who are overweight or obese is increasing rapidly. Both conditions are associated with serious health consequences, such as cardiovascular diseases, pulmonary disorders, metabolic dysfunction, and psychological conditions.

Signs and Symptoms of Obesity

Body mass index (BMI) is traditionally used to quantify healthy body weight. It is calculated by dividing a patient's weight in kilograms by the square of his height in meters:

$$BMI = weight \; (kg) \div height^2 \; (m^2)$$

A BMI between 19 and 25 is considered a healthy body weight. **Overweight** is defined as a BMI of 25 or greater, and **obesity** is defined as a BMI of 30 or greater. A BMI of 30 is roughly equal to being 30 pounds over a healthy body weight. **Extreme obesity** is defined as a BMI of 40 or greater.

BMI is a reliable indicator of body fatness for most adults, and it serves as a guideline for assessing weight-related disorders. However, BMI is not appropriate for every patient. For example, BMI may be overestimated for people who have a high proportion of muscle mass; they may be considered overweight in spite of having a healthy percentage of body fat. Edema also affects BMI measurements, as do muscle-wasting syndromes or extremely short stature. In these cases, clinical judgment, a complete medical history, and a physical examination must be used together to determine whether a weight-related disorder exists.

Additionally, BMI is not effective in determining weight status in children, adolescents, or adults younger than 20 years of age because body composition and body fat proportions change during growth and development. For these patients, BMI is calculated using the standard formula, but then converted to a percentage based on height- and weight-for-age charts, resulting in BMI-for-age guidelines. Children who fall under the fifth percentile of BMI-for-age are considered underweight; those between the fifth and 85th percentiles are healthy weight; those between the 85th and 95th percentiles are overweight; and those above the 95th percentile are obese.

One BMI unit is equivalent to approximately seven pounds in men and six pounds in women.
© auremar/ShutterStock, Inc.

Childhood obesity is a serious public-health crisis. It leads directly to adult obesity and its resultant health consequences.

Alternatively, waist circumference can be used to identify overweight and obese individuals. A patient may have excess body fat if the waist circumference is equal to or greater than 35 inches in women or 40 inches in men.

Treatment of Obesity

When patients are determined to be overweight or obese, dietary management and behavior modification are the first steps to losing excess body fat. Lifestyle choices that support sustained weight loss are essential to maintaining a healthy body weight and avoiding the health consequences associated with obesity. A well-balanced diet containing proteins, fats, and carbohydrates, along with regular physical activity, are the most effective weight-control methods available. Severely calorie-restricted diets or extremely limited food choices do not show long-term benefit in health status or weight loss. If six months of dietary and behavior modifications are not effective in reducing body weight, pharmacological therapy may be initiated. These agents should be reserved for patients with a BMI of 30 or greater. In the presence of other complicating disease states, weight-loss agents may be used in patients with a BMI of 27 or greater.

No herbal products or supplements are approved by the FDA for the treatment of those who are overweight or obese. The content, safety, and effectiveness of such products cannot be guaranteed, and patients should be advised to use caution with these agents.

Weight loss of as little as 5 percent of total body weight significantly reduces the cardiovascular and metabolic risks associated with being overweight or obese.
© auremar/ShutterStock, Inc.

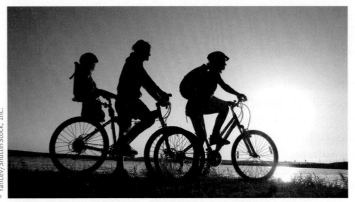
Staying active as a family can be effective for prevention and treatment of obesity.

Pancreatitis

Pancreatitis is an acute or chronic inflammation of the pancreas. In this condition, the enzymes and digestive substances normally excreted by the pancreas remain in the organ and destroy the pancreas itself. If the islets of Langerhans (the cells that produce insulin) are destroyed, diabetes mellitus will result. Acute pancreatitis is usually caused by gallstones. Alcoholism, trauma to the pancreas, certain medications, and pancreatic cancer can cause chronic pancreatitis.

Signs and Symptoms of Pancreatitis

Epigastric pain, persistent vomiting, and a rigid abdomen are symptoms of pancreatitis. Fever and rapid heart rate may also occur. Hemorrhage can occur with rapidly progressing disease, which can lead to shock, coma, and death.

Treatment of Pancreatitis

The goals of treatment of pancreatitis are to relieve pain and prevent complications associated with the inflammation. Severe acute attacks of pancreatitis are often emergency situations. Maintaining fluid and electrolyte balance and decreasing pancreatic secretions are the cornerstones of treatment. Pain management and nutrition changes are the mainstays of treatment. Alcohol avoidance and smoking cessation are also indicated.

Peptic Ulcer Disease

Peptic ulcer disease (PUD) is characterized by the frequent recurrence of **peptic ulcers**, which are lesions in the mucosal lining of the stomach (gastric ulcer) or in the first part of the small intestine (duodenal ulcer) **FIGURE 16.14**. The three most common types of peptic ulcers include *Helicobacter pylori*–associated peptic ulcers, NSAID-induced peptic ulcers, and stress-related peptic ulcers. Often, the presence of the bacteria *H. pylori* combined with acidic conditions alter the mucosal lining of the GI tract, allowing erosions and ulcerations to occur. Other causes of ulcers include increased acid secretion and pepsin activity, reduced mucus and bicarbonate secretion, imbalanced bile salt secretion, increased gastric contractions, and decreased blood flow in the GI tract. The duodenum receives the highest concentration of acid from the stomach and is prone to ulcers.

As many as 10 percent of Americans will develop peptic ulcer disease in their lifetime.

Signs and Symptoms of Peptic Ulcer Disease

The signs and symptoms of PUD vary depending on the cause of the ulcers and their severity. In general, patients present with abdominal pain that may be described as burning, fullness, or cramping. Nocturnal pain related to PUD often awakens patients in the middle of the night. Heartburn, belching, and bloating often accompany PUD pain. Nausea, vomiting, and loss of appetite are seen more often with gastric ulcers than duodenal ulcers; these symptoms may also signal the onset of ulcer-related complications, such as bleeding, perforation, or obstruction.

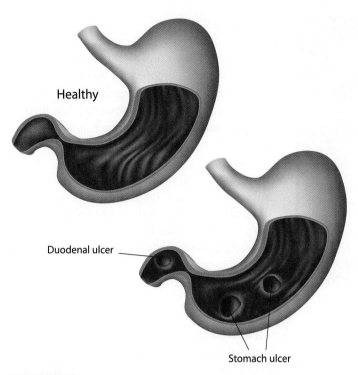

Healthy

Duodenal ulcer

Stomach ulcer

FIGURE 16.14 Peptic ulcers can occur in the gastric or duodenal mucosa.
© Alila Sao Mai/ShutterStock, Inc.

Treatment of Peptic Ulcer Disease

The goal of PUD treatment is to relieve pain and discomfort associated with the ulcer, heal the ulcer, and prevent its recurrence. Common drug regimens include antimicrobial therapy to eliminate *H. pylori* infections and acid-reducing agents to decrease the symptoms of PUD. H2RAs and PPIs used to treat GERD are also used to treat PUD. Lifestyle modifications are also important in PUD. Eliminating aggravating foods from the diet, reducing stress, and smoking cessation will promote ulcer healing and reduce pain.

Diagnostic Procedures and Therapeutic Modalities of the Digestive System

The symptoms of many GI diseases and disorders overlap with each other and involve multiple body systems, so a thorough medical history and physical examination are required to accurately diagnose conditions of the GI tract. Symptom onset, factors that worsen or relieve symptoms, and the precise presentation of symptoms will aid in assessing the patient's condition. Diagnostic procedures and imaging studies also help visualize the GI tract and evaluate disorders. MRI studies, CT scans, and ultrasound evaluations can also be applied to examinations of the digestive system.

Many diagnostic procedures are uncomfortable and require significant patient preparation. A medical assistant may be responsible for providing complete instructions and patient support to ensure safe and accurate testing. Several of the diagnostic tests used to evaluate GI diseases are discussed in Chapter 12.

Colonoscopy

A **colonoscopy** is a procedure used to visualize the inside of the colon and rectum. The examination can

The American Cancer Society recommends a colonoscopy every 10 years, beginning at age 50, as a screening for colorectal cancer.
© auremar/ShutterStock, Inc.

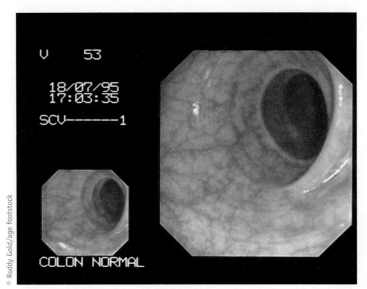

COLON NORMAL

A colonoscopy visualizes the inside of the colon.

identify inflammation, ulcers, and abnormal growths in the colon. A colonoscopy is indicated for routine colorectal cancer screenings and to diagnose changes in bowel habits, abdominal pain, and bleeding from the GI tract. Tissue samples can be obtained for further analysis and **polyps**, which are small, usually harmless growths, can be removed during a colonoscopy.

Prior to a colonoscopy, all solid material must be emptied from the large intestine. Patients are required to consume a clear liquid diet for one to three days before the procedure. Beverages with red or purple dyes should be avoided during this time, because the dyes can mimic the appearance of blood in the colon. A laxative or enema may be provided the night before the colonoscopy. An **enema** is a water or soap solution that is flushed into the anus to remove solid material from the rectum and colon.

During a colonoscopy, a flexible endoscope is inserted through the anus and guided into the rectum and colon. The patient is sedated during the procedure and positioned on his or her left side. Bleeding and puncture of the intestine are possible, but uncommon, complications of a colonoscopy.

Gastroscopy

Gastroscopy, also called **esophagogastroduodenoscopy (EGD)**, is the visualization of the esophagus, stomach, and duodenum with a flexible, fiber-optic endoscope. The endoscope is inserted into the patient's mouth and guided into the esophagus, stomach, and duodenum to identify or evaluate tumors, ulcers, bleeding, structural abnormalities, and other damage to the upper GI tract. Foreign objects can be removed and tissue samples for biopsy can be obtained during an EGD. Endoscopic evaluations can also be used to control bleeding in the GI tract with the application of heat, chemicals, or lasers to the affected area or the placement of a clip or band to the affected blood vessel.

The patient must remain awake during an EGD in order to swallow the scope. The back of the throat is first sprayed with a local anesthetic to inhibit the gag reflex. A mild sedative is given to induce drowsiness.

Radiological Studies

X-rays are used to visualize areas of the GI tract and can be used to diagnose a variety of conditions such as inflammation, ulcers, abnormal growths, abnormal narrowing of the GI tract, and abnormalities in the blood vessels of the GI tract. Radiological studies are indicated for abdominal pain, nausea and vomiting, swallowing difficulties, GERD, and unexplained weight loss. Radiological examinations are less accurate than endoscopic evaluations.

An upper GI series helps diagnose disorders of the upper GI tract, including the esophagus, stomach, and duodenum. To complement an upper GI series, a patient may swallow a liquid that contains barium (a procedure called a barium swallow), which coats the GI tract and allows enhanced visualization through a specialized camera called a fluoroscope. The patient may be asked to change position several times during an upper GI series to allow visualization of the GI tract from different angles. Prior to an upper GI series, no eating or drinking is allowed for eight hours in order to empty the upper GI tract. Smoking and chewing gum are also prohibited. An X-ray series is not painful, but the barium liquid is chalky and unpleasant, and patients may experience nausea, vomiting, and bloating for a short time after the examination. A laxative may be ordered to facilitate the removal of the barium.

A lower GI series examines the large intestine. To examine the lower GI tract, a liquid containing barium is administered as an enema. Preparation similar to that used for a colonoscopy is ordered prior to a lower GI series. A clear liquid diet and a laxative or enema is required to clear all solid material from the colon and rectum. As with an upper GI series, patients are asked to change positions during a lower GI series to allow the barium liquid to coat all parts of the GI tract. A water-based enema may be ordered to facilitate the removal of the barium after the examination.

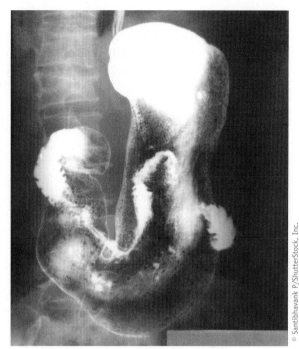

A barium swallow visualizes the upper GI tract.

© Santibhavank P/ShutterStock, Inc.

Occult Blood Test

A **fecal occult blood test (FOBT)** is used to identify the presence of blood in the feces that is not visible to the naked eye. Fecal occult blood is a sign of colorectal cancer.

Blood in the stool has characteristic coloration that indicates the location of the bleeding. The closer the bleeding is to the end of the GI tract, the brighter red the blood. Black, tarry blood in the stool indicates bleeding in the stomach or esophagus. Maroon blood indicates bleeding in the ileum or jejunum. When blood is not visible or identifiable, an FOBT is performed by applying a small amount of fecal material to an occult blood slide. Within one minute, a change of color on the slide will indicate the presence of blood. Two samples are usually obtained by the patient from three separate stools.

An FOBT requires specific patient preparation to avoid false positive results. Patients must avoid red meat and certain vegetables, including turnips, broccoli, cauliflower, and radishes, for three days prior to testing. They must also avoid iron-containing medications for three days and NSAIDs for seven days. Digital rectal exams are prohibited within three days prior to the FOBT. False negative results are prevented by advising patients to avoid vitamin C for three days prior to testing. Also, testing dehydrated fecal samples may give a false negative result.

Colostomy

A **colostomy** is an artificial opening of the colon that allows fecal material to be excreted from the body through the abdominal wall. An opening is made in the colon and a tube is connected to the opening through the abdominal wall. A pouch is connected to the tube outside the body that collects material from the colon.

A colostomy can be temporary or permanent, depending on the disease or condition that necessitates the colostomy. Colostomies may be indicated if a disease or condition of the colon requires the colon to rest and heal. A colostomy may also be indicated when an obstruction such as a tumor prevents the passage of feces through the colon. In this case, fecal matter is removed from the GI tract prior to the diseased or obstructed area.

Colostomies require immense emotional and physical adjustments for patients. Elimination of fecal matter is no longer a voluntary process and the need to wear a pouch containing fecal material is unappealing. Luckily, many support groups exist for colostomy patients and diet and lifestyle changes can mitigate many of the ill effects of colostomies.

Ileostomy

Similar to a colostomy, an **ileostomy** is an artificial opening in the ileum that allows chyme in the small intestine to empty through a tube in the abdominal wall **FIGURE 16.15**. Chyme is very acidic and could damage the skin. An ileostomy must, therefore, be attached to a tightly sealed collection bag that surrounds the opening in the abdominal wall. A protective adhesive covers the opening to prevent skin damage.

Ileostomies are indicated for patients with severe UC or Crohn's disease. The emotional and physical adjustment required for an ileostomy often outweigh the pain and emotional stress associated with living with one of these conditions. An ileostomy may offer patients more freedom and better health than they had prior to the ileostomy.

Therapeutic Diets

Diets can be designed to correct or compensate for disease states, including malnutrition, diabetes mellitus, cardiovascular disease, and even cancer. The total number of calories consumed can be adjusted, as can the specific combination of nutrients, to control various conditions. The consistency and texture of food can be adjusted and the frequency of consumption can be altered.

Weight loss is a common goal of dietary changes. To lose weight, individuals must consume fewer calories than they expend. Patients can engage in low-calorie and low-fat diets in addition to increasing physical activity levels to begin the process of losing weight. Weight loss should be restricted to approximately one to two pounds per week to prevent nutritional deficiencies that accompany rapid weight loss. Slow, steady weight loss will often lead to long-term weight control. Significant weight loss

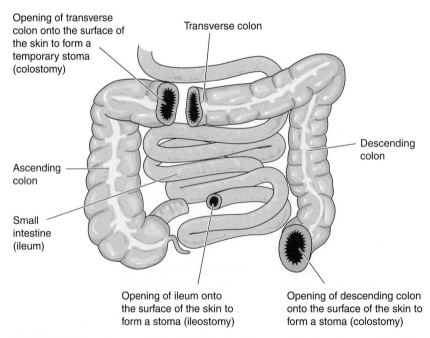

Opening of transverse colon onto the surface of the skin to form a temporary stoma (colostomy)

Transverse colon

Descending colon

Ascending colon

Small intestine (ileum)

Opening of ileum onto the surface of the skin to form a stoma (ileostomy)

Opening of descending colon onto the surface of the skin to form a stoma (colostomy)

FIGURE 16.15 Colostomies and ileostomies are artificial openings in the colon and small intestine, respectively.

involves lifestyle changes and behavior modification. Support from friends and family is essential to continued success in maintaining a healthy way of life.

Patients with diabetes mellitus (DM) must adhere to strict diets to control blood glucose levels. The total number of calories does not need to be altered in DM unless the patient is overweight or underweight, but the proportion of carbohydrates in the diet must be controlled. Simple sugars should be avoided because these undergo fast digestion by the GI system, resulting in spikes in blood glucose levels. Complex carbohydrates, on the other hand, lead to slower, steadier rises in blood glucose levels. High dietary fiber also aids in digestion, prolonging absorption of carbohydrates and preventing spikes in blood sugar. Refer to Chapter 15 for a complete discussion of the pathophysiology of DM.

Hypertension and atherosclerosis are two common cardiovascular conditions that can be controlled, at least partially, with dietary changes. Restricting dietary sodium is helpful in controlling high blood pressure because sodium influences water retention in the body. Increased water retention increases pressure on the walls of the blood vessels. Many foods contain sodium because it is often used as a preservative for packaged foods. The recommended daily intake of sodium is less than 2.4 grams, the equivalent of 1 teaspoon of table salt from all sources. For individuals with a diagnosis of hypertension, sodium intake of less than 1.5 grams daily can reduce blood pressure significantly, both with and without the help of antihypertensive medications.

Atherosclerosis is caused, in part, by a lack of physical activity and increased consumption of dietary fat and cholesterol. A low-fat diet in which fewer than 20–30 percent of total Calories come from fat, as part of an overall healthy, active lifestyle, can reverse signs of atherosclerosis. Less than one-third of fat calories should come from saturated fats. Cholesterol consumption should be limited to 200mg daily. Refer to Chapter 13 for a complete discussion of the pathophysiology of hypertension and atherosclerosis.

Cancer risk can be mitigated by dietary habits. Stomach and esophageal cancers are associated with the intake of nitrates, which are found in bacon and smoked meats; breast, uterine, and colon cancers are associated with high fat intake. High-fiber diets protect against colon cancer, while vitamins A and C protect against stomach, lung, and bladder cancers. Fruits and vegetables, as well as soy-containing foods, are associated with a decreased risk of many types of cancer. In general, an active, healthy lifestyle, including a nutritious, balanced diet, defends the body against many types of cancer.

Patients with cancer will have specific nutritional requirements. Total caloric needs tend to increase during cancer because tumors take nutrients away from the rest of the body. Chemotherapy also destroys rapidly growing cells in the body, and increased nutrients are needed to repair and replace damaged tissues. Loss of appetite, nausea, and vomiting usually accompany cancer and its treatments, so efforts should be made to make food as appealing as possible for cancer patients. Small, frequent meals are often better tolerated than large meals. Patients may also be sensitive to taste, texture, or consistency of food, so patient preference should be observed when developing diets for patients with cancer.

What Would You Do?

A 25-year-old female presents to the physician's office where you work for her annual physical. Her examination indicates that she has gained 15 pounds in the last year. She admits to you that she has not been eating well due to a new job that requires a lot of travel and presents her with quite a bit of stress. She also says that she is feeling sluggish and tired more often than she previously did. What would you tell the patient?

© NorthGeorgiaMedia/ShutterStock, Inc.

Skills for the Medical Assistant

As a medical assistant, you will have the opportunity to participate in several procedures relating to the digestive system. A significant task is instructing the patient in collecting a stool sample, an often unappealing task. If tests are not completed in accordance with specific instructions, the results may be useless and the test will need to be conducted again. Your confidence will ease the patient's apprehensions and allow for safe and accurate testing.

Instructing a Patient to Collect a Stool Sample

Stool samples may be necessary to test for a variety of GI disorders and diseases. Analysis of the stool can detect infections of the GI tract, deficiencies in nutrient absorption, or cancer. Stool can be assessed for color, consistency, volume, shape, odor, and the presence of mucus, blood, bile, or white blood cells. Depending on the type of analysis that needs to be conducted, the patient may need to avoid certain foods and medications prior to collecting the sample. Also, several samples from different stools may need to be collected. In this exercise, you will learn how to instruct a patient to collect a stool sample at home.

Equipment Needed

- Specimen container with lid
- Tongue depressors or commercially available stool sample collection kit with stick or spoon

Steps

1. Introduce yourself and identify the patient. Explain the provider's instructions and rationale for collecting a stool sample. Explain that you will be teaching the patient how to collect a stool sample. Answer the patient's questions and ensure he or she is calm and comfortable before proceeding with the instruction. Provide written instructions if necessary.

2. Instruct the patient to obtain 3–4 tablespoons of stool from his or her next bowel movement and place it in the specimen cup. Emphasize that nothing else should be in the specimen cup other than the stool sample, such as toilet paper or urine. Stool that has come in contact with cleaning solutions in the toilet bowl should not be used for analysis.

To obtain a stool sample, patients may defecate onto a paper plate or use a tongue depressor to scrape a stool sample from the toilet bowl.

Stool samples should not be collected during a woman's menstrual cycle or while a patient has actively bleeding hemorrhoids.

3. Instruct the patient to attach the lid of the specimen container securely and write the time and date of collection on the container. The specimen should be delivered to the designated lab or office

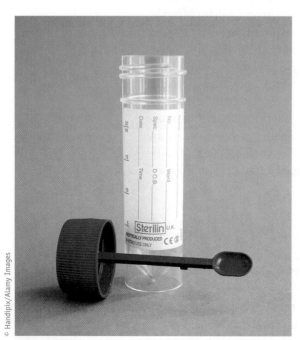

© Handipix/Alamy Images

Stool collection containers are available in a variety of sizes.

within two hours of collection. If it cannot be delivered within two hours, the stool sample should be refrigerated.

4. Record in the patient's chart that instructions were provided. For example, write "1015: Verbal and written instructions for collecting a stool sample provided to patient. Patient acknowledged understanding. J. Jones, CMA."

If a patient is collecting stool samples for a fecal occult blood test, the patient should keep the test slides at room temperature and away from sunlight. A small smear of stool sample should be placed on the slide's labeled boxes. The slide should be allowed to dry overnight before closing the cover. The process should be repeated with the next two bowel movements, and a total of three slides should be returned for testing.

Performing a Fecal Occult Blood Test

An FOBT is used to test for the presence of blood in the stool. Special commercially available slides and kits are available for performing an FOBT. A patient will provide three slides with samples from three separate stool samples. In this exercise, you will learn how to complete an FOBT, provided with sample slides prepared by a patient.

Equipment Needed

- Hemoccult or other commercially available FOBT slides prepared by patient
- Developer solution
- Timer or timepiece
- Disposable gloves

Steps

1. Wash your hands and assemble the materials and equipment. Check the expiration dates on the slides and the developer solution. Apply gloves.
2. Open the cover on the test side of the slide.
3. Remove the cap from the developer solution and apply two drops on each section of the slide.
4. Begin timing. At 30 seconds, begin to watch for a color change on the slides.
5. At 60 seconds, observe the results. A positive result, indicated by a blue color change, means that blood is present in the stool. A negative result means that no blood is present.
6. To test the quality of the materials, place one drop of developer solution between the positive and negative controls. Read the results within 10 seconds. If the positive control does not turn blue or the negative control does not remain neutral, the test supplies are faulty and the test should be repeated.
7. Discard the test slides in the biohazard waste container. Remove the gloves and wash your hands.
8. Record the results in the patient's chart. For example, write "1235: Hemoccult slides: 1. Negative 2. Positive, 3. Positive. J. Jones, CMA."

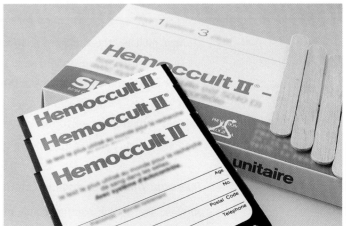

Hemoccult slides and developing solution are commercially available for ease of testing.

Math Practice

Question: **Metoclopramide is available as an oral solution in a concentration of 5mg per 5mL. A physician orders 10mg by mouth four times daily to improve GI symptoms associated with diabetes mellitus. What volume of metoclopramide will be administered at each dose?**

Answer: Step 1: Multiply the number of milligrams ordered by the number of milligrams in each 5mL. To do this, first convert the number of milligrams in each dose to a fraction: $10mg = {}^{10mg}/_{1\ dose}$. Therefore, $10mg \times {}^{5mL}/_{5mg} = {}^{10mg}/_{1\ dose} \times {}^{5mL}/_{5mg}$

   Now, multiply the numerators: $10mg \times 5mL = 50mg \times mL$

   Then, multiply the denominators: $1\ dose \times 5mg = 5\ dose \times mg$

   The result is ${}^{50mg\times mL}/_{5\ dose} \times mg$

Step 2: Cancel the units and divide the fraction: $50mg \times {}^{mL}/_{5\ dose} \times mg = {}^{10mL}/_{dose}$

Question: **A nutrition label includes the following information regarding nutritional content:**

   Total Calories: 210

   Total fat: 7g

   Saturated fat: 4g

   Total carbohydrates: 23g

   Protein: 14g

   How many Calories are provided by the total fat content?

Answer: Step 1: Multiply the number of grams of total fat by the number of Calories per gram. To do this, first convert the number of grams of fat to a fraction: $7g = {}^{7g}/_{1}$

   Therefore, $7g \times {}^{9\ Calories}/_{1g} = {}^{7g}/_{1} \times {}^{9\ Calories}/_{1g}$

   Now, multiply the numerators: $7g \times 9\ Calories = 63g \times Calories$

   Then, multiply the denominators: $1 \times 1g = 1g$

Step 2: Cancel the units and divide the fraction: $63g \times {}^{Calories}/_{1g} = 63\ Calories$

Question: **What percentage of Calories is provided by saturated fat?**

Answer: Step 1: Multiply the number of grams of saturated fat by the number of Calories per gram. To do this, first convert the number of grams of saturated fat to a fraction: $4g = {}^{4g}/_{1}$

   Therefore, $4g \times {}^{9\ Calories}/_{1g} = {}^{4g}/_{1} \times {}^{9\ Calories}/_{1g}$

   Now, multiply the numerators: $4g \times 9\ Calories = 36g \times Calories$

   Then, multiply the denominators: $1 \times 1g = 1g$

Step 2: Cancel the units and divide the fraction: $36g \times {}^{Calories}/_{1g} = 36\ Calories$

Step 3: Divide the number of Calories provided by saturated fat by the total Calories: 36 Calories saturated fat ÷ 210 total Calories = 0.17

Step 4: Multiply by 100% to convert the decimal to a percentage: $0.17 \times 100\% = 17\%$

Question: **What percentage of Calories is provided by carbohydrates?**

Answer: Step 1: Multiply the number of grams of saturated fat by the number of Calories per gram. To do this, first convert the number of grams of carbohydrates to a fraction: $23g = {}^{23g}/_{1}$

Therefore, $23g \times {}^{4\ Calories}\!/_{1g} = {}^{23g}\!/_1 \times {}^{4\ Calories}\!/_{1g}$

Now, multiply the numerators: $23g \times 4\ Calories = 92g \times Calories$

Then, multiply the denominators: $1 \times 1g = 1g$

Step 2: Cancel the units and divide the fraction: $92g \times {}^{Calories}\!/_{1g} = 92\ Calories$

Step 3: Divide the number of Calories provided by carbohydrates by the total Calories: 92 Calories carbohydrates ÷ 210 total Calories = 0.44

Step 4: Multiply by 100% to convert the decimal to a percentage: $0.44 \times 100\% = 44\%$

Question: **Ranitidine is available as an oral syrup in a concentration of 15mg per 1mL. A physician orders 300mg ranitidine by mouth at bedtime for the treatment of a duodenal ulcer. What volume of syrup will the patient consume each day?**

Answer: Step 1: Multiply the number of milligrams ordered by the number of milligrams in each mL. To do this, first convert the number of milligrams in each dose to a fraction: $300mg = {}^{300mg}\!/_{1\ dose}$

Therefore, $300mg \times {}^{1mL}\!/_{15mg} = {}^{300mg}\!/_{1\ dose} \times {}^{1mL}\!/_{15mg}$

Now, multiply the numerators: $300mg \times 1mL = 300mg \times mL$

Then, multiply the denominators: $1\ dose \times 15mg = 15\ dose \times mg$

The result is $300mg \times {}^{mL}\!/_{15\ dose} \times mg$

Step 2: Cancel the units and divide the fraction: $300mg \times mL \div 15\ dose \times mg = 20mL/dose$

Question: **A 33-year-old female is 5 ft 4 inches tall and weighs 113 lb. What is her BMI? Is this considered a healthy BMI?**

Answer: Step 1: Calculate the patient's weight in kilograms. Remember that 1kg equals 2.2 lb. Convert this to a fraction: ${}^{1kg}\!/_{2.2\ lb}$

Next, convert the number of pounds to a ratio in fraction form: ${}^{113\ lb}\!/_1$

Multiply the number of pounds by the number of kilograms per pound: ${}^{113\ lb}\!/_1 \times {}^{1kg}\!/_{2.2\ lb}$

Now, multiply the numerators: $113\ lb \times 1kg = 113\ lb \times kg$

Then, multiply the denominators: $1 \times 2.2\ lb = 2.2\ lb$

The result is $113\ lb \times {}^{kg}\!/_{2.2\ lb}$

Cancel the units and divide the fraction: $113\ lb \times {}^{kg}\!/_{2.2\ lb} = 51.4kg$

Step 2: Calculate the patient's height in inches. Remember that there are 12 inches in 1 foot. Convert this to a ratio in fraction form: ${}^{12\ inches}\!/_{1\ foot}$. Next, convert the total number of feet to a fraction: ${}^{5\ ft}\!/_1$

Multiply the height in feet by the number of inches per feet: $5\ ft \times {}^{12\ inches}\!/_{1\ foot} = {}^{5\ ft}\!/_1 \times {}^{12\ inches}\!/_{1\ ft}$

Now, multiply the numerators: $5\ ft \times 12\ inches = 60\ ft \times inches$

Then, multiply the denominators: $1\ ft \times 1 = 1\ ft$

The result is $60\ ft \times {}^{inches}\!/_{1\ ft}$

Cancel the units and divide the fraction: $60\ ft \times inches \div 1\ ft = 60\ inches$

Now, add the additional 4 inches of her height: 60 inches + 4 inches = 64 inches

Now, remember that 1 inch equals 0.0254 meters. Convert this to a ratio in the form of a fraction: ${}^{0.0254\ meters}\!/_{1\ inch}$

Next, convert the number of inches of height to a fraction: ${}^{64\ inches}\!/_1$

Multiply the number of inches by the number of meters per inch: ${}^{64\ inches}\!/_1 \times {}^{0.0254\ meters}\!/_{1\ inch}$

Now, multiply the numerators: 64 inches × 0.0254 meters = 1.63 inches × meters

Then, multiply the denominators: 1 × 1 inch = 1 inch

The result is 1.63 inches × $^{\text{meters}}\!/_{1\ \text{inch}}$

Cancel the units and divide the fraction: 1.63 meters

Step 3: Insert the patient's weight in kilograms and height in meters into the formula for BMI:

BMI = wt (kg) ÷ ht (m)^2 = 51.4kg ÷ (1.63)^{2}m = 51.4kg ÷ (1.63 × 1.63)m^2 = 19.35kg/m^2

Step 4: Note that a BMI between 19 and 25 is considered healthy

WRAP UP

Chapter Summary

- The gastrointestinal (GI) system includes the structures and organs that store and digest food, eliminate waste, and utilize nutrients. It includes the mouth, esophagus, stomach, small intestine, large intestine, liver, gallbladder, and pancreas.

- The entire digestive process takes place in four steps: ingestion, digestion, absorption, and elimination.

- The mouth is the point at which food enters the body. The teeth break food into smaller pieces and saliva moistens the food and begins the process of digestion. Food is chewed and formed into a bolus in the mouth, then swallowed into the esophagus.

- The esophagus is a muscular tube that connects the mouth and the stomach. It begins peristalsis, which involves coordinated muscle movements that propel food through the digestive tract.

- The stomach stores and digests large particles of food. The lining of the stomach secretes digestive enzymes and proteins. After three to five hours in the stomach, food is churned into a semiliquid substance called chyme.

- The small intestine is a long tube that is connected to the stomach. The first section of the small intestine, the duodenum, receives chyme from the stomach and completes the process of digestion. The remaining sections of the small intestine, the jejunum and the ileum, are the sites of absorption. Villi line the small intestine and facilitate the absorption of nutrients and water from the chyme.

- After nutrients are absorbed in the small intestine, chyme travels to the large intestine. Excess water is absorbed from the chyme and solid waste products are collected and prepared for elimination from the body.

- The liver produces bile, which digests fats, and contributes to carbohydrate and protein metabolism. The liver also stores blood, body fluids, vitamins, and iron, and filters waste products from the abdominal organs.

- The gallbladder stores and concentrates bile. When small stones form from the minerals in bile, they can block the ducts that transport bile to the duodenum.

- The pancreas secretes several enzymes required for digestion. The pancreatic juices are delivered to the duodenum through the common bile duct.

- Nutrition is essential for the proper functioning of the digestive tract. Consuming too many or too few nutrients results in significant health consequences.

- Macronutrients provide energy for the body and include carbohydrates, fats, and protein. Micronutrients regulate body processes and include vitamins, minerals, trace elements, and water.

- Carbohydrates are the body's main source of energy. Monosaccharides are one-sugar carbohydrates; disaccharides are two-sugar carbohydrates. Polysaccharides are long-chain carbohydrates that take longer for the body to digest than monosaccharides and disaccharides. Fiber is an indigestible polysaccharide derived from plants.

- Fats are classified as saturated or unsaturated. Saturated fats are solids at room temperature and tend to increase cholesterol levels in the body. Unsaturated fats are liquids at room temperature and tend to be healthier than saturated fats. Trans fats are not naturally occurring fats and are not required in the diet. Intake of trans fats should be limited as much as possible.

- Proteins are chains of amino acids that serve as building blocks for body functions or structures. Proteins can be used as an energy source when carbohydrates or fats are not available.

- Vitamins are molecules that regulate body processes. Vitamin B complexes and vitamin C are water soluble. Vitamins A, D, E, and K are fat-soluble.

- Minerals are inorganic substances that regulate body processes. They cannot be manufactured by the body and must be consumed in the diet. Trace elements are also required for body processes, but in minute quantities related to other minerals.

- Water is essential for human life. The human body is composed of approximately 50 percent water. Water must be continuously consumed and replenished.

- The amount of energy provided by nutrients is measured in calories. The basal metabolic rate is the amount of energy needed for the body's activities while at rest.

- Dietary supplements may be used as part of a holistic, integrative healthcare approach. Dietary supplements are not regulated by the FDA and patients should inform their healthcare providers if they are taking supplements.

- Diseases and disorders of the GI system commonly cause nausea, vomiting, diarrhea, epigastric pain, loss of appetite, weight loss, fatigue, and blood in the vomit or feces.

- Appendicitis is an inflammation of the appendix. Surgical removal of the appendix is the only treatment.

- Cirrhosis is a progressive, irreversible destruction of the liver caused by chronic inflammation. Cirrhosis is frequently caused by malnutrition associated with alcoholism, as well as hepatitis or diseases of the bile ducts. Mortality associated with cirrhosis is high.

- Constipation is the decreased frequency of bowel movements or difficulty defecating. An increase in dietary fiber usually relieves constipation.

- Diarrhea is an increased frequency and decreased consistency of stools. It may be caused by infectious organisms, disease states, medications, or food intolerances. Dehydration is a complication of diarrhea. Maintaining hydration and electrolyte balance is the most important aspect of diarrhea treatment.

- Gastroenteritis is an inflammation of the stomach or intestines. It may be caused by an infection, diarrhea, food poisoning, allergies, drug reactions, or ingestion of a toxin or poison. Most cases of gastroenteritis are self-limiting and resolve within a few days.

- Gastroesophageal reflux disease (GERD) is a condition in which gastric and duodenal contents flow back into the esophagus due to a dysfunction in the lower esophageal sphincter. Behaviors and medications that reduce the production of acidic content in the stomach can prevent the symptoms of GERD.

- Hepatitis is an inflammation of the liver caused by a viral infection. The three most common types of hepatitis are hepatitis A, hepatitis B, and hepatitis C. Permanent liver damage may occur if hepatitis is not treated properly. Vaccines to prevent hepatitis A and B infections are available.

- Irritable bowel syndrome (IBS) is a GI syndrome characterized by abdominal pain and altered bowel habits. IBS may be diarrhea-predominant or constipation-predominant. Dietary and pharmacological interventions to correct bowel function usually relieve IBS symptoms.

- Inflammatory bowel disease (IBD) includes ulcerative colitis (UC) and Crohn's disease. UC is characterized by lesions in the mucosa and submucosa of the rectum and colon. Crohn's disease may cause lesions at any point in the GI tract. Nutritional interventions to prevent or correct malnutrition are indicated as part of a treatment regimen for IBD.

- Obesity is defined as body mass index of more than 30, roughly 30 pounds or more overweight. Obesity can lead to significant health consequences that affect multiple disease states. Long-term maintenance of a healthy weight and an active lifestyle that includes regular physical activity are critical to avoiding weight-related disorders.

- Pancreatitis is the acute or chronic inflammation of the pancreas. Pain relief and maintenance of fluid and electrolyte balance are essential in the treatment of pancreatitis.

- Peptic ulcers are lesions in the lining of the stomach or small intestines. They are usually stress-related, NSAID-induced, or related to the presence of an infectious bacterium, *H. pylori*. Medications that decrease acidic conditions in the stomach and eradicate infectious organisms can prevent and treat peptic ulcers.

- Several diagnostic and imaging techniques are available to visualize the inside of the GI tract.

MRIs, CT scans, ultrasound, endoscopy, and X-rays can detect structural and functional abnormalities of the GI tract. A fecal occult blood test identifies the presence of blood in the stool, which may be a sign of colorectal cancer.

- When a disease or obstruction prevents the passage of chyme through the entire digestive tract, a colostomy or ileostomy can be inserted in the colon or ileum, respectively, to allow the elimination of fecal material or chyme through the abdominal wall.

- Dietary interventions can be applied to prevent and treat disease, including obesity, diabetes, hypertension, and atherosclerosis.

- As a medical assistant, you will have the opportunity to assist in procedures related to the diagnosis and evaluation of disorders of the digestive system, including teaching a patient how to obtain a stool sample and performing an occult blood test. You should be calm, confident, and professional throughout the procedures to maintain the safety and comfort of the patient. You also have the opportunity to promote healthy lifestyle choices to patients and encourage lifestyle modifications to manage risk factors for multiple diseases and complications.

Learning Assessment Questions

1. Which of the following is *not* a component of the digestive process?
   A. Ingestion
   B. Absorption
   C. Filtration
   D. Elimination

2. What is the function of saliva?
   A. To initiate peristalsis
   B. To sense taste
   C. To form a bolus
   D. To moisten food and cleanse the mouth

3. What is the function of the stomach?
   A. To absorb nutrients from food
   B. To store and digest food
   C. To promote glycogen synthesis
   D. To concentrate bile

4. Where does most absorption of nutrients occur?
   A. Mouth
   B. Small intestine
   C. Large intestine
   D. Rectum

5. Which sphincter in the body is controlled by voluntary muscle?
   A. External anal sphincter
   B. Pyloric sphincter
   C. Cardiac sphincter
   D. Ileocecal valve

6. Which of the following is *not* a function of the liver?
   A. Synthesizing amino acids
   B. Storing glycogen
   C. Filtering waste products
   D. Removing excess water from chyme

7. Which of the following substances or enzymes is not received by the duodenum?
   A. Bile
   B. Pancreatic amylase
   C. Chyme
   D. Intrinsic factor

8. Which nutrient is the main source of energy for the body?
   A. Carbohydrates
   B. Fats
   C. Vitamins
   D. Water

9. Which of the following is a consequence of insufficient fiber intake?

   A. Diarrhea

   B. Flatulence

   C. Constipation

   D. Colon polyps

10. Which of the following are true regarding saturated fats?

    A. They tend to be liquids at room temperature.

    B. They are more common from animal sources than from plant sources.

    C. They are produced by a process known as hydrogenation.

    D. They tend to decrease levels of cholesterol in the body.

11. Which of the following vitamins is fat-soluble?

    A. Vitamin A

    B. Vitamin B_6

    C. Vitamin C

    D. Vitamin H

12. Which B vitamin is used to lower cholesterol levels?

    A. Folate

    B. Niacin

    C. Pyridoxine

    D. Cyanocobalamin

13. What is the primary extracellular cation in the body?

    A. Chloride

    B. Calcium

    C. Potassium

    D. Sodium

14. What percentage of total dietary calories should come from fat?

    A. 10–20 percent

    B. 50–60 percent

    C. Less than 30 percent

    D. 9 percent

15. Which of the following is *not* a common cause of cirrhosis?

    A. Alcoholism

    B. Hepatitis

    C. Diseases of the bile ducts

    D. Excess intake of vitamin C

16. How much fiber should adults consume each day?

    A. 25–30g

    B. 2.4g

    C. 200mg

    D. 4g

17. Which of the following signs of GERD indicates a potentially serious complication that needs prompt medical attention?

    A. A sore throat

    B. Worsening symptoms when lying down

    C. Recurrent ear infections

    D. Difficulty swallowing

18. Which of the following is true regarding ulcerative colitis?

    A. Inflammatory lesions occur in any part of the GI tract, from the mouth to the anus.

    B. Bloody diarrhea is the most common symptom.

    C. Chronic constipation can lead to nutritional deficiencies.

    D. It is caused by an infectious virus.

19. Which of the following behaviors can lead to a false positive result on a fecal occult blood test?

    A. Vitamin C intake

    B. Steroid use

    C. Eating red meat

    D. Testing dehydrated samples

20. Which of the following is *not* an important factor in long-term weight control?

    A. Limiting weight loss to 1–2 lb per week

    B. Family support in establishing a healthy, active lifestyle

    C. Increasing regular physical activity levels

    D. Restricting the intake of carbohydrates

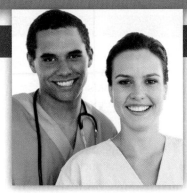

Urinary and Reproductive Systems

OBJECTIVES

After reading this chapter, you will be able to:

- Identify combining word forms of the urinary and reproductive systems and their role in the formation of medical terms.
- Define the structures and functions of the urinary and reproductive systems.
- List abbreviations related to the urinary and reproductive systems.
- Identify common diseases of the urinary and reproductive systems and their treatment, as well as diagnostic procedures related to the urinary and reproductive systems.
- Explain the process of urine formation.
- Describe the importance of proper collection and preservation of 24-hour urine specimens.
- Describe methods for chemical examination of a urine specimen.
- Explain the importance of prenatal care, and discuss what examinations will be performed as part of the initial visit.
- List signs and symptoms and their possible corresponding conditions for which the provider searches during the prenatal history and physical examination.
- Describe what takes place during the postpartum examination.
- Describe common sexually transmitted diseases.
- Explain the medical assistant's responsibilities related to a gynecologic examination.
- Describe breast self-examination and a method of teaching patients breast self-examination.
- Describe testicular self-examination and a method of teaching testicular self-examination to a male patient.

KEY TERMS

Abortion
Abstinence
Acute renal failure (ARF)
Afterbirth
Albuminuria
Amenorrhea
Amnion
Amniotic fluid
Amniotic sac
Areola
Bacteriuria
Benign prostatic
    hypertrophy (BPH)
Bilirubin
Bowman's capsule
Breast cancer
Breast milk
Breast self-examination
    (BSE)
Calyx
Casts
Cervical cancer
Cervix
Cesarean delivery
Chain of custody
Chancre
Chlamydia
Chorion
Chronic renal failure
    (CRF)
Circumcision
Clitoris
Colostrum
Colposcopy
Conception
Contraception
Corona
Corpora cavernosa
Corpus luteum
Corpus spongiosum
C-section
Cystitis
Dialysis
Dysuria
Eclampsia
Ejaculatory duct
Embryo
Endometriosis
Endometrium
End-stage renal disease
    (ESRD)
Epididymis
Estimated date of
    confinement (EDC)

Fallopian tubes
Fetus
Fibroids
Follicular phase
Foreskin
Gametes
Genital herpes
Genitourinary (GU)
    system
Gestation
Glans
Glomerulonephritis
Glomerulus
Gonorrhea
Gravidity
Gynecologist
Hematuria
Hemodialysis
Hemodialyzer
Hilum
Hormonal contraceptives
Human chorionic
    gonadotropin (hCG)
Hyperkalemia
Hysterectomy
Hysteroscopy
Incontinence
Ketones
Ketonuria
Kidney
Lumpectomy
Luteal phase
Mammary glands
Mammogram
Mastectomy
Meatus
Menarche
Menopause
Menorrhagia
Menstruation
Miscarriage
Multigravida
Myometrium
Nephrolithiasis
Nephrologist
Nocturia
Nullipara
Obstetrician
Oliguria
Oophorectomy
Orchidectomy
Ovarian cancer
Ovarian cyst
Ovum

Papanicolaou test
Parity
Parturition
Pelvic inflammatory
    disease (PID)
Penis
Perimetrium
Perineum
Peritoneal dialysis
Peritonitis
Placenta
Polycystic kidney disease
Postpartum
Postpartum depression
    (PPD)
Preeclampsia
Premenstrual syndrome
    (PMS)
Prepuce
Proctitis
Prostate
Prostate cancer
Prostatectomy
Prostate-specific antigen
    (PSA)
Proteinuria
Pyelonephritis
Pyuria
Renal calculi
Renal corpuscle
Renal cortex
Renal failure
Renal medulla
Renal tubule
Salpingectomy
Scrotum
Semen
Seminal fluid
Seminal vesicles
Seminiferous tubules
Sertoli cells
Sexually transmitted
    diseases (STDs)
Specific gravity
Sperm
Spermatogenesis
Sterility
Syphilis
Testicular cancer
Testicular self-
    examination (TSE)
Trimester
Ureter
Ureteritis

Urethra	Urine	Vas deferens
Urinalysis	Urologist	Vasectomy
Urinary bladder	Uterine cancer	Viability
Urinary catheterization	Uterine leiomyomas	Vulva
Urinary tract infection (UTI)	Uterus	Zygote
	Vagina	

Chapter Overview

The urinary system, sometimes called the **genitourinary (GU) system**, filters and removes waste products from the blood. The waste products are excreted from the body in the **urine**. Ultimately, the urinary system determines the fluid volume, composition, and distribution within the body. The urinary system is a critical and hard-working system of the human body. It continuously filters and excretes waste because these waste products quickly become toxic if they remain in the body. The urinary system works closely with the digestive system, the endocrine system, the muscular system, the integumentary system, and the respiratory system. A medical specialist who studies the kidneys, the primary organ of the urinary system, is called a **nephrologist**.

The reproductive organs are necessary to generate offspring. The reproductive process involves a series of coordinated and interrelated events of the male and female reproductive systems. A **urologist** specializes in disorders of the male urinary tract and reproductive system **FIGURE 17.1**. A healthcare provider who specializes in the female

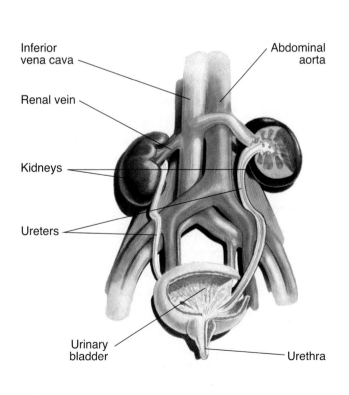

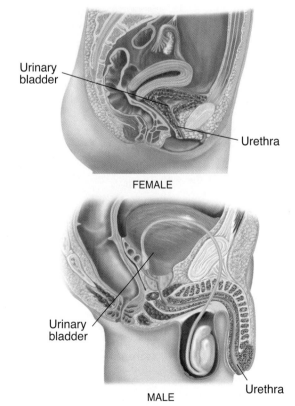

FIGURE 17.1 The urinary and reproductive systems are closely related.

reproductive system is a **gynecologist**. A gynecologist nearly always also serves as an **obstetrician**, caring for a woman during pregnancy, delivering the baby, and caring for the mother after the delivery.

As a medical assistant, you will have the opportunity to interact with patients with a variety of disorders and conditions of the urinary and reproductive systems, as well as participate in diagnostic and treatment-related procedures.

Terminology

TABLE 17.1 lists word roots and terms used in the study of the urinary and reproductive systems.

Structure and Function of the Urinary System

The urinary system consists of two kidneys, two ureters, a bladder, and a urethra. Blood enters the kidneys by way of arterioles that branch from the abdominal aorta. The urinary system removes nitrogenous waste products, salts, and excess water from the blood. The urinary system also constantly evaluates the acid-base balance of the blood and selectively reabsorbs or eliminates products to maintain the proper ratio and support homeostasis. The urinary system has distinct main functions or processes: removal of waste products and other elements from the blood, urine production, and elimination of urine from the body.

Table 17.1   Word Roots of the Urinary and Reproductive Systems

Word Root or Term	Meaning	Example
Balan/o	Penis	Balanitis (inflammation of the penis)
Colp/o	Vagina	Colposcopy (visual examination of the vagina)
Cyst/o	Bladder	Cystoscopy (visual examination of the bladder)
Gravid/o	Pregnancy	Multigravida (multiple pregnancies)
Hyster/o	Uterus	Hysterectomy (removal of the uterus)
Lith/o	Stone	Nephrolithiasis (formation of kidney stones)
Mast/o	Breast	Mastitis (infection and inflammation of breast tissue)
Men/o	Menstruation	Menopause (cessation of menstruation)
Mict/o	Urine	Micturition (the act of passing urine)
Nat/o	Birth	Prenatal (the period prior to birth)
Nephr/o	Kidney	Nephrectomy (removal of a kidney)
Oophor/o	Ovary	Oophorectomy (removal of an ovary)
Orchi/o or orchid/o	Testes	Orchialgia (pain in the testes)
Para	Offspring	Nulliparous (having not given birth to offspring)
Ren/o	Kidney	Renal artery stenosis (narrowing of the arteries that carry blood from the heart to the kidneys)
Salping/o	Fallopian tubes	Salpingorrhaphy (suturing of the fallopian tubes)
Ur/o	Urine	Dysuria (painful urination)

Abbreviations Related to the Urinary and Reproductive Systems

The following are abbreviations related to the urinary and reproductive systems:

- ADH—Antidiuretic hormone
- AH—Abdominal hysterectomy
- ARF—Acute renal failure
- BPH—Benign prostatic hypertrophy
- BUN—Blood urea nitrogen
- CIS—Carcinoma in situ
- CRF—Chronic renal failure
- C&S—Culture and sensitivity test
- CS or C-section—Cesarean section
- cysto—Cystoscopic examination
- DUB—Dysfunctional uterine bleeding
- EDC—Estimated date of confinement
- Grav 1, Grav 2, etc.—First pregnancy, second pregnancy, etc.
- GU—Genitourinary
- hCG—Human chorionic gonadotropin

- HD—Hemodialysis
- HSO—Hysterosalpingo-oophorectomy
- I&O—Intake and output
- IUD—Intrauterine device
- LMP—Last menstrual period
- OB—Obstetrics
- PAP—Papanicolaou test
- Para 1, Para 2, etc.—First delivery, second delivery, etc.
- PID—Pelvic inflammatory disease
- PMS—Premenstrual syndrome
- PSA—Prostate-specific antigen
- TAH—Total abdominal hysterectomy
- UA or U/A—Urinalysis
- UC—Urine culture
- UTI—Urinary tract infection

Kidney

The main organ of the urinary system is the **kidney** FIGURE 17.2. The kidneys are bean-shaped organs that are situated toward the back of the lumbar region of the abdominal cavity on either side of the spinal column. The left kidney is located slightly higher than the right due to the location of the liver, and the left kidney is usually slightly larger than the right. Kidneys are necessary for life. Humans have two kidneys. However, when a kidney is lost or damaged from disease, trauma, or surgery, life can be sustained with only one healthy kidney. The adrenal glands sit on top of each kidney. The structure and function of the adrenal glands are discussed in Chapter 15.

The kidney is covered by a thick, fibrous capsule. The concave border of the capsule is called the **hilum**. The renal artery and the renal vein enter and exit the kidney near the hilum. Inside the protective capsule, the kidney is composed of two distinct sections: the outer **renal cortex** and the inner **renal medulla**. The renal cortex is reddish-brown in color and has a grainy appearance. The cortex acts as a shell for the kidney. The renal medulla is lighter in color and has a striped appearance due to the parallel arrangement of blood vessels and specialized collecting ducts and tubules.

The kidney can be divided into approximately 12 lobes, each containing a pyramid of medullary tissue covered by cortical tissue. The tip of each pyramid faces the hilum. The renal pelvis is the center area of the kidney.

Urine is formed as a result of three processes within the kidney: filtration, reabsorption, and secretion. All these processes occur inside the microscopic nephrons. The hormones that control the amount of urine that the kidneys produce are ADH and aldosterone, which are produced by the pituitary gland and the adrenal cortex, respectively.

Each adult kidney is about the size of a fist. The kidneys are each roughly 4.5 inches long, 2–3 inches wide, and 1 inch thick. They weigh less than half a pound each.

© auremar/ShutterStock, Inc.

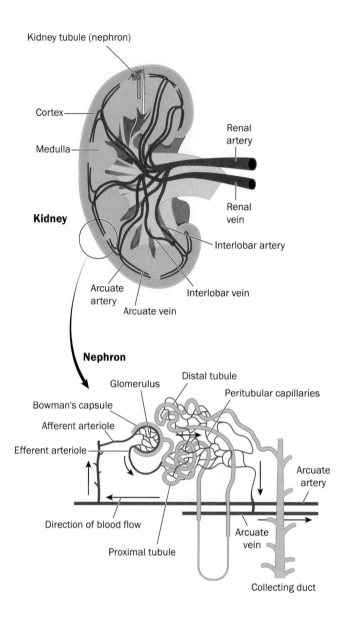

FIGURE 17.2 The kidney is the main organ of the urinary system.
© Blamb/ShutterStock, Inc.

The nephron is the basic functional unit of the kidney (refer to Figure 17.2). Each kidney has roughly one million nephrons. Each nephron consists of a **renal corpuscle** and a **renal tubule**. The renal corpuscle consists of a bed of capillaries, known as the **glomerulus**, surrounded by a cuplike structure called **Bowman's capsule**. Together, the glomerulus and Bowman's capsule filter blood delivered to the kidney. Blood that flows through the nephron contains water, electrolytes, nutrients, soluble waste, and toxins. The water, nutrients, and electrolytes are returned to the blood and the waste and toxins are eliminated from the body. The renal tubule is divided into several anatomical segments: the proximal convoluted tubule, the loop of Henle, the distal tubule, and the collecting tubule. Reabsorption of water, electrolytes, and some amino acids takes place in the renal tubule.

Secretion is the final stage of urine production and occurs when the cells of the collecting tubules secrete ammonia, uric acid, and other substances into the tubule. Once formed, urine collects in the **calyx**, which are cavities that collect urine from the collecting tubules. Urine then moves from the calyx to the renal pelvis and, ultimately, to the ureter. Waves of muscle contractions, called peristalsis, facilitate the movement of urine from the kidney to the ureter to the bladder.

Each kidney filters more than 1L of blood every minute and produces 60mL of urine every hour. The average adult consumes 2.5L of fluid every day and produces 1.5L of urine. Fluid is also eliminated from the body through feces, respiration, and sweat.

Ureter

Each kidney has a **ureter** that drains urine from the renal pelvis into the urinary bladder. The ureter is a narrow tube that exits the kidney near the center of the kidney. Each ureter measures less than ¼ inch wide and is 10–12 inches long. Mucous membrane lines the ureter. Urine travels through the ureter every few seconds, entering the bladder in small amounts.

Bladder

The **urinary bladder** is a muscular sac that holds urine produced by the kidneys. The bladder sits behind the pubic symphysis. The kidneys are constantly producing urine, and the bladder is an elastic organ that can hold roughly one quart of urine.

Similar to the stomach of the GI tract, which stores variable amounts of food, the bladder is composed of three layers of smooth muscle and the inside of the bladder is lined with rugae that can unfold and expand. When the bladder is full, an urge to empty the bladder is felt. Involuntary muscles cause the bladder to contract and the internal sphincter that controls the opening between the bladder and urethra to relax. Voluntary muscles control the external sphincter that directs the act of urinating or voiding the bladder.

Urethra

The tube that drains the bladder is called the **urethra**. The urethra facilitates the elimination of urine from the body. The opening of the urethra to the outside of the body is called the **meatus**. The **perineum** is the area in between the urinary meatus and the anus.

The urethra is approximately 1½ inches long in adult females and 8 inches long in adult males. Mucous membrane lines the inside of the urethra. In females, the urethra is located in the front wall of the vaginal muscle and its only function is to eliminate urine from the body. In males, the urethra extends the length of the penis and is the outlet for urine and the pathway for reproductive fluids.

Diseases and Disorders of the Urinary System

The urinary system is critical to life. Without kidney function, a patient will die. Any disease or disorder that involves an abnormality in the urine or the ability to urinate must be addressed and corrected promptly. Many symptoms describe conditions of the urinary system, often relating to the appearance or characteristics of urine: **dysuria** (painful urination), **proteinuria** (protein in the urine),

More than 10 percent of American adults have impaired renal function and many cases are undiagnosed.
© auremar/ShutterStock, Inc.

hematuria (blood in the urine), **pyuria** (pus in the urine), urinary frequency, urinary urgency, **oliguria** (scant urine production), and **nocturia** (excessive urination at night).

Urinary Tract Infections

A **urinary tract infection (UTI)** is an infection of any part of the urinary tract, but is usually confined to the urinary bladder or the kidney. UTIs are the most common disorders affecting the urinary system. **Cystitis** is an inflammation of the bladder. **Pyelonephritis** is an inflammation of the kidney and the renal pelvis. Pyelonephritis usually occurs after signs and symptoms of cystitis or **ureteritis** (inflammation of the ureter). An infection at any point in the urinary tract puts the entire system at risk for infection.

The cause of a UTI is usually infectious bacteria that are introduced into the urinary tract through the urinary meatus. UTIs are most common among women who are sexually active. The most common cause of UTIs is *E. coli* that moves from the rectum to the meatus due to improper cleaning following defecation. *E. coli* are gram-negative rod-shaped bacteria that are normally located in the intestines. UTIs are rarely caused by a virus or fungus. Women should cleanse from front to back when washing, wiping, or drying the perineal area. Bacteria from the vagina may also cause cystitis.

Women have a shorter urethra than men, so they are more prone to fecal contamination of the urinary tract. Also, prostatic fluid present in the urinary tract of men has antibacterial properties, conferring protection against infections of the urinary tract. UTIs also occur more frequently among women who are pregnant and patients (men and women) who have been catheterized. In men, UTIs are often associated with prostatic hypertrophy and urinary retention.

Signs and Symptoms of Urinary Tract Infections

Frequent urination and pain on urination, especially at the end of voiding, are the most common symptoms of a UTI. Severe UTIs may also lead to a feeling of urinary urgency. Bacteria, white blood cells, red blood cells, and pus are found in the urine during a UTI. Fever also frequently accompanies a UTI. Nausea, vomiting, chills, and low back pain may occur. Symptomatic presentation and the presence of infectious organisms in the urine confirm a diagnosis of a UTI.

Treatment and Prevention of Urinary Tract Infections

The goals of treatment of cystitis are to relieve the pain and symptoms associated with the infection and eradicate the offending organism from the urinary tract. Because the cause of cystitis is usually bacterial, antibiotics are the treatment of choice. Antibiotics are usually administered for three to seven days. A repeat culture of the urine after the course of antibiotics is completed should show no presence of bacteria. Patients should also be instructed to drink plenty of water to mechanically flush the kidneys of bacteria and dilute the urine.

Women are particularly vulnerable to infections of the urinary tract, and steps can be taken to prevent the occurrence of infections. First, drink plenty of water to dilute the urine and mechanically flush bacteria from the urinary tract. Urine should be a light straw color. Second, drinking 4 ounces of cranberry juice reduces the occurrence of infections of the urinary tract. If a woman is prone to repeat UTIs, she should not use a diaphragm for birth control, as it is an easy reservoir for bacteria and increases the risk for recurrent infections. Also, women should be advised to urinate immediately following sexual intercourse. Bacteria from the vagina and perineum can enter the bladder during sexual activity and urinating expels the bacteria, reducing the likelihood of infection.

Glomerulonephritis

Glomerulonephritis is the inability of the glomerulus to function normally. It is a group of symptoms caused by a noninfectious factor. Most cases of glomerulonephritis are acute and self-limiting, causing no long-term damage. Patients completely recover in one to two years. However, some cases may progress slowly to chronic renal failure, and other cases may progress rapidly to renal failure and result in death.

Glomerulonephritis can be acute or chronic. Acute glomerulonephritis usually follows bacterial infections of the respiratory tract, urinary tract, or bloodstream. The symptoms of acute glomerulonephritis are caused by an accumulation of the antibodies created in response to the infection, not from the infectious bacteria. Acute glomerulonephritis is most commonly seen in boys between the ages of three and seven years. Most children and adults with acute glomerulonephritis recover fully with no long-term consequences.

Chronic glomerulonephritis is a progressive disease that leads to scarring and hardening of the affected glomeruli. Eventually, this will lead to renal failure. The onset of symptoms is so slow and gradual that chronic glomerulonephritis is often not diagnosed until the damage is irreversible. Chronic glomerulonephritis usually occurs as a result of other renal syndromes or conditions.

Signs and Symptoms of Glomerulonephritis

Hematuria and **albuminuria** (albumin in the urine) are the two hallmark symptoms of glomerulonephritis. The degree of hematuria can range from microscopic amounts of red blood cells not visible to the naked eye to completely red urine. The urine of a patient with glomerulonephritis will also contain protein, usually in the form of albumin. White blood cells and **casts** (molds of the renal tubules created by protein deposits) are also found in the urine when examined under a microscope.

The patient may experience tenderness in his or her back. Generalized edema develops due to salt and water retention. This retention can, in turn, lead to hypertension and congestive heart failure. Increased blood urea nitrogen (BUN) and serum creatinine levels will be evident in laboratory evaluations of the blood.

In advanced stages of glomerulonephritis, patients may experience nausea, vomiting, pruritis, shortness of breath, fatigue, and anemia. Extreme hypertension and edema can lead to congestive heart failure.

Treatment of Glomerulonephritis

The treatment of glomerulonephritis is symptomatic. A salt-restricted diet will reduce signs and symptoms of high blood pressure and edema. Fluids may be restricted due to decreased urine output. In chronic glomerulonephritis, drugs may be administered to lower blood pressure, correct electrolyte imbalances, or reduce edema.

Incontinence

Incontinence is the uncontrollable or involuntary loss of urine. Most people who suffer from incontinence are women. Incontinence interferes with sleep, physical and sexual activity, travel, and daily routines. Extreme cases of incontinence require patients to be homebound for fear of urinating in public.

Incontinence is divided into three categories:

- Stress incontinence is the most common form of incontinence and occurs when a person laughs, coughs, sneezes, or otherwise places stress on the urinary tract. Exercise or even standing up from a seated position can place stress on the muscles of the urinary tract and cause urine to leak from the bladder.

- Overflow incontinence is a condition in which the bladder never completely empties and it becomes full. The constant fullness causes leakage.
- Urge incontinence is the strong, uncontrollable urge to void the bladder. It requires immediate voiding to prevent accidental leakage of urine.

The incidence of incontinence increases with age, but age is not the only factor. Any condition that affects the physical structure or function of the bladder or urethra can cause incontinence. Hysterectomy in females and prostate surgery in males can cause incontinence. Also, alpha blockers used for hypertension, antihistamines, and sedatives can cause incontinence. Smoking and obesity increase the risk for incontinence.

Signs and Symptoms of Incontinence

Loss of urine is the primary symptom of incontinence. It may be accompanied by urinary urgency, increased urinary frequency, and nocturia. Incontinence significantly affects quality of life, but is an underreported and underdiagnosed disorder. Patients with incontinence may experience depression and a loss of self-confidence. Perineal dermatitis, pressure ulcers, and UTIs may accompany incontinence.

Treatment of Incontinence

The goals of incontinence treatment are to improve quality of life and decrease the symptoms of involuntary urinary leakage. Behavioral modifications are effective in managing some cases of incontinence. Wearing sanitary napkins, incontinence pads, adult diapers, or waterproof underwear allows patients to conceal urine leakage. Exercises of the pelvic floor, called Kegel exercises, strengthen the muscles supporting the urinary tract. To perform Kegels, contract and hold the muscles of the pelvic floor several times a day. To target the correct muscles, imagine trying to stop the flow of urine.

Bladder training and behavioral changes may be useful in controlling incontinence. Scheduling frequent bathroom trips and limiting fluid intake before bedtime can mitigate some symptoms of stress and urge incontinence. Self-catheterization to remove urine can improve symptoms of overflow incontinence. Drug therapy with agents that relax the bladder muscles are effective for treating cases of incontinence not controlled with behavioral or lifestyle modifications.

Nephrolithiasis

Nephrolithiasis, commonly called kidney stones or **renal calculi**, is a condition characterized by the formation of stones or calculi in the kidney or urinary bladder **FIGURE 17.3**. Kidney stones can range in size from a grain of sand to a golf ball. Small stones can pass out of the body in the urine, but large stones may obstruct urine flow and lead to retention of urine in the renal pelvis.

Young to middle-aged men are the most frequent group affected by kidney stones. The cause of kidney stones is not always clear, but several factors can

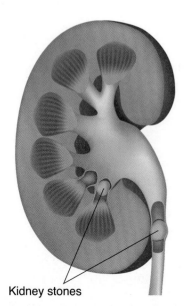
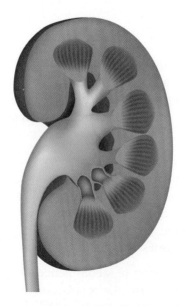

Kidney stones

FIGURE 17.3 Kidney stones (left) can block the outflow of urine.
© Alila Sao Mai/ShutterStock, Inc.

increase the risk of stone formation: not drinking enough fluid, chronic UTIs, mechanical obstruction of the urinary tract, prolonged periods of limited activity, certain medications and foods, and a genetic predisposition or metabolic disease.

Signs and Symptoms of Nephrolithiasis

Pain may occur as a result of kidney stones. The pain may be severe and radiate the entire length of the urinary tract. The pain may last from minutes to hours, and it may subside for periods of relief. Nausea and vomiting, burning on urination, urinary frequency and urgency, and blocked urine flow are symptoms of nephrolithiasis.

An infection may accompany the kidney stones and a fever may be present. Red blood cells may be present in the urine due to the trauma caused by the stone. The urine may also appear cloudy or foul-smelling.

Treatment of Nephrolithiasis

Pain relief is essential in the treatment of kidney stones. Patients may be prescribed narcotic analgesics until the stone has passed out of the kidney. Acute pain will resolve once the stones have passed out of the kidney. Once the stones have passed, a special diet may be prescribed to prevent future stones from forming.

For kidney stones that do not pass on their own, an endoscopic procedure can be performed to manually remove the stones or a laser or shockwave procedure can be performed to break up the stones. Following laser or shockwave treatment, the tiny stone fragments pass naturally out of the kidney in the urine. In the case of large stones or patients with conditions that make endoscopy or laser or shockwave treatment inappropriate, surgical removal of the stone from the kidney is indicated.

Polycystic Kidney Disease

Polycystic kidney disease is an inherited disorder characterized by the presence of grapelike clusters of fluid-filled cysts in the kidneys **FIGURE 17.4**. The cysts replace normal renal tissue and reduce kidney function. The cysts gradually enlarge, replacing all of the renal tissue and resulting in renal failure. When polycystic kidney disease occurs in newborns, a stillbirth or early neonatal death occurs. Rarely, a baby will survive up to two years before developing renal failure. When polycystic kidney disease occurs in adults, the symptoms appear gradually between the ages of 30 and 50 years. The kidney will deteriorate slowly and progressively.

Signs and Symptoms of Polycystic Kidney Disease

In adults, polycystic kidney disease usually begins with generalized symptoms, including hypertension, increased urination, and UTIs. Eventually, back pain, a widened body, and a swollen, tender abdomen will occur. Recurrent hematuria, bleeding from cyst rupture, protein in the urine, and pain from renal calculi accompany advanced disease.

Treatment of Polycystic Kidney Disease

There is no cure for polycystic kidney disease. Eventually, dialysis or a kidney transplant will

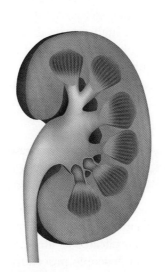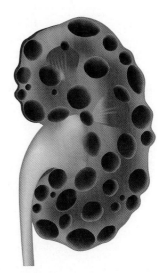

FIGURE 17.4 Polycystic kidney disease, shown on the right, results in the gradual loss of renal function.
© Alila Sao Mai/ShutterStock, Inc.

be required. Patients with polycystic kidney disease must control hypertension and prevent UTIs, either through behavioral and lifestyle interventions or medications.

Renal Failure

Renal failure or renal insufficiency is a condition in which the kidneys are not able to perform their function of filtering waste products from the blood and maintaining the balance of water, electrolytes, and other vital substances. Renal failure may be acute or chronic in nature.

Acute renal failure (ARF) is the sudden loss of kidney function. ARF is a critical illness. It may result from a mechanical obstruction in the kidney or urinary tract, such as a tumor, an enlarged prostate, renal calculi, or blood clots; poor circulation or inadequate blood flow; or damage to the nephrons. ARF often occurs as a complication in hospitalized patients. It is associated with a high mortality rate. Advanced age, chronic kidney disease, chronic cardiovascular or respiratory disease, dehydration, and acute infection increase the risk for ARF.

Chronic renal failure (CRF) is the end result of a progressive loss of kidney function. Chronic infections, obstructions of the kidney or urinary tract, vascular disease, endocrine disease, and hypertension can cause CRF.

Signs and Symptoms of Renal Failure

A change in urination patterns is often one of the first signs of renal failure. Patients will notice a need to void in the middle of the night. Patients will produce more dilute urine and will experience increased thirst. A patient with renal failure is more susceptible to dehydration following episodes of vomiting or diarrhea.

A patient with renal failure will likely appear pale and weak and will tire easily. Loss of appetite and nausea may accompany renal failure. Blood tests will show increased BUN and serum creatinine values. Because the kidneys cannot excrete potassium from the body, it accumulates in the blood; a high level of potassium (**hyperkalemia**) will also be observed in patients with renal failure. Hyperkalemia can cause cardiac arrhythmias. Anemia may also be present.

Treatment of Renal Failure

The goal of treatment of renal failure is to allow the patient to live as normal a life as possible. Other goals include correcting electrolyte imbalances and maintaining appropriate volume status. Most treatments are symptomatic and supportive. In acute renal failure, a high-calorie diet that is low in protein, sodium, and potassium will correct electrolyte imbalances. Fluids are restricted to control urine output. Dialysis may be required in ARF.

Most cases of CRF progress to **end-stage renal disease (ESRD)**. Once ESRD is diagnosed, the patient must receive dialysis to sustain life.

Diagnostic and Treatment-Related Procedures of the Urinary System

Countless techniques are available to analyze, diagnose, and treat disorders of the urinary system. Techniques may be as simple as visual inspection of the color of urine or as complicated as life-sustaining dialysis. Visualization techniques, including X-rays, and endoscopic procedures such as a cystoscopy (visualization of the bladder) can evaluate the size, placement, and function of organs of the urinary system, as well as evaluate the presence of inflammation, polyps, calculi, and tumors inside the urinary tract.

Examination of the Urine

Healthy urine is composed of 95 percent water. Dietary or metabolic waste products make up the remaining fraction of urine. Mostly, these are dissolved substances including urea, uric acid, creatinine, sodium, potassium, ammonium, sulfate, and chloride. Healthy urine should not contain bile, blood, fat, glucose, protein, or microorganisms. Normal urine is considered sterile. Changes in the composition or characteristics of urine can signal an underlying disease process.

A **urinalysis** is a test that provides chemical and physical information about the quality of urine. It is a quick, inexpensive test that can be completed in large part by visual inspection. Urinalysis is one of the most frequently performed tests in a medical office setting.

The physical characteristics of urine that can be assessed with a urinalysis include color, clarity, volume, and odor. Normally, urine is yellow or straw-colored. If it is lighter or darker than normal, or is not yellow, this may be the result of blood in the urine, certain medications, or underlying disease. Normal urine should also be clear. If it is not clear, urine may be described as slightly hazy, hazy, cloudy, or turbid.

Volume is an important assessment for a 24-hour urine collection, but random samples for routine testing do not require notation of volume. Although the odor of urine is not normally recorded on a urinalysis report form, it may provide clues to abnormal conditions or diseases of various body systems. For example, a strong odor of ammonia may indicate a UTI, while a sweet, fruity odor is indicative of diabetes. Certain foods, such as garlic, can alter the smell of urine, but this does not signify an underlying pathology.

Chemical properties of urine can also be assessed by urinalysis: pH, specific gravity, and the presence of substances that should not be in healthy urine. Healthy urine should have a pH of 5.0–7.0, indicating its slight acidity. The acidic environment prevents the growth of bacteria, which are not able to survive in acidic environments.

Specific gravity indicates how concentrated or dilute the urine is. It is measured with special reagent sticks. Specific gravity uses distilled water as a reference for all other substances. Distilled water should have no substances dissolved in it; its specific gravity is 1.000. Healthy urine contains a small amount of dissolved particles, so its specific gravity should be slightly higher than that of water; a normal value for the specific gravity of urine is 1.005–1.030. The higher the reading, the more dissolved particles and the more concentrated the urine; the lower the reading, the fewer dissolved particles and the less concentrated the urine. Color is a qualitative assessment of the specific gravity of urine. A very light-colored urine sample will likely have a low specific gravity, and a dark urine sample will likely have a high specific gravity.

Healthy urine should not contain protein, ketones, bilirubin, blood, nitrite, or glucose. Protein, primarily albumin, is normally reabsorbed by the nephron tubules. In cases of kidney disease or infection, protein may be found in urine samples. A reagent that precipitates protein can be added to a urine sample to detect the presence of protein.

Ketones are by-products of fat metabolism. Ketones are not present in healthy urine. **Ketonuria** is the abnormal presence of ketones in the urine and results in

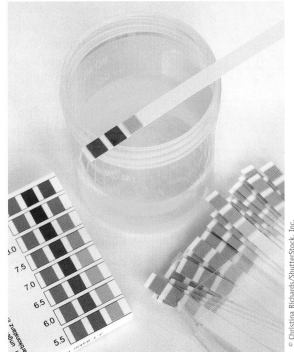

Urine can be examined for color, clarity, pH, specific gravity, and the presence of drugs or other substances.

a characteristic fruity odor. Any disease or condition that includes the metabolism of large amounts of fats can lead to ketonuria. In uncontrolled diabetes mellitus and anorexia or starvation, ketone bodies are undesirable. However, if patients are on a calorie-restricted diet to promote weight loss, ketone bodies may be desirable and indicate that the body is metabolizing stored fat for energy. To test for the presence of ketones, a drop of urine is placed on a reagent strip, timed, and observed for a color change.

Bilirubin is a yellow-orange pigment that is produced during the liver's degradation of hemoglobin. A healthy liver removes old or damaged red blood cells from circulation and uses some of the still-healthy parts to build new red blood cells. When the liver is unable to perform this function, bilirubin is found in the urine. Bilirubin in the urine often precedes more overt signs of liver disease such as jaundice and ascites. Observation of the color of urine is a qualitative assessment of the presence of bilirubin. If bilirubin is present, urine will appear orange to green in color and will produce green foam when shaken. Most commonly, the definitive test for the presence of bilirubin in the urine is performed by placing several drops of urine on a reagent mat and adding water to observe a color change.

Hematuria is the presence of red blood cells in the urine. Unless a woman is menstruating, red blood cells should not be found in urine. A reagent strip is used to detect the presence of red blood cells in the urine during urinalysis.

Nitrites are present in urine that contains microorganisms. When bacteria are present in urine, nitrates are converted to nitrites. The nitrites produce a characteristic ammonia smell. Bacterial growth may occur in a urine sample that has been at room temperature for an extended period of time and produce a false positive test result when evaluating for the presence of nitrites. A definitive diagnosis of bacteria in the urine (**bacteriuria**) must be made by microscopic evaluation or culture and sensitivity testing.

Glucose is normally reabsorbed by the nephron tubules in the kidney. When there is too much glucose for the nephrons to reabsorb, such as in diabetes mellitus, it is excreted in the urine. The level of glucose in the blood at which the nephrons cannot reabsorb glucose varies among individuals, but the normally accepted level for most individuals is 180mg/dL. That is, when the blood glucose level exceeds this threshold, glucose will appear in the urine. A simple reagent strip that tests for the presence of sugar in the urine can diagnose glycosuria.

Special instructions are required to collect urine samples for testing to preserve the integrity of the sample and avoid false positive and negative results. Samples are collected in plastic disposable containers that may be either sterile or nonsterile. The container should be labeled with a patient's name, date and time of collection, and the tests that need to be performed.

Urine should be analyzed within one hour of collection. If the sample cannot be tested within one hour, it should be refrigerated. If refrigerated, the sample should be allowed to come to room temperature before performing the analysis.

The most concentrated urine is the first morning urine, because it has been collecting in the bladder overnight. However, a random sample—meaning that it is unscheduled and requires no preparation—may be easier for patients to provide. A midstream clean-catch urine sample provides the best specimen for urine examination. To instruct a patient to provide a midstream specimen, remember a few key points:

- Instruct the male patient to clean the tip of his penis with soap and water, then with an antiseptic wipe. Tell him to start the urine stream and, without stopping, begin the specimen collection by moving the container into the urine stream. For an uncircumcised male, remind him to retract the foreskin to clean the urinary meatus more effectively and to keep it retracted during voiding.
- Instruct the female patient to clean her genital area with soap and water and then to sit far back on the toilet or to sit backward on the toilet. It may be easier for her to strip from the waist down in order to spread her legs far enough apart. With an antiseptic wipe, instruct her to wipe first down one side, then down the other side, and finally down the middle of the labial folds, vulva, and urinary meatus. Stress the importance of wiping from front to back to avoid fecal contamination. Instruct the patient to begin voiding into the toilet and to keep the labial folds separated during the specimen collection. Tell her to start the stream and, without stopping, begin collecting the specimen in the middle of the stream by moving the specimen container into the stream.
- The patient should not touch the inside of the collection container or the inside of the lid.
- The patient should then begin voiding into the collection container, collecting roughly 3 ounces of urine, or the quantity specified by the provider.
- The patient may then finish voiding into the toilet.
- The patient should replace the lid onto the container and wipe any residual urine from the outside of the container.

A 24-hour urine specimen is ordered to assess urine output over a 24-hour period. Because the composition of urine changes throughout the day due to circadian rhythms and food and water intake, a 24-hour sample will allow for better assessment of long-term renal function compared with a random, one-time sample.

Printed and verbal instructions should be provided to a patient to ensure proper collection technique and storage of a 24-hour urine sample. A single, large, dark-colored container will be provided for the patient to collect all voids in a 24-hour period. The patient begins timing the 24-hour period with the first void of the day, but this first void is not collected for testing. The patient should collect and record the time of each subsequent void for the next 24 hours. The final void collected will be the first morning urine on the second morning. This collection should take place within 10 minutes of the start time of the test the previous day. Usually, the patient keeps the sample refrigerated for the length of the collection period and until he or she is able to return it to the laboratory or office for analysis. Preservatives may be added to the collection container to prevent the degradation of substances in the urine.

Catheterization

Urinary catheterization is a procedure in which a small, sterile, flexible tube is inserted into the urethra and threaded to the bladder **FIGURE 17.5**. Catheterization may be performed to collect a urine sample when completely sterile conditions are required or when the patient is not able to follow cleansing or collection procedures. Catheterization is a sterile procedure and should be performed only under the authority of a healthcare provider by professionals who have been adequately trained. An improper catheterization procedure can introduce bacteria into the patient's urinary tract. As

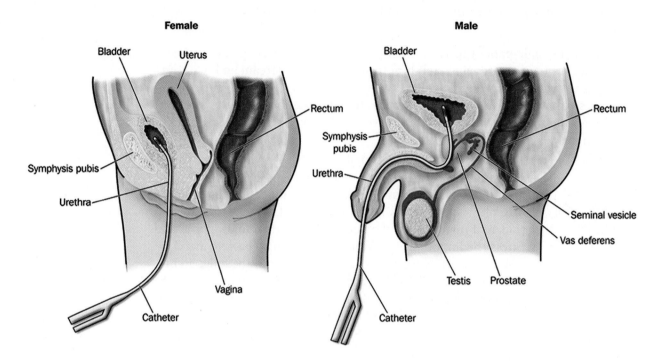

Female

Bladder

Uterus

Symphysis pubis

Urethra

Vagina

Catheter

Rectum

Male

Bladder

Rectum

Symphysis pubis

Urethra

Seminal vesicle

Vas deferens

Testis   Prostate

Catheter

FIGURE 17.5   Catheters are inserted into the urethra and threaded to the bladder.
© Blamb/ShutterStock, Inc.

a medical assistant, your primary role in catheterization procedures is to assist the healthcare provider as necessary.

Catheterization can be used if medication must be instilled into the bladder. Catheterization is also used when patients are unable to empty their own bladders due to physical or mental limitations. The use of catheters may be recommended in cases of uncontrollable urinary incontinence, urinary retention, genital or prostate surgery, multiple sclerosis, spinal-cord injury or deformity, and dementia.

Catheters may be employed for short-term use, in which case they are straight tubes. Such intermittent catheters are placed into the bladder just long enough to remove the urine. Once the urine has stopped flowing, the catheter is removed.

An in-dwelling catheter is one that is intended for long-term use, such as a Foley catheter. In-dwelling catheters have a small balloon that is inflated with saline once in place in the bladder. This prevents the catheter from sliding out of place. In-dwelling catheters increase the risk of UTIs because bacteria can travel up the catheter into the bladder. In-dwelling catheters collect urine from the bladder in a collection bag attached to the end of the catheter that is outside the body.

Catheter diameters are described in French units, denoted as F. The most common catheters range from 10F to 28F. The higher the unit, the larger the diameter of the catheter.

Dialysis

Dialysis is a process that filters the blood and removes harmful waste products when the kidneys are unable to perform this function. Dialysis is often initiated once 85–90 percent of kidney function is lost. In ARF, dialysis may be used for short-term treatment until the kidneys heal and regain normal function. Most cases of dialysis, however, are permanent and will be required for the remainder of a patient's life.

Two types of dialysis can be performed:

■ **Hemodialysis** uses a machine to remove blood, filter it, and return it to the body.
■ **Peritoneal dialysis** uses the lining of a patient's own abdomen to filter the blood.

Both types of dialysis require significant lifestyle changes; patients often have trouble coping with the emotional aspects of dialysis. Significant changes in diet, mobility, daily routine, and sleep patterns may be observed. Many medications are removed from the body by dialysis, and these must be monitored or changed to provide optimal care for patients.

The hemodialysis equipment (**hemodialyzer**) is essentially an artificial kidney. Blood is removed from the body through a catheter or a fistula and passed through thin membranes. A dialysate solution surrounds the membranes, and substances in the blood pass through the membranes into the lesser-concentrated dialysate by simple diffusion. Additionally, minerals, electrolytes, and other substances are diffused into the blood. Dialysate is individualized for each patient.

Hemodialysis is also individualized with regard to length of treatment, frequency of treatment, and location of procedures. Many patients receive dialysis in a clinic setting, but hospitals can provide hemodialysis. It can also be performed at home for some patients. Factors that influence hemodialysis include the function of the kidneys, fluid weight gained in between dialysis sessions, the amount of waste products in the blood, and the size of the patient. Most hemodialysis sessions last between three and four hours and occur three times per week. As kidney disease and damage progress, hemodialysis needs will change.

Peritoneal dialysis does not require a machine; instead, it uses the patient's own body to filter the blood. The peritoneum, the lining of the abdominal cavity, acts as the filter in this case. The dialyzing solution is placed in the abdominal cavity through a permanent catheter inserted into the abdomen **FIGURE 17.6**. In continuous ambulatory peritoneal dialysis, gravity is used to instill the solution by hanging a bag of dialyzing solution higher than the patient's abdomen. The empty bag is then rolled and tucked into the patient's clothing. In the abdomen, the dialyzing solution comes in contact with the blood vessels. Approximately 2L of solution is introduced for dialysis. The dialyzing solution collects waste products and water from the blood through diffusion and osmosis. After four to six hours, the dialyzing solution is removed from the abdomen—again, by gravity. The bag is unrolled and placed lower than the patient's abdomen and drained from the patient's body. The entire process is repeated every four to six hours during the day and for an eight-hour period overnight.

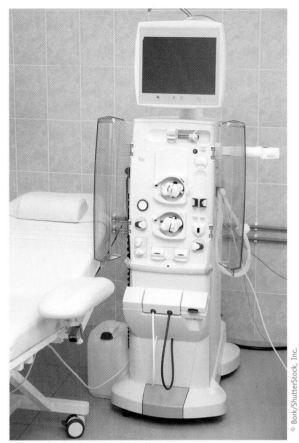

A hemodialyzer is essentially an artificial kidney.

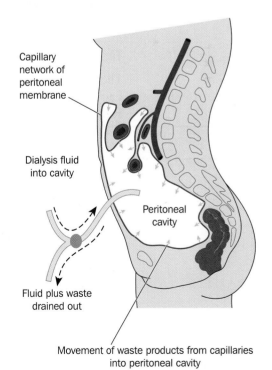

FIGURE 17.6 Solution is instilled into a patient's abdomen for peritoneal dialysis.
© Blamb/ShutterStock, Inc.

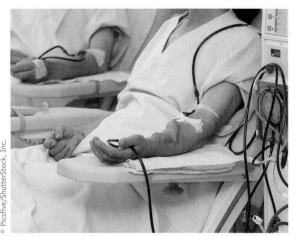

Patients may receive hemodialysis in a hospital, a clinic, or a home setting.

Continuous cycler-assisted peritoneal dialysis is performed only overnight. This type of peritoneal dialysis provides patients more freedom during daily activities and is well-suited for children. Dialyzing solution is again placed in the abdomen, but it is cycled three to five times by means of the automated cycler instead of gravity. In the morning, one instillation of solution is performed, and this will stay in the abdomen all day.

Nocturnal intermittent peritoneal dialysis is similar to cycler-assisted peritoneal dialysis in that it is performed at night. But, nocturnal dialysis does not involve instillation of fluid during the day. Patients who can appropriately receive only nightly dialysis still have some renal function remaining or will have a peritoneum that can rapidly remove waste products from the blood.

Peritonitis (an inflammation of the peritoneum) is a complication of peritoneal dialysis. If sterile procedures are not followed for connecting and disconnecting tubing and instilling and draining solution, contamination of the peritoneum can occur. Peritonitis can lead to scarring of the peritoneum, which will render it useless for dialysis. Peritonitis can be fatal.

Structure and Function of the Male Reproductive System

The male reproductive system **FIGURE 17.7** is closely related to the urinary system. In both genders, the reproductive system produces, nourishes, and transports the cells required for reproduction. The male reproductive system is composed of glands and a series of ducts.

Testes

The testes, or testicles, are the two glands that produce sperm and male sex hormones. Each testis is an oval-shaped gland that is approximately 2 inches long, 1 inch wide, and 1 inch thick. They are located in a muscular sac called the scrotum, which is suspended from the perineum. The **scrotum** can contract and relax to maintain optimal temperatures for **spermatogenesis** (the production of sperm).

Sperm are male **gametes**, the cells required for reproduction. Unlike all other cells of the human body, which contain 46 chromosomes, gametes contain 23 chromosomes. When two gametes (a sperm from a male and an egg from a female) combine during **conception**, the newly formed embryo will have 46 total chromosomes. Sperm are produced in miles of **seminiferous tubules** in the testes. Surrounding the tubules are **Sertoli cells**, which produce hormones that direct male characteristics such as patterns of hair distribution, large muscle mass, long bone structure, and enlargement of the larynx. Testosterone is a major product of Sertoli cells and also plays a large role in sexual desire.

The functions of the testes begin around age 10, when the hypothalamus releases a hormone that initiates puberty. Mature sperm are usually not produced until age 14.

Sperm development takes 74 days.

Epididymis

The **epididymis** sits on top of the testes and is another large collection of tiny, coiled tubes. It extends and straightens to enter the abdominal cavity through

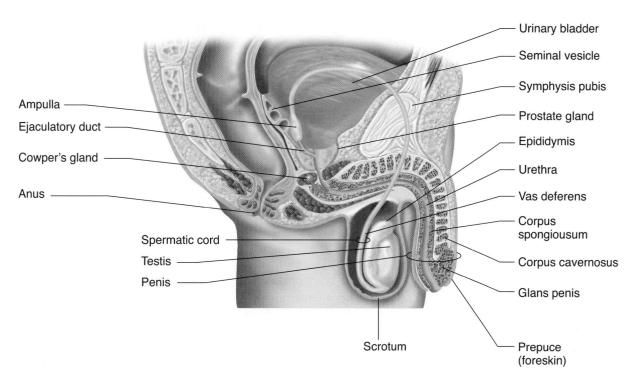

Ampulla

Ejaculatory duct

Cowper's gland

Anus

Spermatic cord

Testis

Penis

Scrotum

Urinary bladder

Seminal vesicle

Symphysis pubis

Prostate gland

Epididymis

Urethra

Vas deferens

Corpus spongiousum

Corpus cavernosus

Glans penis

Prepuce (foreskin)

FIGURE 17.7 The male reproductive system contains the organs and cells required for reproduction.
© Jones & Bartlett Learning

the **vas deferens**. The vas deferens sits behind the urinary bladder. The vas deferens from each epididymis joins with a duct from a seminal vesicle to form the **ejaculatory duct**, which passes through the prostate gland and eventually joins with the urethra. The epididymis stores sperm for approximately 18 hours. If sperm are not expelled from the body, they die and are reabsorbed into the body.

A **vasectomy** is a procedure that prohibits the release of sperm from the body **FIGURE 17.8**. It is an effective form of sterilization for males and is commonly used as a method of birth control. A small incision is made in each side of the scrotum. Each vas deferens is located and pulled through the incision. A small portion of the vas deferens is removed and the ends are sutured closed. The remainder of the vas deferens is returned to the scrotum. The incision in the scrotum is closed with sutures.

A vasectomy does not interfere with the production of testosterone or normal sexual function. Sperm is still produced, but its exit from the body is impeded. It collects in the epididymis until it dies and is reabsorbed by the body.

Seminal Vesicles

The **seminal vesicles** are muscular tubes that produce a thick secretion. This secretion, or **seminal fluid**, is a vehicle for sperm. It provides

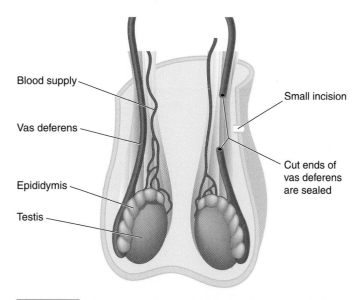

Blood supply

Vas deferens

Epididymis

Testis

Small incision

Cut ends of vas deferens are sealed

FIGURE 17.8 A vasectomy prevents sperm from leaving the body.
© Blamb/ShutterStock, Inc.

nourishment for sperm, mostly in the form of glucose. It also provides most of the liquid that is expelled during ejaculation. Seminal fluid is slightly alkaline, which neutralizes the acidic environment created in the epididymis by sperm.

Prostate Gland

The **prostate** is a donut-shaped muscular gland that surrounds the top of the urethra where it joins the bladder. During ejaculation, sperm is propelled through the vas deferens, the seminal vesicles, and the prostate gland. The prostate gland contains roughly 40 small ducts through which sperm and seminal fluid (now called **semen**) pass during ejaculation. The prostate also produces a fluid that is added to semen to improve its mobility.

Penis

The **penis** is a vascular, muscular, cylindrical structure that surrounds the urethra. The **corpus spongiosum** is the layer of the penis that contains the urethra. The other two layers are called the **corpora cavernosa** **FIGURE 17.9**. The entire penis is covered in a layer of subcutaneous tissue and skin. The ridge of tissue near the end of the penis is called the **corona** and the tip of the penis is called the **glans**. Males are born with a **foreskin** or **prepuce** covering the glans, which may be removed during a process called circumcision.

Circumcision is the surgical removal of the foreskin of the penis. It is a centuries-old practice that is performed for religious ceremonies and social acceptance. There is debate on whether it is necessary for the health of the male, but many reports indicate a lower incidence of penile cancer in men who have been circumcised. Also, women who are married to circumcised men have a lower incidence of cervical cancer.

The urethra extends through the penis and opens at the urinary meatus in the glans. In males, the urethra serves two purposes: to remove urine from the body and to expel semen.

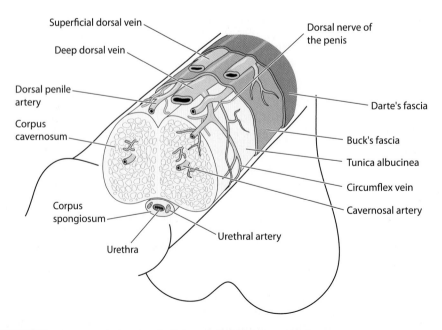

FIGURE 17.9 The penis is composed of three cylindrical layers of tissue.
© Blamb/ShutterStock, Inc.

The appearance and function of the male reproductive system change during sexual activity. The corpora cavernosa are erectile tissue and engorge with blood during sexual arousal. The erectile tissue becomes large and firm. Stimulation of the glans leads to stimulation of the seminal vesicles. At the height of arousal and stimulation, orgasm occurs, which is a series of rhythmic contractions of the muscles surrounding the vas deferens, seminal vesicles, ejaculatory ducts, and prostate gland. Any secretions produced and stored in these structures, as well as sperm, are forcefully expelled through the urethra during orgasm. The engorgement of the erectile tissue gradually subsides after orgasm.

Diseases and Disorders of the Male Reproductive System

Because the male urinary and reproductive systems are closely related, a disorder of one will likely affect the other. Cancers and disorders related to the prostate are common reasons for men to seek medical care. In general, the risk of both types of diseases increases with age, but some cancers appear almost exclusively in young men. Adequate, routine screenings are critical to early identification of diseases of the male reproductive system. Early diagnosis often leads to complete cure of the disease.

Benign Prostatic Hypertrophy

Prostatic hypertrophy is the enlargement of the prostate gland. This enlargement is common in men over 50 years of age. **Benign prostatic hypertrophy (BPH)** is nonmalignant, but may result in significant consequences. The prostate may enlarge so much that it restricts the flow of urine through the urethra **FIGURE 17.10**. BPH is likely due to changes in hormone levels as men age. The prevalence of BPH is 50 percent at age 60 and 90 percent at age 85. However, the prevalence of symptoms associated with BPH is 50 percent by age 75.

Signs and Symptoms of Benign Prostatic Hypertrophy

A reduced urine stream, in both size and force, is a notable sign of BPH. Difficulty starting a urine stream, dribbling, incomplete voiding, straining to void, nocturia, and frequent urination are also common among BPH sufferers. The severity of the symptoms is correlated with the size of the prostate. As the prostate grows larger, the symptoms will become more pronounced. Hematuria and urinary retention will eventually develop.

The International Prostate Symptom Score self-evaluation is a useful tool for identifying BPH. A digital rectal examination of the prostate will definitively diagnose prostatic hypertrophy. A **prostate-specific antigen (PSA)** blood test, urinalysis, and cystoscopy can also assess the presence and progression of BPH. PSA is a protein produced by the prostate gland; a PSA test measures the level of PSA in the blood. An elevated PSA indicates abnormal function of the prostate gland due to cancer, inflammation, or hypertrophy. A PSA level of 2.5mg/mL is considered the upper limit of normal, although levels can vary among individuals.

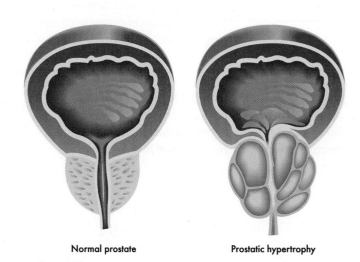

Normal prostate   Prostatic hypertrophy

FIGURE 17.10 An enlarged prostate can impede urine flow from the bladder to the urethra.
© rob3000/ShutterStock, Inc.

Treatment of Benign Prostatic Hypertrophy

The goals of treatment of BPH are to relieve the signs and symptoms of prostatic hypertrophy and improve a patient's quality of life. Medications are available that improve urinary flow and relax the bladder. Hormone-based therapies can shrink the size of the prostate. The results of medication therapy are gradual and confer side effects that may be undesirable for some men, including the inability to achieve an erection or engage in sexual activity, decreased interest in sexual activity, and breast enlargement. Surgical removal of the prostate (a **prostatectomy**) will eliminate symptoms of BPH, but this procedure should be reserved for men who have failed medication therapy or have severe, advanced cases of BPH.

Prostate Cancer

Prostate cancer is a malignancy that starts in the prostate. Men at high risk for prostate cancer include African American men, men over 60 years old, and men with a family history of prostate cancer. Also, men who have been around agent orange (an herbicide used by the United States during the war in Vietnam), men who drink excessive amounts of alcohol, farmers, and men who eat a high-fat diet are at increased risk for the disease. Prostate cancer is less common in vegetarians than in men who eat meat. Cadmium, a metal, is a well-known environmental toxicant and carcinogen and has been associated with an increased risk of prostate cancer. Tire-plant workers, painters, welders, and machine operators are at risk for occupational exposure to cadmium.

Signs and Symptoms of Prostate Cancer

Signs and symptoms of prostate cancer may mimic those of BPH. Because a malignancy of the prostate can cause the gland to enlarge, the same urinary symptoms experienced with BPH will occur with prostate cancer. A PSA test is recommended as a screening tool for prostate cancer for men over 50 years old, but its use has limitations and its results are controversial.

Treatment of Prostate Cancer

The goals of treatment of prostate cancer are to remove the malignancy and restore normal function and quality of life to the patient. Today, early treatment of prostate cancer results in a high cure rate in developed countries. If the malignancy is advanced or aggressive, metastasis to the spine or pelvis may occur.

Treatment of prostate cancer is determined by overall clinical assessment, remaining life span, stage of disease, and tolerance for treatment. Options may include a prostatectomy, radiation therapy, hormone therapy with estrogen, removal of the testes (an **orchidectomy**) to stop the production of testosterone, and freezing the cancer cells with liquid nitrogen (cryotherapy). Several regimens offer effective treatment but also present the patient with undesirable side effects such as erectile dysfunction, incontinence, cystitis, and **proctitis** (inflammation of the rectum).

Prostate cancer is the leading cause of cancer death in men over 75 years old. It is the third leading cause of cancer death among all men. Prostate cancer is rarely diagnosed in men younger than 40.

© auremar/ShutterStock, Inc.

Testicular Cancer

Testicular cancer is a malignancy that begins in the testicles. It is the most common form of cancer in men aged 20–35 years. It is rarely seen in other age groups. Abnormal testicular development, an undescended testicle, a history of mumps, or Klinefelter syndrome increases the risk of testicular cancer. White men are more likely to develop testicular cancer than African-American or Asian-American men.

Signs and Symptoms of Testicular Cancer

Testicular cancer may cause no symptoms. Or, patients may experience discomfort or pain in the testicle or a feeling of heaviness in the scrotum, as well as low back pain, an enlarged testicle, or the development of excess breast tissue. A lump or swelling of either testicle may be felt on palpation. Self-examinations should be performed once a month by men at risk for testicular cancer to detect abnormalities in the testicles that may signify a cancerous growth.

Treatment of Testicular Cancer

The goals of treatment of testicular cancer are to remove the malignancy and restore normal function and quality of life to the patient. Treatment is determined based on the type, location, and stage of the tumor. Surgical therapy, radiation therapy, and chemotherapy are effective at curing most cases of testicular cancer.

Structure and Function of the Female Reproductive System

The female reproductive system **FIGURE 17.11** involves organs and cells responsible for conception, pregnancy, childbirth, and lactation. The female reproductive system is controlled by a much more sophisticated and integrated system of hormones than the male reproductive system.

Ovaries

The ovaries are a pair of small organs in the pelvic cavity, located on either side of the uterus. Each ovary is supported by ligaments and loosely attached to the outside of the uterus. An ovary sits next to the open ends of a tube that extends from each side of the uterus (**fallopian tubes**). The primary functions of the ovaries are to produce

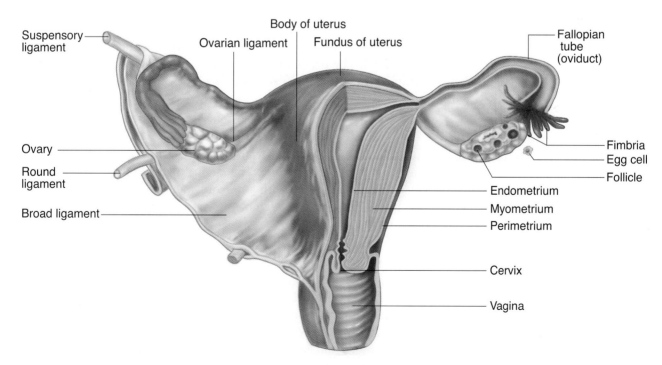

FIGURE 17.11 The female reproductive system includes the cells and organs required for reproduction.
© Jones & Bartlett Learning

the female gamete (the **ovum**, or egg) and produce hormones. The ovaries secrete estrogen and progesterone in response to signals from the pituitary gland. Estrogen is responsible for the maturation of the reproductive organs, including the fallopian tubes, uterus, and vagina. Estrogen also causes the appearance of female characteristics such as the broadening of the pelvis, the development of soft and smooth skin, the growth of pubic hair, and deposits of fat in the breast tissue, buttocks, and thighs. Estrogen also affects sexual desire. Progesterone is responsible for maintaining pregnancy when conception occurs.

At birth, a female's ovaries contain all the eggs, although in immature form, that she will have in her life. Between 200,000 and 400,000 immature ova are present at birth, but most of these will disappear by puberty. During her reproductive life, the ovaries will mature and release 375 eggs. By age 50, nearly all of the eggs will be gone.

Fallopian Tubes

A fallopian tube extends approximately four inches from each side of the uterus. The ovaries are situated near the ends of the tubes, which have funnel-like ends, and are the passageway for an egg to move from the ovary to the uterus. The fallopian tubes have muscular layers and mucosal layers with cilia. The funnel-like end of the tube with its fingerlike projections, along with the movement of cilia, facilitates the movement of the egg.

Conception takes place in the outer third of the fallopian tube. The newly formed **zygote** (a one-celled union of egg and sperm) begins to multiply and travel to the uterus.

Uterus

The **uterus**, sometimes called the womb, sits between the urinary bladder and the rectum. The uterus is a pear-shaped hollow, muscular organ with thick walls. Before pregnancy, a normal uterus measures approximately three inches tall, two inches wide, and two inches thick, but it possesses an enormous capacity for expansion.

The uterus is lined with a mucous membrane that has a rich supply of blood vessels called the **endometrium**. The **myometrium** is the thick, muscular layer surrounding the endometrium. The muscles of the myometrium run in three distinct layers: circular, longitudinal, and diagonal. The **perimetrium** is the outermost layer of the uterus.

The lower portion of the uterus is called the **cervix**. The cervix connects the uterus to the vagina.

Vagina

The **vagina** is a muscular tube that extends from the uterus to the vulva. The primary function of the vagina is as the birth canal. The vagina also receives semen during sexual intercourse. The vagina is lined with a mucous membrane that is oriented in folds. The vagina is also capable of considerable expansion. The vagina opens to the exterior of the body in the perineum.

Vulva

The **vulva** includes the external female genitalia, including the clitoris, the labia minora, and labia majora. The mons pubis is the pad of fat that lies over the pubic symphysis and is covered in coarse pubic hair. The **clitoris** is a small, round structure composed of erectile tissue. The clitoris is very sensitive and provides arousal for sexual activity. The clitoris becomes engorged and enlarged when aroused and participates in orgasm. The labia minora and majora are fatty folds of skin surrounding the vulva.

Mammary Glands

The **mammary glands** in the breasts of the female consist of lobes of connective tissue. Clusters of cells that secrete milk are embedded into each lobe **FIGURE 17.12**. The clusters drain into minute ducts that converge into larger ducts. Eventually, all milk leaves each lobe through one duct. Each breast has 12 to 15 ducts, arranged like the spokes of a wheel and meeting at the nipple. The ducts exit the body through tiny openings in the **areola**, the area around the nipple.

In late pregnancy and immediately after childbirth, the mammary glands secrete **colostrum**, concentrated milk that nourishes the newborn in the first few days of life and is rich in antibodies from the mother. About three days after childbirth, the glands begin producing **breast milk** in response to the release of prolactin from the pituitary gland. Oxytocin, also produced in the pituitary gland, allows milk to be expelled from the breasts in response to infant suckling.

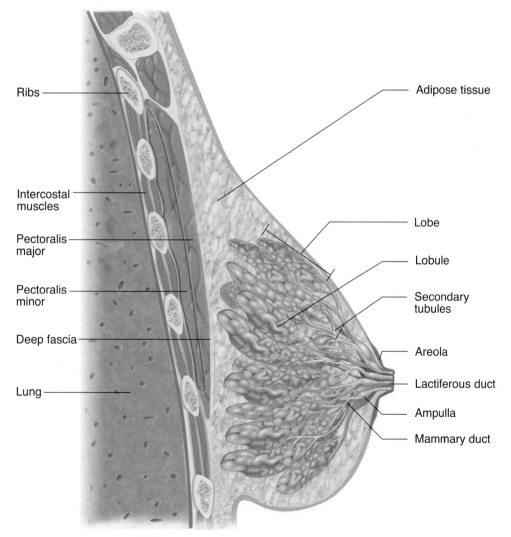

FIGURE 17.12 The mammary glands produce breast milk.

© Jones & Bartlett Learning

Breast Milk: Nature's Nutrition

Breast milk provides the perfect nutritional support for a newborn and infant. When breast feeding is not possible or not desired, commercial formulas are available that mimic the components of breast milk as closely as possible.

Breast milk contains proteins, lactose, vitamins, minerals, fat, water, antibodies, and lymphocytes. In addition to providing nourishment, breast milk provides immune-system components to act in place of an infant's underdeveloped immune system.

The American Academy of Pediatrics recommends breast milk exclusively for nutrition in the first six months of life. Ideally, a mother will continue to provide breast milk for her infant for at least 12 months. However, any amount of breast feeding is beneficial to a baby. Mothers should be supported to select the feeding method that works best for her, her baby, and her family.

Menstrual Cycle

Menstruation is the process by which the lining of the uterus is shed and discharged from the body in the absence of pregnancy. The onset of menstruation is called **menarche**, and usually begins around age 12 or 13. **Menopause** is the cessation of menstruation and usually occurs around age 50. The average menstrual cycle is 28 days, though normal variations range from 21–35 days and are highly variable among women. Menstruation occurs from days 1–5 during the menstrual cycle. This marks the beginning of the **follicular phase**. The entire menstrual cycle is illustrated in FIGURE 17.13.

Beginning on the fifth day, the follicular phase of the menstrual cycle allows for the development of an ovarian follicle. During this time, the pituitary gland secretes high levels of follicle-stimulating hormone (FSH). A follicle matures an egg and begins the process of ovulation. The mature follicle secretes estrogen. Around day 10, the pituitary gland secretes luteinizing hormone (LH) in response to the growth of the follicle. FSH production declines.

At ovulation, the follicle releases the mature egg from the ovary. The estrogen level is high, and FSH declines just prior to ovulation. The estrogen stimulates additional LH secretion from the pituitary, which causes the follicle to rupture and release the egg around day 14 of the menstrual cycle.

During the follicular phase, the endometrium also undergoes changes. In response to estrogen production, the endometrium undergoes proliferation, becoming thicker and preparing to receive a fertilized egg.

After the egg is released, the **luteal phase** begins. LH stimulates the rapid change of the ruptured follicle. It becomes a mass called the **corpus luteum** and releases progesterone and estrogen. Progesterone from the corpus luteum encourages the endometrium to produce nourishing substances for a fertilized egg. The corpus luteum will secrete progesterone until day 26 of the cycle.

Rising levels of progesterone during the luteal phase inhibit the production and release of LH. When LH levels fall, the corpus luteum degenerates and progesterone and estrogen levels fall sharply.

Without an implanted fertilized egg, the lining of the uterus sheds. Menstruation signifies the beginning of another cycle. Estrogen and progesterone levels are low, but FSH is slowly rising to prepare for the follicular phase once again. Menses is the term that identifies the actual flow of blood out of the uterus. Most women have menses or menstrual periods that last between four and seven days.

Several disorders related to menstruation can occur. **Menorrhagia** is heavy, prolonged, or irregular bleeding. This may be caused by bleeding disorders, uterine cancer, hormone therapy, changes in diet or exercise, infections of the pelvic organs,

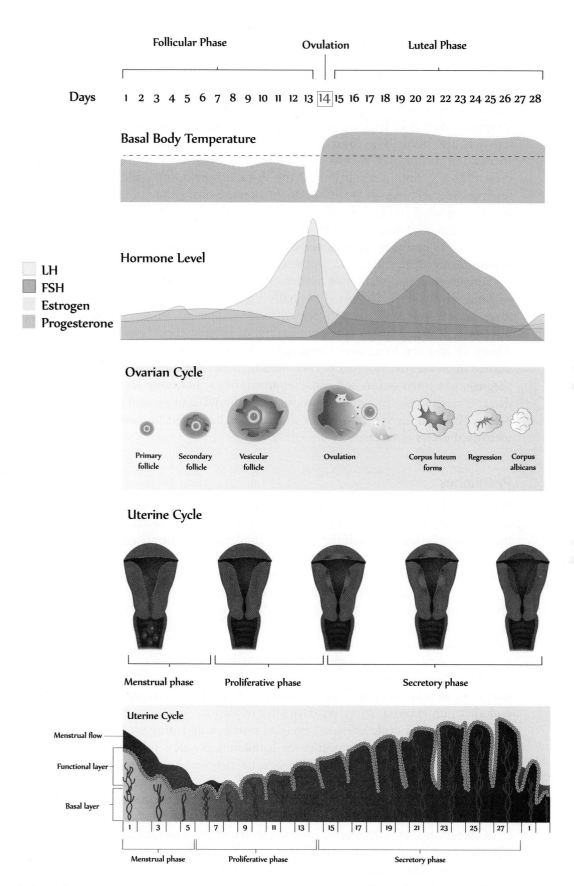

FIGURE 17.13 During the menstrual cycle, hormone levels fluctuate and induce changes in the ovaries and uterus.

endocrine abnormalities, or recent trauma or stress. Treatment of menorrhagia will depend on the underlying cause of the bleeding.

Dysmenorrhea is pain associated with menstruation. It is common among young females. Its incidence tends to decrease with age and, particularly, after pregnancy. The pain of dysmenorrhea begins 12–14 hours before the onset of menses and includes symptoms such as nausea, vomiting, fatigue, and diarrhea. Pain in the back and upper legs may also occur. The cause of dysmenorrhea is unknown, but hormonal imbalances and psychological factors play a role in its occurrence. Dysmenorrhea may be present as a symptom of an underlying disorder, including endometriosis, uterine tumors, incorrect uterine position, or inflammation of pelvic organs. Pain relievers and heat applied to the area of discomfort are simple, cost-effective treatments for most women who suffer from dysmenorrhea. Drugs that control hormone fluctuations, such as **hormonal contraceptives** (birth control pills), can regulate symptoms of extreme dysmenorrhea.

Amenorrhea is the absence of menstruation for at least six months in a woman who has previously menstruated normally. Causes of amenorrhea can include obesity, excessive exercise, less than 15 percent body fat, severe anxiety, or sudden weight loss. Also, pituitary tumors, ovarian failure, or thyroid conditions may cause amenorrhea. In addition to missed menstrual cycles, a woman may experience headache, change in breast size, changes in body weight, acne, and increased hair growth. After pregnancy is ruled out as the cause of amenorrhea, hormone levels are assessed to detect abnormalities in estrogen production, thyroid activity, and pituitary function. Normally, the underlying cause of the amenorrhea must be corrected for normal menstrual cycles to return.

Pregnancy

Fertilization occurs following sexual intercourse if one sperm is able to penetrate the outer protective covering of an egg. Sperm travels from the vagina, through the cervix, into the uterus, and through the fallopian tube. Usually, the sperm will meet the egg during its travels from the ovary to the uterus in the outer third of the fallopian tube. Only the strongest sperm are able to survive the acidic environment of the vagina.

Sperm must continually attack the outer protective layer of the egg. Once a single sperm penetrates the egg, the membrane covering the egg seals to prevent additional sperm from entering. The nucleus of the sperm travels to meet the nucleus of the egg and a zygote is formed. A zygote is the one-celled product of fertilization. At this point, the chromosomal composition of the individual is determined.

The zygote will begin to divide and grow, becoming an **embryo** approximately one week after conception. The embryo travels to the uterus and implants into the endometrium approximately six days after ovulation. At this point, a change in the normal menstrual cycle occurs. Levels of estrogen and progesterone are high, and FSH and LH are low. This prevents the formation of a new follicle and prevents the shedding of the endometrium. Progesterone also encourages development of the mammary glands. The developing **placenta** (the organ that connects the developing embryo to the uterine wall) **FIGURE 17.14** secretes **human chorionic gonadotropin (hCG)** to maintain the corpus luteum during the initial stages of pregnancy.

Once the placenta develops enough to secrete its own progesterone, approximately 12 weeks after the last menstrual period, hCG production ceases and the corpus luteum disintegrates. The placenta continues to produce estrogen and progesterone throughout the pregnancy. It is connected to the growing embryo by the umbilical cord. The umbilical cord has three blood vessels: two small arteries that carry blood to the placenta and one vein that returns blood to the fetus. The placenta is connected to the **amniotic sac**, which is filled with **amniotic fluid** in which the embryo floats. The amniotic sac is a tough, transparent pair of membranes. The inner membrane is the **amnion**. The outer later, the **chorion**, is part of the placenta. The fetus "breathes" amniotic fluid as its respiratory system develops.

The embryo continues to grow during pregnancy **FIGURE 17.15**. By the end of the 10th week of pregnancy, all body systems are completed, although immature. At this point, the embryo is now called a **fetus**. By the 20th week of pregnancy, movement can be felt by the mother and a heartbeat can be heard with a specialized fetal stethoscope. A fetus must be carried at least 23 weeks of gestation to have a chance at survival. A fetus born at 23 weeks' gestation will weigh less than two pounds and have a one in 10,000 chance of survival. Odds of survival increase every week of gestation after this point. During the final weeks of pregnancy, a fetus grows rapidly in size and assumes a head-down position to prepare for childbirth.

The loss of a pregnancy prior to 20 weeks' gestation is termed an **abortion**. It may be either spontaneous (unforced) or elective or therapeutic (induced). A spontaneous abortion is also called a **miscarriage**. A spontaneous abortion usually results from the defective implantation of the fetus in the endometrium or the defective development of the embryo. A premature separation of the placenta may

FIGURE 17.14 The placenta connects the developing embryo and fetus to the uterine wall and provides nutrients and eliminates waste for the fetus.
© Jones & Bartlett Learning

Placenta
Umbilical cord
Amniotic cavity
Uterus
Lumen of uterus

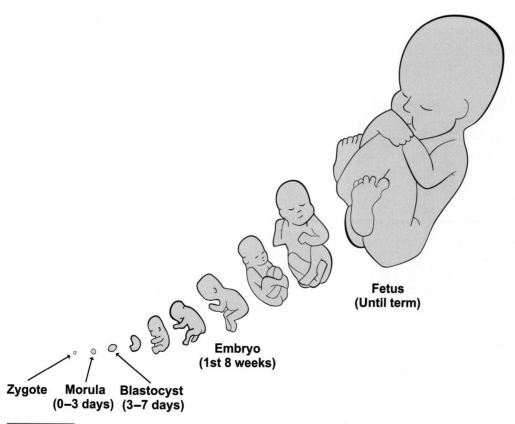

Fetus
(Until term)

Embryo
(1st 8 weeks)

Zygote   Morula   Blastocyst
(0–3 days) (3–7 days)

FIGURE 17.15 Enormous fetal growth and development takes place during pregnancy.
© udaix/ShutterStock, Inc.

also induce the loss of a pregnancy. Maternal factors such as poor nutrition, trauma, or blood-group incompatibility can also cause a loss of a pregnancy. Miscarriages are common and occur in approximately 25 percent of pregnancies. An abortion may be induced if a woman does not wish to carry a child to term or to preserve her physical or mental health.

A missed menstrual period is the first sign of pregnancy for many women. A urine test to detect hCG is often performed by many women to determine if pregnancy has occurred. As pregnancy progresses, a women will experience a variety of symptoms related to pregnancy. Breast tenderness and nausea (often called by the misnomer "morning sickness") are common during the first six to eight weeks for most women. Fatigue and frequent urination are also common complaints. Shortness of breath, indigestion, hemorrhoids, and edema are common in later pregnancy. Psychological stress and emotional instability are common during pregnancy.

Prenatal Care

Gestation is the carrying of an embryo or fetus or, more simple, a pregnancy. A pregnancy is divided into three **trimesters**, each approximately 13 weeks long. A full-term pregnancy is one that lasts 37 to 42 weeks. The estimated date of delivery or **estimated date of confinement (EDC)** is calculated by counting 40 weeks from the date of the last menstrual period. Early confirmation of pregnancy and initiation of prenatal care will help ensure a healthy baby. Proper nutrition is essential, including adequate intake of vitamins and minerals—particularly folic acid.

Pregnant women should refrain from alcohol, illegal drugs, and tobacco, which may harm the developing fetus. Exercise is important during pregnancy to maintain a healthy body weight and relieve stress. Maternal weight gain will continue during pregnancy as the fetus grows and the mother's caloric needs increase. Excessive weight gain during pregnancy can lead to cardiovascular and endocrine complications for the mother and fetus. The recommended weight gain for women of normal weight is 25 to 35 pounds. Underweight women should gain 30 to 40 pounds, and overweight women should gain no more than 25 pounds.

Ideally, prenatal care should commence before a woman becomes pregnant. However, the first prenatal visit usually takes place after a second missed menstrual period or a positive home pregnancy test. This visit will establish rapport with the patient and assess risk factors for pregnancy-related complications. Health promotion should occur as early in pregnancy as possible. A thorough health history and physical examination should be completed at the first prenatal visit. Breast, pelvic, and abdominal examinations should be included. Pelvic measurements can be obtained to assess whether there is room for a fetus to pass through the vagina. A complete list of all the woman's medications, vitamins, and herbal supplements should be reviewed. Laboratory tests should include hemoglobin, blood type and screen, platelet count, and screening for hepatitis B and HIV. Genetic counseling can be offered based on patient history or risk factors.

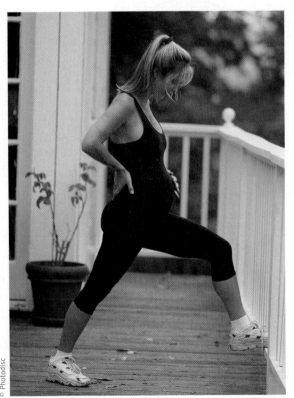

© Photodisc

Women should maintain an active, healthy lifestyle during pregnancy.

Folic Acid in Pregnancy

Folic acid, also known as vitamin B9 or folate, prevents neural tube defects in a developing embryo. Women should consume at least 400mcg of folic acid daily prior to conception to ensure the health of her baby. Folic acid is found in orange juice, leafy green vegetables, and enriched grains. It is also available as an OTC supplement for women who do not achieve adequate dietary intake.

An obstetrical history will include a notation of the number of previous pregnancies, or **gravidity**. **Parity** is the number of pregnancies carried to **viability** (the ability to grow and develop after birth). Multiple births, such as twins and triplets, count as one pregnancy and one birth. **Nullipara** identifies a woman who has not carried a pregnancy to viability. **Multigravida** identifies a woman who has been pregnant more than once. For example, a women who miscarried a pregnancy, then had one child delivered at 40 weeks, would be gravida 2, para 1 (or G2 P1). A woman who is pregnant for the first time is gravida 1, para 0.

Prenatal visits occur throughout pregnancy, with increasing frequency toward the end of gestation. The growth of the fetus and the health of the mother are assessed continually. The obstetrician monitors for conditions such as gestational diabetes, UTIs, anemia, and high blood pressure, which can pose serious risks to the mother and fetus. **Preeclampsia** is high blood pressure, usually greater than 140–90mmHg, in the second or third trimester of pregnancy. Preeclampsia may be caused by an autoimmune disorder, cardiovascular diseases or disorders, obesity, diet, or genetic factors. Edema of the hands, ankles, and face, as well as sudden and extreme weight gain, are signs of preeclampsia. Severe preeclampsia may also present with a headache, pain on the right side of the body, decreased urine output, nausea, vomiting, and vision changes. Preeclampsia must be managed by medication or by delivery of the baby if the gestation has reached at least 37 weeks. If not treated, preeclampsia may progress to **eclampsia**, which is characterized by maternal seizures and extreme high blood pressure. Both preeclampsia and eclampsia can be fatal for the mother and fetus.

An ultrasound is a common procedure used in obstetrics. The test uses high-frequency sound waves to produce an image of the fetus. Ultrasounds can be performed through the vagina in early pregnancy or through the abdomen in later pregnancy. Ultrasound can be used to assess the number of fetuses, assess the gestational age, and detect fetal abnormalities. If abnormalities are suspected, an amniocentesis can be performed. An amniocentesis is a procedure that obtains a sample of amniotic fluid,

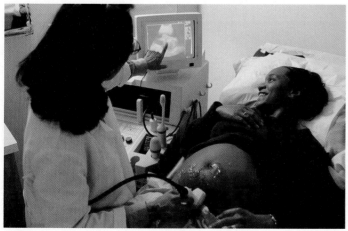

An ultrasound creates images of the developing fetus.

which contains fetal cells. Fetal cells can then be analyzed for chromosomal abnormalities and genetic defects.

A lack of financial resources, a lack of social support, a lack of transportation, and poor communication contribute to many women being unable to receive prenatal care. This places both the mother and the fetus at risk for complications before, during, and after birth.

Labor and Delivery

The birth process, or **parturition** **FIGURE 17.16**, begins with the release of mucus from the cervix that was in place during the pregnancy to protect the fetus from organisms in the vagina. Amniotic fluid that surrounds the fetus may also begin to leak from the mother's body. Contractions of the uterus will begin, usually as irregular, infrequent cramps.

Labor begins when contractions are regular and frequent. The cervix thins and dilates to a diameter of approximately 10 centimeters (four inches). Contractions become forceful, frequent, and exhausting during the first stage of labor. This stage can last from two to 24 hours.

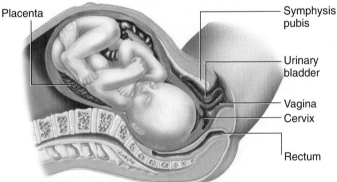

Placenta — Symphysis pubis

Urinary bladder

Vagina
Cervix

Rectum

Early first-stage labor

Ruptured amniotic sac

Later first-stage labor: the transition

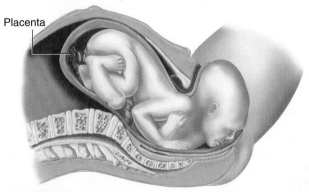

Placenta

Early second-stage labor

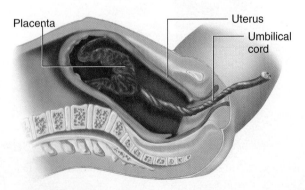

Placenta — Uterus
Umbilical cord

Third-stage labor: delivery of afterbirth

FIGURE 17.16   Parturition takes place in three distinct stages.
© Jones & Bartlett Learning

The next stage of labor begins when the fetus's head (or other body part) enters the vagina. Continued contractions and pushing by the mother propels the baby through the vagina until the entire body is delivered.

A few minutes after the baby is delivered, the placenta and its membranes detach from the uterine wall and are expelled through the vagina. This is known as **afterbirth**. This process is accomplished with several more contractions of the uterus. After the entire birth process is complete, the uterus will continue to contract to close open blood vessels and control bleeding.

When a fetus is unable to pass out of the uterus through the birth canal due to the improper positioning of the fetus, inadequate pelvic space, a large fetus, labor that is ineffective or not progressing, or other complications, a baby may need to be delivered through a surgical opening in the abdomen. A **cesarean delivery** or **C-section** involves cutting through the abdomen and uterus to remove the baby and afterbirth. Today, roughly one-third of deliveries are cesarean deliveries.

Postpartum Care

The **postpartum** period begins after delivery and continues until the infant is six to eight weeks old. The hormonal, physical, and physiological changes that occurred during pregnancy will return to normal during this time. Evaluation and management of chronic medical conditions, as well as those that occurred during the pregnancy or delivery, should be addressed during the postpartum period. Mothers should be advised of circumstances that necessitate prompt medical attention such as high fever or depression during the postpartum period. Prevention of pregnancy during this period should be discussed with patients, as short periods between pregnancies leads to high infant mortality rates. Open communication with healthcare providers during the postpartum period is essential for new mothers. The postpartum period is a time of great physical and emotional stress; support and encouragement from knowledgeable providers will help maintain the health of mothers and newborns.

Postpartum depression (PPD) is a serious issue that may be seen by obstetricians, gynecologists, and family practitioners. PPD is moderate to severe depression that occurs after a woman gives birth. Usually, PPD appears within three months after giving birth, but symptoms may not appear for up to a year. Symptoms of PPD are consistent with other depressive disorders and may include agitation and irritability, changes in appetite, feelings of guilt or worthlessness, feeling withdrawn, lack of energy, negative feelings toward the baby, lack of interest in once enjoyable activities, and thoughts of suicide or death.

PPD adversely affects mothers, children, and families. PPD prevents a mother from adequately caring for herself or her baby and interferes with her ability to bond with her baby. Women should be supported by family, friends, and healthcare providers during the postpartum period. By routine mental-health screenings at postpartum visits, early diagnosis and treatment of PPD is possible. Cognitive behavioral therapy and medication therapy are available to treat PPD. Mothers should be encouraged to ask for help whenever they are feeling overwhelmed or are afraid they might hurt their babies.

Contraception

Many women, due to financial, social, medical, or family-related reasons, desire not to conceive or undergo a pregnancy. Therefore, many patients will seek counseling and advice on contraceptive methods. The best method of **contraception** (the prevention of pregnancy) for each woman will depend on efficacy, safety, personal preferences, and cost. **Abstinence** (refraining from sexual activity) is the only com-

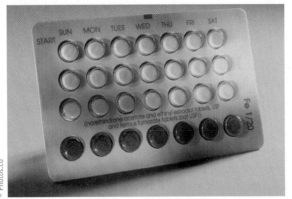

Birth control pills are a common choice for contraception.

© Photos.co

pletely effective means to prevent pregnancy, but many other pharmacological and mechanical options exist that decrease the occurrence of pregnancy. Combined estrogen and progesterone methods are available in oral pills, transdermal patches, and vaginal rings. These hormonal contraceptives not only prevent pregnancy with nearly 100 percent effectiveness, but they can also be used to control menstrual cycles and decrease the risk of **pelvic inflammatory disease (PID)**, an inflammation of any of the female reproductive organs. Estrogen therapy has been associated with an increased risk of deep vein thrombosis, myocardial infarction, and stroke, but these incidents are rare.

Nonhormonal barrier-style contraceptive methods are also available. Male and female condoms, female diaphragms, cervical caps, and cervical sponges are generally low-cost and easy-to-use methods of contraception. They are not hormone-based therapies and are completely reversible if contraception is no longer desired. Permanent surgical methods of contraception or sterilization are also available for both men and women. A vasectomy, as previously discussed, is effective sterilization for men. Removal of the female reproductive organs or the occlusion of the fallopian tubes with cautery or a band or clip is effective sterilization for women.

Diseases, Disorders, and Conditions of the Female Reproductive System

Disorders related to menstruation and the structure and function of the female reproductive tract are common reasons that women seek medical care. Premenopausal women are advised to receive an annual gynecologic examination, which includes routine screenings for many cancers and conditions of the reproductive system. Early screening and diagnostic tools offer effective treatment options for many gynecologic disorders, but many factors must be considered when initiating treatment. A woman's desire to bear children after treatment should be of utmost concern when considering various treatment options.

Cancers of the Female Reproductive System

Cancers of the female reproductive system are, unfortunately, common. Malignancies can occur in any part of the female reproductive system. The incidence of most gynecologic cancers increases with age. Early screening and diagnosis have improved outcomes of cancer treatment.

Breast cancer, a malignancy of the breast tissue, is the most common cancer among females, affecting one in nine women who survive to 90 years of age. The average age of diagnosis in the United States is 64 years. Breast cancer is rare in women younger than 35. Estrogen is believed to play a role in the development of breast cancer, but the exact cause is not known. A family history of breast cancer, long menstrual cycles, early menarche or late menopause, a first pregnancy after 30, obesity, heavy alcohol consumption, and a high-fat diet are all risk factors for the development of breast cancer. Breast cancer can occur in men, but males account for less than one percent of all breast cancer cases.

Cervical cancer is a malignancy of the cervix of the uterus. Early age of intercourse, multiple sexual partners, multiple pregnancies, and infectious bacterial or viral diseases increase the risk for cervical cancer. Human papillomavirus (HPV) has recently been identified as a causative factor in 70 percent of cervical cancers. A preventive vaccine is now available for adolescent boys and girls to prevent the spread of HPV during sexual intercourse.

Ovarian cancer, a malignancy on an ovary, is a common cause of cancer death among women. This form of cancer has a low survival due to the fact that is it often detected at advanced stages, which limits treatment options and confers a poor prognosis. Ovarian cancer also metastasizes rapidly. Women who have never had children, women who have had breast cancer, and women with a family history of breast or ovarian cancer are at an increased risk of ovarian cancer. Living in an industrialized country and being of a high socioeconomic status also increases the risk.

Uterine cancer, a malignancy of the uterus, usually affects postmenopausal women between the ages of 50 and 60 years. High estrogen exposure, accumulated over a lifetime, is the primary risk factor for uterine cancer. Estrogen exposure may come from hormone therapy, early menarche, late menopause, never having children, or a history of ovulatory dysfunction. Infertility, diabetes, gallbladder disease, hypertension, and obesity are also risk factors for uterine cancer.

Signs and Symptoms of Cancers of the Female Reproductive System

Signs that may signal breast cancer include a lump or mass in breast tissue; a change in the size, shape, or appearance of the breast or nipple; a change in skin temperature; or discharge from the breast in a nonnursing woman. Pain is not usually associated with early symptoms of breast cancer.

A monthly breast self-examination is indicated for women over 18 years old. A **mammogram** is a visualization technique that uses low-energy X-rays to examine the breast tissue. Early mammography is the best and most reliable form of screening for breast cancer. Annual or biannual mammograms should begin between age 40 and 50, depending on a patient's individual risk for breast cancer. A definitive diagnosis of breast cancer is made with a mammogram, an ultrasound, or a surgical biopsy.

Early symptoms of cervical cancer include abnormal vaginal bleeding, pain or bleeding after sexual intercourse, or persistent vaginal discharge. Early signs of cervical cancer and precancerous cells can be detected with a **Papanicolaou test**, more commonly known as a Pap smear. This routine screening test is performed at annual gynecological examinations. A **colposcopy** (visual examination of the vagina) is used to screen and test for abnormal cells in the cervix if a Pap smear indicates the need for further investigation. Due to the success and prevalent nature of cervical cancer screening, the survival rate of precancerous lesions of the cervix is 100 percent. The five-year survival rate for cervical cancer that is detected early is 92 percent. Cervical cancer is still a global health problem in underdeveloped countries, however.

Vague symptoms associated with ovarian cancer contribute to its difficult diagnosis, including abdominal discomfort and mild gastrointestinal disturbances. Urinary frequency, constipation, and pelvic discomfort occur with disease progression. Diagnosis is confirmed with a surgical biopsy.

Uterine enlargement and unusual bleeding are the earliest signs of uterine cancer. A biopsy of uterine tissue will usually diagnose uterine cancer.

Treatment of Cancers of the Female Reproductive System

All cancer treatment plans are individualized and consider a patient's overall health status, her age, her personal preferences, the stage of disease, and confounding medical circumstances. Fear and apprehension surround many surgical options related to gynecologic cancers because the surgeries may result in permanent disfigurement or the loss of function of part of the urogenital or reproductive tract. Surgical options may be coupled with chemotherapy and/or radiation therapy, depending on the type of cancer.

A **lumpectomy** (the removal of the tumor only) is appropriate for breast cancer treatment when only a small tumor is present and there is no evidence that the cancer has metastasized to the lymph nodes. If larger portions of the breast are involved in the tumor, a **mastectomy** (complete removal of the breast) is indicated. A radical mastectomy removes the breast and underlying tissue and axillary lymph nodes. A prosthetic breast or reconstructive surgery is often indicated after a mastectomy.

If cervical cancer is not invasive, cryotherapy or the use of an electrical current to remove malignant tissue can be used. For invasive cancer, a combination of chemotherapy, radiation therapy, and surgery is appropriate.

The treatment of ovarian cancer involves surgical removal of all reproductive organs, lymph nodes, and the appendix. Chemotherapy may extend survival time if initiated in the early stages of the disease.

Like ovarian cancer, uterine cancer is treated by surgically removing reproductive organs. A **hysterectomy** is the removal of the uterus. An **oophorectomy** is the removal of the ovaries. A **salpingectomy** is the removal of the fallopian tubes.

Endometriosis

Endometriosis is one of the most common gynecological disorders seen in practice. It is defined as the presence of endometrial tissue outside of the uterus, usually on the ovaries, ligaments, and peritoneum. The cause of endometriosis in unknown, but recent uterine surgery, inflammation of the endometrium, and endometrial fragments expelled through the fallopian tubes during menstruation may play a role in its development. Endometriosis likely has a genetic component.

Endometriosis occurs almost exclusively in reproductive-aged women. Early menarche, frequent menses, long menses, few pregnancies, late first pregnancy, and less breast-feeding increase a woman's risk for endometriosis. Endometriosis is not life threatening, but pain and anemia decrease quality of life.

Signs and Symptoms of Endometriosis

Dysmenorrhea is the primary symptom of endometriosis. Menorrhagia, hematuria, rectal bleeding, nausea, vomiting, and abdominal cramps may also occur, depending on the location of the endometrial tissue. Infertility and painful sexual intercourse may occur. Laparoscopic surgery is the diagnostic method of choice for endometriosis. Ultrasound and MRI offer some ability to visualize and diagnose endometriosis, but the techniques offer a risk of false positives.

Treatment of Endometriosis

Endometriosis may be treated by controlling pain with analgesic agents and controlling symptoms with hormone therapy. Definitive treatment is only accomplished with a hysterectomy. If a woman no longer desires to have children, a hysterectomy, with or without a salpingo-oophorectomy, is appropriate treatment.

Fibroids

Uterine leiomyomas are more commonly referred to as **fibroids**. These are benign, smooth tumors of the muscle cells of the uterus. Estrogen increases fibroid growth.

Signs and Symptoms of Fibroids

Menorrhagia is the primary symptom of fibroids. Pain or a feeling of heaviness in the abdomen may occur if the fibroid is large. Anemia due to heavy blood loss during menstruation also appears with fibroids. Urinary frequency, urinary urgency, and constipation may occur, depending on the location and size of the fibroid. Infertility and lethargy may also occur. A **hysteroscopy** (an endoscopic visualization of the inside of the uterus) can be used for the diagnosis of fibroids.

Treatment of Fibroids

Only symptomatic fibroids require treatment. Hormone therapy may control the growth of fibroids, but surgical removal may be necessary. To preserve a woman's child-bearing ability, only the fibroid may be removed. Or, if no children are desired, a hysterectomy may be performed.

Premenstrual Syndrome

Premenstrual syndrome (PMS) is a group of emotional, behavioral, and physical symptoms that occur seven to 14 days before the onset of menses. The symptoms usually subside with the onset of menses. PMS affects an estimated 30–50 percent of women, mostly between the ages of 25 and 40 years.

Signs and Symptoms of Premenstrual Syndrome

PMS includes a combination of several symptoms that are clinically significant and affect quality of life or daily activities. Symptoms may include irritability, anxiety, confusion, social withdrawal, depression, bloating, swelling, breast tenderness, headache, fatigue, dizziness, tingling in the extremities, respiratory infections, allergic rhinitis, asthma, constipation, diarrhea, change in appetite, acne, and palpations.

A full medical history to determine if underlying medical conditions are causing the symptoms and rule out substance use is required to diagnose PMS. Premenstrual dysphoric disorder (PMDD) is a severe form of PMS.

No definitive test is used to diagnose PMS or PMDD. Women suspected of either condition should maintain a log of symptoms, activities, and their menstrual cycles for at least two months to assess a pattern of symptom occurrence.

Treatment of Premenstrual Syndrome

Treatment of PMS is symptomatic. Pain relief may assuage the physical symptoms and antidepressants may control the emotional symptoms of PMS. Hormone therapy to control hormonal fluctuations may mitigate symptoms of PMS. Maintaining a healthy lifestyle by eating a balanced diet, engaging in regular physical activity, and getting an adequate amount of sleep also helps control PMS.

Ovarian Cysts

An **ovarian cyst** is a fluid-filled or semisolid mass on an ovary. It is usually small and benign and produces no symptoms. Cysts may occur in response to hormone fluctuations in the follicular or luteal phases of the menstrual cycle. Cysts grow from an ovarian follicle that failed to properly release an egg or dissolve completely at the end of the cycle.

Signs and Symptoms of Ovarian Cysts

Large cysts or multiple cysts may cause pelvic pain or discomfort, low back pain, or uterine bleeding. Pain during sexual intercourse, weight gain, nausea, vomiting, and breast tenderness may also occur. Ovarian cysts are diagnosed with a pelvic examination or an ultrasound.

Treatment of Ovarian Cysts

Ovarian cysts that cause no symptoms may not require treatment. Hormone therapy may be helpful in controlling hormone fluctuations associated with the development of cysts. If changes in the size of the cyst occur, or symptoms develop, surgical removal of the cysts may be necessary. If the cyst is small and child bearing is still a concern for a woman, only the cyst may be removed. If the cyst is large and the woman no longer desires children, the entire ovary may be removed.

Sexually Transmitted Diseases

Sexually transmitted diseases (STDs) are a taboo subject in society, but they are still significant to urinary and reproductive health of both men and women. There is a wide variety of pathogens spread by sexual contact and a large number of infected individuals worldwide. Generally, the incidence of STDs is higher in men, but complications occur more often in women. More than two-thirds of STDs occur among individuals in their late teens or early adulthood. Demographic, socioeconomic, and cultural factors contribute to the occurrence and transmission of STDs. The single greatest risk factor for STDs is the number of sexual partners. STD rates are also higher among homosexual men than heterosexual men and women.

Unfortunately, many STDs are becoming resistant to antibiotic therapy, which poses challenges to the future of sexual, reproductive, and urinary health. There are several STDs for which curative therapy is not available. In addition to the physical complications related to STDs, psychological, social, and emotional consequences significantly affect the lives of those infected with STDs.

The most frequently occurring STDs in the United States are chlamydia, gonorrhea, herpes, and syphilis. STDs can be completely prevented through sexual abstinence. If abstinence is not a desired choice, maintaining a mutually monogamous sexual relationship with an uninfected partner is also effective at preventing STDs. Safe sex practices, including the use of condoms, vaginal sponges, and spermicides, alone or in combination, will decrease the risk of STDs. Notifying one's partner about one's infection status is crucial to maintaining a healthy sexual relationship.

Chlamydia

Chlamydia is the most frequently reported STD in the United States. It is caused by *Chlamydia trachomatis*, a bacterium that lives as an intracellular parasite. Chlamydia can cause irreversible damage to the female reproductive system and result in **sterility** (the inability to reproduce) if left untreated. Young women are more vulnerable to chlamydia infections.

A majority of people infected with chlamydia have no symptoms. If symptoms do appear, they appear one to three weeks after infection. Symptoms may include discharge from the vagina or penis or burning or irritation while urinating. Women may also experience abdominal pain, back pain, nausea, fever, and pain during intercourse.

If untreated, chlamydia infects the uterus and fallopian tubes of women and causes PID. This can lead to permanent damage to the reproductive system. Chronic pelvis pain and infertility are the most significant consequences of chlamydia. Men may have no lasting effects from a chlamydia infection, but they may still be able to spread the infection to a sexual partner.

If a woman is infected with chlamydia during pregnancy, it will likely be passed to her baby during the birth process. Chlamydia is a frequent cause of conjunctivitis and pneumonia among newborns.

Chlamydia is treated with antibiotics, usually azithromycin or doxycycline. Differentiating chlamydia from other STDs will determine the appropriate course of treatment.

Gonorrhea

Gonorrhea is caused by the bacteria *Neisseria gonorrhoeae*. This bacterium is fragile and survives only in moist, dark, warm areas. It is spread only through sexual contact. Humans are the only known host of *N. gonorrhoeae*. Gonorrhea has a rapid incubation period. There are large numbers of infected individuals worldwide, making gonorrhea difficult to control from a public-health standpoint.

Symptoms of a gonorrhea infection vary between males and females. Males experience burning, itching, and pain on urination. A sore throat, anal discharge, and penile drainage may also occur. Women usually experience no symptoms of a gonorrhea infection. However, women may develop a yellow discharge from the cervix. Swollen glands and lower abdominal pain may also occur.

High doses of antibiotics, usually penicillins or tetracyclines, are necessary to treat gonorrhea. Untreated, gonorrhea can spread to other organs of the pelvis and cause extensive damage to the urinary and reproductive system, including chronic urethritis, long-term urinary tract inflammation, and sterility.

Women who are infected with gonorrhea when giving birth present a significant risk to their newborn. If *N. gonorrhoeae* infects the newborn's eyes during delivery, permanent blindness can occur. Most newborns receive erythromycin ointment to their eyes immediately following birth to prevent gonorrhea infections.

Herpes

Genital herpes is an acute inflammatory condition of the genitals. It is a common infection, but most people do not even know they are infected by the herpes simplex virus. Type 1 herpes simplex virus causes cold sores around the mouth and type 2 herpes simplex virus causes genital sores. Herpes is passed through direct skin-to-skin contact with the lesions. More than 50 million Americans have genital herpes.

Once infected, the lesions will appear in three to seven days. In women, lesions appear on the cervix, labia, vulva, vagina, or perineum. In men, lesions appear on the glans, foreskin, and shaft of the penis. Normally, the lesions are painless, but they may erupt and develop into shallow ulcers accompanied by edema and redness.

After the lesions heal, the virus becomes dormant and the lesions may never recur. However, most people will experience outbreaks of lesions several times during the first year after infection. The outbreaks decrease in frequency over time. There is no cure for herpes, but antiviral medications can shorten and prevent outbreaks. Daily therapy can help reduce the risk of transmission to another person.

Herpes infections can be passed to babies during vaginal delivery. If a woman has active lesions at the time of delivery, a C-section is indicated. Herpes can cause an infection of the brain in newborns, which is usually fatal.

Syphilis

The incidence of **syphilis** is rising in the United States. It is a highly contagious disease caused by the bacterium *Treponema pallidum*. Syphilis occurs most frequently among men aged 35–39 years and women aged 20–24 years. Most cases are seen among homosexual men.

The signs and symptoms of syphilis are often indistinguishable from other diseases (resulting in the nickname "the great imitator") and vary with disease stage. During the primary stage, people may remain asymptomatic for several years. Transmission of the infectious bacteria can still occur during this stage, even if an individual does not know he or she is infected. There may be a single sore or multiple sores on the genitalia of the infected individual; many sores go unrecognized. The sore, or **chancre**, is firm, round, small, and painless and appears on the body at the point where the *T. pallidum* entered the body. The chancre usually lasts three to six weeks and will progress to the secondary stage if not treated promptly.

The secondary stage is characterized by a skin rash and lesions of the mucous membranes. The rash, which does not usually itch, appears one to six months after the chancre has healed. The characteristic syphilis rash appears as red, rough patches on the palms of the hands and soles of the feet. Fever, swollen lymph nodes, sore throat, patchy hair loss, headaches, weight loss, muscle aches, and fatigue also occur during the secondary stage of syphilis.

The third stage is a latent period of syphilis. Symptoms completely disappear, but the person is still infected with the bacteria. This stage can last for several years. Symptoms can reappear 15–20 years after the infection initially occurred. Late symptoms of syphilis include inflammation in virtually every body system. Cardiovascular symptoms and neurological symptoms are the most damaging, including difficulty coordinating muscle movements, paralysis, numbness, blindness, and dementia. Late symptoms of syphilis can be fatal.

If a woman is pregnant while infected with syphilis, *T. pallidum* can cross the placenta and infect the fetus. If the mother is in the primary or secondary stages, the risk for disease transmission is higher than if she is in the latent stage of the disease. The infection can cause fetal death, prematurity, or congenital syphilis. Congenital syphilis can cause symptoms of syphilis in childhood and adolescence. If a mother is treated for syphilis early in her pregnancy, the disease may not be passed to her fetus. Routine testing for syphilis takes place as part of most prenatal screenings.

A blood test is the only definitive diagnostic tool available, as medical history and physical examination may reveal no signs or symptoms of the disease. Penicillin is the treatment of choice for syphilis. Syphilis remains fairly responsive to antibiotic treatment. Treatment is easier in early stages of the disease.

Tuskegee Syphilis Study

Much of what is known about the long-term effects of untreated syphilis come from a study of African American men conducted at Tuskegee University in Alabama. In 1932, the United States Public Health Service enrolled 600 impoverished black men in Macon County, Alabama, in a program that the men were told would provide them with free health care. Nearly 400 of the men already had syphilis. The men were provided with medical care, meals, and burial insurance, but were never told they had syphilis, nor were they ever treated for the disease.

By the mid-1940s, penicillin had become standard treatment for syphilis, but the men in the study were never provided with antibiotic treatment. The study continued until 1972, when a whistle-blower revealed the study's ethical failures. The victims of the study include hundreds of men who died of syphilis, wives who contracted the disease, and children born with congenital syphilis.

The Tuskegee Syphilis Study is one of the most notorious ventures in modern medicine. Its failings led to drastic changes in the way clinical trials are conducted and the way informed consent is provided by patients. It also contributed greatly to the distrust of the medical establishment by racial minorities—a problem that still plagues some communities today.

Skills for the Medical Assistant

As a medical assistant, you will have the opportunity to participate in several procedures relating to the urinary and reproductive systems. You may assist with diagnostic or treatment-related procedures or instruct patients to conduct self-examinations for screening purposes. The urinary and reproductive systems are private and intimate elements, both physically and emotionally, of the human body. Take care to make your patients comfortable and at ease during examinations or procedures related to the urinary or reproductive systems. Always maintain the highest standards of professionalism when encountering patients under these circumstances.

Instructing a Patient in Testicular Self-Examination

Males should begin monthly self-examinations of the testicles at about 15 years of age. The **testicular self-examination (TSE)** is a simple procedure that can lead to early diagnosis and treatment of testicular cancer. The more often a man performs a TSE, the more familiar he will become with the normal feel and appearance of his testes. In this exercise, you will learn how to instruct a patient to conduct a TSE.

Equipment Needed

- Mirror

Steps

1. Introduce yourself and identify the patient. Explain the provider's instructions and rationale for performing a TSE. Explain that you will be teaching the patient how to perform a TSE. Answer the patient's questions and ensure he is calm and comfortable before proceeding with the instruction. Provide written instructions if necessary.
2. Advise the patient that the TSE should be performed after a warm shower or bath because the scrotal sac will be relaxed, allowing easier palpation of the testes. He should stand in front of a mirror while performing the test.
3. The patient should examine each testis. One testis may be larger than the other. This is a normal finding.
4. Explain that he should hold the testes in between the thumb and fingers, with a thumb on top and an index and middle finger underneath each testis **FIGURE 17.17**.
5. Instruct the patient to gently roll the testes between the thumb and index finger. He should feel for lumps or nodules.
6. Advise the patient to contact his healthcare provider if any abnormal findings are noted on his TSE.
7. Document the procedure in the patient's chart. For example, write "1325: Provided written and verbal instruction for testicular self-examination. Patient acknowledged understanding. J. Jones, CMA."

Instructing a Patient in a Breast Self-Examination

Females should begin monthly self-examinations of the breasts in early adulthood or when they begin

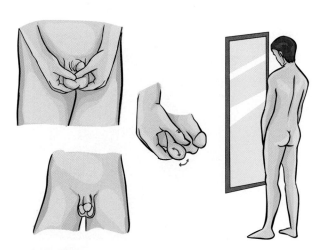

FIGURE 17.17 A man should examine his testes for abnormal lumps or nodules.
© Jones & Bartlett Learning

having annual gynecological examinations. The **breast self-examination (BSE)** is a simple procedure that can lead to early diagnosis and treatment of breast cancer. The more often a woman performs a BSE, the more familiar she will become with the normal size, shape, and feel of her breasts. In this exercise, you will learn how to instruct a patient to conduct a BSE.

Equipment Needed

- Pillow or blanket
- Mirror

Steps

1. Introduce yourself and identify the patient. Explain the provider's instructions and rationale for performing a BSE. Explain that you will be teaching the patient how to perform a BSE. Answer the patient's questions and ensure she is calm and comfortable before proceeding with the instruction. Provide written instructions if necessary.

2. Advise the patient that the BSE should be performed on the same day every month, seven to 10 days after the start of menses.

3. For the first part of the test, the patient should lie down with a pillow or blanket underneath the side of the body of the breast she will examine. She should place the hand on the same side of the body underneath her head. Instruct her to use the tips of the middle, index, and ring fingers of the opposite hand to press the breast tissue toward the chest wall and feel for any lumps or thickening of the breast tissue. Starting at the nipple and working out, she should move her fingers in a circular pattern around the breast. Or, she may prefer to work in a wedge pattern around the breast. Advise her to use the same pattern each month. Repeat the examination on the other side.

4. Instruct the patient to stand in front of a mirror and observe the breasts for asymmetry, deformities, or changes in appearance. Have the patient observe her breasts with her arms raised and with her arms down by her sides.

5. An additional BSE may be conducted while showering. A woman can take time to examine the breasts in the same manner as when lying down. Wet, soapy hands will allow lumps and thick tissue under the skin to be felt more easily **FIGURE 17.18**.

6. Advise the patient to contact her healthcare provider if any abnormal findings are noted on her BSE.

7. Document the procedure in the patient's chart. For example, write "1615: Provided written and verbal instruction for breast self-examination. Patient acknowledged understanding. J. Jones, CMA."

Assisting With a Gynecological Examination

A woman should receive an annual gynecological examination when she becomes sexually active or when she turns 21, whichever is sooner. A gynecological examination is divided into four parts: evaluation of the external genitalia, a pelvic examination that includes a Pap smear, a rectal examination, and a breast examination. The medical assistant will be responsible for preparing the

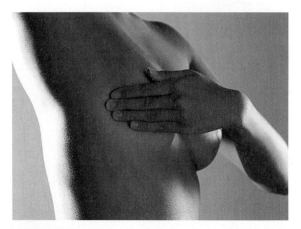

FIGURE 17.18 A woman should compress her breast tissue to feel for lumps.
© LiquidLibrary

patient, assembling the equipment, and organizing the room before the healthcare provider arrives. In this exercise, you will learn how to assist with a gynecological examination using the ThinPrep method for the Pap smear.

Equipment Needed

- Patient gown
- Two pairs of disposable gloves (one for the healthcare provider and one for you)
- ThinPrep bottle
- Vaginal speculum
- Basin of warm water
- Cervical broom
- Light source
- Drape sheet
- Lubricant
- Biohazard waste container

An empty bladder facilitates examination of the uterus.
© auremar/ShutterStock, Inc.

Steps

1. Introduce yourself and identify the patient.
2. Wash your hands and assemble all the necessary equipment.
3. Instruct the patient to empty her bladder. If a urine specimen is requested by the healthcare provider, obtain this now.
4. Provide the patient with a gown and ask her to undress completely.
5. When the patient is undressed, have her sit at the end of the examination table. Drape her lower body to provide privacy. Label the ThinPrep bottle to prepare for the Pap smear.
6. Assist the patient to lay down, with feet in stirrups and knees relaxed. Her thighs should be rotated out as much as is comfortable. Instruct her to breathe slowly and deeply during the examination to relax the muscles of the pelvis and allow for easier examination of the external and internal organs **FIGURE 17.19**.
7. Warm the speculum in water, if necessary. Do not lubricate the speculum. Hand the cervical broom to the healthcare provider as directed. Hold the ThinPrep bottle for the provider as he or she swishes the broom in the solution 10 times. Cap the ThinPrep bottle.
8. If instructed, apply lubricant to the healthcare provider's gloved fingers. Take care not to touch the gloves. The healthcare provider will use two fingers inside the vagina and the other hand on the lower abdomen to palpate the uterus. He or she will also insert one finger into the rectum to assess pelvic and rectal muscle tone.
9. Assist the patient in wiping her genitalia and rectum clean.
10. Help the patient to a sitting position. Assess her for any signs of distress.
11. Discard of used supplies and equipment as directed.
12. Remove the gloves and wash your hands.

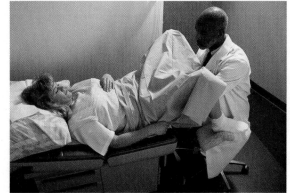

FIGURE 17.19 The woman should relax and breathe deeply during the gynecological examination.
© Photodisc

13. Help the patient down from table and instruct her to dress. Inform her of when the results of the examination and tests will be available.

14. Document the procedure in the patient's chart. For example, write "0830: Assisted with annual gynecological examination. Patient appeared comfortable with no apparent signs of distress. Advised patients of when lab results will be ready. J. Jones, CMA."

Assisting With a Routine Prenatal Visit

Prenatal visits occur throughout a pregnancy, with increasing frequency toward the end of gestation. A mother and fetus should be continually evaluated and monitored for growth and development. In this exercise, you will learn the general principles involved in assisting with a routine prenatal examination. The actual roles and responsibilities of a medical assistant will vary among practice settings, so always follow the instructions of your employer or supervisor.

Equipment Needed

- Patient drape

Steps

1. Introduce yourself and identify the patient. Explain the provider's instructions and rationale for performing a prenatal examination. Answer the patient's questions and ensure she is calm and comfortable before proceeding with the examination.

2. Before the healthcare provider sees the patient, interview the patient to determine whether she has experienced any problems or has any concerns that have developed since the last visit. Obtain a urine specimen from the patient.

3. Obtain a blood sample, if requested by the provider. Refer to Chapter 13 for instruction on collecting blood specimens.

4. Measure the patient's weight and vital signs. Record the results in the patient's chart FIGURE 17.20 .

5. Check the patient's chart to ensure that all reports or lab results ordered since the last prenatal visit are in the chart.

6. Prepare the patient for the provider's examination by asking her to undress from the waist down. Provide her with a drape to cover her lower body. Assist her to lie down on the examination table.

7. You will continue to assist the provider during the examination as directed. You may be asked to record results or make notations in the patient's chart as the provider conducts the examination.

8. After the examination is complete, offer to answer any other questions the patient may have, as you are able. Encourage her to schedule her next prenatal visit.

9. Clean the examination room. Discard all waste in the appropriate containers. Restock or replenish supplies in the examination room as necessary. Prepare the room for the next patient.

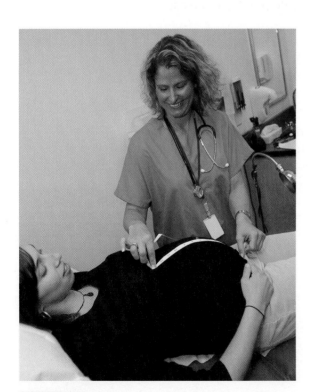

FIGURE 17.20 The medical assistant may be asked to obtain measurements of fetal growth.
© C. Docken/ShutterStock, Inc.

Testing Urine With Reagent Strips

Reagent strips, or dipsticks, can be used to measure many qualities of urine, including pH, protein, glucose, ketones, blood, bilirubin, and specific gravity. In this exercise, you will learn how to perform the chemical and physical assessments of a urinalysis using reagent strips.

Equipment Needed

- Reagent strips
- Fresh urine specimen
- Disposable gloves
- Watch or timepiece
- Tongue depressor

Blood pressure is extremely important to assess at each prenatal visit. High blood pressure in pregnancy is indicative of potentially serious and life-threatening complications.
© auremar/ShutterStock, Inc.

Steps

1. Gather the equipment and supplies. Check the expiration date on the reagent strips and ensure that the strips have not expired.
2. Wash your hands and apply gloves.
3. Stir the urine sample with the tongue depressor. This distributes any solutes evenly in the urine sample.
4. Remove a reagent strip from the bottle, taking care not to touch the testing end of the strip.
5. Dip the strip into the urine sample. Pull the strip across the inside of the opening of the urine collection cup to remove excess urine from the strip. A saturated test strip can produce inaccurate results.
6. Begin timing the test.
7. Hold the reagent strip bottle on its side in your left hand and the test strip in your right hand. Hold the strip so that it is lined up with the color strip on the reagent bottle.
8. Read the results of the test strip, in accordance with the standard timings of the tests **FIGURE 17.21**:

    10 seconds: glucose (qualitative)

    30 seconds: glucose (quantitative)

    30 seconds: bilirubin

    40 seconds: ketone

    45 seconds: specific gravity

    50 seconds: blood

    60 seconds: pH

    60 seconds: protein

    60 seconds: urobilinogen

    60 seconds: nitrite

    2 minutes: leukocytes

9. Discard the used reagent strip, gloves, and other disposable materials. Wash your hands.
10. Record the results in the patient's chart. For example, write "0825: Clean catch urine specimen tested with dipstick; clear yellow urine tested positive for blood. J. Jones, CMA."

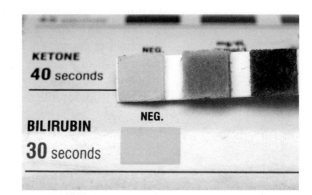

FIGURE 17.21 Compare the urine test strip to the colors on the reagent bottle.
© Keith A Frith/ShutterStock, Inc.

Performing a Urine Pregnancy Screening

The healthcare provider will likely order a urine test in the office to confirm the pregnancy when a patient presents to an obstetrician's office for her first prenatal visit. Pregnancy tests screen for the presence of hCG in the urine. In this exercise, you will learn how to perform a urine pregnancy screening.

Equipment Needed

- Disposable gloves
- Urine specimen
- Quality control materials
- Reagents

Steps

1. Wash your hands and apply gloves.
2. Perform quality-control tests on two reagent cards: one positive and one negative. Record the results of the quality control tests in a log, if applicable. Do not continue with the urine pregnancy screening unless the quality-control tests report accurate results.

Quality-control samples should be tested once a day and when a new box of reagents is opened.
© auremar/ShutterStock, Inc.

3. Prepare the reagent for patient testing and perform the test according to the manufacturer's instructions.
4. Dispose of waste in the appropriate containers.
5. Remove gloves and wash your hands.
6. Record the results of the screening in the patient's chart. For example, write "1545: Pregnancy test positive. J. Jones, CMA."

Performing a Urine Drug Screening

Urine testing may be required to screen for the presence of drugs. This is a common practice for employment and legal issues. The test is simple, but detailed legal documentation must be maintained. The chain of custody must be observed and documented to reduce specimen tampering and preserve the integrity of the sample. The **chain of custody** is the legal documentation of the possession, control, transfer, and analysis of a sample. The chain of custody is extremely important in legal cases of custody, paternity, or drug use. In this exercise, you will learn the criteria for collecting a urine sample for a drug screening.

Equipment Needed

- Consent forms
- Urine collection cup
- Thermometer
- Test strips (optional)

Steps

1. When the individual arrives for the urine test, ask for his or her photo identification. Copy the identification and sign the copy.
2. Ask the patient to complete a consent form.
3. Instruct the patient to leave all coats, bags, and other personal items with the office personnel. Secure these items.
4. Inspect the bathroom and the patient to ensure that no chemicals or urine samples that do not belong to the patient are present.
5. Provide the individual with a urine collection cup and instruct him or her to provide a urine sample. In some cases, the urine collection must be monitored. Refer to the policies of your employer and the requirements for the urine test.
6. After the individual provides the urine sample, record the temperature of the urine. Some collection containers have thermometers built in to the cup. You may also use a thermometer.
7. Seal the sample and secure it for transport to another laboratory facility, if applicable.
8. If immediate testing is required, a test strip for a variety of substances can be dipped into the urine and observed for positive, negative, or inconclusive results. Inconclusive results will require further testing.

Math Practice

Question: **A 25-year-old man is prescribed penicillin for syphilis that he acquired more than one year ago. He is prescribed 2.4 million units in two injection sites once weekly for three weeks. How many units will he receive in each injection site? If the suspension for injection is supplied in a 4mL vial with a concentration of 600,000 units/mL, what is the total volume of penicillin he will receive in each injection site?**

Answer: Step 1: Divide the total number of units by the number of injection sites: 2.4 million units ÷ 2 injection sites = 1.2 million units per injection site

Step 2: Multiply the number of units ordered by the number of units in one milliliter. To do this, first convert the number of units to a fraction: 1.2 million units = $\frac{1.2 \text{ million units}}{1}$

Therefore, 1.2 million units $\times \frac{1mL}{600,000 \text{ units}} = \frac{1.2 \text{ million units}}{1} \times \frac{1mL}{600,000 \text{ units}}$

Now, multiply the numerators: 1.2 million units × 1mL = 1.2 million units × mL

Then, multiply the denominators: 1 × 600,000 units = 600,000 units

The result is 1.2 million units $\times \frac{mL}{600,000 \text{ units}}$

Cancel the units and divide the fraction: [1.2 million units × mL ÷ 600,000 units] = 2mL

Question: **A 32-year-old female is prescribed ciprofloxacin for a UTI. Her healthcare provider orders 250mg every 12 hours for three days. What is the total dose of ciprofloxacin she will receive in her course of treatment?**

Answer: Step 1: Multiply the number of milligrams per dose by the number of doses in one day. To do this, first convert the dose to a fraction: 250mg = $\frac{250mg}{1}$. Then, convert the dose frequency to a fraction: $\frac{1 \text{ dose}}{12 \text{ hours}}$

Remember that there are 24 hours in one day: $\frac{24 \text{ hours}}{1 \text{ day}}$. Therefore, 250mg every 12 hours equals $\frac{250mg}{1} \times \frac{1 \text{ dose}}{12 \text{ hours}} \times \frac{24 \text{ hours}}{1 \text{ day}}$

Now, multiply the numerators: 250mg × 1 dose × 24 hours = 6,000mg × dose × hours

Then, multiply the denominators: 1 × 12 hours × 1 day = 12 hours × day

The result is $\frac{6,000mg \times dose \times hours}{12\ hours \times day}$

Step 2: Cancel the units and divide the fraction: 6,000mg × dose × $\frac{hours}{12\ hours}$ × day = 500mg/day

Step 3: Multiply the daily dose by the total number of days of therapy: 500mg/day × 3 days = 1,500mg

---

Question: **A 54-year-old woman is prescribed carboplatin for ovarian cancer. Her body-surface area is 1.6m² and she weighs 125 pounds. Her oncologist orders 360mg/m² every four weeks. What dose of carboplatin will she receive with each round of treatment?**

Answer: Step 1: Multiply the dose ordered by the body-surface area. To do this, first convert the body-surface area to a fraction: 1.6 = $\frac{1.6}{1}$

Therefore, 1.6m² × $\frac{360mg}{m^2}$ = $\frac{1.6m^2}{1}$ × $\frac{360mg}{m^2}$

Now, multiply the two numerators: 1.6 m² × 360mg = 576 m² × mg

Then, multiply the denominators: 1 × 1m² = 1m²

The result is 576 m² × $\frac{mg}{1m^2}$

Step 2: Cancel the units and divide the fraction: 576 m² × $\frac{mg}{1\ m^2}$ = 576mg

WRAP UP

Chapter Summary

- The urinary system, also referred to as the genitourinary system, filters blood and removes waste products from the body through urine. The reproductive system is required to produce offspring. Both systems work closely together and are integrated with other body systems.

- The main organ of the urinary system is the kidney. Each kidney contains millions of nephrons, which are the basic functional unit of the kidney. The nephron is the site of filtration of the blood and reabsorption of water and electrolytes.

- Each kidney has a ureter, which drains urine formed in the kidney to the urinary bladder. The bladder is a muscular sac that stores urine. The urethra drains urine from the bladder to the outside of the body.

- A UTI is the most common disorder affecting the urinary system. A UTI is an infection in any part of the urinary system. UTIs are effectively treated with antibiotics.

- Glomerulonephritis is the inability of the glomerulus to function normally. Glomerulonephritis may be acute or chronic, and treatment of glomerulonephritis is symptomatic, primarily to prevent high blood pressure, edema, and electrolyte imbalances.

- Incontinence is the involuntary or uncontrollable loss of urine from the bladder. The incidence of incontinence increases with age, but any factor that affects the structure or function of the bladder can cause incontinence. Behavioral changes, lifestyle adjustments, and medications can treat incontinence.

- Nephrolithiasis is the formation of small stones in the kidney or bladder. Pain is the primary symptom associated with nephrolithiasis. Some stones pass out of the body naturally in the urine, but others required surgical removal or mechanical destruction.

- Polycystic kidney disease is an inherited disorder characterized by the formation of fluid-filled cysts in place of normal renal tissue. It is a progressive disease and, eventually, kidney transplant or dialysis will be necessary to sustain life.

- Renal failure is the inability of the kidneys to function normally. Renal failure may be acute or chronic. Acute cases require supportive treatment while chronic cases progress to end-stage renal disease and require dialysis.

- Urinalysis is a test to measure physical and chemical properties of urine. It is an easy test that is useful for discerning underlying causes of disorders of the urinary system.

- Urinary catheterization is a means of inserting a small, flexible tube into the bladder to drain the bladder or instill medication into the bladder. Catheters may be used for short periods or long-term treatment.

- Dialysis is the process of filtering the blood and removing waste products when the kidneys cannot perform this function. It can be accomplished with hemodialysis, in which a machine is used to filter blood, or peritoneal dialysis, in which the patient's own abdomen is used to filter blood.

- The male reproductive system is closely related to the urinary system. It consists of glands and a series of ducts and tubes that produce, nourish, and transport the cells required for reproduction.

- Sperm is produced in the testes. The epididymis stores sperm. The seminal vesicles and the prostate gland produce secretions that provide nourishment for sperm and improve its mobility. Sperm and semen travel to the urethra to be expelled from the body during sexual activity.

- Disorders of the prostate and cancers of the male reproductive system are common reasons for men to seek care. An enlarged prostate can be a sign of a benign condition or prostate cancer. A PSA test can assess prostate function. Testicular cancer is common among young men and self-examinations are effective screening tools.

- The female system contains the organs and cells required for reproduction. The ovaries produce eggs, which are necessary for reproduction. The fallopian tubes transport an egg to the uterus, which will act as a womb during pregnancy. The vagina acts as the birth canal during parturition and receives semen during sexual intercourse. The vulva contains the external genitalia. The mammary glands produce breast milk, which provides nourishment for a newborn.

- The female reproductive system is controlled by a sophisticated and integrated hormone cycle. The menstrual cycle is divided into menstruation, the follicular phase, and the luteal phase. The average menstrual cycle is 28 days.

- Pregnancy, or gestation, is 40 weeks long. During this time, a zygote will grow to an embryo and, finally, a fetus. Prenatal care is important throughout the pregnancy to maintain the health of the mother and child. Preeclampsia is a serious complication of pregnancy.

- Postpartum care is important to maintain the physical and mental health of the mother and child. Obstetricians, as well as family healthcare providers, should screen for signs of postpartum depression.

- Cancers can occur in any part of the female reproductive system. The frequency of most gynecological cancers increases with age and many are believed to be related to hormone exposure. Cervical cancer can be caused by a virus; a vaccine is now available to prevent infection and transmission of the virus.

- Disorders related to the structure and function of the female reproductive system, such as fibroids, cysts, and endometriosis, often produce vague and overlapping signs and symptoms, making diagnosis difficult. Emotional and behavioral symptoms are also a component of premenstrual syndrome.

- Sexually transmitted diseases (STDs) are caused by pathogens spread through sexual contact. Chlamydia, gonorrhea, herpes, and syphilis are the most common STDs in the United States. The incidence of most STDs is higher among men, but complications occur more frequently among women. STDs during pregnancy can cause significant, sometimes fatal, consequences to the fetus. Abstinence and a mutually monogamous relationship with a noninfected partner are the only means of complete protection against STDs.

- As a medical assistant, you will have the opportunity to participate in procedures related to the urinary and reproductive system, including routine examinations, prenatal care, screening tests, and patient instruction in self-examinations. The urinary and reproductive systems are intimate and private areas of the human body and care should be taken to maintain the comfort, modesty, and respect of the patient at all times.

Learning Assessment Questions

1. What is the main functional unit of the kidney?
   A. Nephron
   B. Glomerulus
   C. Renal cortex
   D. Bowman's capsule

2. Where does glomerular filtration take place?
   A. Hilum
   B. Renal tubule
   C. Renal corpuscle
   D. Urinary meatus

3. What is the most common cause of a UTI?
   A. *N. gonorrhoeae*
   B. *E. coli*
   C. *T. pallidum*
   D. *C. trachomatis*

4. What is the specific gravity of distilled water?
   A. 1.000
   B. 1.030
   C. 5.0
   D. 95 percent

5. Which of the following substances is *not* normally present in healthy urine?

   A. Uric acid

   B. Sodium

   C. Chloride

   D. Bilirubin

6. What is a potentially fatal complication of peritoneal dialysis?

   A. End-stage renal disease

   B. Diabetes mellitus

   C. Peritonitis

   D. Cystitis

7. What are the two functions of the testes?

   A. Store sperm and produce progesterone

   B. Produce sperm and produce testosterone

   C. Store urine and produce seminal fluid

   D. Control body temperature and facilitate urination

8. How many chromosomes are present in one zygote?

   A. 2

   B. 23

   C. 46

   D. 92

9. What is the function of the urethra in females?

   A. To transport urine from the kidney to the bladder

   B. To remove urine from the body

   C. To act as the birth canal

   D. To allow the ovum to travel to the uterus

10. Which of the following men are at increased risk for BPH?

    A. Men aged 20–35 years

    B. Vegetarians

    C. Men with folic acid deficiency

    D. Men who consume a high-fat diet

11. Which hormone expels breast milk from the breast?

    A. Oxytocin

    B. Prolactin

    C. Estrogen

    D. Luteinizing hormone

12. What are the stages of the menstrual cycle?

    A. Filtration, reabsorption, secretion

    B. First trimester, second trimester, third trimester

    C. Primary stage, secondary stage, latent stage

    D. Menstruation, follicular phase, luteal phase

13. A urine pregnancy test assesses the presence of what hormone?

    A. Progesterone

    B. Human chorionic gonadotropin

    C. Luteinizing hormone

    D. Estrogen

14. How is the estimated date of confinement calculated?

    A. From the date of the mother's first prenatal visit

    B. From the age of menarche

    C. From the date of the mother's last menstrual period

    D. By measuring blood pressure

15. Which of the following is *not* used for an ultrasound during pregnancy?

    A. To analyze chromosomal defects

    B. To assess the gestational age

    C. To determine the number of fetuses

    D. To observe fetal abnormalities

16. Which of the following identifies the early symptoms of ovarian cancer?

    A. Vaginal bleeding, pain after intercourse, and a persistent vaginal discharge

    B. Abdominal discomfort and gastrointestinal disturbances

    C. Difficulty urinating, urinary retention, and frequent urination

    D. Acute right lower quadrant pain, blood in the urine

17. Kegel exercises can treat symptoms of which condition?

    A. Endometriosis

    B. Renal calculi

    C. Incontinence

    D. Fibroids

18. Which of the following individuals is *not* at elevated risk for contracting an STD?

    A. A homosexual man

    B. A woman in a mutually monogamous relationship

    C. A teenaged male with multiple sexual partners

    D. A 21-year-old female with an infected partner

19. Which of the following is *not* a routine part of an annual gynecological examination?

    A. Breast examination

    B. Rectal examination

    C. Pap smear

    D. Colposcopy

20. For which of the following tests would the chain of custody be particularly important?

    A. A pregnancy urine test

    B. A thyroid function blood test

    C. A DNA test to determine paternity

    D. A breast biopsy

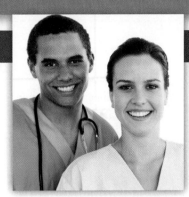

18

Medical Insurance and Coding

OBJECTIVES

After reading this chapter, you will be able to:

* Explain the basics of health insurance in the United States.
* Understand the process of procedure and diagnosis coding.
* Recognize common errors in completing insurance claim forms.
* Explain the difference between the CMS-1500 and the UB-04 forms.
* Discuss legal and ethical issues related to coding and insurance claims processing.

KEY TERMS

Advance beneficiary notice (ABN)
Annual premium
Bundling
Children's Health Insurance Program (CHIP)
The Civilian Health and Medical Program of the Department of Veterans Affairs (CHAMPVA)
CMS-1500
Coding

Co-insurance
Consumer-driven health plan (CDHP)
Coordination of benefits
Co-pay
Current Procedural Terminology (CPT)
Deductible
Diagnosis-related group (DRG)
Downcoding
Encounter form
Flexible spending account (FSA)

Healthcare common procedure coding system (HCPCS)
Health insurance
Health maintenance organization (HMO)
Health savings account (HSA)
International classification of diseases (ICD)
Managed care
Medicaid

Medicare	Preferred provider	Reimbursement
Network	organization	TRICARE
Patient Protection and	(PPO)	UB-04
Affordable Care Act	Primary care provider	Unbundling
(PPACA)	(PCP)	Upcoding

Chapter Overview

Medical care is undeniably expensive. Payment is required for hospitalizations, physician visits, diagnostic procedures, treatments, and prescription medications. Payment is received by providers through several mechanisms, including private health-insurance programs, consumer-driven health plans, and government health coverage plans. Each program requires extensive documentation and procedural and diagnostic coding to ensure adequate coverage of fees and to expedite **reimbursement** (monetary compensation for medical care provided).

As a medical assistant, you will likely participate in reviewing health-insurance coverage for patients and processing claim forms. An understanding of the rules and regulations surrounding coding, billing, and payments will facilitate the timely provision of care and receipt of fees.

Terminology

TABLE 18.1 lists terms used in medical insurance and coding.

Table 18.1   Terms Used in Medical Insurance and Coding

Term	Meaning
Annual premium	The amount an individual pays to purchase health-insurance coverage each year
Coding	The process of assigning alphanumeric designations to diagnoses, procedures, and services
Co-insurance	A percentage of the total cost of care that an individual must contribute
Co-pay	A fixed fee that is received from the patient each time care is provided
Deductible	The amount an individual must pay before the insurance provider will begin paying for services
Network	The group of providers who are contracted by a managed care organization to provide care at negotiated rates
Reimbursement	The monetary compensation for care provided

Abbreviations Related to Medical Insurance and Coding

The following are abbreviations related to the medical insurance and coding:

- ABN—Advance beneficiary notice
- CPT—Current Procedural Terminology
- DRG—Diagnosis-related group
- ECT—Electronic claims tracking
- FSA—Flexible spending account
- HCPCS—Healthcare common procedure coding system
- HMO—Health maintenance organization
- HSA—Health savings account
- ICD—International classification of diseases
- NPI—National provider identifier
- PBM—Pharmacy benefit manager
- PCP—Primary care provider
- PPO—Preferred provider organization
- YTD—Year-to-date

Health Insurance

Health insurance protects people from the high costs associated with medical care. It is a system in which individuals prepay for medical coverage so they do not have to pay the entire cost of the care received at the time of service. Originally, health insurance was designed to protect individuals from payment associated with catastrophic illness or injury. Today, health insurance has evolved into a program that encourages preventive and routine care.

Most people in the United States who have private health insurance receive this coverage from their employers. People are often able to choose the plan that suits their needs the best. Now, people can participate in consumer-directed plans that provide increased autonomy and control in the care they receive.

Other people receive medical coverage from government plans. Special programs are conducted by federal and state governments that provide healthcare services for the elderly, the indigent, children, veterans, and those receiving dialysis.

Still other people choose to receive healthcare services on a fee-for-service basis. That is, they pay for care received at the time of service. This type of self-pay system requires individuals to pay sometimes high out-of-pocket costs, but they have increased flexibility and choice in providers and treatment plans compared with those who have insurance coverage.

The **Patient Protection and Affordable Care Act (PPACA)** of 2010 will reform health insurance and the provision of health care. The goal of the PPACA is to expand coverage and improve access to health care for more Americans and make insurance companies more accountable for their coverage decisions. The debate continues regarding how the PPACA will affect individuals and, specifically, private insurance providers and the

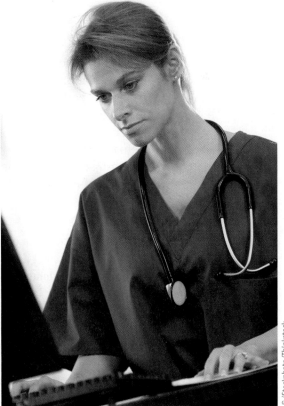

Medical assistants often assist in processing health insurance claims.

long-term ramifications of the plan are still unknown. Most changes will begin in 2014. The following discussion presents the state of the healthcare insurance industry as of 2012.

Managed Care

Managed care is a system in which an organization contracts with providers to provide comprehensive healthcare services to its subscribers or enrollees at a reduced cost. The providers who are contracted to provide services are termed the **network**. The primary goal of managed care is to reduce costs, due to the large volume of patients enrolled in the program. Also, managed care focuses on preventive services and helps patients obtain routine care and screening assessments. By identifying risk factors and diagnosing conditions early, quality of life is increased and treatment outcomes are improved. Most employers in the United States offer some type of managed care plan to their employees.

Commercial Insurance Programs

Commercial insurance programs are privately owned and managed health-insurance providers. These plans vary in their benefits and costs, but most include limits on annual benefits and require patients to pay an annual premium, a deductible, a co-pay, or co-insurance. An **annual premium** is the amount an individual pays to purchase the insurance coverage each year. A **deductible** is the amount that an individual must pay on his or her own before the insurance provider will begin paying for services. A **co-pay**, or co-payment, is the amount that an individual must pay toward each service provided. A co-pay is a fixed fee that is paid up front each time a service is provided. For example, an individual might have a $25 co-pay for each routine physician visit. **Co-insurance** is a percentage of the total cost that an individual must contribute toward each service. For example, an individual might be required to pay for 20% of services provided and the insurance provider will pay the remaining 80%.

In general, the higher the annual premium, the lower the out-of-pocket costs throughout the year. Individuals can choose the plan that serves their needs by evaluating the affordability, their average healthcare use, and their projected healthcare needs. Several types of commercial insurance plans are available, including health maintenance organizations (HMOs) and preferred provider organizations (PPOs), and many providers facilitate consumer-directed plans. UnitedHealth, WellPoint, Aetna, Blue Cross Blue Shield, CIGNA, and Kaiser are among the largest private health-insurance providers in the United States, providing coverage for hundreds of millions of Americans.

Health Maintenance Organizations

A **health maintenance organization (HMO)** is a commercial insurance plan that requires individuals to select a **primary care provider (PCP)**—often a general practitioner, family practice physician, or internist who acts as a "gatekeeper" for all of the individual's medical care. The PCP must be part of the program's network. The PCP is responsible for providing referrals to specialists to obtain additional medical care.

HMOs tend to have lower costs for subscribers than other types of commercial insurance coverage, but they provide less flexibility and choice than other plans. HMOs do encourage comprehensive and preventive health care by providing coverage for annual physicals and screening assessments.

HMOs may be staff-model or group-model. Staff-model HMOs are organizations in which all the providers in the network are employees of the HMO. All services, such as laboratory tests, physical therapy, or screenings, are provided by the practice. Group-model HMOs, on the other hand, contract with providers who are not employees of the HMO, but rather receive reimbursement from the HMO after services are rendered to a patient. The providers may be reimbursed based on capitation, which is a set monthly fee per patient, regardless of how many times the patient is seen, or a fee-for-service structure in which the providers are reimbursed based on actual services provided.

Preferred Provider Organizations

A **preferred provider organization (PPO)** is another type of commercial insurance plan that contracts with a network of providers to provide services to patients. PPOs do not require an individual to select a PCP or to obtain referrals before seeing a specialist. PPOs offer patients more freedom in choosing providers, but costs tend to be higher than those associated with HMOs.

Consumer-Driven Health Plans

A **consumer-driven health plan (CDHP)** enables consumers to make more choices regarding how their healthcare dollars are spent. CDHPs were created in 2003 with the establishment of the health savings account (HSA). A **health savings account (HSA)** is a savings account that can be used to pay for medical expenses. The funds deposited in the HSA are not subject to income tax until the time of withdrawal.

> *HSAs and FSAs can be used to pay for services not covered by the health-insurance provider. Examples include ambulance services, orthodontia, equipment to assist a hearing or visually impaired person, or home improvements to assist a person with disabilities.*
>
> © auremar/ShutterStock, Inc.

Any amount not used in the HSA stays in the account and accrues interest year after year. An HSA must be used in conjunction with a qualified high-deductible healthcare plan. Contributions to an HSA can be made by an individual or an employer. As of 2012, the maximum annual contribution toward an HSA is $3,100 for an individual and $6,250 for a family.

A **flexible spending account (FSA)** is another means of paying for medical expenses. The account is funded with pretax dollars by an employee. Unlike an HSA, funds in as FSA do not roll over to the next year. If money in the account is not spent by the end of the year, the funds are lost. An FSA is considered a use-it-or-lose-it plan.

Government Health Plans

Federal and state government programs are available to provide medical care to patients who do not have private health-insurance coverage. Plans are available for children, veterans, the elderly, and low-income individuals.

Medicare

Medicare is a federal program that provides health insurance for individuals older than 65 years of age. Medicare also provides health care for people diagnosed with ESRD who are receiving dialysis, people who are disabled, and people receiving Social Security benefits. Medicare is divided into four distinct programs:

- Medicare part A provides coverage for hospitalization expenses. Medicare part A requires an annual deductible, which increases every year.
- Medicare part B pays for medical expenses such as office visits, laboratory tests, and diagnostic services. A patient must see a provider who accepts Medicare insurance in order to receive treatment from that provider. The patient must pay an annual premium and shares some of the cost associated with the care.
- Medicare part C is also known as Medicare Advantage. This coverage allows patients to select a private health-insurance provider as their primary coverage.

Medicare Advantage plans usually provide additional services compared with traditional Medicare plans.

■ Medicare part D provides prescription drug coverage. It is provided through Medicare itself or through a specific Medicare Advantage plan. All Medicare plans require some level of cost-sharing, whether it is an annual premium, co-pays, or deductibles. The out-of-pocket costs vary among specific plans.

All providers who accept Medicare for services rendered are required to complete and submit claims for patients. All claims must be completed on a **CMS-1500** claim form `FIGURE 18.1`. This is a standardized health-insurance claim form that applies to universal medical services. As of 2005, all Medicare claims are required to be submitted electronically. Businesses with fewer than 10 full-time employees are exempt from this requirement and may still submit claims on paper forms.

Medicare will only pay for medically necessary services and procedures. No coverage is provided for cosmetic surgery or experimental or investigational services. Limited preventive services and screenings are available from Medicare. If a service is not covered by Medicare, a patient must be informed in advance and he or she must sign an **advance beneficiary notice (ABN)** of noncoverage `FIGURE 18.2`. The ABN must list the cost of the services and the fee for which the patient will be responsible.

Medicaid

Medicaid is a state-administered program that provides health-insurance coverage for low-income individuals, uninsured pregnant women, and individuals with disabilities. Medicaid also provides coverage for children in low-income families through the **Children's Health Insurance Program (CHIP)**.

The eligibility requirements for Medicaid vary from state to state. Eligible individuals may receive coverage with no out-of-pocket costs, or they may pay co-pays based on income. Patients must receive care from a Medicaid provider to receive subsidized care. Some people qualify for both Medicare and Medicaid. They are termed *dual eligible*.

TRICARE and CHAMPVA

The Department of Defense coordinates the Civilian Health and Medical Program of the Uniformed Services (CHAMPUS) **TRICARE** program to provide health-insurance coverage for active and retired military personnel and their dependents (spouses and children). **The Civilian Health and Medical Program of the Department of Veterans Affairs (CHAMPVA)** provides coverage for the dependents of military personnel who have permanent service-related disabilities.

Government Health Coverage

For more information on government health-insurance coverage programs, visit these Web sites:

■ Centers for Medicare and Medicaid Services—www.cms.gov

■ Medicare—www.medicare.gov

■ Medicaid—www.medicaid.gov

■ TRICARE—www.tricare.osd.gov

Uninsured Individuals

Nearly 50 million Americans do not have health-insurance coverage. They are termed *uninsured*. When these patients are seen in a provider's office, they are expected to pay for services provided at the time services are received. Systems for collecting payments

1500

HEALTH INSURANCE CLAIM FORM

APPROVED BY NATIONAL UNIFORM CLAIM COMMITTEE 08/05

PICA | PICA

CARRIER

1. MEDICARE (Medicare #) | MEDICAID (Medicaid #) | TRICARE CHAMPUS (Sponsor's SSN) | CHAMPVA (Member ID#) | GROUP HEALTH PLAN (SSN or ID) | FECA BLK LUNG (SSN) | OTHER (ID)

1a. INSURED'S I.D. NUMBER (For Program in Item 1)

2. PATIENT'S NAME (Last Name, First Name, Middle Initial)

3. PATIENT'S BIRTH DATE MM | DD | YY SEX M F

4. INSURED'S NAME (Last Name, First Name, Middle Initial)

5. PATIENT'S ADDRESS (No., Street)

6. PATIENT RELATIONSHIP TO INSURED Self Spouse Child Other

7. INSURED'S ADDRESS (No., Street)

CITY STATE

8. PATIENT STATUS Single Married Other

CITY STATE

ZIP CODE TELEPHONE (Include Area Code) ( )

Employed Full-Time Student Part-Time Student

ZIP CODE TELEPHONE (Include Area Code) ( )

9. OTHER INSURED'S NAME (Last Name, First Name, Middle Initial)

10. IS PATIENT'S CONDITION RELATED TO:

11. INSURED'S POLICY GROUP OR FECA NUMBER

a. OTHER INSURED'S POLICY OR GROUP NUMBER

a. EMPLOYMENT? (Current or Previous) YES NO

a. INSURED'S DATE OF BIRTH MM | DD | YY SEX M F

b. OTHER INSURED'S DATE OF BIRTH MM | DD | YY SEX M F

b. AUTO ACCIDENT? PLACE (State) YES NO

b. EMPLOYER'S NAME OR SCHOOL NAME

c. EMPLOYER'S NAME OR SCHOOL NAME

c. OTHER ACCIDENT? YES NO

c. INSURANCE PLAN NAME OR PROGRAM NAME

d. INSURANCE PLAN NAME OR PROGRAM NAME

10d. RESERVED FOR LOCAL USE

d. IS THERE ANOTHER HEALTH BENEFIT PLAN? YES NO *If yes*, return to and complete item 9 a-d.

READ BACK OF FORM BEFORE COMPLETING & SIGNING THIS FORM.

12. PATIENT'S OR AUTHORIZED PERSON'S SIGNATURE I authorize the release of any medical or other information necessary to process this claim. I also request payment of government benefits either to myself or to the party who accepts assignment below.

SIGNED ____ DATE ____

13. INSURED'S OR AUTHORIZED PERSON'S SIGNATURE I authorize payment of medical benefits to the undersigned physician or supplier for services described below.

SIGNED ____

PATIENT AND INSURED INFORMATION

14. DATE OF CURRENT: MM | DD | YY ILLNESS (First symptom) OR INJURY (Accident) OR PREGNANCY(LMP)

15. IF PATIENT HAS HAD SAME OR SIMILAR ILLNESS. GIVE FIRST DATE MM | DD | YY

16. DATES PATIENT UNABLE TO WORK IN CURRENT OCCUPATION MM | DD | YY FROM MM | DD | YY TO

17. NAME OF REFERRING PROVIDER OR OTHER SOURCE

17a.

17b. NPI

18. HOSPITALIZATION DATES RELATED TO CURRENT SERVICES MM | DD | YY FROM MM | DD | YY TO

19. RESERVED FOR LOCAL USE

20. OUTSIDE LAB? YES NO $ CHARGES

21. DIAGNOSIS OR NATURE OF ILLNESS OR INJURY (Relate Items 1, 2, 3 or 4 to Item 24E by Line)

1. ___ . ___ 3. ___ . ___

2. ___ . ___ 4. ___ . ___

22. MEDICAID RESUBMISSION CODE ORIGINAL REF. NO.

23. PRIOR AUTHORIZATION NUMBER

24. A. DATE(S) OF SERVICE From MM DD YY	To MM DD YY	B. PLACE OF SERVICE	C. EMG	D. PROCEDURES, SERVICES, OR SUPPLIES (Explain Unusual Circumstances) CPT/HCPCS MODIFIER	E. DIAGNOSIS POINTER	F. $ CHARGES	G. DAYS OR UNITS	H. EPSDT Family Plan	I. ID. QUAL.	J. RENDERING PROVIDER ID. #
1									NPI	
2									NPI	
3									NPI	
4									NPI	
5									NPI	
6									NPI	

PHYSICIAN OR SUPPLIER INFORMATION

25. FEDERAL TAX I.D. NUMBER SSN EIN

26. PATIENT'S ACCOUNT NO.

27. ACCEPT ASSIGNMENT? (For govt. claims, see back) YES NO

28. TOTAL CHARGE $

29. AMOUNT PAID $

30. BALANCE DUE $

31. SIGNATURE OF PHYSICIAN OR SUPPLIER INCLUDING DEGREES OR CREDENTIALS (I certify that the statements on the reverse apply to this bill and are made a part thereof.)

SIGNED DATE

32. SERVICE FACILITY LOCATION INFORMATION

a. NPI b.

33. BILLING PROVIDER INFO & PH # ( )

a. NPI b.

NUCC Instruction Manual available at: www.nucc.org

APPROVED OMB-0938-0999 FORM CMS-1500 (08/05)

FIGURE 18.1 Form CMS-1500.

Courtesy of the Centers for Medicare & Medicaid Services

Patient's Name: _____   Medicare # (HICN): _____

ADVANCE BENEFICIARY NOTICE (ABN)

NOTE: You need to make a choice about receiving these laboratory tests.

We expect that Medicare will not pay for the laboratory test(s) that are described below. Medicare does not pay for all of your health care costs. Medicare only pays for covered items and services when Medicare rules are met. The fact that Medicare may not pay for a particular item or service does not mean that you should not receive it. There may be a good reason your doctor recommended it. Right now, in your case, **Medicare probably will not pay for the laboratory test(s) indicated below for the following reasons:**

Medicare does not pay for these tests for your condition	Medicare does not pay for these tests as often as this (denied as too frequent)	Medicare does not pay for experimental or research use tests

The purpose of this form is to help you make an informed choice about whether or not you want to receive these laboratory tests, knowing that you might have to pay for them yourself. Before you make a decision about your options, you should **read this entire notice carefully.**
- Ask us to explain, if you don't understand why Medicare probably won't pay.
- Ask us how much these laboratory tests will cost you (**Estimated Cost: $_____**), in case you have to pay for them yourself or through other insurance.

PLEASE CHOOSE **ONE** OPTION. CHECK **ONE** BOX. **SIGN & DATE** YOUR CHOICE.

☐ **Option 1. YES.   I want to receive these laboratory tests.**
I understand that Medicare will not decide whether to pay unless I receive these laboratory tests. Please submit my claim to Medicare. I understand that you may bill me for laboratory tests and that I may have to pay the bill while Medicare is making its decision. If Medicare does pay, you will refund to me any payments I made to you that are due to me. If Medicare denies payment, I agree to be personally and fully responsible for payment. That is, I will pay personally, either out of pocket or through any other insurance that I have. I understand I can appeal Medicare's decision.

☐ **Option 2. NO.   I have decided not to receive these laboratory tests.**
I will not receive these laboratory tests. I understand that you will not be able to submit a claim to Medicare and that I will not be able to appeal your opinion that Medicare won't pay. I will notify my doctor who ordered these laboratory tests that I did not receive them.

_____   _____
Date   **Signature of patient or person acting on patient's behalf**

NOTE: Your health information will be kept confidential. Any information that we collect about you on this form will be kept confidential in our offices. If a claim is submitted to Medicare, your health information on this form may be shared with Medicare. Your health information which Medicare sees will be kept confidential by Medicare.

OMB Approval No. 0938-0566   Form No. CMS-R-131-L   (June 2002)

FIGURE 18.2 Advance beneficiary notice.
Courtesy of the Centers for Medicare & Medicaid Services

from self-paying patients vary among practice settings, but systems to reduce delays in reimbursement are often implemented to ensure collection of fees.

Secondary Insurance Coverage

Patients may have more than one insurance provider. For instance, each spouse may have a separate plan to cover the family's medical needs. Most insurance plans include a coordination of benefits clause to prevent duplicate payment for services. Each patient must select a primary provider, to be billed first, and a secondary provider, to provide payment after the primary insurer has provided coverage. **Coordination of benefits** is the method for determining which insurance carrier pays what portion of the medical-care costs. The total amount of benefits received by an individual cannot be more than 100% of the medical costs.

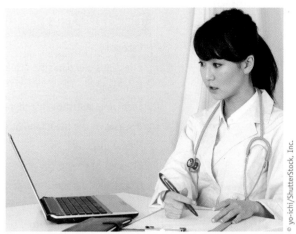

In an office setting, diagnostic and procedural codes are documented on a patient's encounter form.

© yo-ichi/ShutterStock, Inc.

Diagnostic and Procedural Codes

To ensure accurate reimbursement from insurance providers, proper coding is essential. **Coding** is the process of assigning alphanumeric designations to diagnoses, procedures, and services. If incorrect or incomplete codes are provided on claim forms, insurance coverage could be delayed or denied. The system of codes is complex and time consuming to learn, but it becomes manageable with practice. In an office setting, codes will be documented on a patient's **encounter form**, which usually contains the most common diagnoses and procedures used in that practice. A sample patient encounter form is shown later in the chapter.

International Classification of Diseases

More than a century ago, healthcare providers and their representative professional organizations recognized the need for a universal system of classification and record-keeping. By 1938, such a system had evolved into the **International Classification of Diseases (ICD)**. The ICD codes became a means of classifying deaths, statistically assessing diseases, categorizing illnesses, and retrieving records.

ICD codes have been revised and expanded many times since their inception. In 1978, the World Health Organization published the ninth version of the codes (ICD-9). The United States still uses the clinical modification of the ICD-9 codes (ICD-9-CM) to report all medical care and services on claim forms for Medicare, Medicaid, and private health-insurance providers. Further, ICD codes are used to assign a **diagnosis-related group (DRG)** to each service provided at a hospital. Medicare uses DRGs to determine the amount of reimbursement provided for related procedures.

ICD-9 codes, presented in **TABLE 18.2**, describe the disease and condition of a patient. These codes establish the medical necessity for services that will be provided. Other codes are used to specify what care was provided to a patient. The diagnosis must justify the service or procedures performed.

ICD-9 codes are available in a three-volume manual. Volume I contains 17 chapters that list conditions by body system and by cause. Volume II is an alphabetic list of diseases and injuries (section 1), drugs and chemicals (section 2), and external causes of injuries and poisons (section 3). Volume III is a list of procedure codes used by hospitals.

Table 18.2 ICD-9-CM Categories and Codes	
Category	**ICD-9-CM Codes**
Infectious and parasitic diseases	001–139
Neoplasms	140–239
Endocrine, nutritional, and metabolic diseases, and immunity disorders	240–279
Diseases of the blood and blood-forming organs	280–289
Mental disorders	290–319
Diseases of the nervous system	320–359
Diseases of the sensory organs	360–389
Diseases of the circulatory system	390–459
Diseases of the respiratory system	460–519
Diseases of the digestive system	520–579
Diseases of the genitourinary system	580–629
Complications of pregnancy, childbirth, and the puerperium	630–679
Diseases of the skin and subcutaneous tissue	680–709
Diseases of the musculoskeletal system and connective tissue	710–739
Congenital anomalies	740–759
Conditions originating in the perinatal period	760–779
Symptoms, signs, and ill-defined conditions	780–799
Injury and poisoning	800–999

Several general principles apply to the use of ICD codes:

- Code correctly and completely.
- Apply the minimum number of codes that accurately describes the patient's condition or care.
- Code each problem to the highest level of specificity.
- Code the primary reason for the visit first and list all other issues in decreasing order of importance.

The 10th revision of the ICD codes (ICD-10) is scheduled for adoption in the United States on October 1, 2014. Most of the rest of the world implemented the use of ICD-10 codes in the 1990s. The upgraded ICD-10 codes allow for increased capacity that reflects changes in technology and the need for more specific data collection. It includes more than 68,000 alphanumeric codes, compared with 13,000 numeric codes in the ICD-9. ICD-10 codes, presented in **TABLE 18.3**, will likely help reduce errors associated with coding and accommodate future expansion of the codes.

Healthcare Common Procedure Coding System

The **healthcare common procedure coding system (HCPCS)** is a set of codes that identifies healthcare procedures. HCPCS is often referred to by its acronym, pronounced "hick picks." It was established in 1978 to standardize the identification of medical services, supplies, and equipment.

Level I HCPCS codes are **Current Procedural Terminology (CPT)** codes and Level II HCPCS codes identify durable medical equipment, prosthetics, orthotics, and supplies not included in Level I. Level I codes are five-digit numeric codes. Level II codes

Table 18.3 ICD-10 Categories and Codes	
Category	**ICD–10 Codes**
Infectious and parasitic diseases	A00–B99
Neoplasms	C00–D48
Diseases of the blood and blood-forming organs and disorders of the immune system	D50–D89
Endocrine, nutritional, and metabolic disorders	E00–E90
Mental and behavioral disorders	F00–F99
Diseases of the nervous system	G00–G99
Diseases of the eye and adnexa	H00–H59
Diseases of the ear and mastoid process	H60–H95
Diseases of the circulatory system	I00–I99
Diseases of the respiratory system	J00–J99
Diseases of the digestive system	K00–K99
Diseases of the skin and subcutaneous tissue	L00–L99
Diseases of the musculoskeletal system and connective tissue	M00–M99
Diseases of the genitourinary system	N00–N99
Complications of pregnancy, childbirth, and the puerperium	O00–O99
Conditions originating in the perinatal period	P00–P96
Congenital anomalies	Q00–Q99
Symptoms, signs, and ill-defined conditions	R00–R99
Injury and poisoning	S00–T98
External causes of morbidity and mortality	V01–Y98
Factors influencing health status and contact with health services	Z00–Z99
Codes for special purposes	U00–U99

are five-digit alphanumeric codes; the first digit is always a letter and the remaining four digits are numbers.

Current Procedural Terminology

CPT codes were first published by the American Medical Association in 1970. As shown in TABLE 18.4, the codes are divided into six sections: evaluation and management, anesthesiology, surgery, radiology, pathology and laboratory, and medicine. A majority of providers use evaluation and management codes, which are subdivided into 17 categories, to report most of their services.

Table 18.4 CPT Categories and Codes	
Category	**CPT Codes**
Evaluation and management	99201–99499
Anesthesiology	00100–019999, 99100–99140
Surgery	10021–69990
Radiology	700010–79999
Pathology and laboratory	80047–89398
Medicine	90281–9199, 99500–99607

ICD-9 codes describe the disease and condition of the patient. HCPCS and CPT codes identify what was done for the disease or condition.
© auremar/ShutterStock, Inc.

Coding Accuracy

Accurate coding is required, not only to guarantee appropriate reimbursement but to maintain a high standard of ethical conduct as a healthcare professional. Several fraudulent activities are associated with medical coding and billing. In such cases, fines and penalties may be levied against the offending employee and his or her professional future could be placed at risk. Also, insurance providers engage in dishonest practices by changing codes to decrease reimbursement. It is the responsibility of the person submitting the claims and receiving payment to verify that codes have been entered, billed, and reimbursed appropriately.

Reporting multiple codes when only one is appropriate, termed **unbundling**, is a fraudulent practice. Likewise, assigning additional codes that do not match patient documentation, or **upcoding**, is fraudulent. Insurance providers sometimes engage in **bundling**, in which they only pay for certain claim codes and ignore others. Or, they engage in **downcoding** and pay for a lower level of care than what was actually provided.

Under the False Claims Act of 1986, a person charged with fraud can be fined between $5,500 and $11,000 per claim.
© auremar/ShutterStock, Inc.

Claim Forms

Claim forms must be submitted to insurance providers for providers to receive reimbursement. Today, most claims are submitted electronically. Form CMS-1500 is the standard medical insurance claim form submitted by most office practices and is accepted by Medicare, Medicaid, and other insurance providers. Form CMS-1450, also called **UB-04**, is the claim for use by a facility, such as a hospital or clinic, to claim reimbursement for services provided.

Errors

When errors are detected on a claim form, the claim for reimbursement is rejected and coverage is delayed or denied until the error is corrected. (Remember, it is imperative to complete forms correctly the first time.) Several common errors lead to delayed payment. First, the patient may be identified incorrectly. The patient's identification number (often the Social Security number or the insurance plan ID) might be entered incorrectly. Or, the spelling of his or her name or his or her birth date might be wrong. Second, the information provided might be incomplete. The coordination of benefits section might not be completed or the required reports might not be attached to the submission. Third, the use of incorrect or outdated ICD or CPT codes will cause the claim to be rejected.

Tracking Claims

Each provider will have a system for monitoring the status of submitted claims. Tracking claims, usually by an electronic filing system, will ensure prompt follow-up for any issues that might delay payment. Many claims can be tracked online in real time.

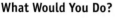

What Would You Do?

You are the newest employee at a family medical practice. During your training, the office manager explains that you may be doing some medical coding and submitting insurance claims. To ensure maximum reimbursement, she advises you to use as many codes as possible that apply to a patient's condition, even if the physician did not document that care was provided. What would you do?

© NorthGeorgiaMedia/ShutterStock, Inc.

If a claim that was submitted electronically has not been processed and paid within three weeks, follow up with the insurance company. Allow six weeks if a claim was submitted on paper.

When payment is received, proper documentation of the date, the amount received, and the check number should be included in the patient's account. Computerized accounting and billing systems facilitate such data collection and ensure accuracy in patient billing.

Skills for the Medical Assistant

As a medical assistant, you will have the opportunity to participate in medical insurance coding and billing. You must maintain accurate and complete records and submit factual claims reflecting the patient's diagnoses, treatments, and procedures.

Using Medical Coding to Reflect Care Provided

When completing and submitting a claim form, you must be able to accurately locate and assign medical codes to reflect the care provided to a patient. You may need to work with the provider to clarify any uncertain terms and guarantee maximum reimbursement. In this section, you will learn how to assign a CPT code based on a patient encounter form **FIGURE 18.3**. The principles are similar for locating assigned ICD or HCPCS codes.

Equipment Needed

- Patient encounter form
- CPT manual or online access to coding resources

Online Coding Resources

CPT and HCPCS codes are available online from several organizations:

- www.icd9data.com
- www.drchrono.com/public_billing_code_search/
- www.icd10data.com
- www.who.int/classifications/icd/icdonlineversions/en/index.html

---

Steps

1. Review the encounter form and clarify any uncertain terms or descriptions.

2. Identify the procedure on the encounter form and determine the main term for the procedure performed.

3. Look up the main term in the alphabetic index of the CPT manual or browse the online coding database. Locate the subterm in the index that applies to the procedure. Turn to the identified code in the manual and read its description. Verify that the description matches the procedure.

4. Indicate the correct CPT code on the encounter form next to the procedure.

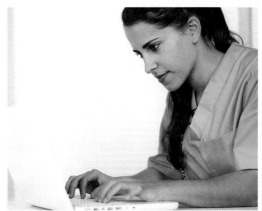

Look up the main term in the CPT manual index or browse the online coding database.

© Pablo Calvog/ShutterStock, Inc.

ENCOUNTER FORM

( ) Johnson ( ) Martinez ( ) Chin
555-38-1234　555-37-1234　555-78-1234

Name: _____

ID: _____

DATE OF SERVICE: _____ ☐ NO SHOW

Please circle (or record) those services provided

OFFICE & OUTPATIENT VISITS:

New Pts.	Established Pts.		
99202			
99203	99212		
99204	99213		
99205	99214		
	99215	Home Visit _____	
		Emer. Room _____	

OFFICE CONSULTATIONS:

New or Established
99241
99242
99243
99244
99245

DIAGNOSIS:

Abdominal	789.0	Muscular/Skeletal Injury	848.8
Acne	706.1	Newborn Care	V30*+
Allergy	995.3	Obesity	278.00
Angina	413.9	Otitis Media	380.10
Anxiety	300.00	Otitis Extrema	380.1
Arthritis	716.9+	Pharyngitis	462
Asthma	493.9+	Pneumonia	486
Back Pain	724.5	Pyrexia (FUO)	780.6
Behavior Disturbance	312.9	Pregnancy	V22.2+
Bronchitis	490	Rash (dermatitis)	782.1
Burns	949.0+	Seizure Disorder	780.39
Chest Pain	786.5	Syncope	780.2
Conjunctivitis	372.30	Sinusitis	473.9
Depression	311	Suture Removal	V58.3
Diabetes	250.0	Trauma	959.5
Dizziness	780.4	U.R.I.	465.9
Emergency	V72.9	U.T.I.	599.0
Fatigue	780.7	Vaginitis	616.10
Feeding Problems	783.3	Viral Infection	079.99
Gastroenteritis	558.9	Well Adult	V70.9
G.I. Bleeding	578.9	Well Baby	V20.2
Headache	784.0	Well Child	V20.2
Hypertension	401.1		

Other Dx _____ _____ _____　Code _____

* Needs 4th digit
\+ Needs 5th digit

IMMUNIZATIONS:

*DPT (A CEL)	W0350	Influenza Virus	90724
*DPT	90701	*MMR	90707
DT (Adult)	90718	*Measles	90705
*DT (PED)	90702	*OPV	90712
*Hepatitis B	90744	*PV (inj)	90713
Indicate Dosage _____		Pneumo-vax	90732
*HIB	90737	Administration	90782
Other _____			

INJECTIONS: IM, Subcutaneous, IV

Adrenaline	J0170	Demerol	J2175
Allergy, aq	J1200	Depo-medrol, 40 mg	J2920
Ampicillin	J0290	Hydrocort, up to 50 mg	J1710
Aristocort Forte	J3301	Kenalog-40	J3301
B-12	J3420	Penicillin	J2510
Benadryl, 10 mg	W0485	Phenobarbital	J2560
Celestone	J0702	Poison Ivy Extract	W2615
Compazine, 5 mg/cc	W0775	Rocephin	J0696
Cortisone	J0810	Susphrine	W3025
Decadron	W0888	Wycillin	J2510
Other _____			

LABORATORY:

Comprehensive Metabolic	80054	Pregnancy Test (blood)	84703
Blood Sugar	82947	Pregnancy Test (urine)	84702
CBC	85022	Smear (gram stain)	87205
Cholesterol	82465	Stool Occult Blood	
Hct	85014	(hemoccult)	82270
Hgb	85018	Throat Culture (strep)	87069
Mono Test	86406	Triglyceride	84478
Pap Test	88150	Urinalysis Routine	81000
Phlebotomy	36415	Urine Culture	Z8712
Other _____			

DIAGNOSTIC STUDIES:

Anoscopy	46600	Rigid Procto	45300
Audiometry	92551	Tine PPD	86580
EKG	93000	Tonometry	92100
PPD	86580	Tympanometry	92567
Other _____			

OFFICE PROCEDURES:

Arthrocentesis	206_ _	Nebulizer	94640
Avulsion of Nail	X11_ _	Removal of Foreign Bodies	10120
Burn Care	160_ _	Routine Venipuncture	36415
Control of Nasal		Suture Removal	X1070
Hemorrhage	30901; 30903	Treatment of Sprains/	
I&D of Abscess	10_ _ _	Dislocations	29_ _ _
Other _____			

FIGURE 18.3 A sample patient encounter form.

© Jones & Bartlett Learning

Never code straight from the index. Always read the full procedure description.

Completing a Medical Insurance Claim Form

As a medical assistant, you may be asked to complete a medical insurance claim form. Most often, this will be form CMS-1500 (refer to Figure 18.1). You will often complete this form on a provider-specific computer program and submit the claim electronically. In this section, you will learn the principles behind completing a CMS-1500 form.

Equipment Needed

- Form CMS-1500
- Patient record
- Patient account information or ledger

Steps

1. Check the patient's record for a copy of his or her insurance card.
2. Check the patient's file for a signature that allows the release of information and assignment of benefits.

According to requirements from the Health Insurance Portability and Accountability Act, patients must have a signature on file for the provider to release data to the insurance company for benefit or payment information.

3. Complete the boxes on form CMS-1500. **FIGURE 18.4** shows a sample completed form CMS-1500.

- In box 1, check the appropriate type of coverage.
- In box 2, enter the patient's name, exactly as it appears on the insurance card.
- In box 3, use eight digits to write the date. For example, write 05-13-2000 for May 13th, 2000.
- In box 4, enter the insured person's name.

The patient might not be the insured person. For example, if a spouse or parent provides coverage for his or her dependents, this person's name will be placed in box 4.

- In box 5, enter the patient's full address and telephone number.
- In box 6, check the box identifying the patient's relationship to the insured.
- In box 7, enter the insured person's address and telephone number.
- In box 8, enter the patient's marital status.
- In box 9, enter any other insured person's name and identifying information.
- In box 10, check the box identifying the patient's condition.
- In box 11, enter the insured person's policy and employer information.
- In boxes 12 and 13, obtain the patient's and insured person's signature, or note "signature on file."
- In box 14, enter the date that the illness began.
- In box 15, enter the date that the patient was treated for the same or a similar illness.
- In box 16, enter the dates that the patient will be unable to work.
- In box 17, enter the name and identifying number of the referring provider, if applicable. Otherwise, leave blank.
- In box 18, enter the dates of hospitalization, if applicable. Otherwise, leave blank.
- Leave box 19 blank.
- In box 20, check the box identifying laboratory services.
- In box 21, enter the ICD diagnosis codes, using a separate line for each entry.

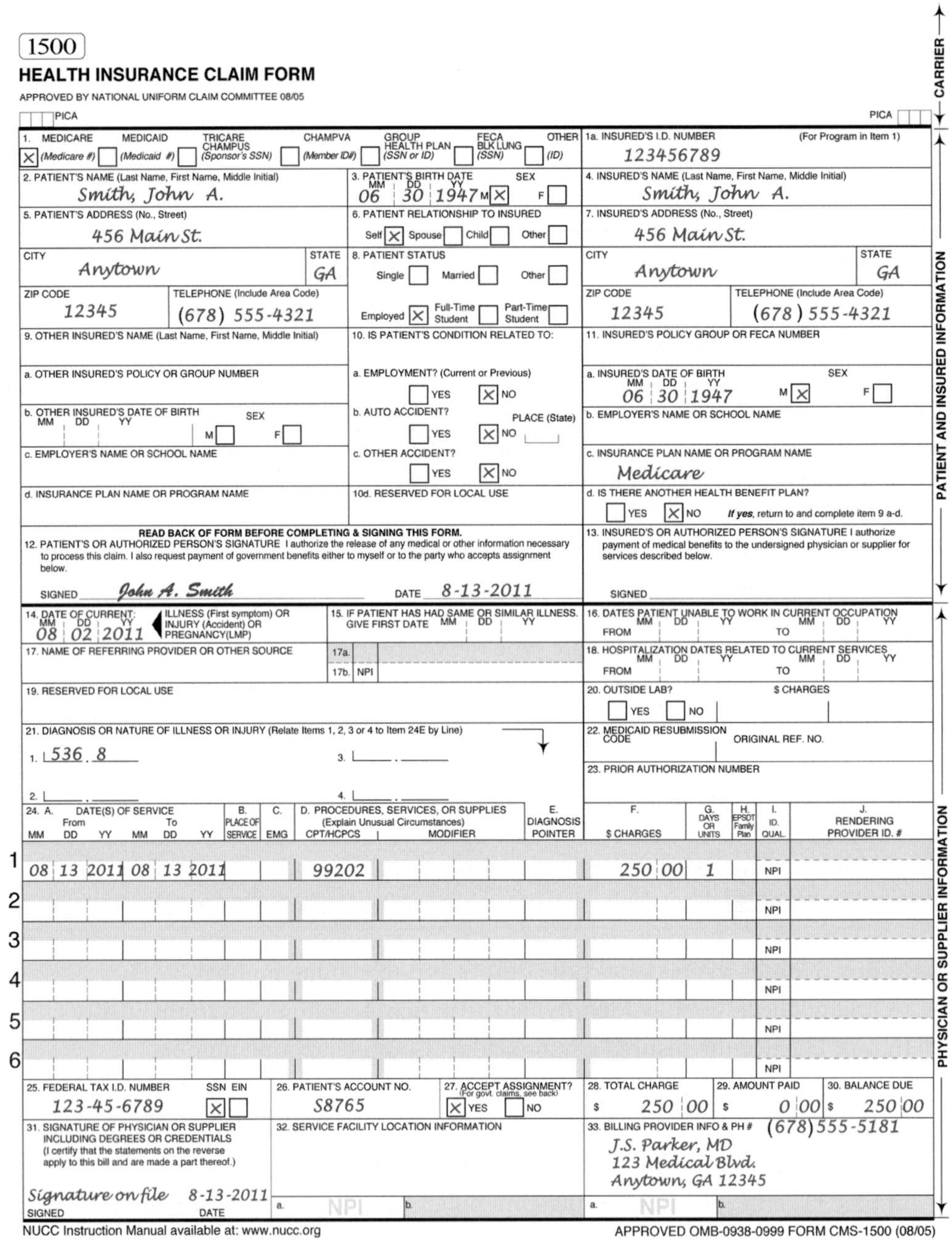

1500
HEALTH INSURANCE CLAIM FORM
APPROVED BY NATIONAL UNIFORM CLAIM COMMITTEE 08/05
PICA PICA

1. MEDICARE [X] (Medicare #) MEDICAID (Medicaid #) TRICARE CHAMPUS (Sponsor's SSN) CHAMPVA (Member ID#) GROUP HEALTH PLAN (SSN or ID) FECA BLK LUNG (SSN) OTHER (ID)
1a. INSURED'S I.D. NUMBER (For Program in Item 1): 123456789
2. PATIENT'S NAME (Last Name, First Name, Middle Initial): Smith, John A.
3. PATIENT'S BIRTH DATE MM DD YY: 06 30 1947 SEX M [X] F
4. INSURED'S NAME (Last Name, First Name, Middle Initial): Smith, John A.
5. PATIENT'S ADDRESS (No., Street): 456 Main St.
6. PATIENT RELATIONSHIP TO INSURED: Self [X] Spouse Child Other
7. INSURED'S ADDRESS (No., Street): 456 Main St.
CITY: Anytown STATE: GA
8. PATIENT STATUS: Single Married Other
CITY: Anytown STATE: GA
ZIP CODE: 12345 TELEPHONE (Include Area Code): (678) 555-4321
Employed [X] Full-Time Student Part-Time Student
ZIP CODE: 12345 TELEPHONE (Include Area Code): (678) 555-4321
9. OTHER INSURED'S NAME (Last Name, First Name, Middle Initial)
10. IS PATIENT'S CONDITION RELATED TO:
11. INSURED'S POLICY GROUP OR FECA NUMBER
a. OTHER INSURED'S POLICY OR GROUP NUMBER
a. EMPLOYMENT? (Current or Previous) YES [X] NO
a. INSURED'S DATE OF BIRTH MM DD YY: 06 30 1947 SEX M [X] F
b. OTHER INSURED'S DATE OF BIRTH MM DD YY SEX M F
b. AUTO ACCIDENT? YES [X] NO PLACE (State)
b. EMPLOYER'S NAME OR SCHOOL NAME
c. EMPLOYER'S NAME OR SCHOOL NAME
c. OTHER ACCIDENT? YES [X] NO
c. INSURANCE PLAN NAME OR PROGRAM NAME: Medicare
d. INSURANCE PLAN NAME OR PROGRAM NAME
10d. RESERVED FOR LOCAL USE
d. IS THERE ANOTHER HEALTH BENEFIT PLAN? YES [X] NO *If yes, return to and complete item 9 a-d.*

READ BACK OF FORM BEFORE COMPLETING & SIGNING THIS FORM.
12. PATIENT'S OR AUTHORIZED PERSON'S SIGNATURE I authorize the release of any medical or other information necessary to process this claim. I also request payment of government benefits either to myself or to the party who accepts assignment below.
SIGNED John A. Smith DATE 8-13-2011
13. INSURED'S OR AUTHORIZED PERSON'S SIGNATURE I authorize payment of medical benefits to the undersigned physician or supplier for services described below.
SIGNED

14. DATE OF CURRENT: ILLNESS (First symptom) OR INJURY (Accident) OR PREGNANCY(LMP) MM DD YY: 08 02 2011
15. IF PATIENT HAS HAD SAME OR SIMILAR ILLNESS. GIVE FIRST DATE MM DD YY
16. DATES PATIENT UNABLE TO WORK IN CURRENT OCCUPATION FROM TO
17. NAME OF REFERRING PROVIDER OR OTHER SOURCE 17a. 17b. NPI
18. HOSPITALIZATION DATES RELATED TO CURRENT SERVICES FROM TO
19. RESERVED FOR LOCAL USE
20. OUTSIDE LAB? YES NO $ CHARGES
21. DIAGNOSIS OR NATURE OF ILLNESS OR INJURY (Relate Items 1, 2, 3 or 4 to Item 24E by Line)
1. 536.8 2. 3. 4.
22. MEDICAID RESUBMISSION CODE ORIGINAL REF. NO.
23. PRIOR AUTHORIZATION NUMBER

	24. A. DATE(S) OF SERVICE From MM DD YY	To MM DD YY	B. PLACE OF SERVICE	C. EMG	D. PROCEDURES, SERVICES, OR SUPPLIES (Explain Unusual Circumstances) CPT/HCPCS	MODIFIER	E. DIAGNOSIS POINTER	F. $ CHARGES	G. DAYS OR UNITS	H. EPSDT Family Plan	I. ID. QUAL.	J. RENDERING PROVIDER ID. #
1	08 13 2011	08 13 2011			99202			250 00	1		NPI	
2											NPI	
3											NPI	
4											NPI	
5											NPI	
6											NPI	

25. FEDERAL TAX I.D. NUMBER SSN EIN: 123-45-6789 [X] SSN
26. PATIENT'S ACCOUNT NO.: S8765
27. ACCEPT ASSIGNMENT? (For govt. claims, see back) [X] YES NO
28. TOTAL CHARGE: $ 250 00
29. AMOUNT PAID: $ 0 00
30. BALANCE DUE: $ 250 00
31. SIGNATURE OF PHYSICIAN OR SUPPLIER INCLUDING DEGREES OR CREDENTIALS (I certify that the statements on the reverse apply to this bill and are made a part thereof.)
Signature on file 8-13-2011
SIGNED DATE
32. SERVICE FACILITY LOCATION INFORMATION
a. NPI b.
33. BILLING PROVIDER INFO & PH # (678) 555-5181
J.S. Parker, MD
123 Medical Blvd.
Anytown, GA 12345
a. NPI b.
NUCC Instruction Manual available at: www.nucc.org
APPROVED OMB-0938-0999 FORM CMS-1500 (08/05)
CARRIER
PATIENT AND INSURED INFORMATION
PHYSICIAN OR SUPPLIER INFORMATION

FIGURE 18.4 A sample completed CMS-1500 form.

Courtesy of the Centers for Medicare & Medicaid Services

- Complete box 22 if the claim will be submitted to Medicaid.
- Complete box 23 if a prior authorization code was received.
- In box 24, enter CPT or HCPCS codes. List each code separately, in order of decreasing importance.
- In box 25, enter the provider's identification number for tax purposes.
- In box 26, add the patient's account number that is used by the provider.
- In box 27, check the box to identify acceptance of assignment. By accepting assignment, a provider agrees to accept the amount of reimbursement assigned by Medicare and agrees not to charge the patient an additional fee for the service.

- In box 28, enter the total amount charged for the services.
- In box 29, enter the amount the patient paid.
- In box 30, enter the remaining account balance.
- In boxes 31 through 33, enter the provider's signature and facility and location information.

The provider's signature may be stamped. Alternatively, the provider's typed name and credentials can be submitted in place of a signature.

The insurance claim will be rejected if the claim form is not completed accurately and in its entirety.

WRAP UP

Chapter Summary

- Health insurance protects individuals from the high costs associated with medical care. Through private health-insurance programs, consumer-driven health plans, and government health coverage, individuals prepay for medical care so they do not have to pay the entire cost of care at the time of service.

- Most people in the United States receive medical insurance from their employers. Others receive assistance from government-sponsored programs. Some individuals choose to self-pay for medical care on a fee-for-service basis. Individuals must weigh the costs and benefits of each type of plan, as well as assess their medical care needs, when choosing insurance coverage.

- Managed care is a system in which an organization contracts with providers to provide healthcare services to its enrollees. Managed care plans require some out-of-pocket expenses on the part of the enrollee, usually through an annual premium, a deductible, a co-pay, or co-insurance.

- Managed care may be provided through a health maintenance organization (HMO) or a preferred provider organization (PPO). An HMO requires individuals to choose a primary care provider (PCP) to coordinate medical care. Costs associated with HMOs are usually lower than PPOs, but HMOs offer less flexibility and freedom of choice.

- Consumer-driven health plans, including health savings accounts (HSAs) and flexible spending accounts (FSPs), give individuals more control over how their medical care money is spent. The money may be contributed by an employee or an employer, and it can be used to pay for medical and health-related expenses not covered by traditional insurance coverage.

- The government provides medical care for select groups of individuals. Medicare is the federal program that provides care for senior citizens, people receiving dialysis, people who are disabled, and people receiving Social Security benefits. Medicaid is a state-administered program that provides care for low-income individuals, uninsured pregnant women, and people with disabilities. TRICARE and CHAMPVA are programs that provide care for military personnel and their families.

- When filing insurance claims, codes are used to reflect the diagnoses, treatments, and procedures for each patient. International Classification of Diseases (ICD) codes are used to describe the disease and condition of a patient. The healthcare common procedure coding system (HCPCS) and Current Procedural Terminology (CPT) are used to describe what was done for the disease or condition.

- Accurate coding ensures prompt reimbursement from the insurance company. Common errors on claim forms include excluding patient identification information and assigning incorrect codes to diagnoses or treatments.

- Electronic submission of insurance claims allows for real-time tracking of claim status and prompt follow-up of rejected claims.

- As a medical assistant, you will have the opportunity to participate in verifying medical insurance coverage for individuals and completing and submitting claim forms. Attention to detail and accuracy in completing forms will ensure that the maximum insurance benefits are received in a timely manner.

WRAP UP

Learning Assessment Questions

1. What was the original intent of health-insurance programs?
   A. To encourage preventive care
   B. To promote good nutrition during childhood
   C. To protect individuals from payment associated with catastrophic injuries or illnesses
   D. To treat service-related injuries among military veterans

2. How do most Americans receive their health insurance?
   A. Through their employers
   B. Through their state government
   C. Through pharmacy benefit managers
   D. Through fee-for-service programs

3. What is a goal of the Patient Protection and Affordable Care Act of 2010?
   A. To decrease the reimbursement for Medicare services
   B. To improve access to health care
   C. To decrease the accountability of insurance providers for coverage-related decisions
   D. To encourage wellness exams for children and the elderly

4. What is the definition of a *network*, as related to health-insurance coverage?
   A. The group of providers that are contracted with an insurance company to provide coverage at a negotiated rate
   B. An individual's primary care provider and all the specialists he or she sees on a regular basis
   C. The group to which a diagnosis belongs that determines Medicare reimbursement
   D. All of the insurance providers available in a geographic area

5. What is a deductible?
   A. The amount of money that an individual must pay each year to purchase health-insurance coverage
   B. The percentage of the total cost of care that an individual must contribute toward his or her care
   C. The monetary compensation for medical care
   D. The amount of money that an individual must pay before an insurance provider will cover medical services

6. Which of the following accurately describes a preferred provider organization?
   A. An insurance plan that allows complete freedom for patients to choose their own providers and pay for services out of pocket
   B. A system of insurance coverage in which all the providers are employees of the insurance company
   C. A system of insurance coverage that allows patients to choose primary care providers and specialists within a network without a referral
   D. An entity that organizes consumer-driven health plans

7. A health savings account *cannot* be used to pay for which of the following services?
   A. Childcare services
   B. Ambulance services
   C. Equipment for a visually impaired person
   D. Home improvement to assist a person in a wheelchair

8. Which Medicare program provides coverage for prescription drugs?
   A. Medicare part A
   B. Medicare part B
   C. Medicare part C
   D. Medicare part D

WRAP UP

9. What government program provides insurance coverage for children in low-income families?

   A. Medicare

   B. Medicaid

   C. TRICARE

   D. CHAMPVA

10. What government program provides health insurance for active members of the military?

    A. Medicare

    B. Medicaid

    C. TRICARE

    D. CHAMPVA

11. What is a coordination of benefits?

    A. The process of accepting Medicare assignment

    B. The process of preventing duplication of insurance coverage

    C. The process of assigning ICD codes and coordinating CPT codes

    D. The entire process of completing, filing, and tracking an insurance claim

12. Which of the following is *not* a principle of medical coding?

    A. Code with the minimum number of codes that reflect a patient's condition

    B. Code correctly and completely

    C. Code each problem as specifically as possible

    D. Code only the primary reason for the visit

13. What are the benefits of ICD-10 codes compared with ICD-9 codes?

    A. The ICD-10 codes include the use of technology in medicine.

    B. There are fewer ICD-10 codes.

    C. Only numeric codes are used for ICD-10.

    D. The United States will be the first to adopt ICD-10.

14. What category of CPT codes is used to report a majority of services?

    A. Evaluation and management

    B. Anesthesiology

    C. Surgery

    D. Medicine

15. How many categories of CPT codes exist?

    A. 3

    B. 6

    C. 17

    D. 13,000

16. Which set of codes is used to identify a patient's diagnosis for insurance claims?

    A. CPT

    B. DRG

    C. HCPCS

    D. ICD-9

17. Which of the following is an example of fraud in completing insurance claims?

    A. Listing multiple diagnoses on one claim form

    B. Reporting multiple codes for one procedure

    C. Submitting a claim to a secondary insurance provider

    D. Misspelling the patient's surname on the claim form

18. Which form is required for submitting claims to Medicare and Medicaid?

    A. UB-04

    B. ICD-9-CM

    C. ACA 2012

    D. CMS-1500

19. Which of the following is an example of a common error on claim forms?

    A. Providing only a stamped provider signature

    B. Providing an insured person's name that is different from that of the patient

    C. The use of incorrect medical codes

    D. Including additional reports with the claim form

20. What does it mean to accept assignment?

    A. A patient agrees to only see providers in his network.

    B. A provider agrees to accept reimbursement determined by Medicare.

    C. A specialist agrees to see patients referred by a primary care provider.

    D. A patient verifies that diagnosis codes are correct on his or her claim form.

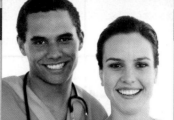

CHAPTER

19

Working With Pediatric and Geriatric Clients

OBJECTIVES

After reading this chapter, you will be able to:

- Describe pediatric care, including measuring height, weight, head, chest circumference, and vital signs.
- Explain the process of collecting a urine specimen from a pediatric patient.
- Explain the process of screening for hearing and visual impairments in pediatric patients.
- Explain the importance of immunizations for pediatric patients and the immunization schedule.
- Describe infant holds for injections and procedures.
- Identify expected physiological changes that occur as part of the aging process.
- List five common functional changes that can occur with age.
- Explain the importance of communication with older adults.
- Identify several techniques or strategies to communicate with visually and hearing-impaired older adults.

KEY TERMS

Activities of daily living
   (ADLs)
Adolescents
Beers criteria
Children
Elderly
Failure to thrive (FTT)

Geriatricians
Geriatrics
Gerontology
Growth charts
Infants
Neonates
Pediatricians

Pediatrics
Polypharmacy
Prescribing cascade
Recumbent length
Vaccine information
   statement (VIS)

Chapter Overview

As a medical assistant, you may have the opportunity to work with special patient populations. Pediatrics and geriatrics are two distinct patient groups that deserve special attention due to their physiology, functional abilities, cognitive status, and risk factors for certain diseases and conditions. Special skills are needed to gain the trust and confidence and to provide for the emotional, physical, and psychological needs of these patients.

When working with pediatric or geriatric patients, you may also be asked to work with caregivers such as parents, spouses, adult children, or other family members. Even in these circumstances, maintaining patient confidentiality is important. Patients should be treated with dignity, privacy, and respect. Access to medical information should be limited only to those who need to know the information in order to provide care or make medical decisions for the patient.

Terminology

TABLE 19.1 lists terms used in working with pediatric and geriatric patients.

Table 19.1   Terms Used in Working With Pediatric and Geriatric Patients

Term	Meaning
Assisted living	A facility in which a geriatric patient resides and maintains some independence, but receives assistance with medication administration or activities of daily living
Long-term–care facility	A residential facility for patients with chronic illnesses or disabilities that do not require hospitalization, but cannot complete their activities of daily living
Percentile	A comparison of a child's growth compared with national averages for children of the same age and gender
Skilled nursing facility	A long-term–care facility that participates in and is reimbursed for Medicare services and is subject to staffing requirements imposed by Medicare

Abbreviations Related to Pediatric and Geriatric Patients

The following are abbreviations related to pediatric and geriatric patients:

- ADHD—Attention-deficit/hyperactivity disorder
- ADLs—Activities of daily living
- BSA—Body-surface area
- DTaP—Diphtheria toxoid, tetanus toxoid, and acellular pertussis vaccine
- FTT—Failure to thrive
- Hib—*Haemophilus influenza* type B
- IPV—Inactivated polio vaccine
- LGA—Large for gestational age
- LTCF—Long-term-care facility
- MAI—Medication appropriateness index
- MMR—Measles, mumps, and rubella
- NBS—Newborn screening
- PCV—Pneumococcal conjugate vaccine
- RV—Rotavirus
- SGA—Small for gestational age
- SNF—Skilled nursing facility
- UTD—Up-to-date (used for childhood vaccines)
- VAERS—Vaccine adverse events reporting system
- VIS—Vaccine information statement

Pediatric Patients

Pediatrics is the branch of medicine that studies and cares for the patient under 18 years of age. This group includes newborns, infants, children, and adolescents. Newborns or **neonates** are babies between one day and one month old. **Infants** are babies who are between one month and one year old. **Children** are between one year and 11 years old, and **adolescents** are between 12 and 18 years old. **Pediatricians** are the physicians who care for pediatric patients.

Pediatric patients encompass diverse stages of growth and development. Special training is needed to accurately diagnose and treat disorders and conditions associated with pediatric patients. Well-child exams are important components of pediatric care and represent an opportunity to promote healthy living for patients and their families and to prevent common childhood illnesses.

Physiology of Pediatric Patients

Pediatric patients are not just small adults. They have different physical, emotional, and psychological needs than adult patients. The physiology of pediatric patients is also markedly different from that of adults; pediatric patients require different diagnostic tools, strategies for disease prevention, choices for drug therapy, and methods of treatment. The rate and development of organ growth varies not just between pediatric and adult patients, but also among pediatric patient groups.

In terms of body composition, pediatric patients have a larger proportion of body water than adults. Newborns have the highest proportion of water, and the percentage gradually decreases as a child grows. Also, due to their smaller size, pediatric patients have a larger body-surface area than adults. Children have an increased ratio of skin to body size, placing them at risk for excessive loss of fluids and heat. Also, the skin of pediatric patients is thinner and less keratinized, which places them at risk for increased absorption of drugs or chemicals that are absorbed through the skin.

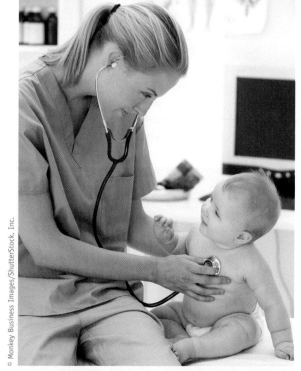

Pediatric patients also have an increased heart rate and respiratory rate compared with adults. Overall, they have less circulating blood volume than adults and the increased respiratory rate places them at risk for increased inhalation of toxic substances. Pediatric patients also have an increased metabolic rate compared with adults. They need more calories per body size than adults. Pediatric patients have slower gastric emptying than adults and reduced gastric acidity.

Pediatric immune systems are not mature, which places them at risk for contracting contagious illnesses. Many organ systems are also not mature, including the kidneys, which affects drug metabolism and elimination. Drug doses must be calculated carefully because drugs affect pediatric bodies differently than adult bodies. Often, pediatric doses are based on body weight or body-surface area.

Caring for Pediatric Patients

Pediatric patients have many fears related to unknown people and places. A physician's office, clinic, or hospital setting can make a child anxious and fearful. Any pro-

Use a smile and maintain eye contact to ease a child's or infant's fears.

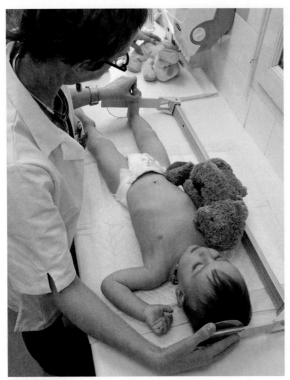

FIGURE 19.1 Assess an infant's or child's height using recumbent length.
© BSIP/Corbis

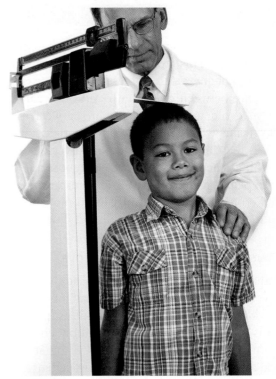

FIGURE 19.2 Older children can stand on a balance-beam scale to measure height.
© forestpath/ShutterStock, Inc.

viders working with pediatric patients should be alert to the patient's comfort level. Speak directly to the child and maintain a caring, positive attitude. Show interest and care for the patient and be attentive to his or her questions and concerns. This will gain the child's cooperation and facilitate examinations and procedures.

Physical Examination of Pediatric Patients

Precise and accurate measurements are essential to caring for pediatric patients. Normal growth and development can be monitored; in addition, diseases and conditions of growth and development can be diagnosed based on routine measurements. Common parameters for assessment include height or length, weight, head circumference, and chest circumference. If any of these values falls out of the normal ranges of measurements for children of the same age and gender, or if the measurements change at an abnormal rate, an underlying disease or disorder could be the cause.

Until a child is about three years old, height is assessed by **recumbent length** **FIGURE 19.1**. That is, the child is placed in a supine position on a table and his or her length from head to feet is measured. Once a child is three years old, he or she can likely cooperate with instructions and stand on a regular balance-beam scale and the height can be assessed in the same manner as for adults **FIGURE 19.2**.

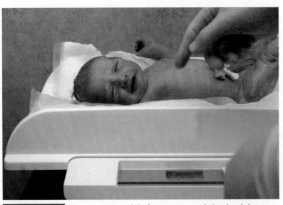

FIGURE 19.3 Neonates and infants are weighed without clothing or diapers.
© Francois Etienne du Plessis/ShutterStock, Inc.

For improved accuracy, infants are usually weighed without clothes or diapers **FIGURE 19.3**. An infant who is too young to sit on his or her own can be placed in a pediatric scale lying down. If an infant can sit up on his or her own, keep your hand close to the infant while obtaining the measurement to prevent a fall.

Head circumference is measured by placing a flexible tape measure around the head of the child or infant **FIGURE 19.4**. Measure across the largest part of the head, approximately one inch above the ears. Head circumference should be measured at every well-child exam until the child is three years of age.

Chest circumference is measured by placing a flexible tape measure around the chest, just above the nipples. If assistance is needed to keep an infant or child still while obtaining measurements, do not hesitate to ask another healthcare provider or the child's caregiver for help.

FIGURE 19.4 Head circumference is measured until a child is three years old.
© Marlon Lopez/ShutterStock, Inc.

Measurements of physical growth and development are placed in the patient's chart and compared with **growth charts** **FIGURE 19.5**. The National Center for Health Statistics publishes normal childhood growth and development patterns. The charts are gender- and age-specific. Take care to reference the correct chart when assess-

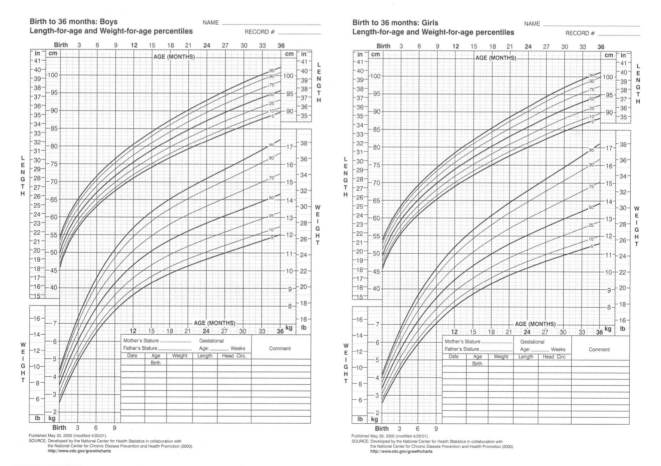

FIGURE 19.5 Length-for-age and weight-for-age growth chart shown for (A) boys and (B) girls.
Kuczmarski RJ, Ogden CL, Guo SS, et al. 2000 CDC growth charts for the United States: Methods and development. National Center for Health Statistics. *Vital Health Stat 11*(246). 2002

Chest circumference is measured and recorded in the patient's chart, but is not included on standardized growth charts.
© auremar/ShutterStock, Inc.

ing a patient's growth. The patient's growth can be compared with the growth of other children as a percentile. That is, the growth of the child is related to the national averages for growth and the percentile indicates how the child compares to 100 percent of other children. For example, if a child's weight corresponds to the 75th percentile, he or she weighs more than 75 percent of children of the same age and gender. Growth charts are available to compare length or height, weight, and head circumference from birth to age 20 years.

Failure to thrive (FTT) is often defined as poor physical growth, often falling below the fifth percentile. Normally, FTT is defined by weight—either extremely low weight for a child's age and gender or a low rate of weight increase. FTT does not necessarily imply poor emotional, social, or intellectual development; it may be caused by metabolic errors, nutritional deficiencies, structural abnormalities of organ systems, or psychosocial factors.

Vital signs, including temperature, pulse, respiratory rate, and blood pressure, are also important in evaluating a child's health. Temperature can be measured by several routes, depending on the age of the child. The rectal route is the preferred route for measuring temperature in infants and in young children when other routes are not appropriate. The axillary route is preferred for young children. The aural route is used for patients more than two years old. The oral route is appropriate for children more than five years old.

To measure the heart rate in a patient under five years old, listening to the pulse with a stethoscope is the preferred method. The apical pulse should be assessed by listening to the apex of the heart between the fifth and sixth ribs at the mid-clavicular line. When listening to heart rate, note whether the rate is regular or irregular. Heart rates for most pediatric patients are much higher than they are for adults. Heart rate will decrease with age, with newborns having an average heart rate of 140 beats per minute and adolescents having an average heart rate of 85 beats per minute. **TABLE 19.2** lists normal heart rates for each age group.

Respirations are assessed in older children and adolescents by counting the number of breaths in the same manner as in adults. In younger children and infants, however, respirations are counted by observing the rise and fall of the abdomen or chest. Each time the abdomen or chest falls is counted as one respiration. Count respirations for one full minute. The respiratory rate of pediatric patients varies considerably and decreases with age. Newborns have a normal respiratory rate of 30–60 breaths per minute and adolescents have a normal respiratory rate of 12–20 breaths per minute.

Table 19.2 Normal Heart Rates by Age Group	
Age	**Heart Rate**
Birth	90–190 beats per minute
0–6 months	80–180 beats per minute
6–12 months	75–155 beats per minute
1–2 years	70–150 beats per minutes
2–6 years	68–138 beats per minute
6–10 years	65–125 beats per minute
10–14 years	55–115 beats per minute
14 years–adult	60–100 beats per minute

Blood pressure might not be taken at every infant exam, unless directed by the provider. After a child turns three years old, however, blood pressure should be assessed at each well-child exam. Take care to use the correct size blood-pressure cuff. Pediatric cuffs can be placed on the arms or the leg. An electronic or manual blood-pressure cuff and stethoscope can be used for pediatric patients. If the cuff is too large, the blood pressure will be falsely low. If the cuff is too small, it will be falsely high.

Collecting urine from a pediatric patient may be required for laboratory testing. The clean catch bag is useful for collecting specimens for urinalysis. The bag is a clear plastic bag with adhesive strips that attaches to the perineum of the infant. The procedure can be time consuming because infants and young children cannot control urination, and the bag poses risks for contamination. A quicker and less time-consuming method is catheterization, in which a small catheter is inserted into the urethra and threaded to the patient's bladder. A sterile specimen is withdrawn from the bladder and the catheter is removed.

Health Screenings for Pediatric Patients

Vision and hearing screenings are recommended by the American Academy of Pediatrics (AAP) as part of preventive child health care. Due to limited cognitive and motor skills in very young infants and children, vision and hearing abnormalities can be difficult to detect. Rely on caregiver's reports of a child's history to note any changes or monitor for irregularities in vision or hearing. Symptoms that might indicate a vision problem are frequent eye rubbing, excessive blinking, looking cross-eyed, straining to see, turning the head to look at objects, sitting close to a television, or holding a book unusually close to the face. When children are old enough to cooperate and understand a test, vision can be assessed with Snellen charts, either with big Es or with shapes.

In infants and young children, hearing is assessed by monitoring the child's reaction to sounds. Parents or caregivers will likely be the first to notice a hearing change. Symptoms that hearing may be impaired include not responding to normal auditory stimuli and increasing the volume on televisions or media devices.

Hearing is normally assessed in newborns using specialized sensory equipment that measure a newborn's response to sounds. The screening must be performed in a quiet environment to avoid extraneous sounds that may invalidate the results.

Immunizations

Immunizations against potentially serious and life-threatening diseases are recommended by the AAP and the Centers for Disease Control and Prevention (CDC) as part of disease-prevention and routine child-wellness programs FIGURE 19.6. Documentation of immunizations is required by law. Immunizations must be up to date before a child is eligible to enter public school.

A **vaccine information statement (VIS)** should be provided with each vaccination FIGURE 19.7. A VIS provides details about the type of vaccine received and side effects of which caregivers should be aware. The CDC provides a VIS for every available vaccine in multiple languages. Provide all patient information in the language and format that is appropriate for each patient and caregiver.

Caregivers must sign consent forms prior to immunization administration. Allow plenty of time during a child's appointment for caregivers to ask questions about the vaccine. Many myths and fears surround vaccinations; as a result, parents may be apprehensive about their administration. Parents may refuse vaccination for their children by providing legal documentation of their refusal.

<table>
<tr><th>VACCINE ▼ AGE ▶</th><th>Birth</th><th>1 mth</th><th>2 mths</th><th>4 mths</th><th>6 mths</th><th>9 mths</th><th>12 mths</th><th>15 mths</th><th>18 mths</th><th>19-23 mths</th><th>2-3 years</th><th>4-6 years</th></tr>
<tr><td>Hepatitis B</td><td>HepB</td><td colspan="2">HepB</td><td></td><td colspan="5">HepB</td><td></td><td></td><td></td></tr>
<tr><td>Rotavirus</td><td></td><td></td><td>RV</td><td>RV</td><td>RV</td><td></td><td></td><td></td><td></td><td></td><td></td><td></td></tr>
<tr><td>Diphtheria, tetanus, pertussis</td><td></td><td></td><td>DTaP</td><td>DTaP</td><td>DTaP</td><td></td><td></td><td colspan="2">DTaP</td><td></td><td></td><td>DTaP</td></tr>
<tr><td>Haemophilus influenzae type b</td><td></td><td></td><td>Hib</td><td>Hib</td><td>Hib</td><td></td><td colspan="2">Hib</td><td></td><td></td><td></td><td></td></tr>
<tr><td>Pneumococcal</td><td></td><td></td><td>PCV</td><td>PCV</td><td>PCV</td><td></td><td colspan="2">PCV</td><td></td><td></td><td colspan="2">PSSV</td></tr>
<tr><td>Inactivated poliovirus</td><td></td><td></td><td>IPV</td><td>IPV</td><td colspan="5">IPV</td><td></td><td></td><td>IPV</td></tr>
<tr><td>Influenza</td><td></td><td></td><td></td><td></td><td colspan="8">Influenza (yearly)</td></tr>
<tr><td>Measles, mumps, rubella</td><td></td><td></td><td></td><td></td><td></td><td></td><td colspan="2">MMR</td><td></td><td></td><td></td><td>MMR</td></tr>
<tr><td>Varicella</td><td></td><td></td><td></td><td></td><td></td><td></td><td colspan="2">VAR</td><td></td><td></td><td></td><td>VAR</td></tr>
<tr><td>Hepatitis A</td><td></td><td></td><td></td><td></td><td></td><td></td><td colspan="4">Dose 1</td><td colspan="2">HepA series</td></tr>
<tr><td>Meningococcal</td><td></td><td></td><td></td><td></td><td></td><td colspan="7">MCV4</td></tr>
</table>

Range of recommended ages for all children | Range of recommended ages for certain high-risk groups | Range of recommended ages for all children and certain high-risk groups

FIGURE 19.6 Recommended vaccine schedule for infants and children.

Courtesy of the CDC

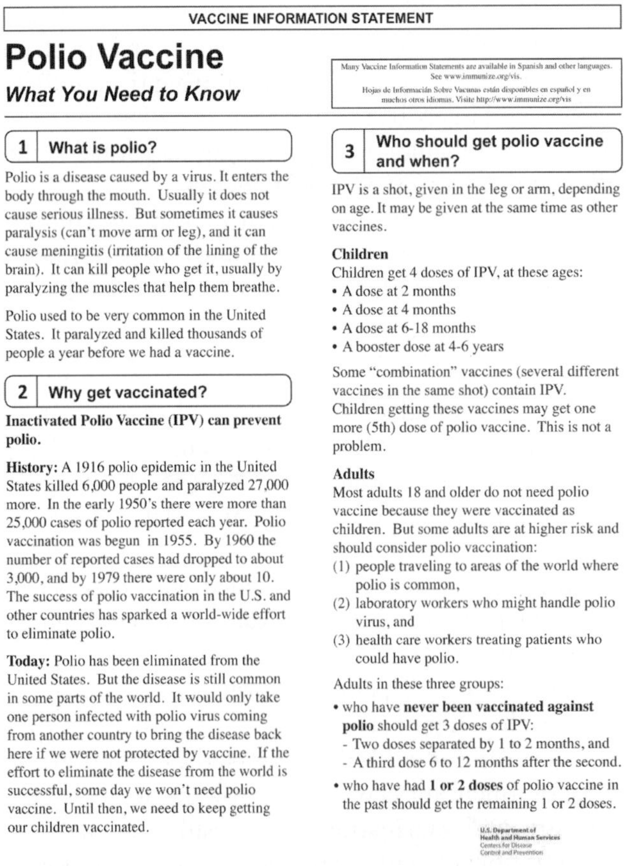

VACCINE INFORMATION STATEMENT

Polio Vaccine

What You Need to Know

Many Vaccine Information Statements are available in Spanish and other languages. See www.immunize.org/vis.

Hojas de Información Sobre Vacunas están disponibles en español y en muchos otros idiomas. Visite http://www.immunize.org/vis

1 What is polio?

Polio is a disease caused by a virus. It enters the body through the mouth. Usually it does not cause serious illness. But sometimes it causes paralysis (can't move arm or leg), and it can cause meningitis (irritation of the lining of the brain). It can kill people who get it, usually by paralyzing the muscles that help them breathe.

Polio used to be very common in the United States. It paralyzed and killed thousands of people a year before we had a vaccine.

2 Why get vaccinated?

Inactivated Polio Vaccine (IPV) can prevent polio.

History: A 1916 polio epidemic in the United States killed 6,000 people and paralyzed 27,000 more. In the early 1950's there were more than 25,000 cases of polio reported each year. Polio vaccination was begun in 1955. By 1960 the number of reported cases had dropped to about 3,000, and by 1979 there were only about 10. The success of polio vaccination in the U.S. and other countries has sparked a world-wide effort to eliminate polio.

Today: Polio has been eliminated from the United States. But the disease is still common in some parts of the world. It would only take one person infected with polio virus coming from another country to bring the disease back here if we were not protected by vaccine. If the effort to eliminate the disease from the world is successful, some day we won't need polio vaccine. Until then, we need to keep getting our children vaccinated.

3 Who should get polio vaccine and when?

IPV is a shot, given in the leg or arm, depending on age. It may be given at the same time as other vaccines.

Children

Children get 4 doses of IPV, at these ages:

- A dose at 2 months
- A dose at 4 months
- A dose at 6-18 months
- A booster dose at 4-6 years

Some "combination" vaccines (several different vaccines in the same shot) contain IPV. Children getting these vaccines may get one more (5th) dose of polio vaccine. This is not a problem.

Adults

Most adults 18 and older do not need polio vaccine because they were vaccinated as children. But some adults are at higher risk and should consider polio vaccination:

(1) people traveling to areas of the world where polio is common,

(2) laboratory workers who might handle polio virus, and

(3) health care workers treating patients who could have polio.

Adults in these three groups:

- who have **never been vaccinated against polio** should get 3 doses of IPV:
  - Two doses separated by 1 to 2 months, and
  - A third dose 6 to 12 months after the second.
- who have had **1 or 2 doses** of polio vaccine in the past should get the remaining 1 or 2 doses.

U.S. Department of Health and Human Services
Centers for Disease Control and Prevention

FIGURE 19.7 A sample vaccine information statement (VIS).

Courtesy of the CDC

Vaccine Safety

In recent years, parental fears have proliferated regarding a link between autism, attention-deficit/hyperactivity disorder, and speech and language delays and preservatives used in vaccines. Many studies have been conducted to evaluate such claims, and no links have been confirmed. Vaccines are safe when administered properly and parents should be educated about the validity of warnings against routine vaccination.

In 2010, the landmark journal article that incited the debate about vaccine safety was retracted by the distinguished journal *The Lancet*. The retraction bolstered support for practitioners who repeatedly claimed that vaccines were safe.

Vaccines are provided for hepatitis A and B, polio, measles, mumps, rubella, pertussis, diphtheria, tetanus, *Haemophilus influenza* type B, pneumonia, chicken pox, influenza, rotavirus, meningitis, and human papillomavirus. Vaccine schedules are published by the CDC to ensure adequate protection of pediatric populations. These are based on the theory that repeat immunization is required to ensure complete immunity against diseases. "Catch-up" schedules are available for patients who did not receive vaccines at the recommended time. Not only should pediatricians maintain documentation of a child's vaccinations, parents and caregivers should also be aware of when a child received each immunization.

> *Do not tell a child that an injection is not going to hurt. Be honest and tell him or her that it will sting for a short time, but then it will feel better. Provide a bright-colored or fun adhesive strip to place over the injection site.*
> © auremar/ShutterStock, Inc.

When administering an injectable vaccine to a child, it is important to follow the same infection-control practices and preparation procedures as for any other injection. When administering vaccines to children, holding them is the most difficult part. The child must be held in such a way as to prevent injury to the child as well as to provide access to the injection site. Because infants and young children are not always able to cooperate, this can be a difficult task. See Chapter 11 for a complete discussion of techniques used for administering immunizations and injections.

The vastus lateralis is the preferred injection site for IM and subQ injections in infants. After a child's first birthday, IM injections can be administered in the deltoid and subQ injections can be administered to the back of the arm. To administer an injection to the vastus lateralis, an infant or young child can be laid supine on an examination table and held in place by a caregiver. This provides access to the injection site and offers limited mobility for the child **FIGURE 19.8**. Alternatively, a caregiver can hold the child securely on his or her lap. The

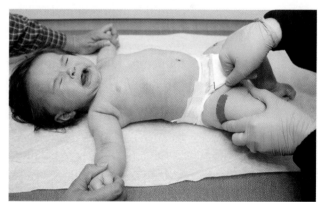

FIGURE 19.8 Have the caregiver help hold the child while administering a vaccine.
© Darren Brode/ShutterStock, Inc.

What Would You Do?

A mother brings her five-year-old son to the pediatrician's office where you work for a well-child exam. You tell her that the child is due for four vaccines. She refuses, stating that her neighbor's child got a vaccine and was then diagnosed with autism. She tells you she will not give her child any more vaccines. What do you tell her?

© NorthGeorgiaMedia/ShutterStock, Inc.

caregiver can place the child's legs in between his or her own legs to prevent the child from moving and provide access to the vastus lateralis and the deltoid.

Geriatric Patients

Geriatrics is the branch of medicine that studies and cares for older patients. There is no set age for geriatric patients, but the classification is determined by the needs of the patient. Generally, patients older than 65 years of age are considered geriatric or **elderly. Gerontology** is the study of the aging process itself. **Geriatricians** are physicians who care for geriatric patients. Many geriatricians seek interdisciplinary involvement in the care of their patients; a comprehensive approach to geriatric patients improves outcomes in every discipline.

Aging is a natural and progressive process. It happens at a different rate for every individual and the changes are not related to a disease process. It is difficult to predict when these changes will occur, so careful monitoring of geriatric patients will prevent problems in diagnosing and treating older patients. Geriatric patients often suffer from the same diseases, conditions, and ailments as younger patients, but more time is often required for healing. In addition, rehabilitation may be necessary to maintain independence and function. Aging does not only include physical and functional changes, but also changes in hobbies, interests, monetary resources, and family structure. Lifestyle, genetics, diet, and experience all influence how a person ages.

Activities of daily living (ADLs) are the normal self-care functions that people perform in order to live, including eating, ambulating, dressing, bathing, and grooming. Routine assessment of ADLs evaluates the functional status of an elderly person. If ADLs are limited due to physical or cognitive disabilities, physical, occupational, and recreational therapists can provide exercises to maintain a patient's independence.

Geriatric patients should be advised to maintain an active, healthy lifestyle. Engaging in physical activity, as well as social and creative outlets, will help maintain cognitive function and enhance well-being. While the aging process will continue, quality of life and functional ability will be increased. Thanks to advances in medical care, people are living longer, healthier lives than ever before. It is not uncommon for people to live well into their 80s, 90s, or even 100 years. Ideally, habits of healthy living should be initiated in childhood to build a successful, balanced, healthy life.

Physical and Physiological Changes in Geriatric Patients

Changes occur in nearly every body system as a result of aging. Visual changes occur as the lens of the eye becomes less elastic and more dense. Pupil size also decreases. Eyes may be red, dry, and itchy, and there is usually an increased sensitivity to glare. Reading small print can be difficult; many older people wear glasses specifically for reading. Decreased visual acuity coupled with a loss of balance and coordination place elderly patients at increased risk for falls.

Hearing loss occurs, as well as delays in auditory processing. Hearing loss is usually gradual and occurs over many years. Inattention and confusion are signs that hearing may be abnormal.

Esophageal and gastric motility decrease, leading to symptoms of gastroesophageal reflux disease. Saliva production decreases, which can lead to mouth pain and decreased intake of food and drink. Metabolism also slows; as a result, fewer calories are required than when patients were younger. The senses of taste and smell also diminish with age. Food is less appealing because it does not taste as good as it used to; therefore, older patients may add more salt and sugar to their food to improve its palatability. A decreased sense of smell not only affects appetite, but also poses a safety concern, as elderly people cannot smell fires or noxious fumes.

The blood contains more carbon dioxide and less oxygen. Increased rigidity in the chest wall decreases the maximum inhalation and exhalation volumes during respiration. Both issues affect the heart's ability to deliver oxygen to the rest of the body.

Kidney function decreases with age, including a decreased glomerular filtration rate. The kidneys are not able to excrete drugs from the body as effectively, and drug doses may have to be decreased for geriatric patients.

Hormone levels change, which alters countless body systems and functions. The reproductive system is notably affected by the aging process. In females, a decreased level of estrogen after menopause leads to a decrease in

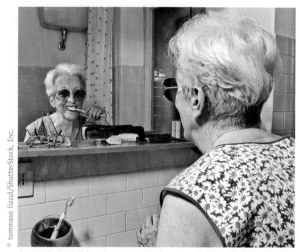

Grooming and hygiene are activities of daily living.

the size of the vulva and genitalia. The vagina atrophies due to a lack of estrogen. Testosterone levels decline in men, leading to prostatic hypertrophy.

Changes in the overall composition of the body, including a decrease in lean muscle and an increase in body fat, affects the distribution of drugs in the body. Due to a loss in body water, skin is drier and more fragile. Also, less connective and subcutaneous tissue is present in the skin. Sweat glands decrease in size and the body is less able to respond to temperature extremes. Fingernails thicken and hair thins and loses its pigment. Decreased muscle strength and flexibility limit mobility. Osteoporosis and arthritis are common conditions in the elderly.

Mental health is of great concern in elderly patients. Depression is common in this population, often due to life changes, loss of loved ones, loss of independence, financial difficulties, and chronic medical conditions. Signs of depression in older adults include lack of self-care, poor hygiene, insomnia, excessive sleep, crying, intense feelings of sadness or worthlessness, inability to concentrate, and excessive alcohol consumption.

Aging also affects memory and cognition, placing geriatric patients at risk for misunderstanding instructions related to medical care and failure to comply with prescribed therapy. Problems with balance, coordination, insomnia, and pain sensation occur with aging. Elderly patients are also at risk for accidents due to their inability to hear or see warning signs, decreased reaction time, and decreased pain sensations.

Drug-Related Problems in Geriatric Patients

Age-related changes in physiology alter the way drugs are absorbed, metabolized, distributed, and eliminated from the body. Additionally, elderly patients tend to take multiple drugs, which poses an increased risk for drug interactions and side effects. **Polypharmacy** describes the practice of taking multiple medications. Patients may simply require several drugs for multiple disease states, or they may take more drugs than are clinically necessary. A **prescribing cascade** is a scenario in which a medication is prescribed to treat the side effects of another medication. One tool used by clinicians who treat geriatric patients is the **Beers criteria**. It is a list of drugs that should be avoided in elderly patients due to the risk of side effects and inappropriate use. Medication therapy should be individualized to meet the needs of each patient. Particularly in geriatric patients, it is important to weigh the benefits with the known risks of medication therapy before initiating any new medication.

Potentially Inappropriate and Unsafe Medication Use in Older Adults

The Beers criteria, published by the American Geriatrics Society, provides a list of medications that may be used inappropriately or unsafely in elderly patients. The following list includes some of the most common medications that appear on the 2012 Beers criteria.

- Alprazolam
- Amiodarone
- Amitriptyline
- Benztropine
- Brompheniramine
- Butabarbital
- Butalbital
- Carisoprodol
- Chlordiazepoxide
- Chlorpheniramine
- Clomipramine
- Clonazepam
- Clonidine
- Cyclobenzaprine
- Cyproheptadine
- Diazepam
- Diphenhydramine
- Dipyridamole
- Dofetilide
- Doxazosin
- Doxylamine
- Estazolam
- Eszopiclone
- Flecainide
- Flurazepam
- Glyburide
- Guanfacine
- Hydroxyzine
- Ibuprofen
- Imipramine
- Indomethacin
- Ketorolac
- Lorazepam
- Meloxicam
- Meperidine
- Meprobamate
- Metaxalone
- Methocarbamol
- Methyldopa
- Metoclopramide
- Naproxen
- Nifedipine
- Nitrofurantoin
- Oxazepam
- Pentazocine
- Pentobarbital
- Phenobarbital
- Prazosin
- Procainamide
- Promethazine
- Quinidine
- Scopolamine
- Sulindac
- Terazosin
- Thioridazine
- Ticlopidine
- Triazolam
- Zaleplon
- Zolpidem

Also, geriatric patients may be seeing multiple healthcare providers and specialists, all of whom may prescribe medication therapy. Geriatric patients should be advised to share a complete list of all medications, herbal supplements, and vitamins that they take with all physicians and pharmacists. This will decrease duplicate therapy, minimize drug interactions, and optimize care.

Communicating With Geriatric Patients

Good communication skills are essential for treating geriatric patients. As a medical assistant, you must be respectful of patients and be aware of their emotions, fears, and apprehensions. Allow time for patients to express their concerns and address them as

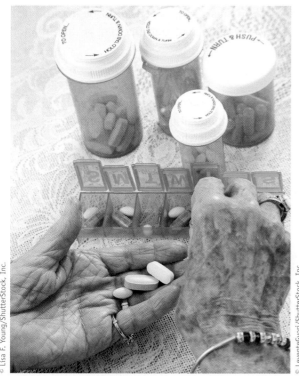

Geriatric patients often see multiple healthcare providers and take multiple medications.

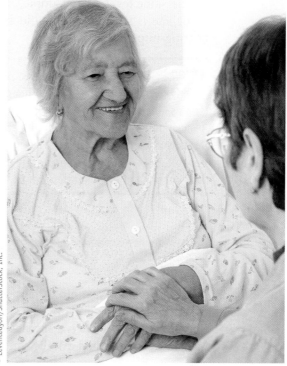

Use nonverbal communication with geriatric patients.

adequately as you can. Empathize with patients and validate their anxieties. Be professional and courteous. Speak slowly and clearly and always look at the patient when you are speaking. Provide written and verbal instructions if necessary.

Conduct examinations in a quiet place with no distractions. Because many geriatric patients have trouble hearing or seeing, eliminate as much extraneous sensory input as possible to facilitate concentration and attention. Always identify yourself and orient the patient. Address the patient in a respectful manner by his or her preferred name or title. Do not talk down to any patient and maintain a warm and pleasant tone of voice. Use nonverbal cues to express interest in the patient, such as a smile or touching the person's hand. Also, be aware of social or cultural preferences when addressing older patients.

If working with a visually or hearing-impaired patient, special strategies can be used to maintain the patient's comfort and safety. If you enter a room where a visually impaired person is present, verbally identify yourself and others in the room. Do not approach the individual until he or she acknowledges your presence. For hearing-impaired individuals, keep your hands away from your face while speaking. Eliminate extraneous noise as much as possible and use clear, well-enunciated words. Speak to the patient face-to-face and

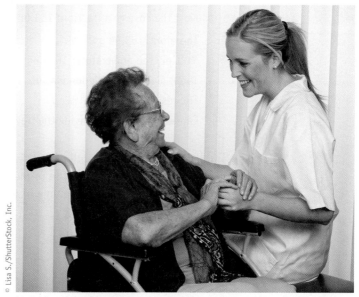

Listening to your patients can establish rapport and teach life lessons.

on the same level. For example, if he or she is standing, you should be standing; if he or she is sitting, you should be sitting. Written instructions can be helpful for hearing-impaired patients.

Listen to Your Patients

Elderly patients can offer fascinating narratives about their life experiences. Listen to these stories—not only as a backdrop for medical care and representing social pleasantries, but as a means for obtaining valuable information about their preferences, their medical history, their fears, and their social support. Being attentive to the stories of elderly patients establishes rapport and encourages a supportive environment. And, the life lessons you receive from the wisdom of another generation can be invaluable as you begin your career.

Math Practice

Question: **A four-year-old patient weighing 36 pounds is prescribed the antibiotic cefaclor for pharyngitis. The physician orders 10mg/kg by mouth every 8 hours. If the formulation available is a suspension with a concentration of 125mg/5mL, what volume of medication will the child receive for each dose?**

Answer: Step 1: Remember that 1 kilogram equals 2.2 pounds: 1kg = 2.2 lb

Convert this to a ratio in the form of a fraction: $\frac{1kg}{2.2\ lb}$

Next, convert the number of pounds to a fraction: 36 lb = $\frac{36\ lb}{1}$

Multiply the number of pounds by the number of kilograms per pound: $\frac{36\ lb}{1} \times \frac{1kg}{2.2\ lb}$

To do this, multiply the numerators: 36 lb × 1kg = 36 lb × kg

Then, multiply the denominators: 1 × 2.2 lb = 2.2 lb

The result is $\frac{36\ lb \times kg}{2.2\ lb}$

Cancel the units and divide the fraction: $\frac{36\ lb \times kg}{2.2\ lb}$ = 16.36kg

Step 2: Multiply the number of kilograms by dose ordered and cancel the units: 16.36kg × 10mg/kg = 163.6mg

Step 3: Multiply the dose ordered by the concentration of the suspension. To do this, first convert the dose to a fraction: 163.6mg = $\frac{163.6mg}{1}$

Therefore, 163.6mg × $\frac{5mL}{125mg}$ = $\frac{163.6mg}{1} \times \frac{5mL}{125mg}$

Multiply the numerators: 163.6mg × 5mL = 818mg × mL

Then, multiply the denominators: 1 × 125mg = 125mg

The result is 818mg × $\frac{mL}{125mg}$

Cancel the units and divide the fraction: 818mg × $\frac{mL}{125mg}$ = 6.5mL

Question: **A three-year-old patient weighing 28 pounds is prescribed furosemide 1mg/kg by mouth once daily. If the formulation available is a solution with a concentration of 40mg/5mL, what volume of medication will the child receive for each dose?**

Answer: Step 1: Remember that 1 kilogram equals 2.2 pounds: 1kg = 2.2 lb. Convert this to a ratio in the form of a fraction: $\frac{1kg}{2.2\ lb}$

Next, convert the number of pounds to a fraction: 28 lb = $\frac{28\ lb}{1}$

Multiply the number of pounds by the number of kilograms per pound: $\frac{28\ lb}{1} \times \frac{1kg}{2.2\ lb}$

To do this, multiply the numerators: 28 lb × 1kg = 28 lb × kg

Then, multiply the denominators: 1 × 2.2 lb = 2.2 lb

The result is 28 lb × $\frac{kg}{2.2\ lb}$

Cancel the units and divide the fraction: 28 lb × $\frac{kg}{2.2\ lb}$ = 12.7kg

Step 2: Multiply the number of kilograms by dose ordered and cancel the units: 12.7kg × $\frac{1mg}{kg}$ = 12.7mg

Step 3: Multiply the dose ordered by the concentration of the suspension. To do this, first convert the dose to a fraction: 12.7mg = $\frac{12.7mg}{1}$

Therefore, 12.7mg × $\frac{5mL}{40mg}$ = $\frac{12.7mg}{1}$ × $\frac{5mL}{40mg}$

Multiply the numerators: 12.7mg × 5mL = 63.5mg × mL

Then, multiply the denominators: 1 × 40mg = 40mg

The result is 63.5mg × $\frac{mL}{40mg}$

Cancel the units and divide the fraction: 63.5mg × $\frac{mL}{40mg}$ = 1.59mL

Question: **The normal dose of cimetidine for duodenal ulcer prophylaxis is 400mg orally at bedtime. For a geriatric patient with reduced renal function, the recommended dose is 50% of the normal dose. What dose should an elderly man with reduced renal function receive?**

Answer: Step 1: Multiply the normal dose by the recommended decrease. To do this, first convert the dose to a fraction: 400mg = $\frac{400mg}{1}$

Next, convert the percentage to a fraction: 50% = $\frac{50}{100}$

Therefore, 400mg × 50% = $\frac{400mg}{1}$ × $\frac{50}{100}$

Multiply the numerators: 400mg × 50 = 20,000mg

Then, multiply the denominators: 1 × 100 = 100

The result is 2,000mg/100

Step 2: Divide the fraction: $\frac{20,000mg}{100}$ = 200mg

Question: **A normal maintenance dose of digoxin for adults is 0.5mg orally at bedtime. For a geriatric patient with reduced renal function, a physician recommends administering 75% of this normal dose. What dose should the patient receive?**

Answer: Step 1: Multiply the normal dose by the recommended decrease. To do this, first convert the dose to a fraction: 0.5mg = $\frac{0.5mg}{1}$

Next, convert the percentage to a fraction: 75% = $\frac{75}{100}$

Therefore, 0.5mg × 75% = $\frac{0.5mg}{1}$ × $\frac{75}{100}$

Multiply the numerators: 0.5mg × 75 = 37.5mg

Then, multiply the denominators: 1 × 100 = 100

The result is 37.5mg/100

Step 2: Divide the fraction: $\frac{37.5mg}{100}$ = 0.375mg

WRAP UP

Chapter Summary

- Pediatric and geriatric patients have special physical, emotional, and social needs. Special skills are required by medical assistants and other healthcare providers to gain the trust and confidence of these groups and their caregivers.

- Pediatric patients undergo enormous growth and development in a short period of time. In addition to their physical, emotional, and psychosocial needs, which are different from adults, their physiology mandates special tools for diagnosis, disease prevention, and methods of treatment.

- Growth charts are used to compare pediatric growth and development to age- and gender-specific national averages of growth. Abnormal patterns or rates of growth could signify an underlying disease or disorder of many body systems or an external factor that contributes to poor nutrition or development.

- Vision and hearing screenings, as well as routine vaccinations, are recommended by the American Academy of Pediatrics as part of routine child health care. For very young children, parent and caregiver concerns about hearing or vision abnormalities are the most effective screening tool. Vaccines are safe and effective when administered as recommended, but parents may be concerned about the long-term health risks associated with vaccines.

- Aging is a natural, progressive process that involves many physiological changes. Body-composition changes and functional changes dictate the needs of geriatric patients. Assessment of activities of daily living provides insight into a patient's functional status. Many body-system changes place geriatric patients at increased risk for accidents and failure to comply with medical care. Safety is a primary concern for geriatric patients.

- Good communication skills are essential for treating geriatric patients appropriately and effectively. Be respectful of a patient's physical and cognitive limitations, his or her cultural preferences, and his or her fears and anxieties.

Learning Assessment Questions

1. Which of the following pairs correctly matches the patient group with its correct ages?
   A. Adolescents: patients younger than 18 years old
   B. Infants: patients who are one day to one month old
   C. Children: patients who are one year to 11 years old
   D. Neonates: patients who are one month to one year old

2. Which of the following is *not* a significant difference between pediatric and adult patients?
   A. Pediatric patients depend on caregivers for meeting all basic needs.
   B. Pediatric patients cannot always voice their concerns or anxieties.
   C. Pediatric patients are in a period of enormous growth and development.
   D. Pediatric patients do not feel pain.

3. Which of the following is a popular method of calculating pediatric doses of medication?
   A. Weight
   B. Height
   C. Recumbent length
   D. Body mass index

4. Which of the following is *not* a routine measurement that is monitored for pediatric patients?

   A. Height

   B. Chest circumference

   C. Waist circumference

   D. Head circumference

5. Which of the following methods of assessing temperature is preferred for a six-year-old child?

   A. Rectal

   B. Axillary

   C. Aural

   D. Oral

6. Where is the apical pulse observed?

   A. Between the fifth and sixth ribs at the mid-clavicular line

   B. Between the third and fourth ribs close to the sternum

   C. Over the popliteal artery

   D. Over the radial artery

7. What is a normal heart rate for a newborn?

   A. 12–20 beats per minute

   B. 30–60 beats per minute

   C. 60–100 beats per minute

   D. 130–140 beats per minute

8. How often should blood pressure be measured in a pediatric patient?

   A. Only at the newborn screening

   B. Every other year from birth to age 18

   C. Yearly after a child turns three years old

   D. Once a patient reaches adolescence

9. What is the least time-consuming method for obtaining a sterile urine specimen from a young child?

   A. Catheterization

   B. A clean catch bag

   C. Collecting wet diapers

   D. There is no way to collect a urine specimen until a child is toilet trained.

10. What is a reliable method for detecting hearing abnormalities in an infant or young child?

    A. A Snellen chart

    B. Parent or caregiver history

    C. Placing the child in a loud room and observing his or her reaction

    D. Measuring the distance a child sits from the television

11. Which of the following is *not* a routine vaccination recommended for children?

    A. Smallpox

    B. Hepatitis A

    C. Pertussis

    D. Rotavirus

12. Which organization publishes the recommended vaccine schedules for children?

    A. The American Academy of Pediatrics

    B. The World Health Organization

    C. The Centers for Disease Control and Prevention

    D. The Vaccine Information Service

13. What is the preferred route for an IM injection for a nine-month-old infant?

    A. The deltoid

    B. The back of the arm

    C. The gluteus maximus

    D. The vastus lateralis

14. Which of the following is *not* an activity of daily living?

    A. Eating

    B. Dressing

    C. Watching television

    D. Grooming

15. When should promotion of a healthy lifestyle begin?

    A. When a patient turns 65 years old

    B. At the earliest well-child exam

    C. When a patient turns 18 years old

    D. In adolescence

16. Which of the following is *not* a common age-related change in geriatric patients?

    A. Increased tear production

    B. Dry, fragile skin

    C. Memory loss

    D. Decreased flexibility

17. What are common indications of hearing loss in older patients?

    A. Sitting close to the television

    B. Asking frequent questions

    C. Confusion and inattention

    D. Excessive sleep

18. Which of the following is *not* true regarding older people's eating habits?

    A. More calories are required as people age due to an increased metabolic rate.

    B. Decreased senses of smell and taste make food less appetizing.

    C. Many older people add salt and sugar to their food to improve its palatability.

    D. Symptoms of heartburn and indigestion occur frequently.

19. What is one reason that elderly people are at increased risk for accidents?

    A. Increased use of complementary and alternative medicine practices

    B. Heightened body response to extreme temperatures

    C. Decreased balance and coordination

    D. Increased pain sensation

20. Which of the following is an important consideration when communicating with special patient populations?

    A. Speak only to caregivers for pediatric and geriatric patients because they are responsible for making medical decisions.

    B. Greet a visually impaired person by first touching his or her hand or arm.

    C. Maintain a professional relationship with patients by not asking about their personal life experiences or anxieties.

    D. When speaking to a hearing-impaired patient, face him or her and use clear, well-enunciated words.

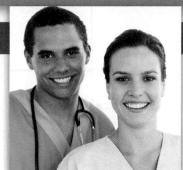

Externship and the Job Search

OBJECTIVES

After reading this chapter, you will be able to:

- Define the term externship.
- Understand externship prerequisites.
- Understand how the externship placement process works.
- Understand the value of a résumé and its role in the job-search process.
- Identify the steps involved in job analysis and research.
- Learn and distinguish accomplishment statements.
- Differentiate chronological, functional, and targeted résumés.
- Identify the purpose and content of a cover letter.
- Demonstrate effective ways to anticipate and respond to an interviewer's questions.
- Describe appropriate overall appearance and dress for an interview.
- Identify and describe the benefits of writing a follow-up letter.
- Understand professionalism as it relates to employment strategies.

KEY TERMS

Accomplishment
    statement
Behavioral interview
    questions
Benefits
Career objective
Chronological résumé
Constructive criticism

Cover letter
Criminal history and
    background check
Drug screen
Employment agency
Employment screening
Externship
Final evaluation

Follow-up letter
Full-time employee
Functional résumé
Gross pay
Interview
Job application
Long-term goals
Net pay

Networking	Professional	Screening interview
Official transcripts	development	Short-term goals
Part-time employee	Professionalism	Site director
Perks	Protocol	Targeted résumé
Portfolio	Reference	Traditional interview
Preceptor	Résumé	questions
	Role model	

Chapter Overview

An externship is a position in which a student applies skills learned with the guidance and supervision of a practicing healthcare provider. Externships involve working on site in a healthcare setting while still enrolled as a student, giving students the opportunity to apply skills learned in their training while under the supervision of other healthcare professionals in real-life scenarios with patients. Externships also give medical assistants firsthand knowledge of how other team members work together to provide superior patient care by using best practices throughout the day.

Your externship experience is probably the most important aspect of your education. If you perform well, your experience could result in an employment recommendation or even a job offer after you graduate.

Upon graduation, it will be time to find a job. An important part of your job search is developing a strong résumé. Networking with people in your field is also crucial. Regardless of where you apply for a job after graduation, any information you submit with an application for employment, either online or in writing, should not be embellished or false. If you are found to have lied on an employment application, it could be cause for automatic dismissal during your employment.

When interviewing for a job, your appearance is very important. Remember that you are selling yourself and putting your best foot forward. If you look sloppy and unpolished, you will more than likely be seen as unprofessional and not be taken seriously during the interview. Discriminatory topics that should be avoided during an interview include a candidate's age, race, ethnicity, religious beliefs, and political beliefs; marital status, number and age of children, and pregnancies; and lifestyle preferences (heterosexual, homosexual, bisexual, transsexual). As a candidate, you should be aware of these and have appropriate responses planned if asked.

Whatever path you choose in medical assisting, make sure you keep your skills sharp as new advancements are made in the field. Medicine is always changing and advancing. Keeping your skills up to date shows that you are a true professional.

Externships

Prior to starting your career as a medical assistant, you must meet eligibility requirements to be placed in an externship in an actual healthcare setting. An **externship** is a position in which a student applies skills learned with the guidance and supervision of a practicing healthcare provider—usually another medical assistant with years of experience. Externships are not paid positions; students in externships are meant to observe and apply their skills, not replace other employees or assume their job responsibilities. Although the experience is not paid, many externs find gainful employment at the end of their externship if a position is available and the student showed exemplary performance.

The United States Department of Labor's *Outlook Handbook, 2010–2011 Edition* projects that the medical assisting field will grow much faster than average for employment in the 2010–2020 decade. Growth is expected to be approximately 31 percent or higher. The job market for medical assistants—62 percent of whom will work in physician offices—is expected to be excellent. This is partly due to the aging baby-boomer population requiring preventive service by physicians.

What Is an Externship and Why Is It Necessary?

An externship is an unpaid, real-life learning experience. For medical assistants, externships involve working on site in a healthcare setting while still enrolled as a student. During your externship, you apply the skills you have learned in your formal training. It is a time to also observe the skills of others, learn how the medical team works as a unit, develop new skills, and gain important experience.

During your time as an externship student, you will be exposed to many different procedures, policies, and issues that may have been discussed only in theory during your education. Many externship program directors require students to keep an ongoing journal of their activities and observations for discussion. This not only helps the student but also gives feedback to the school in seeing the medical site through students' eyes.

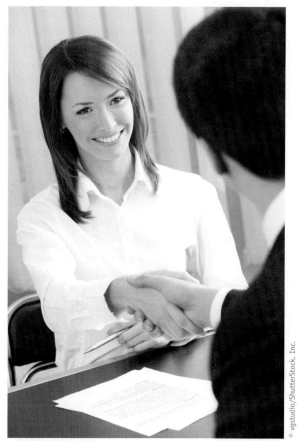

Many externs find gainful employment at the end of their externship if a position is available and the student has had exemplary performance.

Many externship sites hire students after the completion of their hours. If you perform well, you may well receive a positive employment recommendation or even be offered employment if there is an opening for an entry-level medical assistant.

Although this training is not paid, many employers may see your externship as a "working interview." For the hours you attend your externship, employers are going to be watching your performance, your professionalism, and how you fit in the culture of their practice.

Before Your Externship

You have received countless hours of practical instruction and read a wide variety of materials to prepare you for your career as a medical assistant. Now it's time to apply those skills.

Before you begin your externship, you may require clearance with a **criminal history and background check**, which is a review of legal records to determine whether you have been convicted of any crimes. You may also be asked to undergo a **drug screen**, which is a test performed to detect drug use. Drug screens can involve the use of blood, hair, or urine. This is required by many medical offices and hospitals as part of employment screening. **Employment screening** is the process of investigating the background of a potential employee. It is commonly used to verify the accuracy of an applicant's claims and to discover any possible criminal history or employers' negative sanctions. If you feel you may not be able to pass a background check or drug screen, this should be discussed with your externship coordinator prior to your assignment.

In order for you to work in most clinical settings, most practices and programs will also require you to be vaccinated for hepatitis B (or require you to sign a waiver form), mumps, rubella, varicella, measles, tetanus, diphtheria, and pertussis. You also may be required to have a physical and obtain a test for tuberculosis (TB).

Many externship sites invite students to attend a preexternship interview and to meet others prior to starting. This is usually done first with the site director. The **site director** is the person responsible for your assignment at the externship site as well as the person who acts as your manager throughout your externship. Most site directors are practice managers for the medical practice itself. They might be involved in the planning of your experience, but may not see or work with you every day. Instead, you may be assigned to an externship supervisor, who may work with you more on a daily basis.

Your preexternship interview is normally when the site director reviews scheduled hours, discusses your start date and the dress codes, introduces you to the preceptor, and conveys any other detailed information that may help you become more comfortable on your first day of work. A **preceptor** is an instructor, an expert, or a specialist, such as a physician, who gives practical experience and training to a student, especially of medicine or nursing. Be prepared to answer questions about or demonstrate skills essential to the work of a medical assistant.

Before your preexternship interview, it's a good idea to do some research on your assigned site, learning about the specialty, the physicians, and their practice. This is easily done by looking up the practice's website. You will also want to make sure you know where the practice is located. If possible, drive to the practice one or two days prior to your first day to make sure you have the right location. On your first day, arrive at least 15 minutes before your scheduled start time; this will help you feel more at ease and prevent you from appearing unprepared.

Other than passing your clinical medical assisting classes, one of the most important requirements prior to graduating is to successfully complete an externship in a healthcare setting. It should not be taken lightly. View it as a potential stepping stone in your career.

It's Not Wrong, It's Just "Different"

Keep in mind during your externship that you are still a student, there to perfect your skills and learn from others who are also in your chosen profession. Remember: You do not have all the answers. Do not act as though you know everything there is to know about medical assisting. Remain humble and know your place. Many preceptors are chosen by their site directors to work with students because of their expertise and willingness to help and train students just like you.

During your education and training, you were shown the standards according to your school on how to perform certain procedures and tasks. Often, students going through similar training elsewhere will have been shown different techniques or will have learned other techniques on the job to obtain the same results. This doesn't mean they are "wrong." Never correct a peer, your preceptor, or a site supervisor on a procedure or task that you have observed them doing in front of the patient. The statements "That's not how we were taught to do that" and "You're doing that wrong" should never be used when you are observing or receiving instructions to complete a task. It is much better to keep an open mind and learn from others than to feel that your training is the only *right* way.

Keeping It Professional at Your Externship

At your internship, you are an ambassador of your school. How you act and how you are perceived reflects back on you and your school. The site will more than likely have office policies and procedures—also referred to as **protocol**—that will dictate how employees are to handle tasks and procedures. For example, some practices may dictate that employees have their cell phones turned off during working hours or restrict food or coffee from certain work areas. As an extern, you may also be asked to sign a confidentiality statement for HIPAA purposes to protect patients' privacy during your observation at the site.

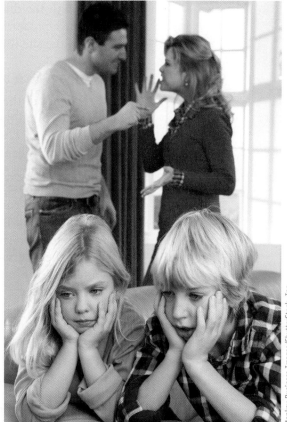

Avoiding the Use of Unprofessional Language

You should never use unprofessional or foul language at your externship site. If you have a bad habit of using foul language on a regular basis, make a conscious effort to delete it from your vocabulary, especially during work hours. Your supervisor, patients, and potential employers will certainly frown upon the use of this type of language. By using it, you diminish your professionalism.

Leaving Personal Issues at Home

The saying "Check your personal problems at the door" holds true for any employee—including you as a student on your externship. If you've had a bad day at school, had a fight with a loved one, or cannot meet your financial commitments, those problems should not follow you into the site. If you come into work upset, you could easily become distracted and make very serious mistakes. Professionals keep personal issues completely away from the workplace.

The saying "Check your personal problems at the door" holds true for any employee—including you as a student on your externship.

People who allow their personal life to affect their work are seen as unprofessional and immature. You can remain friendly and professional at work without divulging all your personal and private information at the site. If you do have personal issues that need to be addressed during your workday, make an effort to speak to your site director or externship coordinator; they may offer to help you schedule some personal time to attend to urgent matters at hand.

Dealing With Patients Who Show Favoritism for Another Employee

Patients sometimes favor one employee over another. It might be as simple as a co-worker going above and beyond by opening a door or helping the patient with a medication, or someone who has seen the patient through multiple medical procedures and hospitalizations, and who knows the patient and his or her prognosis and diagnosis well. If you do have a patient who requests that "Sally" take her vital signs, do not take it personally. This is the patient's preference and should be honored if requested.

Dealing With Office Politics

As an extern, you may be placed in difficult positions at times. You are not an employee, but you will be working one on one with those who are. Some employees may not be happy working for their employer. Hopefully, they will not be assigned to supervise or monitor you. If they are, do not listen to disgruntled employees, spread rumors, get involved in office politics, or encourage gossip during your externship. By engaging with others who may see their employers in a negative light, you will place not only your externship but a possible job reference from the practice at risk.

When faced with the dilemma, simply walk away, start a new assignment, or speak to your externship coordinator. The externship coordinator may need to discuss the situation with the site director or reassign you if warranted.

The Externship Site and the Placement Process

One responsibility of the externship coordinator in your medical assisting program is to assist you in finding proper placement as an extern in a healthcare setting. By carefully matching up the student with the site, the chance for success is increased. The school will establish policies for each site, along with each student's obligations during the externship. A contract will be signed between the school and the site, with the policies and protocols established prior to each student's arrival. The site not only agrees to allow a student to observe its healthcare practices, but it promotes the student by allowing him or her to become part of the staff during the externship. As an extern, you temporarily become part of the site's healthcare team.

Of course, the externship site does want to protect the safety of its patients as well as its reputation for providing care in the community. As a student, remember that you are there to observe and enhance your skills. You cannot and should not act as an employee or speak as though you are an employee of the practice. When patients ask if you're new to the practice, you may identify yourself as such: "My name is [your name]; I am here on my medical assisting externship." If the practice or medical facility has sponsored medical assisting students in the past, many patients may accept that statement and move on. Some may be more curious and ask you about what your training involved and what plans you have for a career after graduation. How you portray yourself and your training during your externship will leave a lasting impression not only on the site, but on the patients it serves.

Many sites do not want to commit to the additional responsibility and training required for most externships. The ones that do have an understanding with the academic program that not only will their students have the skills necessary to perform the most basic tasks at an entry level during their externship (under supervision), but that students will have the initiative, professionalism, and commitment required to complete the assignment. If for some reason the student is found lacking, he or she may be dismissed and the externship canceled. If too many students from the same academic program have similar issues, the site director may refuse to sponsor students in the future. It is important to do your best work at all times during your externship.

Ensuring Excellence During Your Externship

When you are preparing to start your externship, you should treat it no differently from starting a new job, with the same level of commitment as if you were just hired for a position as a medical assistant. By treating your externship with professionalism and showing initiative throughout the assignment, your chances of receiving a good reference or even an employment offer will increase. The following are some criteria that you will want to consider and try to excel in to achieve a successful outcome and reference during your externship.

Dependability

How was your attendance record? Did you call off during your externship or continually show up late? Did you take extended breaks or lunch hours? Employers look at these to assess your dependability, especially in the beginning of their employees' orientation. Showing up late, taking extended breaks, or calling off during your externship may ruin your reputation as a dependable employee.

Professional Appearance

How you appear to your employer and others will make or break you in the medical field. Medicine is traditionally a conservative field. There is no place for multiple piercings, visible tattoos, or trendy hairstyles. By having a more conservative appearance, you will be taken more seriously by employers, staff, and patients alike. Nails should be clean, short, and well kept. Many employers do not allow any color or polish. Hair should be well groomed and away from your face—either pulled back or styled—to promote a neat and professional appearance. Your hair color should be kept as close to your natural color as possible. Makeup should be work-appropriate— not what you would wear out for an evening with friends. Perfume should be avoided during both your interview and work, as it can be unpleasant to ill patients and can cause allergic reactions in some people. Jewelry, if worn at all, should be minimal—one ear piercing, a wedding ring, or a simple necklace. (Some healthcare professionals don't wear any jewelry during work due to safety reasons.) Many employers have policies outlining appropriate jewelry and workplace appearance standards to which you may need to adhere.

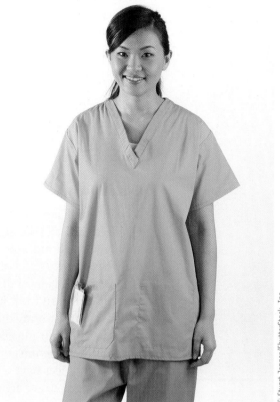

Many healthcare employers have workplace appearance standards to which you may need to adhere.

© Stuart Jenner/ShutterStock, Inc.

Personality and Professional Conduct With Patients

Were you cooperative with your coworkers, supervisors, and physicians? How well were you received by patients? Were you friendly and personable? Did you conduct yourself in a courteous and professional manner? Did you say please, thank you, and you're welcome and address your patients appropriately? How you conduct yourself around staff and patients shows your ability to work as a team player in a busy medical profession.

Working Under Stressful Conditions

Did you tend to look overwhelmed or flustered when involved in a difficult assignment? Were you able to accept assignments and use critical-thinking skills to ask questions when faced with procedures or tasks with which you were unfamiliar? How well you manage yourself under stressful situations will indicate your ability to handle more difficult assignments in the future.

Initiative and Ability to Perform Under Limited Supervision

Did you show initiative and ask for additional assignments, or did you wait to be told what to do on every assignment? Did you accept responsibility for your assignments and finish your duties in the assigned time, or were you found to be sitting around or dawdling with your assignment? When you show initiative, your supervisors and employers will see your potential as a valuable medical staff member.

Positive Attitude and Motivation to Learn

When you were introduced to new procedures, were you motivated? Did you ask appropriate questions? Did you show eagerness and a positive attitude toward different techniques? Your attitude and motivation toward learning new procedures and techniques will show your supervisors that you are open to new teachings and learning experiences. When you are presented with an opportunity to learn something new, make sure to take advantage of enhancing and advancing your skills as much as possible.

Professional Image

Did you convey a professional image at all times, exhibiting dependability, a positive attitude, initiative, and high motivation, with professional appearance and conduct, making the very best impression that you could make with your externship? Were you a model student?

Evaluations in Your Externship

As part of the agreement between the school and the site, the site will be required to give feedback on your skills to your externship coordinator as well as to you. Your site supervisor will monitor your progress. Staff will be assigned to work with you on a daily basis, letting you observe them and practice your skills at the same time. If there is an issue with any skills, these should be addressed and handled immediately so the student can learn from his or her mistake. As a student, if you note that a mistake is made, you must immediately bring it to your preceptor's or physician's attention. Do not cover up your mistake or ignore it. It is very important that you be truthful about how or when the mistake was made; a patient's care and health may be at risk. Most medical practices have a protocol to follow depending on the severity of the error. You will also need to report this to your program director in case there is any follow-up or documentation required.

As the student, you must be open to constructive criticism and remain calm when corrected. **Constructive criticism** is useful criticism or advice given to help or improve something, often with possible solutions shared. Of course, this process should be done in private, away from patients and other staff members unless the patient's safety overrides confidentiality concerns.

The preceptor and site director will be required to perform periodic written evaluations on your performance during the externship. You will be evaluated on your appearance, attitude, maturity, dependability, initiative, interpersonal skills, and ability to perform clinical tasks.

Finishing Your Externship

When your time at your externship is finished, you will likely have a **final evaluation**, usually given by your site supervisor or preceptor, to review your overall experience. If you receive good marks, you may be offered a letter of reference from the site director. Often, externship students will also be offered a position upon graduation or called when positions open up after their externship. As someone who is familiar with the staff, the patients, and the equipment, you make a very good candidate—someone who could fit in very easily if an opening should occur. Make sure your site director has all your contact information in case he or she wants to contact you about employment in the future. If your externship site is not someplace you would like to work in the future, a simple reference letter from the site director is appropriate.

If you have made friends at the site, be sure to keep in contact with them professionally. Sometimes, employees will be the first to find out about openings in different settings. Within a week of ending your externship, a handwritten letter or thank-you note should be sent to the site, thanking them personally for allowing you to be a part of their healthcare team as an extern student.

Your Résumé and Its Role in the Job Search

A **résumé**, also called a curriculum vitae (CV), is a document that summarizes your job qualifications. Your résumé is meant to sell you as a potential candidate and represents the first impression you will make on a potential employer, who has more than likely never met you personally. A great résumé will open many doors for job candidates, while a poor résumé will hinder even the best candidate's chances of finding gainful employment.

If you have kept in contact with your externship host, you may also want to contact that person and ask if you can keep your résumé on file there or if they know of anyone who is currently looking for new hires. Often, practice managers network with other practice managers in the community and will know of potential job openings before they are posted.

While constructing your résumé, keep in mind that it should be a snapshot of your education and experience, and should portray you as a professional. Sloppy grammar, typing errors, and missing information or dates are easily spotted by prospective employers and recruiters. Some managers and recruiters completely dismiss résumés containing errors, never giving the individual a second thought for an initial interview. After all, if the candidate can't take the time to perfect his or her résumé, what kind of employee would he or she be for me? Many candidates ask others to review their résumé to look for glaring errors and mistakes. It's always best to have someone else check your work than to lose a potential interview over a simple mistake.

Résumés should always project a professional appearance. Here are a few points to keep in mind:

- Avoid using colored paper. Use only white or cream for a professional medical résumé.
- Keep your résumé to one page.
- Make sure no smudges, stains, or tears appear on your résumé that you will be submitting.
- Use a standard font. With many résumés now submitted online, it is suggested that you select a font such as Helvetica, Arial, Courier, or Times Roman. Avoid cursive handwriting styles, which cannot be scanned. The font size for the body text should range between 10 and 12 points and be kept consistent throughout.

Even though you may not have any official medical employment, your externship site has provided you with important experience. When seeking a professional position in your new career as a medical assistant, your résumé should highlight your most current education information and your externship experience along with any other accomplishments (leadership roles in school, scholarships, GPA average) to give a snapshot of you as a candidate for the position.

Job Research and Analysis

As a new graduate seeking employment in the field for the first time, you should do some research prior

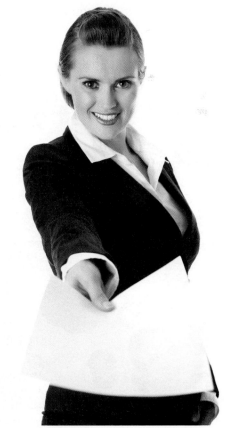

Your résumé is meant to sell you as a potential candidate and represents the first impression you will make on a potential employer.

Any information you submit with an application for employment, either online or in writing, should not be embellished or false. If you are found to have lied on an employment application, it could be cause for automatic dismissal from your employment.
© auremar/ShutterStock, Inc.

to accepting a position. Is it with a large or small employer? Does the employer offer any benefits? How long has the practice been in business? Does the business have more than one location? These are important issues a candidate might want to research prior to interviewing for a position. With the advent of the Internet, it is very easy to find much of this information about a potential employer. By googling pertinent information, you will have a better idea of what type of employer you are dealing with during the interview process. This in turn will help you make a more informed decision at the end.

Researching Employers and Seeking a Position in Your Chosen Field

By the time you are ready to start looking for a position in your chosen field, you should have had some thought as to what type of specialty or facility you would like to work in. Do you like working with children? Do you have an interest in any specialty, such as oncology or orthopedics? Take some time to consider what interested you during your training, as well as any life experiences that have piqued your interest. Maybe you enjoy senior citizens and would like to work in a geriatric or internal medicine practice. Or maybe you would enjoy working in a hospital setting, using your phlebotomy skills. Also, consider the area where you live. Many opportunities exist in communities with teaching hospitals, research programs, or large clinic affiliations. Research them by looking into different practices, clinics, and hospitals. Do you know anyone who works at any of these sites? If so, mention to them that you are in the market for a job and ask them for the name of the manager or human resource director. Networking is one of the most effective ways to gain employment, as discussed later in this chapter.

The Internet has opened many doors for employment candidates. You can use a search engine such as Google or Bing to find information about providers in your state, city, or county. You can develop a list of potential employers simply by searching and creating a set of data on your specified preferences. This will help you determine where you would like to target your employment search.

Online job-search sites such as CareerBuilder (www.careerbuilder.com), Indeed (www.indeed.com), and Monster (www.monster.com) are another great resource for job seekers. They post openings for positions by employers who pay to use their service. They are normally free to candidates. Typically, candidates are required to upload résumés that have been formatted appropriately. (See the section "Your Résumé and Its Role in the Job Search" for more information.)

Many employers enable prospective employees to apply for positions on their company websites. In this case, candidates may

© Luba V. Nel/ShutterStock, Inc.

You can generate opportunities for yourself by networking with other healthcare professionals. Keep in touch with your contacts, letting them know you are seeking employment and ensuring they have your updated contact information.

need to answer questions about their personal and employment history and agree to background, nicotine, and drug testing.

> Often, healthcare professionals will hear of new opportunities before those opportunities are advertised, making it inside information to a candidate like you and increasing your chances for an interview.
> © auremar/ShutterStock, Inc.

Some employers continue with the traditional posting of openings through local newspapers to attract candidates. Although this is becoming less standard, you should not dismiss the prospect of applying in response to an advertisement in the newspaper. Many employers obtain a post office (PO) box to retain anonymity and to avoid countless phone calls and questions from the candidates regarding the opportunity. For the same reason, many others list only an email or fax number to apply, making it anonymous on the employer's end.

Employment agencies offer another route for job seekers. An **employment agency** is an agency that finds people to fill particular jobs or finds jobs for unemployed people. With employment agencies, there is usually a fee involved, either for the candidate or for the employer associated with placement. If you deal with any of these companies, exercise extreme caution. Do not pay any fee prior to obtaining a position, and *never* pay a fee for just an interview.

Networking and the Benefits of Maintaining Connections Within Your Field

During your externship (and even before), you will meet other healthcare professionals who will have some impact on your training and career in medical assisting. Your instructors, your site director, and your supervisor, along with the employees and physicians at your externship site, are excellent connections in the field. By establishing a positive professional relationship with these individuals prior to seeking employment, you will have made contacts who may prove very helpful in the future for your job search.

Networking is connecting with people who can be helpful professionally, especially in finding a position or attempting to advance into another job. When you network, you generate new opportunities for yourself. Be sure to keep in touch with these contacts, letting them know you are seeking either full-time or part-time employment, and making sure they have all of your updated contact information in case they hear of an opportunity in which you may be interested.

In addition to networking in the "real world," you can also network online. Statistics show that 80% of positions are filled through networking contacts, and 65% of adults in a 2011 Pew Research study stated that they use social networking sites such as Twitter, Facebook, and LinkedIn to expand their network. Obviously, this is a number that cannot be ignored.

What Would You Do?

You have just been hired in a new practice. You are making friends quickly and enjoy your work. A coworker asks if you are on Facebook. She wants to become "friends" on the site. You do have a Facebook account, but it is mainly for keeping in touch with friends from high school and college. You have firsthand knowledge that the coworker is also "friends" with the lead physician and the office manager, whom you like, but with whom you do not associate. You are faced with the dilemma of "friending" this coworker on Facebook or keeping your private life private. What would you do?

© NorthGeorgiaMedia/ShutterStock, Inc.

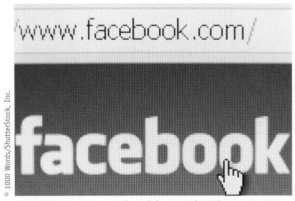

Segregate your personal social network and your professional social network, and use appropriate settings to limit who can see your posts.

Although there are many ways that you as a job candidate can use the Internet as a tool, you must be aware that the Internet can also be used against you. Many employers use a search engine to research potential candidates in order to find behind-the-scenes information that isn't available on a résumé. So, for example, the social network profile you established during high school or college, which might contain comments and pictures that aren't necessarily "professional," may be frowned upon by a potential employer. As long as you post anything to a public networking site, remember that it will forever be connected to you, and is not necessarily considered private. A good rule of thumb is to ask yourself, "Would my parents approve?" You are a professional, and your social networking sites should reflect your professional status. If you must keep up with your friends on a regular basis, segregate your personal social network (such as Facebook) and professional social network (such as LinkedIn) and use appropriate settings to limit who can see your posts (private/friends/connections only). Do not post professional information on your social page or social information on your professional page.

Résumés and Various Formats

In general, your résumé should be a one-page summary of your experience and accomplishments. As you develop your résumé, here are a few points to keep in mind:

- Use clear, concise, and positive statements in your résumé to portray yourself as a confident candidate.
- If the experience you are citing in your résumé occurred more than 10 years ago, you may need to summarize it. If it is not relevant to your current position, leave it off completely.
- Use a 1- to 1.5-inch margin on all four sides of the page to create a frame.
- Capitalize all major headings.
- Use single spacing between lines and double spacing when separating sections.
- When choosing your stationery, find a high-quality bond paper with a weight between 16 and 25 pounds. When you use a higher weight of paper, the résumé will look more professional and will show better when printed. Buff or ivory paper is recommended, with matching envelopes to distinguish your résumé from all the others.

There are three major styles of résumés, each with their own advantages and disadvantages: chronological résumés, functional résumés, and targeted résumés. When choosing a résumé format, you should choose the style that best reflects your strengths, abilities, and accomplishments.

Chronological Résumés

Chronological résumés are the most common. In a chronological résumé, the most recent information is the first thing the reader sees.

A chronological résumé is ideal if:

- You are currently seeking a position in the same field as your prior job.
- Your job history shows that you have had increased growth and professional development.

- Your previous position was in a relevant field such as healthcare, where employers have a higher interest of hiring employees already in the field.
- You held an impressive title at your previous positions.

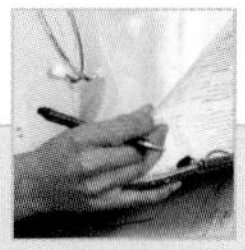

A chronological résumé might *not* be the way to go if:

You may only have 10 seconds or less to impress your prospective employer. If your recent education is your best professional feature, list this information first. If you are stronger in the experience side, then the experience should be listed at the top, followed by your education.

© auremar/ShutterStock, Inc.

- You are in the middle of changing your career (for example, from business to medicine).
- Your work history is incomplete or sporadic.
- You are looking for your first job.
- You have been in the same position for many years.

FIGURE 20.1 shows an example of a chronological résumé.

Molly Ann Maryweather, CMA (AAMA)
12345 Smith Street
Centerville, Ohio 44675
Home: 330-555-1212 Cell: 330-555-3333
Email: MollyCMA@lake.net

WORK EXPERIENCE

October 2009–Present   CENTERVILLE PEDIATRICS
    Clinical responsibilities:
    Patient preparation
    Pediatric immunizations
    EHR experience in AllscriptsPRO
    Ordering and monitoring of medical supplies
    Patient callbacks, chart documentation
    Insurance verification and referral

May 2006–October 2009   VALLEYVIEW MEDICINE, INC.
    Front desk responsibilities:
    Scheduling of patients in NextGen system
    Charge entry, end-of-day closing
    Patient insurance verification, referrals
    Patient education and instruction procedures/hospitals
    Coordinator of physicians' personal appointments

April 2006–May 2006   VALLEYVIEW MEDICINE, INC.
    Medical Assistant Externship, 160 hours
    Administrative and clinical duties with responsibilities utilizing all medical
        assisting skills, including vital signs, patient preparation, patient instruction,
        medical and surgical asepsis, and sterile procedures

EDUCATION/CERTIFICATION

    Certified Medical Assistant (AAMA)   Certification: 268593
    Certificate in Clinical Medical Assisting, May 2006, Boston Reed College,
    Centerville, Ohio 44675

FIGURE 20.1 An example of a chronological résumé.

If you don't have any relevant work history, or you have a limited work history, your résumé will look very short in chronological format. Consider another format unless none of the others fit your needs.

Functional Résumés

A **functional résumé** highlights your accomplishments and strengths. It helps you organize these highlights in an order that supports your career objective.

A functional résumé is ideal if:

- You are attempting to change careers.
- You have work experience that can be segmented into different functional areas (clinical, administrative, supervisory, managerial, etc.).
- You are attempting to reenter the job market after an absence.
- You have had a wide variety of unrelated work experience.

A functional résumé might *not* be the way to go if:

- You need to emphasize a management growth pattern.
- You worked for a highly respected employer and you need to highlight that employer in your résumé.

FIGURE 20.2 shows an example of a functional résumé.

If you need to emphasize a highly respected employer, it will possibly be lost on the bottom part of a functional résumé. A functional résumé calls for the functions of recent employment at the beginning and does not highlight work history until the end.

Targeted Résumés

The **targeted résumé** is best when focus is needed on a clear, specific job target (such as medical assisting). The targeted résumé should contain a **career objective**, which is a statement that gives the reader a quick idea as to what type of job the professional is seeking. The career objective is usually found in a prominent place—typically at the beginning of the résumé, but sometimes at the end. By seeing these objectives, the reader can make a quick decision as to whether the practice or facility can really provide what the health professional is seeking.

A targeted résumé is ideal if:

- You have very clear expectations about your job target.
- You have had a variety of work experiences. You can list the skills gained with each experience and show how they are related to your job target.
- You are considering one area of work versus another. Varied résumés can be used for different employment opportunities (such as administrative targeted résumés versus clinically targeted résumés).
- You have little experience and are just starting your career, but you are clear about your capabilities and you know what you want.

A targeted résumé might *not* be the way to go if:

- You want to use just one résumé for several different types of applications.
- You cannot be clear about your abilities and accomplishments.

FIGURE 20.3 shows an example of a targeted résumé.

Molly Ann Maryweather, CMA (AAMA)
12345 Smith Street
Centerville, Ohio 44675
Home: 330-555-1212 Cell: 330-555-3333
Email: MollyCMA@lake.net

PRACTICE MANAGEMENT

Responsible for daily operations of practice
Headed physician recruitment and human resource management
Determined and oversaw annual budget
Managed over 20 administrative and clinical support staff
Attained collection ratio of 82% in receivables
Developed, implemented, and maintained Allscripts EHR medical record
  and PM system
Managed, maintained, and prepared materials for physicians and staff
  compliance plans, including HIPAA, OSHA, and federal and state regulations

TEACHING

Instructed medical assisting students in certificate program, including
  clinical and administrative theories and applications
Developed class syllabus and instruction materials in conjunction with
  college and NCCMA standards
Counseled students for scheduling and class selection
Served on Advisory Board for Medical Assisting Program
Coordinated student externship program with various medical practices
  and facilities

MEDICAL ASSISTING

Responsible for patient preparation, vitals
Administered pediatric and adult immunizations
EHR experience/Allscripts
Monitored and ordered medical supplies
Proctored medical assisting externship students

WORK HISTORY

2010–2012   Centerville Internal Medicine Specialists, Centerville, Ohio 44215
             Practice Manager

2008–present Centerville Community College, Centerville, Ohio 44215
             Adjunct Instructor, Medical Assisting Division

2003–2008   Valleyview Medicine, Inc., Centerville, Ohio 44215

FIGURE 20.2 An example of a functional résumé.

The targeted résumé is a relatively unusual format. Many people may not like it.

Accomplishment Statements

Accomplishment statements are specific (rather than general) descriptions of experience or tasks that you performed. These experiences or tasks are always things in which you played an active role, even if others worked with you. Accomplishment statements are located within the summary of your work experience. For example, someone who served as the project manager for developing EHR for a medical practice might include

---

Molly Ann Maryweather, CMA (AAMA)
12345 Smith Street
Centerville, Ohio 44675
Home: 330-555-1212 Cell: 330-555-3333
Email: MollyCMA@lake.net

CAREER OBJECTIVE

To obtain a position as a medical assistant in an ambulatory facility that allows use and development of clinical skills

ACHIEVEMENTS

Certified Medical Assistant (AAMA)
Certified Phlebotomist (NPA)
Certificate, Medical Assisting, Boston Reed College, San Diego, California
Experienced in providing assistance in ambulatory setting
Advanced phlebotomy skills
Familiar with both federal and state laboratory regulations as well as blood-borne pathogens and OSHA

SKILLS AND CAPABILITIES

Vital signs
Patient preparation
EKGs
Medical and surgical asepsis
Sterile procedures
Advanced phlebotomy skills, including pediatric butterfly and heelsticks

WORK HISTORY

2008–2012   Centerville Internal Medicine Specialists, Centerville, Ohio 44215
Medical Assistant, Certified Phlebotomist

2003–2008   Valleyview Medicine, Inc., Centerville, Ohio 44215
Medical Assistant

EDUCATION/CERTIFICATION

Certificate, Medical Assisting, Boston Reed College, San Diego, California
Certified Medical Assistant (AAMA)

AFFILIATIONS

American Association of Medical Assistants

FIGURE 20.3 An example of a targeted résumé.

the following accomplishment statement in his or her résumé: "Achieved 100 percent compliance in meaningful use with EHR system after overseeing implementation of system for practice of three physicians and 10 staff members. This in turn returned the federal incentive bonus of $44,000 for the year 2012."

Accomplishment statements contain verbs that convey what you did and how you did it. These often lead and help define the statement. As another example, if you previously worked a job in a fast-food chain and you were responsible for handling money and balancing a cash drawer, you could use words such as achieved, balanced, maintained, operated, or verified in an accomplishment statement. TABLE 20.1 lists verbs commonly used in accomplishment statements, which you may want to consider using to define previous job responsibilities and experience.

Table 20.1	Accomplishment Statements for Use in Résumés			
Accumulated	Achieved	Acquired	Administered	Applied
Assessed	Attained	Attended	Authorized	Balanced
Billed	Budgeted	Calculated	Changed	Charged
Charted	Collected	Composed	Contributed	Coordinated
Delivered	Developed	Directed	Documented	Educated
Established	Expanded	Experienced	Facilitated	Fulfilled
Generated	Greeted	Hired	Identified	Increased
Instructed	Introduced	Invoiced	Issued	Led
Maintained	Measured	Monitored	Negotiated	Notified
Operated	Organized	Participated	Perfected	Prepared
Processed	Produced	Promoted	Purchased	Reconciled
Recorded	Reduced	Reported	Researched	Scheduled
Selected	Summarized	Supervised	Taught	Trained

When including an accomplishment statement on your résumé, do not exaggerate or mislead the reader.

Essential Résumé Information

For potential employers to contact you about a position, they first must know how and where to reach you. You will also want to make sure that you provide them with information about your education, work experience, and skills you possess that are necessary for the job for which you are applying.

Following is essential information to be included on each résumé:

- **Contact information**—This includes your full name, credential, and address, complete with street number, city, state, and ZIP code. Also include a telephone number with area code or a number where a message can be left.
- **Email address**—If you don't already have an email address, create a professional email account. Do not use an email address such as fluffybunnyslippers@ xyz.com on your résumé or as your contact information. You will not be taken seriously. Also, do not use your current employer's email system for correspondence when seeking a new position. This is seen as being in poor taste and unprofessional.
- **Your education**—Begin with the most recent school or college you have attended. Make sure to include the name, address, and graduating date as well as indicating the diploma, certificate, or degree earned.
- **Your work experience**—List the name and address of the practices and companies for which you have worked. Even though you may not have any health-care-related work experience, you no doubt have gained some skills that may apply to your overall career objective.

According to CareerBuilder, you should omit the following information from your résumé:

- Your picture
- Interests and hobbies

Make sure you are prepared for someone to leave a work-related message on your voicemail. Cute, funny messages or messages with music may seem unprofessional, leaving potential employers with the wrong impression before they even meet you.

© auremar/ShutterStock, Inc.

- Personal attributes, such as height, weight, age, race, and religion
- References (unless requested; these can be provided at a later time)
- Detailed irrelevant job information, such as "worked at ice-cream stand during junior year of high school"
- Flair, such as crazy fonts, oddball email addresses, or unusual paper

Also avoid including negative statements. Only positive statements belong on the résumé. In particular, never speak badly about a previous employer. In addition, avoid including selfish objectives—for example, "To gain experience as a medical assistant." Instead, try using a statement that tells the employer what you will bring to the company by using your experience and skills.

Accuracy and Perfecting Your Résumé

When you are ready to distribute your résumé to prospective employers, *make sure* you check, double-check, and triple-check it for accuracy. Your bullet points should line up, a consistent font should be used throughout the document, and no spelling errors should be present on your résumé. Review your résumé for obvious mistakes, such as misspelled words. This type of mistake leads the reader to believe that the person seeking employment either doesn't know how to spell an important word in his or her field or worse that the person put his or her résumé together sloppily and did not check for spelling.

Following are some of the most common errors found on résumés:

- Typographical and grammatical errors
- Lying or exaggerating about your skills, experience, education, or credentials
- Lack of specified work experience or training
- Using objectives that don't focus on the current need of the employer
- Lack of accomplishment statements or verbs
- Not mentioning previous jobs that gave you transferrable skills
- Not highlighting accomplishments
- No credentials listed
- Photos or pictures attached or placed on résumé
- Not following the same font style throughout
- Not following the same format of month/year/day (for example, 06/12/2012 or 06-12-12) throughout the résumé

There is no room for errors on a résumé. Do not rely only on your computer's spell check; many terms common in the medical field do not exist in the database installed in most spell-check software. Asking a friend, an instructor, or someone who is well versed in grammar to proofread your résumé is always a good idea. Others will find small mistakes that your eye might miss. Keep your information consistent and make sure there are no gaps in your dates of employment unless these are explained in your cover letter.

When you are ready to distribute your résumé, *make sure* you check, double-check, and triple-check it for accuracy.

Mass-mailing your résumé, using it for all applications rather than for a specific job, is a no-no. Tailor your résumé for each job for which you apply. Try to go the extra mile and send your résumé to a person, if possible.

Cover Letters

A **cover letter** is an introductory letter sent with a résumé to a potential employer. A well-written cover letter highlights your qualifications and experience and augments the information on the résumé. It should contain a statement that reflects how your skills and experience will meet the current needs of the employer. It should also explain any gaps in your dates of employment. This letter should be no more than one page long **FIGURE 20.4** .

The letter should not just introduce you to the employer; it should also sell you by describing your interest in the position, describing your personality, containing a statement on your skills and experience and how they will relate to the position, and focusing on your career objectives and what you can bring to the company as an employee.

Following are some guidelines for cover letters:

Jane Doe, MA
123 Street, NE
San Francico, CA 55555
555-555-1212   Email: jdoe@xyz.com

June 12, 2012

Mr. Jerry Jones
ABC Medical Clinic
5555 Any Street,
Anytown, California 55555

Dear Mr. Jones:

Please accept this letter in reference to your recent posting of the full-time opportunity for a clinical medical assistant within your facility, posted in the *California Times* on June 7, 2012. I am very interested in this position.

I am a recent graduate of XYZ College and am scheduled to take my certification examination next month. During my schooling, we were taught a well-rounded curriculum that has prepared me to work as a team member in any healthcare facility. I enjoy working with patients and recently completed my externship at Dr. Donald Crystal's office in Anytown, California. I was responsible for preparing and rooming patients for examinations and all other clinical aspects of patient care during my externship. I also observed the central scheduling system and learned how to schedule, instruct, and educate patients on testing and procedures at various hospitals that Dr. Crystal referred to.

I am currently working part-time at a local retail chain, where I have worked throughout my schooling. My current employer is aware that I am seeking a full-time position in the field of medicine and can provide an excellent work reference if requested.

Please feel free to call me anytime at 555-555-1212 or email me at bboop@xyz.com for an interview at your convenience. I look forward to speaking to you.

Sincerely,

Jane Doe, MA

Enclosure (1)

FIGURE 20.4 An example of a cover letter.

What Would You Do?

You have been researching employment options for your career after graduation. After much work, you have found the perfect job. It calls for a certification as a requirement, which you are scheduled to receive but have not yet obtained. Would you still apply? How would you write your résumé and cover letter if you did apply to this job advertisement?

© NorthGeorgiaMedia/ShutterStock, Inc.

- It is best when you can address the letter using the name and title of a supervisory or management employee at the company. You may need to contact the office or department to obtain this information. If you are applying online, check the posting for a name listed, possibly at the beginning or end of the advertisement. If this information is not available to you, addressing the letter "To whom it may concern" is normally appropriate.

- Use standard letter formatting (see the sample letter shown in Figure 20.4), with a formal tone.

- Be concise, using proper grammar with no errors.

- In the first paragraph, state your reason for writing.

- The second paragraph should identify how your education, experience, and qualifications relate to the job opening.

- The last paragraph should contain a closing statement requesting a job interview and information about how and when you can be reached. Be sure to thank the recipient for his or her time and consideration.

- Use an original letter every time. Do not copy and paste cover letters. This will only make it more likely that you will make an error, which will show the employer that you do not put a full effort into your job search.

Interviews

In general terms, an **interview** is a meeting in which a job candidate and an interviewer discuss an employment opportunity with a particular organization or practice. Most interviews are planned, but they may be unplanned, prompted sometimes by the candidate dropping off a résumé or application and being asked to stay to speak to the manager. This is somewhat uncommon in the field of medicine, but not impossible. You should always be prepared for this type of surprise and always dress appropriately when entering prospective employers' worksites to leave applications or résumés.

Screening Interviews

Interviews may be conducted in person or over the telephone. Recently, phone interviews have become more prevalent due to time and financial restraints. If you are offered a phone interview, do not take this any less seriously than a traditional face-to-face interview. Often, when an employer needs to pare multiple equally qualified candidates down to just a few, they will conduct phone interviews as screening interviews. In a **screening interview**, the employer may simply want to assess your demeanor and personality, asking some general introductory questions to see if he or she should schedule you for a face-to-face interview in the future. Unless otherwise indicated, this is more than likely only one of many interviews you may have with the employer.

© Iqoncept/ShutterStock, Inc.

Most interviews are planned, but they may be unplanned, prompted sometimes by the candidate dropping off a résumé or application and being asked to stay to speak to the manager.

During these initial interviews, many candidates make mistakes such as asking inappropriate questions—for example, about the rate of pay and vacation time. You must understand that this early period of the interview process is not the time to discuss benefits. If you place too much emphasis on salary or benefits at this stage, you could be seen as someone who is only interested in the job for money, not for a solid career and position with the practice.

Preparing for a Face-to-Face Interview

When it comes to a face-to-face interview, you must prepare, prepare, and prepare some more. Here are some things you may want to consider along with some research suggestions:

- Do you have voice mail or an answering machine? Is your outgoing message professional in tone or will callers hear a cutesy, funny, or inappropriate message?
- What about your clothes? Do you have a clean, professional interview outfit on hand, or do you need to purchase items or pick them up from the dry cleaner's?
- Do you have young children? Do you have someone who is willing to watch the children on short notice for an interview?

Before you appear for a face-to-face interview, research the practice or company. The practice's or company's website is an excellent place to start. Most websites post the company's philosophy, mission, and vision statements, and give detailed information on services the company provides. Providers are normally highlighted with their training and certifications listed. You can also obtain business hours, office policies, and other information by scanning the website prior to the interview. In this way, you will be able to gain much information and form an initial opinion of the business prior to your interview.

As you research a potential employer, ask yourself the following questions:

- Does the employer seem conservative or more relaxed?
- Is there any information on the website that piques your interest?
- Are there ways for patients to communicate with the office through the Internet?

Answering some of these questions may help you prepare for the interview and have a better understanding of the practice. Remember, you are trying to determine whether this is the right employment setting for you as much as the employer is trying to determine whether you are the right fit for the practice.

When preparing for the actual interview, make it a point to organize your paperwork. Bring copies of your résumé (on professional-grade résumé paper) along with a copy of your original cover letter. Copies of your certifications, **official transcripts** from school, and proof of any additional training (CPR, first aid, etc.) should be kept in a portfolio-style binder for easy access and copying. Also, make sure you bring two forms of identification (driver's license, passport, Social Security card, identification card, etc.) for the verification process. Finally, you will want to have a list of professional references with contact information or a letter of reference to provide to your interviewer when requested. If you know the name of the person with whom you will be interviewing, be sure to include it with your materials for your reference in case you become nervous and forget. You may want to assemble a **portfolio** of your work—that is, materials representing a person's work or accomplishments collected for viewing.

Before the day of the interview, make sure you know where the interview location is and what door you will need to enter. A quick drive to the site a few days prior will enable you to gauge the time required to arrive a few minutes before your scheduled time as well as help reduce any nervousness or apprehension of getting lost. Consider what time of day you will be arriving. Will it be during rush hour? Might there be inclement weather? Do you have to park far away or wait for spaces in a parking garage? Do you have to make sitter arrangements and drop any children off prior to your interview? Are you coming from your current employer, and if so, what factors may cause an issue and delay you? Any factors that may delay your arrival should be taken into careful consideration. Make sure you get plenty of sleep the night before and eat a good meal prior to your appointment. Remember, arriving late for any interview is always seen as a negative sign by the employer and could quickly end any chances you have of securing employment.

Arriving 15 minutes prior to your interview is appropriate. Be aware that as you wait for your interview to start, others may already be observing you. Often, the manager will delay the interview to observe your behaviors before the interview. You should never bring a friend or child to an interview. Make prior arrangements to have these issues covered, and make sure you have a backup plan. Taking calls on your cell phone, playing games, or texting while you are waiting are definite negative signs for employers. Turn your cell phone off or place on vibrate before you enter the interview site. You should not take calls or make them during an interview. Following are a few additional tips:

- Review your résumé, accomplishments, and credentials while you are waiting.
- Consider what you may be asked about your résumé, accomplishments, and credentials, and run through some scenarios ahead of time.
- Prepare yourself mentally by taking deep breaths, sit up straight, and smile. This is your time to shine!

You may be asked to fill out a job application prior to meeting with the interviewer. A **job application**, also called an employment application, is a formal application in which the candidate is asked to supply demographic data about himself or herself as well as any job history and references. Be sure to take your time and answer all questions thoroughly, not leaving any gaps or missing information. If possible, refer to your résumé for dates of employment or schooling. This information should match exactly what you have listed on your résumé.

If you've been convicted of a misdemeanor (a minor offense with fine and/or short jail sentence) or a felony (a major offense with more than one year jail time as penalty), you must disclose this on your application. Most employers will conduct a criminal history and background check as part of the hiring process. Note that not all convictions will eliminate you from consideration. It depends more on the actual offense, when it occurred (possibly when a minor, etc.), and whether you have multiple offenses. If you fail to disclose this information

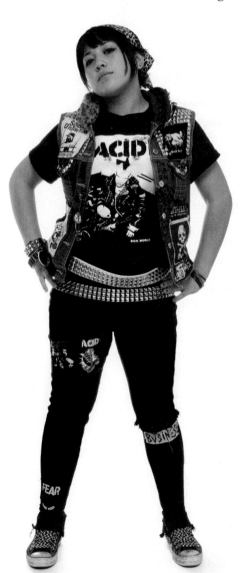

© JamesSteidl/ShutterStock, Inc.

For your job interview, do not dress provocatively or in the latest and newest fad styles. If you look as unprofessional as the model in this picture, an employer may not take you seriously.

when requested and the employer later finds out about it, you could be fired.

Dress for Success: Professional Dress and Appearance for Interviews

In an interview, your personal appearance is very important. When preparing for a face-to-face interview, you should always dress for success. Your appearance is an outward indication of who you are. Remember that you are selling yourself and putting your best foot forward. If you look sloppy and unpolished, you will more than likely be seen as unprofessional and not be taken seriously during the interview.

Following are some recommendations to consider when preparing for a face-to-face interview:

- Conservative colors such as blue, gray, black, tan, and brown are recommended.
- Wear business-dress attire—for example, a suit, a dress, dress slacks, a dress shirt, etc. If you wear a dress or skirt, it should hit just above or below the knee.
- Scrubs are not recommended for interviewing attire unless otherwise indicated.
- Clothes should be clean and pressed, without tears or rips.
- Shoes should be polished and be worn with matching socks. Sandals or shoes without socks are not recommended.
- Nails should be clean with clear or neutral polish (if any) and length appropriate for the job. In a clinical setting, many offices have policies banning long or acrylic nails because they can harbor bacteria.
- Hair should be neat, pulled away from the face, or styled conservatively.
- Makeup should be natural looking.
- Do not wear perfume.
- If you smoke, make sure the odor is not offensive. Many smokers do not realize that their hair, clothing, and skin carry the odor of cigarettes. This can be particularly offensive in the healthcare setting.
- Jewelry should be limited—small and tasteful, not flashy.
- Tongue and facial piercings, tattoos, and other body-altering practices give most employers a negative impression. If you can, remove all piercings and cover tattoos prior to appearing for the interview. A conservative one-piercing earring is acceptable.
- Avoid chewing gum or candies.
- Do not dress provocatively—for example, in mini-skirts or see-through or low-cut blouses—or in the latest and newest fad styles.

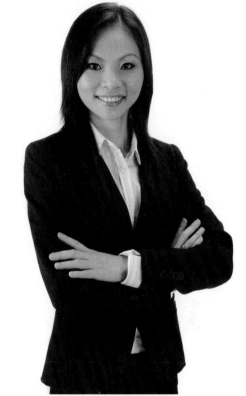

Appearing professional for interviews is imperative.

If you are coming from your current employer or externship and do not have time to change out of your scrubs into business-dress, contact your interviewer, explain the situation, and ask if this is acceptable. The mere fact that you ask this question will show that you know the proper etiquette for the interview.

Anticipating and Responding to Questions During an Interview

Your interview day is finally here. You've picked up your outfit from the dry cleaner's, you've shined your shoes, and you're ready to put your best foot forward. It is going to be a wonderful day. Congratulations; you are halfway there!

Before your interview, practice answering questions to prepare. There are **traditional interview questions**, in which the candidate is asked how he or she *would* behave in certain circumstances, and **behavioral interview questions**, in which the candidate is asked how he or she *did* behave in certain situations. Many interviewers believe the best answers are how a person actually behaved, not how they think they would behave, in a certain situation, which is one of the biggest reasons behavioral interview questions are used. Behavioral interview questions are also thought to be more probing and thought provoking.

Following are some examples of typical questions asked by interviewers, including traditional and behavioral questions:

- What do you consider your greatest strengths and weaknesses? (Traditional)
- What is a weakness you've had in the past and how did you overcome it? (Behavioral)
- What do you see yourself doing in five years? (Traditional)
- What were your goals when starting school and how successful have you been in accomplishing them? (Behavioral)
- How well do you work under pressure? (Traditional)
- Describe a stressful situation you've been in and how you handled it. (Behavioral)
- How do you think a friend or a professor would describe you?
- What qualifications do you have that make you think you would be successful in this position?
- What didn't you like about your last employer? (Trick question)
- Will you be able to work overtime occasionally?
- How would you handle following a procedure with which you do not agree?
- Why should we hire you?
- What attracted you to this practice?
- What are two or three accomplishments that have given you great satisfaction?

Some interviews are formal; others are less structured. Don't be surprised if you are faced with someone saying "Tell me about yourself" from the very beginning of the interview. This is a commonly used tactic by many to break the ice with the candidate and get to know him or her before details of the position are discussed. You should

> *If you are asked in an interview what you didn't like about your last employer, be careful. Offering too much detailed information or speaking too negatively about your past employers may cause your interviewer to view you as someone who complains too much or can't work as a team member. It never looks good to complain about past employers in an interview. If, for example, your hours were changed in your previous position after you were hired and this made you unhappy, you can say so, but stick to the facts, keep it brief, and then move on. Be aware that your words can be considered slanderous if your statements aren't true.*

© auremar/ShutterStock, Inc.

be prepared with an answer that describes yourself professionally (education, experience, career goals, etc.) as well as personally (friendly, energetic, team spirit, etc.).

Another tactic used by many employers is the "group" interview, in which two or more people may sit in on your interview and ask you questions. This can be intimidating if you are not accustomed to interviewing, but try to relax and enjoy meeting the other staff. Remember, how well you react in uncomfortable situations will indicate to your prospective employer how well you work under pressure. This is sometimes used to determine your stress level.

Here are more pointers to help you through your interview:

- Be prepared to describe the skills and abilities that you will bring to the job.
- Project to your prospective employer that you will make a positive contribution to the team as a staff member.
- Be enthusiastic and committed when speaking about the future.
- Always be sincere. Do not say anything just to please the interviewer.
- Try to recognize whether you will be a good match for the position as you learn about it.
- If you decide that the position is not what you thought it was, remain professional throughout the interview and thank the interviewer as you normally would when leaving. You may want to reapply for other positions within the same company down the road in your career.
- If applicable, tell the truth when asked why you were terminated from your last job or why you left school.
- Be prepared to answer questions about your attendance, transportation, and backup plans if something goes wrong.
- Do not talk negatively about former employers.
- Do not broach the subject of salary or benefits in early interviews unless the employer initiates the conversation. It is best to focus on the responsibilities and the job first, then on the pay and benefits.
- Answer questions thoughtfully, thinking before you answer.
- Be prepared to answer technical questions about working as a medical assistant as well as demonstrate skills related to the career.
- Project to the employer that you are interested in learning new skills and can accept change easily.
- Research the practice or the company prior to your interview so you have a basic understanding of what type of patients they treat.

Before your interview, prepare some questions that you might want to ask the prospective employer. These might include the following:

- What potential is there for advancement within the company?
- What characteristics are you looking for in an applicant?
- What are some improvements you would like me to make in this position that have not been achieved before?
- When do you expect to make a decision on your candidate?

You will also want to ask questions if your interviewer was not detailed in reviewing certain information with you. For instance, you will want to know tentative scheduled work hours, if travel is involved, the type of dress required (scrubs, company uniforms), the job description, what training is necessary, etc. If it's your turn to ask questions and the interviewer did not cover these important issues, make sure you ask them before leaving. It will be much more difficult to call back and try to track the interviewer down later to ask questions you should have asked when you were face-to-face.

Most managers who have experience with interviews should be aware of inappropriate questions posed to candidates that could be considered discriminatory. As a candidate, you should be aware of them as well, and have formed answers ahead of time if asked. For example, if asked whether you are married or have children, you might answer, "I have been in school for the past year while working full time supporting my family and feel that I have the skills to manage both very effectively."

Topics that should be avoided during an interview include the following:

- A candidate's age, race, ethnicity, religious beliefs, and political leanings
- Marital status, number and age of children, and pregnancies
- Sexual preferences (heterosexual, homosexual, bisexual, transsexual)

If asked an inappropriate question, do not act rude to the interviewer and assume it is intentional. Still, remain assertive in your answer. Your interviewing manager may be naïve or inexperienced, and likely did not mean any harm by asking the discriminatory question.

Salary Considerations and Benefits

When it is time to discuss the pay rate and benefits for the position you are considering, make sure to consider not just the hourly or yearly pay rate, but also any benefits the practice or company may offer. **Benefits** include any compensation or allowance given to an employee above the employee's regular negotiated pay. These are also sometime referred to as **perks**.

Benefits may vary depending on your position, years of experience, tenure (how long you have been with the company), and whether you are a full-time or part-time employee. A **full-time employee** traditionally works a full workweek (40 hours) while a **part-time employee** works a half workweek (20 hours). Variations on these standards may exist; some businesses consider those who work more than 35 hours per week to be full-time employees those who work 25 hours or less to be part-time employees. Either way, *any* benefit that you are offered is an *increase* in your salary and should be considered.

Examples of benefits include the following:

- Paid vacation
- Sick days and personal days
- Health, dental, and vision insurance
- Continuing education unit (CEU) allowance
- Uniform allowance
- Tuition reimbursement
- Retirement benefits
- Car and phone allowances
- Bonuses (holiday, performance)
- Shared earnings of the company's profit

For example, if your hourly rate of pay is $15 per hour and you work 80 hours per two-week pay period, your gross pay would be $1,200 for the two weeks. Your annual **gross pay**—that is, the amount of money you earn before taxes and employee-paid benefits are deducted; this is in contrast to **net pay**, which is the amount of pay remaining after all taxes and employee-paid benefits are deducted from the gross pay— would be $31,200. In this example, annual gross pay was calculated by multiplying

Table 20.2 Calculating the Total Amount of Benefits	
Benefit	**Value**
10 vacation days ($15 per hour × 8 hours per day × 10 days)	$1,200
5 sick days ($15 per hour × 8 hours per day × 5 days)	$600
8 paid holidays ($15 per hour × 8 hours per day × 8 days)	$960
Holiday bonus	$300
Uniform allowance	$200
Health insurance ($500 per month × 12 months)	$6,000
Total benefit package	**$9,260**

the hourly rate by 2,080 hours. This figure is obtained by multiplying 40 hours per week × 52 weeks per year.

Now suppose that as a full-time employee, you receive health benefits that are worth $500 per month. You also receive 10 paid vacation days, five paid sick days, and eight paid holidays per year; a $300 holiday bonus; and a $200 uniform allowance. The *total* amount of your benefits would be calculated as shown in TABLE 20.2.

Although your annual gross pay before benefits is $31,200 per year (at $15/hour × 2,080 hours), after considering your total benefit package, your real annual gross pay is $40,460 ($31,200 + $9,260 = $40,460). If you break it down to an hourly rate, rather than earning $15 per hour, you are actually earning $19.45 per hour with benefits. ($40,460 ÷ 2,080 hours per year = $19.45 per hour.)

Compare this with what you thought you were making an hour. Quite a difference, isn't it? Now think about comparing two employers, two different rates of pay, and two different benefit packages. You should be able to use the information in this example to formulate a very good idea of your annual salary and benefits.

References and Considerations in Using Them

In the workplace, a **reference** is an endorsement of a person's work ethic, skills, qualities, and ability to excel in a job. Often, as years progress, some references may change, depending on the person and how many other positions he or she has worked over a period of years. It is always best to ask a person you'd like to provide a reference for you before listing him or her on your résumé.

Work references should normally come from a superior—someone who viewed your work from a higher level. Many candidates ask for letters of recommendation from supervisors and other higher ups; that way, they have a letter in writing that gives detailed information about their work. They can give this letter to the interviewer, which helps to avoid any delays.

Your externship site is an excellent resource for a reference. Even though you were not paid for your time at the site, you did work under the physicians, practice managers, site supervisors, and other employees who may be able to vouch for your hard work and dedication during your time at your externship.

There are also personal references from people who may not have worked as your superior, but may have had some contact with you in your position. This might be a vendor with whom you worked on a special project, an accountant, an attorney, or someone who has firsthand knowledge of your work ethic and reputation.

Some students will ask for scholastic references from their instructors, who have had high levels of exposure to the students and their skills. This may be a good idea for someone who has never worked anywhere outside the home and is graduating.

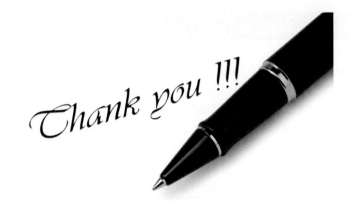

One of the biggest mistakes a candidate can make is to ace an interview and never send a follow-up letter or thank-you note.

Whatever types of references you collect, make sure you ask each person if it is okay for callers to contact them. If you have been in your current position for a while but you are about to embark on a new job search, keep your references in the loop. Make sure their contact information is accurate and that they are willing to take the time necessary for your potential employer.

After the Interview: Follow-Up Letters and Thank-You Correspondence

When it comes to proper business etiquette, ask yourself one question: What would your mother want you to do? One of the biggest mistakes a candidate can make is to ace an interview and never send a follow-up letter or a thank-you note. A **follow-up letter** briefly reviews the interview, and thanks the interviewer for his or her time, and enables the candidate to reiterate his or her interest in the position. The follow-up letter is typically the first point of contact after the interview. A thank-you note is sometimes used in more personal situations, such as if the candidate already knew the interviewer personally or had met the interviewer multiple times before. If the employer has two equally qualified candidates with equal education and experience, and has to choose between someone who sent a follow-up letter or thank-you note and someone who did not, the candidate who shows etiquette and professionalism will be chosen every time.

What Would You Do?

You are a smoker and have been planning to quit. Your prospective employer, with whom you have had a preliminary telephone interview, has a nicotine-free policy, and you may be tested prior to employment. How would you approach this situation?

© NorthGeorgiaMedia/ShutterStock, Inc.

When writing the follow-up letter, thank the person with whom you interviewed as well as any others who may have been part of your interview. Note that you enjoyed speaking to them and learning about the position and that you feel you will make an excellent employee if chosen. Reiterate your contact information and let them know you are willing to discuss any other questions they may have in the future regarding the position. Let them know that you appreciate their time and hope to hear from them soon with regard to the position. Send your thank-you note no more than one week after your interview.

While waiting for an answer, do not be tempted to call the interviewer to ask if a choice has been made. Often, the employer is scheduled to meet with other candidates and will need time to speak to each one.

You may be asked to come in for a second or third interview, depending on the candidates and the position for which you are interviewing. Often, the employer will let the candidate know that the search has been narrowed down to a certain number of candidates. Each time you interview with the same employer, make sure to obtain

Health care is a very conservative industry and centers around customer service and proper treatment of patients. Employers are looking for employees who have the proper skills to deal with the public as professionally as possible at all times.

© auremar/ShutterStock, Inc.

the name of the person with whom you are interviewing and go through the same process of sending thank-you letters as you complete additional interviews.

Employment Strategies and Professionalism

Professional medical assistants will have many opportunities available to them throughout their career. Stay open to employment in different types of settings and situations. Sometimes, after you have completed your schooling, you will find that what you thought you would like isn't what it seemed. Many medical assistants have found a special calling for a certain type of task that they never knew they would like or be particularly good at until they tried something different or outside their comfort zone. Challenging yourself, having the ability to be flexible in your tasks and thinking, and staying professional at all times will put you above the others who won't push themselves to another level.

Employment Strategies

Medical assistants are one of the most versatile healthcare professionals in the field. Some medical assistants choose an administrative path, others choose a clinical path, and still others find themselves working up the management ladder and advancing into a more responsible and challenging position. Whatever path you choose, make sure you keep your skills sharp as new advancements are made in the field. Medicine is always changing and advancing. Much of what you will learn in school is only the groundwork. As time passes, what you've learned will more than likely be replaced with new diagnostic equipment, procedures, and regulations.

Normally, most people just graduating from school have **short-term goals**, or plans for the immediate future. An example of a short-term goal would be to find a good position working as a medical assistant Monday through Friday, full time, with benefits. **Long-term goals** are larger goals that a person sets for himself or herself. For example, a long-term goal for someone just graduating from school might be to someday work as an instructor after he or she has been in the field and gained some experience.

Professional development refers to the skills and knowledge attained for both personal development and career advancement. This is a broad term, encompassing a range of people, interests, and approaches. Those who engage in professional development share a common purpose of enhancing their ability to do their work. At the heart of professional development is the individual's interest in lifelong learning and increasing his or her own skills and knowledge.

Your certification may require that you obtain continuing education units (CEUs) in order to stay current. CEUs are classes or seminars to keep training in the field current and required for most certifications to keep your certifications current. CEUs are important to help you keep up with changes in your field. Any coursework or seminars related to your field after graduation are considered continuing education. Some programs offer credits toward your recertification.

Challenging Assignments

At some point in your career, you will be challenged by an assignment with which you are not familiar or that you do not feel comfortable performing. Unless the assignment is unethical or illegal, you should rise to the challenge and accept it. Change is good. Collect as much information as possible about the assignment, your involvement and responsibilities, the deadline, and anyone else who will be assisting you (or not).

By controlling the situation and gathering all the necessary information required to complete the assignment, you will have already taken the first few important steps.

Answering some additional questions may help you complete your assignment:

- How do you organize yourself at work?
- Do you work better by yourself or in a group?
- Who is training you or helping you with the procedures if you are unfamiliar with them?
- Are there any special certifications or licensures required for this procedure?
- Is there any specific information that you will need to share with patients regarding this assignment?
- Do you have all the necessary tools for the project?
- Is there any research involved?
- Do you have the proper skills to complete this assignment?

Here are a few other points to keep in mind:

- Think of how you want to organize all the materials and data required. Sometimes, using colored folders to designate certain types of files will help you remember what information is located where. Binders will also help organize any loose papers or manuals necessary in your work.
- Create a to-do list. Also keep a list of items you've completed so that you can refer to it at a later date. Seeing items checked off your list will give you a sense of accomplishment throughout the process.
- If you feel overwhelmed, relax. Get up and walk around to clear your mind. Sometimes, just changing the scenery will help you focus when you return.
- If you are running up against a deadline and you more than likely will not complete it on time, notify your manager and ask for help. It is better to admit help is required than to let the deadline pass with nothing mentioned.

Working on a challenging assignment requires hard work, longer hours at times, and the management of stress to meet sometimes impossible deadlines. Keeping everything balanced can be very difficult. Staying organized, directed, and calm as you apply your knowledge to the project at hand will most likely see you through the roughest assignment. After it is completed, you will have a great sense of accomplishment as well as the experience to rely upon in the future.

Developing Leadership Skills

Leadership skills are important for employees who wish to advance. A leader takes pride in his or her work, performs at a high level, and continually seeks ways to improve patient and customer care. Employees who show initiative in growth and development tend to impress employers. It conveys to the employer that you are willing to put forth the additional time and effort to advance within your profession.

Here are some ways to develop your leadership skills:

- Work alongside a skilled leader and observe his or her behavior. Think about what you like about how that person handles himself or herself with others.
- Volunteer for committees at school, work, and other community organizations.
- Participate in professional organizations, school clubs, or athletics.
- Read a book or article about leadership.
- Work on improving your verbal and written communication skills, focusing on conflict resolution.

- Identify your own strengths and weaknesses and make improvements.
- Enhance your skills by taking classes.

Professionalism

Professionalism refers to the status, methods, character, or standards of a person in his or her field. Hopefully by now, you know to project a professional image, attitude, and demeanor. Much can be said for healthcare professionals who take their job seriously, show up on time, and work to complete their assignments on time without complaint.

Do you work with someone who is a true professional? Could this person be a **role model** for you? Professionalism doesn't always come to everyone. Some people see their work as just a job rather than a career. You will find, that over the years, that these people probably won't advance very quickly, if at all.

Professionalism takes a true commitment to your profession. It may mean that you stay late one evening to help a coworker who is overwhelmed with callbacks to patients without being asked. It may mean that your lunch hour sometimes runs short because there is a patient who requires immediate attention in the waiting room. It may mean that you have to put what is best for the practice ahead of what is best for an employee who you need to terminate due to lack of performance. By handling yourself as a professional under stressful circumstances, you are showing others how to react as well by using leadership qualities.

How you decide to handle yourself in your chosen profession as a medical assistant is up to you. You have the tools; now you must decide how you are going to apply them.

WRAP UP

Chapter Summary

- An externship is a position in which a student applies skills learned with the guidance and supervision of a practicing healthcare provider.

- As a prospective medical assistant, it is recommended that you complete an externship as a part of your program. Although the experience is not paid, many externs find gainful employment at the end of their externship if a position is available and the student showed exemplary performance.

- The job market for medical assistants—62 percent of whom will work in physician offices—is expected to be excellent. This is partly due to the aging baby-boomer population requiring preventive service by physicians.

- Many medical sites and hospitals require employment screening prior to hiring candidates. Employment screening is the process of investigating the background of a potential employee. It is commonly used to verify the accuracy of an applicant's claims as well as to discover any possible criminal history or employers' negative sanctions.

- The site director is the person responsible for your assignment at the externship site as well as the person who acts as your manager throughout your externship.

- During your externship, there may be techniques used on the job that are different from the ones you are used to but that obtain the same result. This doesn't mean they are wrong. *Never* correct a peer, preceptor, or site supervisor on a procedure or task that you have observed them doing in front of the patient.

- The externship site will have office policies and procedures—also referred to as protocol—that will dictate how employees are to handle tasks and procedures.

- You should never use unprofessional or foul language at your externship site. Your supervisor, patients, and potential employers will certainly frown upon the use of this type of language. By using it, you diminish your professionalism.

- The saying "Check your personal problems at the door" holds true for any employee—including you as a student on your externship. If you've had a bad day at school, had a fight with a loved one, or cannot meet your financial commitments, those problems should not follow you into the site.

- Do not listen to disgruntled employees, spread rumors, get involved in office politics, or encourage gossip during your externship.

- In the externship placement process, carefully matching the student with the site increases the chance for success. A contract will be signed between the school and the site, with the policies and protocols established prior to each student's arrival.

- To help ensure success during your externship, you should project dependability, good personal appearance and professional image, personality, professional conduct with patients, initiative, ability to work under stressful conditions, ability to perform under limited supervision, a positive attitude, and a desire to learn.

- As a student, you must be open to constructive criticism and remain calm when being corrected. Constructive criticism is useful criticism or advice given to help or improve something, often with possible solutions shared.

- Once your time at your externship has been completed, do not forget to thank everyone at your site. Often, externship students are offered a position upon graduation or called when positions open up after their externship. If you have received good performance reviews, you may also be offered a letter of reference from the site director.

- Upon or prior to graduation, research medical employers and take some time to consider what interested you during your training, as well as any life experiences that have piqued your interest. This should get you moving in the right direction as you start your job search.

- Any information you submit with an application for employment, either online or in writing, should not be embellished or false. If you are found to have lied on an employment application, it could be cause for automatic dismissal during your employment.

- A résumé is a document that summarizes your job qualifications. A great résumé will open many doors for job-seeking candidates, while a poor résumé will hinder even the best candidate's chances of finding gainful employment.

- Accomplishment statements are brief descriptions of your experience or tasks previously performed. Accomplishment statements contain verbs that give a brief description of what you did and how you did it.

- There are three main résumé formats. Chronological résumés are most commonly used. In a chronological résumé, the most recent information is the first thing the reader sees. A functional résumé highlights your accomplishments and strengths. It helps you organize these highlights in an order that supports your career objective. The targeted résumé is best when focus is needed on a clear, specific job target (such as medical assisting). The targeted résumé should contain a career objective, which is a statement that gives the reader a quick idea as to what type of job the professional is seeking.

- Networking is connecting with people who can be helpful professionally, especially in finding a position or attempting to advance into another job. It is not recommended that you post professional information on your social networking websites or social information on your professional networking websites.

- Before you appear for an interview, research the practice or company. If available, the practice's or company's website is an excellent place to start. Also, make sure you know where the interview location is and what door you will need to enter. Allow for any surprises that may happen on your interview day.

- When interviewing, your appearance is very important. Remember that you are selling yourself and putting your best foot forward. If you look sloppy and unpolished, you will

more than likely be seen as unprofessional and not be taken seriously during the interview.

- Discriminatory topics that should be avoided during an interview include a candidate's age, race, ethnicity, religious beliefs, and political beliefs; marital status, number and age of children, and pregnancies; and lifestyle preferences (heterosexual, homosexual, bisexual, transsexual). As a candidate, you should be aware of these and have appropriate responses planned if asked.

- One of the biggest mistakes a candidate can make is to ace an interview and never send a follow-up letter or a thank-you note. Make sure you send your thank-you note no more than one week after your interview.

- You may be required to obtain continuing education units (CEUs) to keep your certification current. CEUs are important to help you keep up with changes in your field.

- Whatever path you choose in medical assisting, make sure you keep your skills sharp as new advancements are made in the field. Medicine is always changing and advancing. Keeping your skills up to date shows that you are a true professional.

- At some point in your career, you will be challenged by an assignment with which you are not familiar or that you do not feel comfortable performing. Unless the assignment is unethical or illegal, you should rise to the challenge and accept it. Change is good.

- Leaders take pride in their work, perform at a high level, and continually seek ways to improve patient and customer care. Employees who show initiative in growth and development tend to impress employers. It conveys to the employer that you are willing to put forth the additional time and effort to advance within your profession.

- Professionalism takes a true commitment to your profession. How you decide to handle yourself and your chosen profession as a medical assistant is up to you.

Learning Assessment Questions

1. Which of the following describes an externship?

   A. A position in which a student applies skills learned as a volunteer

   B. A position in which a student is paid for applying skills learned in school

   C. A period of time during which an employer hires a student as a regular employee

   D. None of the above

2. What has been recommended for cell phones before and during interviews?

   A. If there is an incoming call, it is okay to take the call.

   B. Turn cell phone to off or vibrate.

   C. It is acceptable to check texts and voice mail while waiting.

   D. It doesn't matter if you have a personal cell phone. No one should be restricting its use.

3. Employment screening is the process of which of the following?

   A. Investigating the background of a potential employee's family members to discover a criminal history

   B. Investigating the background of a potential employee; commonly used to verify the accuracy of an applicant's claims and to discover any criminal history

   C. Investigating the background of an employer to discover any criminal history of the business

   D. None of the above

4. Protocol is defined as which of the following?

   A. A list of items requested by the employee for use to perform a task

   B. A list of items the manager uses to order supplies

   C. Coverage of the physician for malpractice claims

   D. The policies and procedures set by the practice

5. Which one of the following styles of dress would be considered appropriate interview attire?

   A. A nice pair of dress jeans and a sweater

   B. A pair of pants or a knee-length skirt with a solid-colored top or blouse

   C. A pair of cropped pants with flip-flops and a comfortable shirt

   D. A stylish black outfit with open-toed four-inch heels

6. Which of the following describes a behavioral interview question?

   A. It asks a candidate how he or she did behave in certain situations.

   B. It asks a candidate how he or she would behave in certain situations.

   C. It asks a candidate how he or she thinks others would behave in certain situations.

   D. It asks a candidate how he or she thinks his or her spouse would behave in certain situations.

7. When is it appropriate to correct another employee or peer while on your externship in front of another employee or patient?

   A. Sometimes

   B. Never

   C. Always

   D. Every once in a while

8. In which circumstances is unprofessional or foul language acceptable in the workplace?

   A. It is never acceptable.

   B. It's okay, as long as patients don't hear you.

   C. It can be used only in extreme situations.

   D. It is only appropriate if someone yells at you.

9. Which of the following describes a chronological résumé?

   A. It highlights your accomplishments and strengths and helps you to organize these highlights in an order that supports your career objective.

   B. The most recent information is the first thing the reader sees.

   C. It is best used when focus is needed on a clear, specific job target.

   D. The oldest information is put first on the résumé for the reader to see.

10. Which of the following describes a functional résumé?

    A. The most recent information is the first thing the reader sees.

    B. It is best used when focus is needed on a clear, specific job target.

    C. It highlights your accomplishments and strengths and helps you to organize these highlights in an order that supports your career objective.

    D. The oldest information is put first on the résumé for the reader to see.

11. Examples of discriminatory interview topics include which of the following?

    A. Who the candidate felt should have won on *American Idol*

    B. A persons' age, sex, and political leanings

    C. Where the candidate went to school and what degree he or she achieved

    D. Whether the candidate has experience using Microsoft software such as Word, Publisher, and PowerPoint

12. Which of the following describes accomplishment statements?

    A. They contain adjectives that explain how you accomplished passing your final exams.

    B. They go into great detail about what you have accomplished in life.

    C. They contain verbs that give a brief description of what you did and how you did it.

    D. They aren't necessary; only candidates with years of experience use them.

13. When in the interview process should you ask about pay and benefits?

    A. Right away, before you even find out the job description. You need to know what you are going to be paid.

    B. After the employer brings up the subject.

    C. After you start on the first day. This is when you fill out the paperwork for applications as well.

    D. After you have worked the first few days and find out whether you like the position.

14. Why is networking so important?

    A. It is one of the most effective ways a candidate can hear about an open position before it is posted or becomes public.

    B. It's not really important.

    C. It guarantees a better wage and benefits when applying for a position.

    D. It helps you attract more friends on Facebook and Twitter so that you can talk to them while working.

15. Why are continuing education credits (CEUs) important to the medical assistant?

    A. If you are terminated, you can request to be reimbursed for your CEUs by your ex-employer.

    B. The field of medicine changes constantly. Keeping your skills up shows that you are a true professional.

    C. The more CEUs you accumulate, the quicker you will be able to take your registered nurse examination.

    D. None of the above

Answer Key

CHAPTER 1

1. D	6. A	11. C	16. C
2. B	7. C	12. C	17. A
3. B	8. D	13. C	18. A
4. B	9. A	14. C	19. A
5. B	10. D	15. D	20. C

CHAPTER 2

1. B	7. A	13. B	19. B
2. A	8. D	14. C	20. B
3. D	9. B	15. A	21. B
4. C	10. C	16. C	22. C
5. B	11. D	17. B	23. B
6. D	12. A	18. D	

CHAPTER 3

1. B	7. A	13. C	19. C
2. A	8. B	14. D	20. C
3. D	9. D	15. A	21. A-1; B-4;
4. B	10. C	16. D	C-7; D-2;
5. B	11. A	17. D	E-3; F-10;
6. D	12. B	18. B	G-8; H-5;
			I-9; J-6

CHAPTER 4

1. C	5. B	9. B	13. B
2. B	6. B	10. D	14. A
3. B	7. A	11. A	15. A
4. A	8. A	12. B	

CHAPTER 5

1. B	6. B	11. A	16. D
2. A	7. A	12. B	17. C
3. C	8. B	13. D	18. A
4. D	9. D	14. A	19. D
5. B	10. C	15. A	20. A

CHAPTER 6

1. B	6. C	11. D	16. A
2. D	7. A	12. A	17. C
3. A	8. B	13. C	18. D
4. B	9. D	14. B	19. B
5. D	10. C	15. D	20. A

CHAPTER 7

1. C	7. D	13. A-5; B-4; C-3; D-6; E-1; F-2	17. C
2. B	8. B		18. A
3. A	9. D		19. C
4. C	10. B	14. B	20. D
5. B	11. A	15. B	
6. A	12. C	16. A	

CHAPTER 8

1. C	6. B	11. C	16. B
2. B	7. C	12. B	17. C
3. B	8. A	13. D	18. A
4. D	9. C	14. B	19. C
5. A	10. B	15. A	20. D

CHAPTER 9

1. A	7. C	13. C	19. B
2. C	8. A	14. A	20. C
3. B	9. B	15. D	21. B
4. C	10. D	16. A	22. A
5. D	11. A	17. C	23. C
6. A	12. C	18. D	

CHAPTER 10

1. B	6. C	11. D	16. D
2. C	7. C	12. B	17. B
3. C	8. D	13. A	18. D
4. A	9. A	14. A	19. D
5. D	10. B	15. D	20. C

CHAPTER 11

1. D	6. D	11. C	16. B
2. A	7. A	12. D	17. D
3. B	8. D	13. B	18. A
4. B	9. D	14. D	19. D
5. D	10. D	15. C	20. A

CHAPTER 12

1. C	6. C	11. A	16. A
2. A	7. B	12. C	17. D
3. D	8. C	13. B	18. C
4. C	9. A	14. D	19. A
5. A	10. C	15. C	20. B

CHAPTER 13

1. B	6. A	11. B	16. A
2. A	7. D	12. C	17. B
3. B	8. B	13. B	18. A
4. D	9. A	14. A	19. D
5. C	10. D	15. C	20. C

CHAPTER 14

1. C	6. B	11. C	16. B
2. D	7. A	12. A	17. D
3. C	8. A	13. A	18. A
4. A	9. B	14. D	19. C
5. C	10. D	15. C	20. C

CHAPTER 15

1. C	6. C	11. C	16. D
2. B	7. D	12. A	17. A
3. A	8. A	13. C	18. C
4. D	9. B	14. A	19. D
5. B	10. D	15. B	20. B

CHAPTER 16

1. C	6. D	11. A	16. A
2. D	7. D	12. B	17. D
3. B	8. A	13. D	18. B
4. B	9. C	14. C	19. C
5. A	10. B	15. D	20. D

CHAPTER 17

1. A	6. C	11. A	16. B
2. C	7. B	12. D	17. C
3. B	8. C	13. B	18. B
4. A	9. B	14. C	19. D
5. D	10. D	15. A	20. C

CHAPTER 18

1. C	6. C	11. B	16. D
2. A	7. A	12. D	17. B
3. B	8. D	13. A	18. D
4. A	9. B	14. A	19. C
5. D	10. C	15. B	20. B

CHAPTER 19

1. C	6. A	11. A	16. A
2. D	7. D	12. C	17. C
3. A	8. C	13. D	18. A
4. C	9. A	14. C	19. C
5. D	10. B	15. B	20. D

CHAPTER 20

1. A	5. B	9. B	13. B
2. B	6. A	10. C	14. A
3. B	7. B	11. B	15. B
4. D	8. A	12. C	

Glossary

A

Abortion—The loss of a pregnancy prior to 20 weeks' gestation.

Absorption—The process by which a drug enters or passes through natural body barriers such as the skin, intestines, stomach, or blood-brain barrier and enters the bloodstream.

Abstinence—Refraining from sexual activity.

Accomplishment statement—A brief description of your experience or tasks previously performed. Accomplishment statements contain verbs to convey what you did and how you did it.

Accreditation—A principle that establishes creditability through formal education with a determined standard.

Accrediting Bureau of Health Education Schools (ABHES)—ABHES is recognized by the United States Secretary of Education for the accreditation of private, postsecondary institutions in the United States offering predominantly allied health education programs and the programmatic accreditation of medical assistant, medical laboratory technician, and surgical technology programs leading to a certificate, diploma, associate of applied science, associate of occupational science, academic associate degree, or baccalaureate degree, including those offered via distance education.

Acculturation—A process by which we learn the rules and values of our society.

Accuracy—The extent of how well a measurement represents the true value.

Acidosis—A condition in which the pH of the blood is below 7.35.

Acquired immunodeficiency syndrome (AIDS)—A disorder of the immune system caused by the human immunodeficiency virus.

Acromegaly—A condition that results from the excess production of growth hormone in adults.

Act—A law passed at the federal level through Congress.

Action potential—A change in the electrical membrane potential of a cell that leads to contraction.

Active listening—A process in which the receiver rewords the original message to verify the message from the sender.

Activities of daily living (ADLs)—Normal self-care functions that people perform in order to live.

Acute renal failure (ARF)—The sudden loss of kidney function.

Acute stage—The stage of infectious disease in which the disease processes reach their peak.

Addison's disease—A condition that results from the decreased production of hormones in the adrenal cortex.

Addition—The process of adding numbers together to obtain a sum.

Adenohypophysis—The anterior portion of the pituitary gland.

Adipose tissue—Fatty tissue that is located in the innermost layer of skin and provides cushioning for the body, maintains food reserves, and facilitates temperature control.

Administrative laws—Laws and legal rules that govern the administration and regulation of both state and federal agencies.

Adolescents—Individuals aged 12 to 18 years.

Adrenal cortex—The outer portion of the adrenal gland that manufactures corticosteroids.

Adrenal glands—A small, triangular gland located above each kidney.

Adrenal medulla—The inner portion of the adrenal gland that produces epinephrine and norepinephrine.

Adrenocorticotropic hormone (ACTH)—A hormone produced by the pituitary gland that stimulates the adrenal cortex to produce hormones.

Advance beneficiary notice (ABN)—A notification of the costs of services that are not covered by Medicare for which a patient will be responsible for paying.

Advance directives—Developed to inform patients of their rights to refuse treatment, choose their advance directives under the state law, and choose the discontinuation of life-sustaining equipment or the refusal of it altogether.

Aerobes—Microorganisms that need oxygen to thrive.

Afebrile—The absence of a fever; a normal body temperature.

Afferent system—The part of the peripheral nervous system that includes all the nerves and sense organs.

Afterbirth—The delivery of the placenta and other membranes after the birth of a baby.

Age-related macular degeneration (AMD)—A disease that affects the macula of the eye and causes loss of central vision.

Airborne precautions—Measures that apply to patients known or suspected to be infected with a pathogen that can be spread via airborne transmission.

Airborne transmission—A route by which infections can be transmitted indirectly via tiny droplets of vapor in the air.

Albuminuria—Albumin in the urine.

Alimentary canal—The continuous chain of organs from the mouth to the anus that makes up the digestive system.

Alkalosis—A condition in which the pH of the blood is above 7.45.

Allergic reaction—A local or general response of the immune system to an antigen.

Alveoli—Air sacs in the lungs where gas exchange occurs.

Alzheimer's disease—A degenerative disorder of the brain that leads to loss of brain function.

Ambulation—Walking.

Amenorrhea—The absence of menstruation in a woman who has been menstruating.

American Association of Medical Assistants (AAMA)—A membership organization that promotes the professional identity and stature of the medical assisting profession.

American Medical Technologist (AMT)—Provides registration for medical assistants. A nonprofit certification agency and professional membership association representing more than 60,000 individuals in allied health care.

Amniocentesis—A medical procedure that removes a small amount of amniotic fluid from the sac that surrounds the baby in the uterus.

Amnion—The inner membrane of the amniotic sac.

Amniotic fluid—The liquid in which the embryo and fetus are sustained during pregnancy.

Amniotic sac—A tough, transparent set of membranes that envelope a developing embryo and fetus during pregnancy.

Amphiarthrosis—A joint that allows very limited movement between the bones it connects; also called a cartilaginous joint.

Ampule—A glass container with a single dose of medication or active ingredient.

Amylase enzymes—Enzymes that break down polysaccharides.

Amyotrophic lateral sclerosis (ALS)—Also known as Lou Gehrig's disease. A progressive neurological disease that attacks the neurons that control voluntary muscles.

Anaerobes—Microorganisms that do not need oxygen or only a little oxygen to grow.

Anal canal—The portion of the colon that connects the rectum to the anus.

Anaphylactic reaction—A severe allergic response to an allergen. This can be an immediate, life-threatening reaction that involves respiratory distress (difficulty breathing) followed by shock.

Anaphylaxis—An extreme, often life-threatening, allergic reaction.

Anatomic position—The position of the body when standing erect, with arms down at the sides and the palms of hands facing forward.

Anatomy—The study of the structures of the human body and its organs.

Androgens—A type of corticosteroid; responsible for male sex characteristics.

Aneroid sphygmomanometer—A manual device for measuring blood pressure that consists of an inflatable cuff attached to rubber tubing and a dial that indicates pressure.

Angina pectoris—Chest pain caused by a decreased oxygen supply to the heart.

Anion—A negatively charged ion.

Annual premium—The amount an individual pays to purchase health insurance each year.

Antecubital space—The area located anterior to the elbow on the inside of the arm; the preferred location for venipuncture.

Anterior (ventral)—The anatomic directional term that describes front.

Antibody—A Y-shaped protein that identifies and neutralizes pathogens.

Antidiuretic hormone (ADH)—A hormone produced by the pituitary gland that facilitates water reabsorption in the kidneys.

Antigen—Any substance or pathogen that elicits the immune system to produce an antibody.

Antineoplastic drugs—Anticancer drugs that inhibit or prevent the development of neoplasms.

Antitussive—Cough suppressant.

Anus—The opening in the body through which waste is expelled from the digestive tract.

Aorta—The largest artery in the body.

Aortic valve—One of four valves in the heart; separates the left ventricle from the aorta.

Apocrine glands—Sweat glands located deep in the skin that produce sweat containing water and organic material.

Aponeurosis—A flat band of connective tissue that connects muscle to bone.

Apothecary system of measurement—An outdated system of measurement that consists of the grain to measure weight and a quart, pint, fluid ounce, dram, and minim to measure volume.

Appendectomy—The surgical removal of the appendix.

Appendicitis—The acute inflammation of the appendix.

Appendicular skeleton—One of two divisions of the human skeleton; composed of 126 bones, including the pectoral girdle, the upper limbs, the pelvic girdle, and the lower limbs.

Arachnoid—The middle layer of connective tissue that is part of the meninges.

Areola—The darker area around the nipple of the breast.

Arrhythmia—A variation in normal heart rate or rhythm.

Arterial blood gases—Tests to determine the presence of oxygen and carbon dioxide in the blood.

Arteries—The vessels that carry oxygenated blood away from the heart to systemic circulation.

Arterioles—The smallest vessels in the arterial system.

Arthroscope—A small instrument containing a lens and illuminating and magnifying systems; used during arthroscopy procedures.

Arthroscopy—An endoscopic procedure that allows for the visualization of a joint.

Articulation—The point at which two bones meet; also called a joint.

Artifact—Any abnormal appearance or interference on an ECG recording.

Ascending colon—The portion of the colon that begins after the cecum and extends up the right side of the abdomen.

Ascites—Fluid retention in the abdomen.

Asepsis—The absence of infection-causing organisms.

Aseptic technique—Practices or procedures performed under sterile conditions.

Assault—Intentional act by a person who threatens bodily harm or attempts to create injury through force, strike, or harm.

Assistive devices—Devices to help people walk or function independently.

Asthma—A chronic inflammatory condition of the airways.

Atherosclerosis—A buildup of fatty deposits in the blood vessels.

Atrioventricular (AV) node—The part of the heart that receives the electrical impulse from the SA node.

Atrioventricular (AV) valves—Two valves in the heart that separate the atria from the ventricles.

Audiometer—An instrument that measures the frequency of sound waves and the ability of the patient to hear various frequencies of sound waves.

Augmented leads—The measurement of the voltage difference between one electrode and a point midway between two other electrodes in an ECG.

Auscultation—An examination technique that involves listening to body sounds to evaluate a patient.

Auscultory gap—A phenomenon in which Korotkoff sounds disappear and reappear at a lower pressure.

Autonomic nervous system—The part of the nervous system that controls involuntary functions, such as breathing, digestion, widening or narrowing of the arteries, and beating of the heart.

Autonomy—In medical ethics, autonomy allows the patient to self-govern and choose his or her course of action, making informed decisions regarding his or her health care and making free and unforced choices.

Axial plane (transverse plane)—A horizontal plane that divides the body or any of its parts into upper and lower parts.

Axial skeleton—One of two divisions of the human skeleton; composed of 80 bones, including the skull and associated bones, the thoracic cage, and the vertebral column.

Axillary crutches—Crutches that fit under a patient's arms.

Axons—Nerve fiber that conducts electrical impulses away from the neuron's cell body.

B

Bacteria—Microorganisms that have only one cell.

Bacteriuria—Bacteria in the urine.

Basal cell carcinoma (BCC)—A cancerous skin lesion that rarely metastasizes.

Basal metabolic rate (BMR)—The level of energy required for the body's activities while at rest.

Basic cardiac life support (BCLS) skills—Basic cardiac life support training enables a caregiver to recognize several life-threatening emergencies, provide CPR to victims of all ages, use an AED, and relieve choking in a safe, timely, and effective manner.

Battery—An action that causes bodily harm. An intentional tort.

Beers criteria—A list of drugs that should be avoided in elderly patients due to the risk of side effects and inappropriate use.

Behavioral interview questions—Questions asked to determine how the interviewee behaved in a certain situation.

Bell's palsy—A disorder of the nerve that controls movement of the facial muscles. Damage to the seventh cranial nerve (facial nerve), the nerve that controls the movement of the muscles of the face, causes muscle weakness or paralysis of facial muscles.

Beneficence—Achieved for the patient when the procedure or test being recommended has focused the intent on what is *best* for the patient.

Benefits—Any compensation or allowance given to an employee above his or her regular negotiated pay. Also known as perks.

Benign prostatic hypertrophy (BPH)—The nonmalignant enlargement of the prostate gland.

Bicuspids—Teeth located toward the back of the mouth that are used for crushing and grinding food.

Bicuspid valve—One of two atrioventricular valves in the heart; separates the left atrium from the left ventricle; also called the mitral valve.

Bile—A bitter liquid that digests fats.

Bilirubin—A pigment produced during the liver's degradation of hemoglobin.

Biohazard materials—Any infectious or dangerous bodily fluids, tissues, or other substances that pose a risk to the health or safety of humans or the environment.

Biopsy—The removal of a small piece of tissue for laboratory examination.

Bipolar leads—A measurement of the voltage difference between two electrodes in an ECG.

Blepharitis—Inflammation of the edges of the eyelids.

Blood-borne transmission—A route by which infected blood enters a susceptible host through blood or body fluids.

Blood pressure—A measurement of the force exerted on the arteries during one heartbeat.

Body language—Unconscious body movements, gestures, and facial expressions that accompany speech.

Body mass index (BMI)—A calculation used to quantify healthy body weight.

Body mechanics—The study or use of proper body form and movement to prevent injury and improve performance.

Body-surface area (BSA)—Calculated surface of a human body.

Bolus—A moist, round mass of chewed food.

Bowman's capsule—A cuplike structure that surrounds the glomerulus.

Brain scan—A diagnostic procedure used to image the brain.

Brain stem—The part of the brain that connects the brain to the spinal cord. It is composed of three sections: the medulla oblongata, the pons, and the midbrain.

Breast cancer—A malignancy of the breast tissue.

Breast milk—Nourishment for newborns and infants produced by the mammary glands.

Breast self-examination—A self-examination to identify early signs of breast cancer.

Bronchi—Major organs of the respiratory system; bronchi branch from the trachea to deliver air to the lungs.

Bronchioles—Major organs of the respiratory system; bronchioles branch from the bronchi to deliver air to the lungs.

Bronchitis—An inflammation of the lining of the bronchi.

Bronchodilator—A medication used to expand the airways.

Bronchoscopy—The technique of using a bronchoscope to visualize the bronchi.

Bundling—A practice by insurance providers in which they pay for only certain claim codes and ignore others.

Bunion—A lateral deviation of the big toe and accompanying enlargement of the first metatarsal head; also known as hallux valgus.

Bursa—A disk-shaped sac filled with fluid that eases movement within a synovial joint.

Bursitis—Inflammation of the bursa.

Business associate—Someone who works with a covered entity that might receive personal healthcare information to help with the operation of the entity.

C

Calorie—The measurement of the amount of energy supplied by a nutrient.

Calyx—Cavities in the kidney that collect urine from the collecting tubules.

Cancellous bone—One of two types of bone; soft, porous, and resembles a sponge; also called trabecular bone or spongy bone.

Candidiasis—A fungal infection caused by *Candida albicans*.

Cane—An assistive device that provides minimal support and balance.

Canines—Pointed teeth that are used to puncture or tear food; also called cuspids.

Capillaries—Tiny vessels between arterioles and venules where gas and nutrient exchange occurs.

Capillary puncture—The technique for collecting only a small sample of blood; also called a finger stick.

Carbohydrates—The body's main source of energy; a macronutrient.

Carbon dioxide—The gas waste product of healthy cellular function; exchanged with oxygen in respiration.

Carbuncle—A group of infected hair follicles.

Cardiac catheterization—The process of inserting a catheter into the blood vessels leading to the heart.

Cardiac cycle—A heartbeat, which involves the electrical activation of the atria and ventricles and the contraction and relaxation of the atria and ventricles.

Cardiac muscle—The type of involuntary muscles found in the heart.

Cardiac output—The amount of blood pumped by the heart in one minute.

Cardiac sphincter—The circular muscle that controls the opening at the top of the stomach.

Cardiologist—An internal medicine specialist who studies diseases and disorders of the human heart.

Cardiovascular system—The body system that includes the heart and blood vessels.

Career objective—A statement that gives the reader a quick idea as to what the professional is seeking.

Carpal tunnel—A hollow tube that contains nerves, blood vessels, and tendons in the wrist.

Carpal tunnel syndrome (CTS)—A painful set of symptoms that occurs among people who regularly use their hands.

Cartilaginous joint—A type of joint in which the bones are attached by cartilage.

Cast—A device used to immobilize a joint or limb to allow a bone to heal.

Casts—Molds of the renal tubules created by protein deposits.

Cataract—A condition in which the normally clear lens of the eye becomes cloudy.

Cation—A positively charged ion.

Cecum—The first segment of the large intestine.

Cell—The basic building block of the human body.

Cellulitis—An infection of the epidermis and dermis that can quickly spread into surrounding tissues and organs.

Central nervous system (CNS)—The body's control center. The CNS includes the brain and spinal cord.

Cerebellum—The part of the brain that lies just beneath the cerebrum. The cerebellum is responsible for motor-movement coordination, balance, equilibrium, and muscle tone.

Cerebral angiogram—A diagnostic test that is used to detect the degree of narrowing of an artery or blood vessel in the brain, head, or neck. It is used to diagnose stroke and to determine the location and size of a brain tumor, aneurysm, or vascular malformation.

Cerebral vascular accident (CVA)—A medical emergency that is caused when blood flow to part of the brain stops.

Cerebrospinal fluid (CSF)—Fluid that acts as a cushion, protecting the brain and spinal cord from injury.

Cerebrospinal fluid analysis—A diagnostic test that involves the removal of a small amount of the CSF by lumbar puncture or spinal tap.

Cerebrovascular accident—The interruption in oxygen supply to an area of the brain; also known as a stroke or brain attack.

Cerebrum—The part of the brain that controls sensory and motor activities.

Certification Commission for Healthcare Information Technology (CCHIT)—A commission developed to enact standards for software and vendors in the medical records industry and to promote greater speed in adaptation of electronic healthcare information.

Certified Clinical Medical Assistant (CCMA)—Medical assistant certified through the National Healthcareer Association (NHA).

Certified Medical Assistant (CMA-AAMA)—Medical assistant who has achieved certification status through the American Association of Medical Assistants. Graduates of medical assisting programs accredited by the Commission on Accreditation of Allied Health Education Programs (CAAHEP) or the Accrediting Bureau of Health Education Schools (ABHES) are eligible to take the CMA (AAMA) certification examination.

Cerumen—Earwax.

Cervical cancer—A malignancy of the cervix.

Cervix—The lower portion of the uterus that connects to the vagina.

Cesarean delivery—The delivery of a baby that involves making an incision through the abdomen and uterus; also called a C-section.

Chain of custody—The legal documentation of the possession, control, transfer, and analysis of a sample.

Chain of infection—Steps or links that must be connected in sequential order for the spread of infection to occur.

Chancre—A lesion caused by a syphilis infection.

CHEDDAR method—Very similar to the SOAP method, but normally much more detailed in nature.

Chief complaint—Usually a very short and to-the-point statement describing the specific reason a patient needs to be seen by the provider.

Children—Pediatric patients aged one year to 11 years.

Children's Health Insurance Program (CHIP)—A program within Medicaid that provides medical coverage for children in low-income families.

Chlamydia—An STD caused by *Chlamydia trachomatis*.

Cholecystectomy—The surgical removal of the gallbladder.

Cholelithiasis—A condition in which small stones are formed from minerals in bile; also called gallstones.

Cholesterol—A component of cell membranes of animals that is necessary for the proper functioning of several body functions and systems.

Chordae tendineae—The ligaments that attach the heart's valves to the chambers of the heart.

Chorion—The outer membrane of the amniotic sac.

Chronic bronchitis—Chronic inflammation of the bronchi; hallmark of COPD.

Chronic obstructive pulmonary disease (COPD)—A progressive disease of airway limitation; includes chronic bronchitis and emphysema.

Chronic renal failure (CRF)—The result of progressive loss of kidney function.

Chronological order—The most recent set of medical records and information is kept at the top of the chart (or in electronic forms, by most recent date) for easy access, allowing an orderly progression.

Chronological résumé—A résumé in which the most recent information is the first thing the reader sees.

Chyme—A semiliquid substance of partially digested food formed in the stomach.

Cilia—Hairlike projections found in epithelial cells.

Circumcision—A surgical procedure to remove the foreskin of the penis.

Cirrhosis—A progressive and irreversible condition in which the liver is destroyed by chronic inflammation.

Civilian Health and Medical Program of the Department of Veterans Affairs (CHAMPVA)—A program administered by the Department of Defense that provides medical coverage for the dependents of military personnel who have permanent service-related disabilities.

Civil laws—Laws that govern certain activities between and among persons or between persons and the government.

Claudication—Fatigue, discomfort, pain, or numbness in the extremities upon exertion.

Clitoris—A small, round structure made of erectile tissue; part of the vulva.

Closed fracture—A fracture that does not include a break in the skin.

CMS-1500—A universal insurance claim form.

Coding—The process of assigning alphanumeric designations to diagnoses, procedures, and services.

Co-insurance—A percentage of the total costs of medical care that an individual must contribute toward each service.

Collagen—A protein fiber found in connective tissue that provides strength and elasticity to the skin.

Colon—The segment of the digestive tract that removes excess water from chyme and facilitates elimination of waste; also called the large intestine.

Colonoscopy—A procedure used to visualize the inside of the colon.

Colostomy—An artificial opening in the colon that allows fecal material to be excreted through the abdominal wall.

Colostrum—Concentrated milk that nourishes a newborn for the first few days of life.

Colposcopy—A visual examination of the vagina.

Combining form—Word roots that have a vowel added to the end to help in connecting suffixes or other word roots and combining forms.

Comedone—A blackhead; occurs when a sebaceous gland becomes blocked.

Commission on Accreditation of Allied Health Education Programs (CAHEEP)—Accreditation through this program is awarded to institutions that meet certain agreed-upon standards. Recognized by the Secretary of Education, programs can lead to a certificate, diploma, associate of applied science, associate of occupational science, academic associate degree, or baccalaureate degree, including those offered via distance education.

Common bile duct—The duct through which bile is transported to the duodenum.

Common denominator—A number into which both denominators can divide evenly.

Communication—The act of transmitting information. An exchange of information between individuals using a common system of signs, symbols, or behavior.

Compact bone—One of two types of bone; densely packed bone that forms a hard, protective shell around cancellous bone.

Complementary and alternative medicine (CAM)—A diverse group of healthcare systems, therapies, and products that includes a philosophy of integrated and holistic treatment.

Complete physical examination—An examination performed to assess the general health status of a patient.

Computed tomography (CT) scan—A diagnostic imaging technique that uses X-rays to create a two-dimensional representation of a patient's anatomy.

Conception—The union of one male gamete and one female gamete.

Condyle—The rounded portion at the end of each long bone.

Conjunctiva—A thin mucous membrane that covers the inner surface of the eyelid and the sclera.

Conjunctivitis—Inflammation of the conjunctiva.

Constipation—The decreased frequency of bowel movements or difficulty defecating.

Constructive criticism—Useful criticism or advice given to help or improve something, often with possible solutions offered.

Consumer-driven health plan (CDHP)—A plan that allows an individual to make choices about how his or her healthcare money is spent; often exists as a flexible spending account or health savings account.

Contact precautions—Measures that apply to patients with stool incontinence, draining wounds, uncontrolled secretions, pressure ulcers, presence of tubes or bags of draining body fluids, or generalized rash.

Continuing education units (CEUs)—Units (credits) given when attending educational conferences and seminars to maintain training and credentials throughout the career.

Contraception—The prevention of pregnancy.

Contract—Exists when two parties meet in agreement. Can be between two parties—individuals or corporations.

Contraindication—A drug, disease, or symptom for which a drug is not indicated or will cause harm.

Contributory negligence—Negligence in which the plaintiff contributed to the injury or loss.

Controlled substance—A drug with the potential for abuse or addiction.

Convalescent stage—The stage of infectious disease in which the patient begins to recover and regain strength.

Coordination of benefits—A clause that prevents duplicate payment by multiple insurance providers.

Co-pay—A fixed-fee that an individual must pay toward each service provided.

Cornea—The clear, dome-shaped surface that covers the front of the eye and allows light into the eye for visual acuity.

Corneal ulcers—A disintegration of the surface of the cornea that results in an open sore that heals very slowly.

Corona—The ridge of tissue near the end of the penis.

Coronal plane (frontal plane)—A vertical plane that divides the body or any of its parts into anterior and posterior portions.

Coronary artery disease (CAD)—Narrowing of the blood vessels in the coronary arteries due to atherosclerosis.

Corpora cavernosa—The two layers of the penis that contain erectile tissue.

Corpus luteum—A mass formed from the ruptured ovarian follicle.

Corpus spongiosum—The layer of the penis that contains the urethra.

Corticosteroids—Hormones produced by the adrenal glands, including mineralocorticoids, glucocorticoids, and androgens.

Cough—A protective reflex that eliminates excess cellular debris, mucus, and foreign bodies from the lower respiratory tract.

Covered entity—A physician, a healthcare provider, a nursing home, a hospital, an insurance company, or other organization that uses electronic transmissions during a transaction under HIPAA standards.

Cover letter—An introductory letter sent with a résumé to a potential employer.

Cranium—The part of the skull that encloses and protects the brain.

Crepitus—A grinding sensation in the joints.

Criminal history and background check—A review of legal records to determine whether a candidate has been convicted of any crimes.

Criminal law—A crime made against the state or government.

Crohn's disease—A type of IBD characterized by lesions throughout the GI tract.

Cross multiplication—Multiplication of the numerator of the first fraction by the denominator of the second fraction, and the multiplication of the denominator of the first fraction by the numerator of the second fraction.

Crutches—Assistive devices that provide moderate support; allow for fast speeds and alternate gait patterns.

Cryotherapy—Therapy using cold.

C-section—The delivery of a baby that involves making an incision through the abdomen and uterus; also called a cesarean delivery.

Culture—The customary beliefs, social norms, and material traits of a racial, religious, or social group.

Current Procedural Terminology (CPT)—Codes that identify the type of procedure or medical care that was provided.

Cushing's syndrome—A condition that results from the excessive production of glucocorticoids from the adrenal cortex.

Cuspids—Pointed teeth that are used to puncture or tear food; also called canines.

Cyst—A fluid-filled sac.

Cystic duct—The duct through which bile is excreted from the gallbladder.

Cystic fibrosis—A genetic disorder characterized by thick, filmy secretions in the respiratory and digestive tracts.

Cystitis—An inflammation of the bladder.

D

Damages—Harm or injury to property or a person resulting in loss of value or the impairment of usefulness.

Deciduous teeth—The first set of teeth; will fall out and be replaced by permanent teeth.

Decimal number—Numbers that are written using place value.

Declining stage—The stage of infectious disease in which the symptoms begin to subside. The infection is still present, but the patient will begin to feel better.

Deductible—The amount an individual must pay before the insurance provider begins paying for services.

Deep vein thrombosis (DVT)—A thrombus in a vein deep inside the body, most often the legs.

Defecation—The act of eliminating solid waste from the body.

Defendant—One who is being charged with the complaint in a lawsuit.

Dehydration—The loss of body water.

Deltoid—The muscle of the upper arm; an injection site for IM injections in adults.

Dendrites—A branched protoplasmic extension of a nerve cell that conducts impulses from adjacent cells inward toward the cell body.

Denominator—The number below the fraction line. The denominator tells you how many equal parts are in the whole.

Depolarization—The process of becoming more positive in the cells of the myocardium.

Dermatitis—An inflammation of the epidermis.

Dermatology—The study of the diseases and disorders of the skin.

Dermatophytoses—Superficial infections of the skin caused by organisms that digest keratin in skin and hair.

Dermis—The second layer of skin. It supports the epidermis and separates it from the lower layers of skin.

Descending colon—The portion of the colon that extends down the abdominal cavity and into the pelvis.

Destructive agent—A drug that destroys or kills abnormal and sometimes normal cells.

Diabetes insipidus—A condition caused by the decreased production of ADH.

Diabetes mellitus (DM)—A condition in which the body either does not have or cannot use insulin.

Diabetic nephropathy—Damage to the kidneys caused by untreated DM.

Diabetic neuropathy—Damage to the nerves caused by untreated DM.

Diabetic retinopathy—A complication of diabetes that affects the blood vessels in the retina. If left untreated, it can lead to blindness.

Diagnosis related group (DRG)—A group of related procedures used by Medicare to determine reimbursement.

Diagnostic agent—Any drug used in the diagnosis or identification of a disease.

Dialysis—A process that filters the blood and removes harmful waste products when the kidneys are not able to perform this function.

Diaphragm—A heavy, dome-shaped muscle that contracts and relaxes during inspiration and expiration.

Diaphysis—The long shaft of a long bone.

Diarrhea—An increased frequency or decreased consistency of bowel movements.

Diarthrosis—A joint that allows for free movement of the bones it connects; also called a synovial joint.

Diastole—The relaxation of the atria and ventricles.

Diastolic blood pressure—The pressure on the arteries during diastole.

Diastolic dysfunction—Any condition that reduces the filling of the ventricles.

Dictate—To say or read aloud information that is recorded or written by another.

Difference—An amount obtained when subtracting numbers.

Digestion—The process of converting food into a form that can be used by the cells of the body.

Digital sphygmomanometer—A device for measuring blood pressure that is automatic and produces a digital display of the result.

Diluent—An inactive solution added to dry powder to prepare it for administration.

Direct transmission—Direct contact between the infectious person or infected body fluids and the susceptible host.

Disaccharides—Two-sugar carbohydrates.

Dislocation—Any displacement of a bone at a joint.

Distal—An anatomic directional term that describes away from or farthest from the trunk or the point of origin of a part.

Distribution—The process by which a drug is distributed to tissues, to other body fluids, and ultimately to organs throughout the body after it is absorbed into the bloodstream.

Division—The operation inverse to multiplication. The process of dividing numbers to find the quotient.

Doctors of osteopathy (DOs)—Physicians who complete four years of undergraduate (premed) classes in college, four years of Osteopathic medical school, and residencies ranging from two to six years, depending on their specialties. They are considered to practice homeopathic medicine, and have an increasingly conservative approach when prescribing medications to their patients due to this philosophy.

Documentation—The provision by healthcare providers of notations and writings about any condition along with changes that occur in the patient, such as medical history, evaluations, testing, and any other pertinent information during patient care and communication and the act or an instance of the supplying of documents or supporting references of record. Documentation must be accurate when placed in the patient's chart.

Do-not-resuscitate (DNR) order—Another example of an advance directive. The patient who chooses this advance directive wishes not to undergo CPR if found to be in cardiac or respiratory arrest.

Dorsal recumbent position—An examination position in which the patient lays on his or her back with feet flat on the examination table.

Dorsogluteal—The muscle at the backside located at the outer, upper quadrant, toward the hip. It is an injection site for IM injections in adults.

Dosage—The entire regimen or schedule of doses.

Dosage form—A system, device, or physical form of a dose by which the drug is delivered or administered to the body.

Dose—The quantity that is intended to be administered, usually taken at one time or during one specified period, such as per day.

Downcoding—A practice by insurance providers in which they pay for a lower level of care than was actually provided.

Droplet precautions—Measures that apply to patients known or suspected to be infected with a pathogen that can be transmitted via a droplet, such as respiratory viruses and bordetella pertussis.

Drug—Any substance used for the diagnosis, cure, treatment, or prevention of a disease or is intended to affect the structure or function of any living system.

Drug dependence—A condition in which the body needs the drug to function normally. Abrupt discontinuation of the drug will lead to withdrawal symptoms.

Drug screen—A test performed to detect drug use. May involve the use of blood, hair, or urine.

Dual energy X-ray absorptiometry (DXA)—A diagnostic technique that uses X-rays to evaluate bone strength.

Duodenum—The first segment of the small intestine.

Dura mater—The layer of meninges farthest from the CNS.

Dysuria—Painful urination.

E

Eccrine glands—Sweat glands that produce sweat containing water and salt.

Echocardiogram (ECHO)—A visualization technique that uses sound waves to create a moving picture of the heart.

Eclampsia—A condition of late pregnancy characterized by seizures and extremely high blood pressure.

Eczema—A chronic dermatitis.

Efferent system—The part of the peripheral nervous system that includes all the nerves and pathways that send information from the CNS to other organs and body systems.

Ejaculatory duct—The duct that is formed from the vas deferens and a duct from the seminal vesicle that passes through the prostate gland and eventually joins with the urethra.

Elderly—Individuals who are over the age of 65; also referred to as geriatric.

Electrocardiogram (ECG or EKG)—A test that measures the electrical activity of the heart.

Electroencephalography (EEG)—A diagnostic test that monitors brain activity through the skull.

Electrolyte—A mineral that exists as an ion when dissolved in water.

Electromyography (EMG)—A diagnostic test that records the electrical activity from the brain and/or spinal cord to a peripheral nerve root found in the arms and legs that controls muscles during contraction and at rest.

Electronic health record (EHR)—Medical records in an electronic format, providing information for planning and decisions about patient care, as well as any ordered testing, medications, letters or communication between other health providers, and statistic information for local or state health departments and/or insurance analysis.

Electronystagmography (ENG)—A diagnostic test used to record involuntary movements of the eye caused by a condition known as nystagmus.

Elimination—1. The removal of the drug from the body. 2. The removal of solid waste products of digestion.

Embolus—A blood clot that travels through the bloodstream.

Embryo—The multicellular form of a zygote during early pregnancy.

Emergency—An unforeseen combination of circumstances or the resulting state that calls for immediate action.

Emollients—An agent that soothes and softens the skin.

Emphysema—Progressive destruction of the alveoli; hallmark of COPD.

Employment agency—An agency that finds people to fill particular jobs or to find jobs for unemployed people.

Employment screening—The process of investigating the background of a potential employee. Commonly used to verify the accuracy of an applicant's claims and to discover any possible criminal history or employers' negative sanctions.

Encephalitis—A severe inflammation of the brain that can destroy nerve cells, cause bleeding in the brain, and cause brain damage.

Encounter form—A form that lists diagnoses and procedures associated with each patient visit.

Endocardium—The inner layer of heart muscle. It has a smooth, pleatlike surface that allows the heart wall to collapse when it contracts.

Endocrine glands—Glands that secrete hormones directly into the bloodstream.

Endocrine system—A system of glands that produce and secrete hormones.

Endocrinologist—A medical specialist who studies the endocrine system.

Endometriosis—The presence of endometrial tissue outside the uterus.

Endometrium—The inner lining of the uterus.

End-stage renal disease (ESRD)—The final stage of kidney failure in which the kidneys have lost all function.

Enema—A solution that is flushed into the anus to remove solid material from the rectum and colon.

Epicardium—The outer layer of heart muscle and inner layer of the pericardium.

Epicondylitis—An inflammation of the forearm extensor tendon; more commonly called tennis elbow.

Epidermis—The outermost layer of skin.

Epididymis—A collection of coiled tubes that stores sperm.

Epilepsy—A neurological condition that is also known as a seizure disorder. It is characterized by sudden and recurring seizures.

Epiphysis—The thick plate at each end of a long bone.

Epistaxis—Nosebleed.

Equivalent ratios—Two ratios that have the same value.

Esophagogastroduodenoscopy (EGD)—A procedure used to visualize the esophagus, stomach, and duodenum; also called gastroscopy.

Esophagus—A tube that connects the mouth to the stomach.

Estimated date of confinement (EDC)—The estimated date of delivery of a baby at the end of a pregnancy.

Ethics—A standard of behavior as well as a personal sense of right and wrong above what is considered legal.

Evoked potentials—Also called evoked responses, these measure the electrical signals to the brain generated by hearing, touch, and sight.

Exocrine glands—Glands that secrete substances through a duct or an organ.

Exophthalmos—A condition in which the eyes protrude dramatically; a symptom of hyperthyroidism.

Expanded precautions—Second-tier guidelines from the CDC that apply to specific categories of patients and that include air, contact, and droplet precautions.

Expectorant—A product that changes the consistency of mucus, allowing it to be more easily expelled with a cough; also called a protussive.

Expiration—The process of exhaling air out.

Expressed contract—An expressed contract between a physician and a patient is in writing and contains a date and signature. An example of this is when the patient signs an agreement for the physician to bill his or her insurance for payment for services.

Extensor—A muscle that extends or straightens a limb or body part.

External anal sphincter—The muscle that controls the junction between the anal canal and the anus.

Externship—A position in which a student applies skills with the guidance and supervision of a practicing healthcare provider. Externships are not paid positions.

Extreme obesity—A BMI of 40 or greater.

Extremes—The two outer numbers within a proportion.

F

Factor—One of two or more numbers that, when multiplied together, produce a product.

Facultative aerobes—Microorganisms that can survive in the presence or absence of oxygen.

Failure to thrive (FTT)—Poor physical growth.

Fallopian tubes—Tubes that extend from each side of the uterus.

Family history—Documentation that provides insight into the patient's current and past medical conditions. The family history contains information necessary for the provider to determine whether the patient is at risk for any familial or hereditary diseases, such as breast cancer, heart disease, diabetes, or if there are other contributing familial factors that may affect the patient. Information about illness or death of grandparents, parents, and siblings can help the provider pinpoint whether the patient may also be at risk for those conditions.

Fasting blood glucose (FBG) test—A blood test that measures the amount of glucose in the bloodstream after a 12-hour fast.

Fat-soluble vitamins—Vitamins that are stored by the body.

Fatty acid—A carboxylic acid with a long hydrocarbon chain.

Febrile—An elevated body temperature; also called pyrexia.

Fecal occult blood test (FOBT)—A test to identify the presence of blood in the feces.

Feces—Solid waste that is eliminated from the body through defecation; also called stool.

Feedback—The last part of the communication cycle. Feedback takes place as the receiver interprets the message and gives back information, giving the sender the opportunity to answer any questions or clear up any misunderstandings about the original message sent.

Felony—A more serious crime that involves punishment of fines and imprisonment for more than one year, and in more severe crimes, such as homicide, death.

Fenestrated drape—A drape with a round or slitlike opening in the center.

Fetus—An embryo that has progressed passed the 10th week of pregnancy.

Fiber—An indigestible polysaccharide derived from plant sources.

Fibroids—Benign tumors of the muscle cells of the uterus; also called uterine leiomyomas.

Fibromyalgia—A syndrome characterized by diffuse, widespread pain.

Fibrous joint—A type of joint that connects bones without allowing any movement.

Final evaluation—Usually given by the site supervisor to review your overall experience during externship.

First-degree burn—A superficial burn that involves only the outer layers of the epidermis.

Five Cs of communication—These are complete (the message must be complete, with all information given); clear (clear information must be communicated to the patient); concise (when speaking to the patient, information should be brief and to the point); cohesive (the message should be logical and organized); and courteous (courtesy should always be shown to the patient).

Fixed joint—A joint that allows no movement between the bones it connects; also called a fibrous joint or synarthrosis.

Flat bones—Bones made of cancellous bone between two layers of compact bone; bones that protect soft, vulnerable organs.

Flexible spending account (FSA)—A savings account that can be used for medical expenses; funded with pretax dollars by an employee.

Flexor—A muscle that contracts and bends a joint or limb in the body.

Flora—Bacteria normally found in or on the body that do not cause disease.

Follicle-stimulating hormone (FSH)—A hormone produced by the pituitary gland that stimulates the ovarian follicle to produce estrogen in females and stimulates the production of sperm in males.

Follicular phase—The phase of the menstrual cycle that allows for the development of an ovarian follicle.

Folliculitis—An inflammation of the hair follicle.

Follow-up letter—A letter or note sent after a job interview to thank the interviewer for his or her time and for reviewing the position with you.

Fomite—An inanimate object or substance that is capable of transmitting an infectious agent from one person to another.

Forced expiratory volume—The volume of air that can be forcibly exhaled in one second after a complete inhalation.

Forced vital capacity—The volume of air that can be forcibly exhaled after a complete inhalation.

Forearm crutches—Short crutches that provide stability and support for patients who need long-term or permanent use of crutches.

Foreskin—A layer of skin that covers the penis glans; also called the prepuce.

Four Ds of negligence—For a malpractice suit to proceed in court, the four Ds of negligence must occur: duty, derelict, damages, and direct cause.

Fowler's positions—Examination positions in which the patient is seated with the back against the examination table and legs resting on the table.

Fractions—A quantity or portion that is used to represent a part of a whole number. It is a ratio of a part to the whole.

Fracture—A broken bone.

Frontal lobe—The part of the cerebrum that seems to be related to motor functions, planning, reasoning, judgment, impulse control, and memory.

Full-time employee—An employee whose job involves 35 or more (usually 40) hours of work during a week.

Functional résumé—A résumé that highlights your accomplishments and strengths. A functional résumé helps you organize these highlights in an order that supports your career objective.

Fundus—The body of the stomach.

Fungi—Plantlike organisms that can grow on cloth, food, showers, or people, or in any warm, moist environment.

Furuncle—An infection of the hair follicle; also called a boil.

G

Gait belt—A device used to assist in lifting and transferring patients.

Gallbladder—A sac under the liver that concentrates and stores bile.

Gallstones—A condition in which small stones are formed from minerals in bile; also called cholelithiasis.

Gametes—Cells required for reproduction.

Ganglia—Clusters of nerve cell bodies.

Gas diffusion—The process by which oxygen and carbon dioxide are transferred from the lungs to the pulmonary blood.

Gas transport—The process by which oxygen and carbon dioxide are carried throughout the body by the blood.

Gastric emptying time—The time it takes for food to pass through the stomach.

Gastroenteritis—The inflammation of the stomach and intestines.

Gastroenterologist—A medical specialist who studies the digestive system.

Gastroesophageal reflux disease (GERD)—A condition characterized by the flow of gastric and duodenal contents into the esophagus.

Gastrointestinal (GI) system—The body system that breaks down food and fluids into small compounds that can be readily absorbed into the bloodstream and used by the body for energy production and protein synthesis, and as enzymes for essential metabolic reactions.

Gastroscopy—A procedure used to visualize the esophagus, stomach, and duodenum; also called esophagogastroduodenoscopy.

General survey—A portion of the physical examination that includes initial assessments of the patient's overall state of health.

Genital herpes—An STD caused by type 2 herpes simplex virus.

Genitourinary (GU) system—The body system that filters and removes waste products from the blood; also called the urinary system.

Geriatricians—Physicians who care for geriatric patients.

Geriatrics—The branch of medicine that studies and cares for older patients.

Germinative layer—The innermost layer of the epidermis; produces new skin cells.

Gerontology—The study of the aging process.

Gestation—The carrying of an embryo or fetus.

Gestures and mannerisms—Forms of body language in which we "talk" with our hands.

Giantism—A condition that results from the excess production of growth hormone in children.

GI transit time—The amount of time it takes for food to pass through the GI tract.

Glans—The tip of the penis.

Glaucoma—A common disorder of the eye characterized by increased ocular pressure.

Glomerulonephritis—The inability of the glomerulus to function normally.

Glomerulus—A bed of capillaries in the renal corpuscle; the site of filtration.

Glucagon—A hormone produced by the pancreas that increases the amount of glucose in the bloodstream.

Glucocorticoid—A type of corticosteroid; controls the formation of glycogen, promotes the metabolism of fats and proteins, and releases fats stored in adipose tissue.

Glucometer—An automated meter for testing blood glucose.

Glucose tolerance test (GTT)—A series of blood tests that measures the body's ability to process a large amount of glucose in a short amount of time.

Glycosuria—Excess glucose in the urine.

Goiter—An enlarged thyroid gland.

Gonads—The endocrine glands that control reproductive functions; they include the ovaries in females and the testes in males.

Goniometer—An instrument that measures joint movement.

Goniometry—The study of joint motion.

Gonorrhea—An STD caused by *Neisseria gonnorrhoeae.*

Good Samaritan laws—Laws designed to protect someone who renders aid in an emergency to an injured person on a voluntary basis.

Gout—A chronic condition of joint pain caused by an accumulation of uric acid.

Gram (g)—The basic unit of measurement in the metric system for measuring dry weight.

Gram-negative—Bacteria that do not retain the crystal-violet dye used in Gram's staining method.

Gram-positive—Bacteria that retain the crystal-violet dye used in Gram's staining method.

Graves' disease—The most common form of hyperthyroidism.

Gravidity—The number of previous pregnancies a woman has had.

Gross pay—The amount of money earned before taxes and employee-paid benefits are deducted.

Growth charts—Gender- and age-specific charts used to assess growth and development patterns.

Gynecologist—The medical specialist who studies the female reproductive system.

H

Hair follicle—Produces and grows hair; located in the dermis and epidermis.

Hallux valgus—A lateral deviation of the big toe and accompanying enlargement of the first metatarsal head; commonly called a bunion.

Healthcare common procedure coding system (HCPCS)—A set of codes that identifies healthcare procedures.

Health history—The clinically relevant information obtained from a patient interview; also called a medical history.

Health insurance—A system in which people prepay for medical care.

Health Insurance Portability and Accountability Act (HIPAA)—An act passed in the 1990s to simplify the administration of health insurance, improve portability of health care from one employer to another, protect and improve patients' rights, enhance patient access to records, and control inappropriate disclosures of patients' information.

Health maintenance organization (HMO)—A commercial insurance plan that requires patients to choose a primary care provider.

Health savings account (HSA)—A savings account that can be used for medical expenses; a tax-deferred account that is funded by the employer and the employee.

Heart—The muscular pump of the circulatory system.

Heart failure (HF)—A condition in which the heart is unable to pump enough blood to meet the body's needs.

Hematemesis—The condition of vomiting blood.

Hematochezia—Bright red blood in the feces.

Hematuria—Blood in the urine.

Hemodialysis—Dialysis that uses a machine to remove blood, filter it, and return it to the body.

Hemodialyzer—Hemodialysis equipment.

Hemoglobin A1c (HbA1c)—A blood test that assesses long-term glucose control by measuring the amount of glycosylated hemoglobin in the blood.

Hemorrhage—The release of blood from a blood vessel.

Hepatic duct—The duct through which bile is excreted from the liver.

Hepatic flexure—The point at which the ascending colon bends to form the transverse colon; located behind the right lobe of the liver.

Hepatitis—Inflammation of the liver.

Herniated disk—A condition in which the gel between the vertebral disks of the spine is forced outside the disk; also known as a ruptured disk.

Herpes simplex virus—The family of viruses that causes cold sores and genital warts.

Herpes zoster—An infection caused by the varicella-zoster virus; also known as shingles.

Hierarchy of needs—Developed by Abraham Maslow, the founder of humanistic psychology. According to Maslow, a person must satisfy one level of need before he or she can move on to the next.

High-density lipoprotein (HDL)—One type of lipoprotein in the body; travels with cholesterol; known as good cholesterol.

Hilum—The concave border of the capsule covering the kidney.

Histamine—The chemical released or produced by the body as an immune response during an allergic reaction.

Hives—*See* urticaria.

Holter monitoring—Ambulatory ECG monitoring; usually performed over 24–48 hours.

Homeostasis—Equilibrium of the body with respect to fluid levels, pH, osmotic pressures, and concentrations of various substances.

Horizontal recumbent position—An examination position in which the patient lays flat on his or her back; also called supine position.

Hormonal contraceptives—Birth control pills.

Hormone—Chemical messenger released into the bloodstream; used by the body to communicate between cells.

Host—A person who is susceptible to infection by a pathogen.

Household system of measurement—A system of measurement that includes drops, teaspoons, tablespoons, fluid ounces, cups, pints, quarts, and gallons for measuring liquid. It also includes ounces and pounds for measuring weight.

Human chorionic gonadotropin (hCG)—The hormone that maintains the corpus luteum during early pregnancy.

Human immunodeficiency virus (HIV)—The retrovirus that causes AIDS.

Human papillomavirus (HPV)—A virus that infects the skin or mucous membranes and causes verrucae, or warts.

Hydrogenation—The process by which trans fats are produced by heating vegetable oil and adding hydrogen.

Hyperglycemia—Excess glucose in the blood.

Hypergonadism—Overproduction of sex hormones.

Hyperkalemia—A high level of potassium in the blood.

Hyperlipidemia—Elevated levels of lipoproteins.

Hyperopia—Also known as farsightedness. A disorder in which people have difficulty focusing on close objects.

Hyperparathyroidism—Overactivity of the parathyroid gland.

Hyperpituitarism—The abnormal increase in hormones produced by the pituitary gland.

Hypertension—Elevated blood pressure; defined as a systolic blood pressure greater than 140mmHg or a diastolic blood pressure greater than 90mmHg.

Hyperthyroidism—Overactivity of the thyroid gland; also called thyrotoxicosis.

Hypodermis—The innermost layer of skin. It contains loose connective tissue and fatty tissue firmly anchored to the dermis. Also called subcutaneous tissue.

Hypoglycemia—Low blood sugar.

Hypogonadism—Decreased function of the gonads.

Hyponatremia—A decreased concentration of sodium in the blood.

Hypoparathyroidism—Underactivity of the parathyroid gland.

Hypopituitarism—The decreased production of hormones in the pituitary gland.

Hypothalamus—An area of the brain that produces hormones that control body temperature, appetite, moods, sex drive, and the release of hormones.

Hypothyroidism—Underactivity of the thyroid gland; also known as myxedema.

Hypoxemia—Insufficient oxygenation of arterial blood.

Hypoxia—The reduction of oxygen supply to a tissue below normal levels despite adequate perfusion of the tissue by blood.

Hysterectomy—The removal of the uterus.

Hysteroscopy—An endoscopic visualization of the inside of the uterus.

I

Ileocecal valve—The sphincter at the junction between the small and large intestines.

Ileostomy—An artificial opening in the ileum that allows chyme to be excreted through the abdominal wall.

Ileum—The third segment of the small intestine.

Immune system—The body's defense mechanism. It protects the body by attacking and destroying invading pathogens.

Impetigo—A superficial infection of the skin, usually caused by *Staphylococcus* or *Streptococcus* bacteria.

Implied consent—Presumed consent, normally in a nonwritten fashion. An example of implied consent is a patient rolling up his or her sleeve for a blood draw ordered by the physician.

Implied contract—A contract created and formed when the physician agrees to see the patient and acts in good faith to the best of his or her abilities to treat the patient. The patient agrees to follow the physician's directions and treatment.

Improper fraction—A fraction with a value equal to or greater than 1.

Incisors—Teeth that have sharp edges that can bite through food.

Incontinence—The uncontrollable or involuntary loss of urine.

Incubation stage—The stage of infectious disease between the exposure to a pathogen and the time the first signs and symptoms of the disease appear.

Indication—When a drug is given according to its labeling and is known to be beneficial for a specific disease, symptom, or condition.

Indirect transmission—An intermediate means that carries the infectious agent to the host.

Infants—Babies between one month and one year old.

Infarction—The death of tissues due to a sudden decrease in blood supply.

Infection control—Precautions taken in a healthcare setting to prevent the spread of disease.

Infectious agents—Pathogens or microorganisms with the ability to cause a disease.

Infectious waste—Any item that has come in contact with blood or body fluids.

Inferior (caudal)—The anatomic directional term that describes away from the head; lower.

Inferior vena cava—Part of the largest vein in the body, which collects blood from the trunk and lower extremities.

Inflammatory bowel disease (IBD)—A condition characterized by inflammation of the GI tract.

Informed consent—Consent in writing that is achieved when the patient has an understanding of what will be involved in a procedure, consents to the treatment, and is advised of the risks involved, expected outcomes, and alternative treatments.

Ingestion—The process by which food is consumed and broken into small pieces.

Insertion—One end at which a muscle attaches to a bone.

Inspection—An examination technique that uses sight to evaluate a patient; also called observation.

Inspiration—The process of breathing air in.

Instillation—The dispensation of a sterile ophthalmic medication into a patient's eye or ear.

Insulin—A hormone produced by the pancreas that decreases the amount of circulating glucose in the blood.

Integumentary system—A body system composed of skin, hair, nails, and glands.

Intentional tort—A civil wrong. May also be criminal. Examples of intentional torts are assault, battery, libel, and slander.

Internal anal sphincter—The muscle that controls the junction between the anal canal and the rectum.

International classification of diseases (ICD)—A system of classifying medical diagnoses.

International unit (IU)—An internationally accepted amount of a substance required to produce a specific response.

Interview—A meeting in which a job candidate and an interviewer discuss an employment opportunity with a particular organization or practice.

Intradermal (ID)—A route of administration by which a parenteral medication is injected into the skin.

Intramuscular (IM)—A route of administration by which a parenteral medication is injected into a muscle.

Intravenous (IV)—A route of administration by which a parenteral medication is injected into a vein.

Intrinsic factor—A protein produced by the stomach that facilitates the absorption of vitamin B12.

Ion—An electrically charged atom or molecule that possesses either a positive charge (cation) or negative charge (anion).

Iris—The part of the eye that filters light and is responsible for the color of the eye.

Irregular bones—Bones that are shaped for a specific purpose or protective function.

Irrigation—Introduction of flushing fluid into the inner corner of the eye or ear to remove foreign objects from the eye or ear.

Irritable bowel syndrome (IBS)—A GI condition characterized by abdominal pain and altered bowel habits.

Ischemia—Decreased blood supply to tissues.

Ischemic heart disease—A condition in which the heart receives a decreased supply of blood.

Islets of Langerhans—The group of cells in the pancreas that produce insulin and glucagon.

Isotope—A form of a chemical element that contains the same number of protons as the regular element, but a different number of neutrons.

Isthmus—The tissue that connects the right and left lobes of the thyroid gland.

J

Jaeger chart—A chart used to screen for near vision acuity.

Jaundice—A yellow discoloration of the skin, mucosa, and sclera.

Jejunum—The second segment of the small intestine.

Job application—A formal application in which the candidate is asked to fill out a form with demographic data about himself or herself as well as any job history and references.

Joint—The point at which two bones meet; also called an articulation.

Joint capsule—The capsule that surrounds the synovial membrane to enclose an entire synovial joint.

Justice—In ethics, when a physician has considered all the benefits and burdens to the patient when weighing new or experimental treatments and helping the patient make informed healthcare decisions.

K

Keratin—A type of protein found in the hair.

Keratoconjunctivitis—Inflammation of the cornea and conjunctiva.

Ketones—By-products of fat metabolism.

Ketonuria—The presence of ketones in the urine.

Kidney—The primary organ of the urinary system.

Kinesics—An area of study that catalogs body movements and attempts to define their meaning. Each culture is believed to possess a separate "language" of kinesics.

Knee-chest position—An examination position in which the patient kneels on the examination table with buttocks elevated and chest resting on the table.

Korotkoff sounds—The sounds heard through a stethoscope during a blood-pressure measurement.

Kyphosis—An abnormal bowing or rounding of the upper back.

L

Laceration—A cut, tear, or puncture in the skin.

Large intestine—The segment of the digestive tract that removes excess water from chyme and facilitates elimination of waste; also called the colon.

Laryngitis—An inflammation of the larynx.

Larynx—A major organ of the respiratory system; the voice box.

Lateral—The anatomic directional term that describes away from the midline of the body.

Lateral position—An examination position in which the patient lays on his or her left side; also called Sims' position.

Laws—Rules of conduct that require everyone to behave the same way or face punishment.

Laxative—A product that softens stools and increases the frequency of bowel movements.

Left atrium—One of two collecting chambers in the heart; receives blood from the pulmonary veins.

Left ventricle—One of two distributing chambers in the heart; pumps blood to systemic circulation.

Libel—A false or defamatory statement in written words.

Lice—Wingless insects with well-developed legs that use humans as a host and receive nourishment from human blood.

Licensed practical nurse (LPN)—A licensed practical nurse (also known as a licensed vocational nurse [LVN] in some states) offers bedside and personal care for patients during hospitalization. LPNs can administer drugs, assess patients, and chart patients' progress when allowed by state law. These nurses usually work in hospitals or nursing homes, but also may be found in physician offices.

Licensed Vocational Nurse (LVN)—*See* licensed practical nurse.

Ligament—Bands of connective tissue that connect bone to bone.

Lipids—A macronutrient; also known as fats.

Lipoproteins—Lipids that are bound to proteins.

Liter (L)—The basic unit of measurement in the metric system for measuring liquid volume.

Lithotomy position—An examination position in which the patient lays on her back and the feet are placed in stirrups attached to the end of the table.

Liver—The digestive organ that produces bile, contributes to protein and carbohydrate metabolism, and filters waste products from the body.

Living will—Expresses the patient's wishes regarding medical treatment and life-sustaining efforts. A living will is a document that speaks for the patient when the patient cannot speak for himself or herself.

Local effect—Describes when the effect of the drug is confined to one area or organ of the body.

Lochia—Discharge after childbirth.

Long bones—Bones that are composed of a long shaft made of compact bone and wide ends made of cancellous bone.

Long-term goals—Larger goals that a person sets for himself or herself.

Lordosis—The abnormal convex curvature of the low back; commonly called swayback.

Low-density lipoprotein (LDL)—One type of lipoprotein in the body; travels with cholesterol; known as bad cholesterol.

Lower respiratory tract—Directs airflow and facilitates gas exchange; consists of the larynx, trachea, bronchi, and lungs.

Lowest common denominator—Lowest multiple for all denominators. The lowest multiple shared by all the denominators in a set of fractions.

Lumpectomy—Removal of a breast tumor.

Lungs—Major organs of the respiratory system; location of gas exchange.

Luteal phase—The phase of the menstrual cycle after ovulation in which the corpus luteum secretes progesterone.

Luteinizing hormone (LH)—A hormone produced by the pituitary gland that stimulates the ruptured ovarian follicle to become a corpus luteum and secrete progesterone in females and stimulates the testes to produce testosterone in males.

Lysozyme—An enzyme in mucus that destroys bacteria.

M

Macronutrients—Nutrients that provide energy.

Magnetic resonance imaging (MRI)—A diagnostic imaging technique that uses a large magnet and radio waves to create two-dimensional images of a patient's anatomy.

Malnutrition—Any nutrition disorder.

Mammary glands—Female breasts that produce and secrete breast milk.

Mammogram—A visualization technique to examine breast tissue.

Managed care—A system in which an organization contracts with providers to provide comprehensive healthcare services to its subscribers at a reduced cost.

Manipulation—An examination technique that uses passive movement of a joint to evaluate a patient.

Massage therapy—A therapeutic modality that manipulates patient's soft tissues to aid in musculoskeletal rehabilitation.

Mastectomy—Complete removal of the breast.

Means—The numbers directly to the left and right of the equal sign within a proportion.

Meatus—The opening of the urethra to the outside of the body.

Medial—The anatomic directional term that describes toward the midline of the body.

Median plane—The sagittal plane through the midline of the body that divides the body or any of its parts into right and left halves.

Mediastinum—The center of the thoracic cavity, where the heart is located.

Medicaid—A state-administered program that provides medical coverage for low-income individuals, uninsured pregnant women, and individuals with disabilities.

Medical asepsis—The use of practices to help contain and prevent the transmission of infectious organisms and to maintain an environment free from contamination.

Medical assistant—Performs both administrative and clinical duties, making them one of the most versatile health professionals in the medical field.

Medical doctors (MDs)—Physicians who complete four years of undergraduate (premed) classes in college, four years of medical school, and residencies ranging from three to eight years, depending on their specialties. They are considered to be allopathic physicians, which are also the most recognized.

Medical history—Documentation that includes all of the patient's health problems, any major illnesses, childbirth information (if female), immunizations, surgeries, allergies, and all current and past medications and reasons if/when their use was discontinued.

Medical liability—A civil wrong, otherwise known as malpractice.

Medical power of attorney—A document that gives the right of making medical decisions to another person who is responsible for carrying out the patient's wishes if the patient is mentally or physically unable to make decisions himself or herself.

Medical transcriptionist—Someone who types medical information spoken by the physician about a patient's examination or testing into a document that becomes a permanent part of the medical record.

Medicare—A federal program that provides medical coverage for people over age 65, people with disabilities, people receiving dialysis, and people receiving Social Security benefits.

Medication order—A prescription for a medication written in a hospital setting.

Medulla oblongata—The part of the brain stem that controls autonomic functions, such as breathing, digestion, heart and blood-vessel function, and sneezing. It helps transfer messages between the spinal cord and various parts of the brain.

Melanin—A pigment responsible for giving skin and hair color.

Melanocytes—The cells in the germinative layer of the epidermis that produce melanin.

Melanocyte-stimulating hormone (MSH)—A hormone produced by the pituitary gland that increases skin pigmentation.

Melanoma—A malignant form of skin cancer.

Melatonin—A hormone produced by the pineal gland that regulates circadian rhythms.

Melena—Blood in the feces.

Menarche—The onset of menstruation.

Meninges—The membranes covering the brain and spinal cord.

Meningitis—Inflammation of the meninges.

Menopause—The cessation of menstruation.

Menorrhagia—Heavy, prolonged, or irregular menstrual bleeding.

Menses—The monthly flow of blood from the female genital tract.

Menstruation—The process by which the lining of the uterus is shed in the absence of pregnancy.

Mensuration—An examination technique that uses measurement to evaluate a patient.

Mesentery—Tissue that attaches to the abdominal wall and supports the small intestine.

Message—Formed during the second part of communication. The message content varies depending on what level of complexity is used to enable the receiver to understand.

Metabolism—The process of biochemical modification or degradation of a drug in the body.

Metaphysis—The wide ends of long bones.

Meter (m)—The basic unit of measurement in the metric system for measuring length or distance.

Metric system—A system of measurement based on the decimal system; all units are described as multiples of 10.

Micronutrients—Nutrients that do not provide energy.

Microorganisms—Microscopic creatures capable of transmission and reproduction in specific circumstances.

Midbrain—The part of the brain stem that is the control center for visual reflexes, such as moving the head and eyes.

Mineral—An inorganic substance that regulates homeostasis or acts as a constituent of an organic molecule.

Mineralocorticoids—A type of corticosteroid; controls the concentration of salt and potassium in the body's fluids.

Miscarriage—A spontaneous abortion.

Misdemeanor—A civil crime that is punishable by imprisonment for less than one year.

Mitral valve—One of two atrioventricular valves in the heart; separates the left atrium from the left ventricle; also called the bicuspid valve.

Mixed nerve—A nerve containing both sensory and motor fibers.

Mixed number—A number that contains both whole numbers and fractions.

Mode of transmission—The means by which a microorganism travels from the portal of exit to another host.

Molars—Teeth located toward the back of the mouth that are used for crushing and grinding food.

Monosaccharides—One-sugar carbohydrates.

Moral values—Learned traits in society, the family, and the culture in which a person lives.

Morphology—Classification based on the shape of a single cell.

Mounting—The process of preparing an ECG tracing for placement in a patient's medical record.

Mucus—Slippery film that lines the respiratory tract and traps foreign bodies and infectious organisms.

Multigravida—A woman who has been pregnant multiple times.

Multiplication—The process of multiplying two or more numbers to find their product.

Musculoskeletal system—A body system that consists of bones and the tissues that connect them, such as tendons, ligaments, and cartilage.

Myelin sheath—Insulating envelope of myelin that surrounds the nerve fiber or axon that facilitates transmission of nerve impulses efficiently and quickly along the nerve cells.

Myelography—An X-ray examination of the spinal canal.

Myocardial infarction (MI)—The death of heart muscle after a prolonged period of decreased oxygen delivery to the heart; also known as a heart attack.

Myocardium—Specialized muscle that is present only in the heart; also called cardiac muscle.

Myometrium—The muscular middle layer of the uterus.

Myopia—Also known as nearsightedness. A disorder in which people have difficulty seeing distant objects and can only see objects close to the eyes.

Myxedema—Underactivity of the thyroid gland; also called hypothyroidism.

N

Nasal speculum—An instrument used to evaluate the nasal passages.

National Healthcareer Association (NHA)—The NHA has two certification boards: the NHA Certification Board and the ExCPT Certification Board. These two entities operate independently to set policy over essential certification activities. They have the responsibility for oversight over all certification and recertification decisions, including governance, eligibility standards, and the development, administration, and scoring of assessment instruments.

Needle—The component that is attached to a syringe that delivers medication.

Needle gauge—The diameter of a needle.

Needle length—The length of a needle.

Needlestick—A wound that pierces the skin, usually caused by a needle or other sharp object.

Negligence—When a professional or his agent does not act in accordance to the standards of his or her profession or makes mistakes and causes injury. Also known as malpractice.

Neonates—Babies between one day and one month old.

Nephrolithiasis—The formation of stones or calculi in the kidney or urinary bladder; also called kidney stones or renal calculi.

Nephrologist—The medical specialist who studies the kidneys.

Nerve—Any of the cordlike bundles of fibers made up of neurons through which sensory stimuli and motor impulses pass between the brain or other parts of the central nervous system and the eyes, glands, muscles, and other parts of the body.

Net pay—The amount of pay remaining after all taxes and employee-paid benefits are deducted from the gross pay.

Network—The group of providers who contract with a managed care organization.

Networking—Connecting with people who can be helpful professionally, especially in finding a position or attempting to advance into another job.

Neurohypophysis—The posterior portion of the pituitary gland.

Neurological examination—An examination that assesses motor and sensory skills, hearing, speech, vision, coordination, balance, mental status, changes in mood or behavior, and the functioning of cranial nerves.

Neuron—The basic functioning unit of the nervous system.

Neurosonography—An ultrasound of the brain and spinal column.

Neurotransmitters—A chemical substance that transmits nerve impulses across a synapse.

Nevus—A chronic, sharply demarcated lesion; commonly called a birthmark or a mole.

Nissl bodies—Large granular bodies found in neurons.

Nocturia—Excessive urination at night.

Nomogram—A graph with several scales arranged so that a straightedge laid on the graph intersects the scales at related values of the variables.

Nonmaleficence—The act of doing no harm to the patient. A physician must not perform acts that risk harm to others.

Nonverbal communication—Body language, gestures, and mannerisms, which may or may not be in agreement with the words a person speaks.

Nose—A major organ of the respiratory system.

Nullipara—A woman who has not carried a pregnancy to viability.

Number—A quantity or amount that is made up of one or more numerals.

Numeral—A symbol or name used to represent a number.

Numerator—The number above the fraction line. The numerator indicates the number of parts out of the whole.

Nurse practitioners (NPs)—Registered nurses with advanced academic training who have obtained a master's degree in nursing. NPs can diagnose and prescribe medications to patients, and focus on preventive care and prevention of disease.

Nutrients—Substances that provide energy for the body or regulate body functions.

Nutrition—The process of taking nutrients into the body.

O

Obesity—A BMI of 30 or greater.

Objective information—Something that can be observed and quantified.

Observation—An examination technique that uses sight to evaluate a patient; also called inspection.

Obstetrician—A medical specialist who cares for a mother before, during, and after pregnancy.

Occipital lobe—The part of the cerebrum that is associated with vision.

Official transcripts—Official school records of students' class grades.

Oliguria—Scant urine production.

Oophorectomy—The removal of the ovaries.

Open fracture—A fracture that involves a break in the skin.

Ophthalmoscope—An instrument used to evaluate the internal structures of the eye.

Orbit—The bony socket that houses the eye.

Orchidectomy—The removal of the testes.

Order—A prescription that is issued and dispensed in an institutional setting.

Ordinance—At the state level, laws passed through the state legislature and local governments.

Origin—One point at which a muscle attaches to the bone.

Orthopedics—The medical field that studies disorders of the musculoskeletal system.

Ossification—The process of the layering of new bone by osteoblasts.

Osteoarthritis (OA)—Degenerative joint inflammation.

Osteoblasts—Cells that deposit new bone during the bone-remodeling process.

Osteoclasts—Cells that erode old bone during the bone-remodeling process.

Osteomyelitis—An infection of the bone and bone marrow.

Osteopathy—A holistic study of medicine that emphasizes the musculoskeletal system and the body as a whole.

Osteopenia—A precursor to osteoporosis, in which the bone begins to lose strength.

Osteoporosis—A condition in which the bone becomes porous and fragile.

Otitis media—Middle ear infection.

Otorhinolaryngology—The medical specialty that studies disorders of the upper respiratory tract.

Otoscope—An instrument used to evaluate the internal structures of the ear.

Ovarian cancer—A malignancy of the ovary.

Ovarian cyst—A fluid-filled or semisolid mass on an ovary.

Ovaries—Female organs responsible for hormones that regulate the menstrual cycle and pregnancy.

Overnutrition—A type of malnutrition characterized by excess nutrient intake.

Over-the-counter drugs—Drugs that can be legally obtained without a prescription and are generally safe for use without medical supervision.

Overweight—A BMI of 25 or greater.

Ovum—The female gamete.

Oxidation—The process of combining a substance with oxygen; the final step of cellular respiration.

Oxygen—The gas needed for healthy cellular function; exchanged with carbon dioxide in respiration.

Oxytocin—The hormone produced in the posterior pituitary, responsible for uterine contraction and milk production in women.

P

Palliative—Treatment that relieves the symptoms of a disease or disorder without curing it.

Palpation—An examination technique that uses touch to evaluate a patient.

Pancreas—An organ found behind the left kidney at the back of the abdominal wall. It aids in digestion and is responsible for the production and secretion of hormones from cells called islets of Langerhans.

Pancreatitis—The acute or chronic inflammation of the pancreas.

Papanicolaou test—A screening test for cervical cancer or precancerous cells; also known as a Pap smear.

Papule—A small, elevated, solid area on the skin.

Parasites—Organisms that benefit at the expense of another living organism.

Parasympathetic nervous system—The part of the peripheral nervous system that returns the body to a normal state.

Parathormone—The hormone produced by the parathyroid gland that promotes the absorption of calcium in the gastrointestinal mucosa; also known as parathyroid hormone.

Parathyroid gland—A gland located slightly behind and above the thyroid gland. It produces parathyroid hormone, which helps maintain calcium levels.

Parathyroid hormone (PTH)—The hormone produced by the parathyroid gland that promotes the absorption of calcium in the gastrointestinal mucosa; also known as parathormone.

Parenteral—A route of administration by which the medication is administered by a needle or catheter into one or more layers of the skin.

Parenteral medications—Injectable medications given intravenously, subcutaneously, intradermally, or intramuscularly.

Parenteral product—A product intended for administration by injection through the skin or another external barrier.

Parietal lobe—The part of the cerebrum associated with cognition, information processing, pain and touch sensation, spatial orientation, speech, and visual perception.

Parity—The number of pregnancies a woman has carried to viability.

Parkinson's disease (PD)—A motor-system disorder caused primarily by progressive degeneration of dopamine-containing neurons in the substantia nigra.

Part-time employee—An employee who works fewer hours than a full-time employee.

Parturition—The birth process.

Past medical history (PMH)—A summary of the patient's health status prior to the present illness.

Patella—The kneecap.

Pathogens—Any microorganism that causes disease.

Pathophysiology—The study of the processes or mechanisms by which an illness or disease occurs, the body's response to this state, and the effects of these processes on normal bodily function.

Patient confidentiality—The patient's rights to privacy and freedom from public release of information that the patient regards as being of a personal nature.

Patient Protection and Affordable Care Act (PPACA)—A federal law passed in 2010 that will reform the provision of health care and insurance in the United States.

Peak expiratory flow—The maximum speed of a forced exhalation.

Peak inflation level—The pressure at which the radial pulse disappears when inflating a blood-pressure cuff.

Pectoral girdle—The bones that connect the upper limbs to the axial skeleton.

Pediatricians—Physicians who care for pediatric patients.

Pediatrics—The branch of medicine that studies and cares for patients under 18 years of age.

Pediculosis—An infection caused by the external parasites *Pediculus humanus capitis*, *Pediculus humanus corporis*, or *Phthirus pubis*; commonly known as lice.

Pelvic girdle—The bones that connect the lower limbs to the axial skeleton.

Pelvic inflammatory disease (PID)—An inflammation of any of the female reproductive organs.

Penis—A vascular muscular structure that surrounds the male urethra.

Pepsin—An enzyme produced by the stomach that aids in digestion.

Peptic ulcer disease (PUD)—The frequent recurrence of peptic ulcers.

Peptic ulcers—Lesions in the mucosal lining of the stomach or duodenum.

Peptidases—Enzymes secreted by the duodenum that digest proteins.

Percentage—A ratio used to express the number of parts of 100.

Percussion—An examination technique that uses tapping on a body part to produce sounds to evaluate a patient.

Pericardium—The connective tissue that surrounds the heart.

Perimetrium—The outer layer of the uterus.

Perineum—The area between the urinary meatus and the perineum.

Perionychium—The soft tissue surrounding the fingernail.

Periosteum—A thin membrane that covers the bone and supplies it with lymph vessels, blood vessels, and nerves.

Peripheral artery disease (PAD)—Narrowing of the blood vessels in the extremities due to atherosclerosis.

Peripheral nervous system (PNS)—The division of the nervous system that contains all the nerves that lie outside the central nervous system.

Peristalsis—Involuntary relaxation and contraction of muscles that move food through the GI tract.

Peritoneal dialysis—Dialysis that uses a patient's own abdominal lining to filter blood.

Peritonitis—An inflammation of the peritoneum.

Perks—*See* benefits.

Peroral (PO)—Commonly referred to as the oral route. A route of administration in which the drug is administered orally through the mouth and swallowed to reach the stomach.

Personal and social history—A summary of the aspects of a patient's personal life that contribute to health status.

Personal protective equipment (PPE)—Gloves, gowns, masks, eye protection, etc. to protect the healthcare professional from blood-borne pathogens.

Personal space—The distance at which we feel comfortable with others while communicating.

Pharmacist (Pharm. D)—A person who distributes drugs prescribed by licensed individuals with prescribing authority.

Pharmacodynamic agent—Any drug that alters bodily functions.

Pharmacology—The study of drugs and their properties and how they interact with the body.

Pharynx—A major organ of the respiratory system; the back of the throat.

Phlebotomist—A person who draws blood.

Phlebotomy—The process of collecting blood samples.

Physician assistants (PAs)—Individuals trained to diagnose and treat patients as directed by the physician. They are licensed and have the authority to write prescriptions in most states with advanced degrees in medicine.

Physiology—The study of the function and physical and chemical processes that take place in cells, tissues, and organs.

Pia mater—The innermost layer of meninges closest to the CNS structures.

Pimple—Raised red lesions that appear in acne vulgaris.

Pineal body—A gland that produces and secretes melatonin, a hormone that regulates the sleep-wake cycle.

Pineal gland—An endocrine gland located in the third ventricle of the brain that produces melatonin.

Pituitary gland—A gland that produces hormones that affect the activity of other endocrine glands and specific organs of the body. It is the control tower of the endocrine system.

Placenta—The organ that connects an embryo and fetus to the uterine wall.

Plaintiff—A complaining party in a court case.

Platform crutches—Crutches for patients who cannot bear weight on their hands.

Plexuses—An area where nerves branch and rejoin.

Pneumonia—An infection in the lungs.

Polycystic kidney disease—An inherited disorder characterized by the presence of fluid-filled cysts in the kidneys.

Polypharmacy—The practice of taking multiple medications.

Polyps—Small, usually harmless, growths in the colon.

Polysaccharides—Carbohydrates composed of three or more sugars; also known as complex carbohydrates.

Pons—The part of the brain stem that serves as the communication center between the two hemispheres of the brain. It is the reflex center for secreting saliva, chewing, and tasting.

Portal of entry—The place where an infectious microorganism enters the host's body.

Portal of exit—The place through which a microorganism leaves the reservoir.

Portfolio—Materials representing a person's work or accomplishments collected for viewing.

Positron emission tomography (PET)—A diagnostic scan that provides two- and three-dimensional pictures of brain activity by measuring radioactive isotopes that are injected into the bloodstream.

Posterior (dorsal)—The anatomic directional term that describes back.

Postpartum—The period after the birth of a baby when the hormonal, physical, and physiological changes that occurred during pregnancy return to normal, lasting six to eight weeks.

Postpartum depression (PPD)—Moderate or severe depression that occurs after a woman gives birth.

Posture—The position of the body or parts of the body.

Precedent—A case that serves as a model for future cases. Laws are based on legal decisions from past cases.

Preceptor—An instructor, an expert, or a specialist, such as a physician, who gives practical experience and training to a student, especially of medicine or nursing.

Precision—The ability of a series of measurements to be consistently reproduced or how close the measurements are to each other.

Precocious puberty—Puberty that occurs at a young age.

Precordial leads—The measurement of electrical activity at one point in an ECG; also called chest leads.

Preeclampsia—Higher blood pressure in the second or third trimester of pregnancy.

Preferred provider organization (PPO)—A commercial insurance plan that does not require a patient to choose a primary care provider and allows patients to see specialists without a referral.

Prefix—A word part that is found at the beginning of a word. It often indicates location, presence or absence, size, frequency, quantity, or position.

Prehypertension—A systolic blood pressure between 120 and 139mmHg or a diastolic blood pressure between 80 and 89mmHg.

Premenstrual syndrome (PMS)—Emotional, behavioral, and physical symptoms that occur 7 to 14 days before the onset of menses.

Premolars—Teeth located toward the back of the mouth that are used for crushing and grinding food.

Prepuce—A layer of skin that covers the penis glans; also called the foreskin.

Prescribing cascade—The practice of prescribing a medication to treat a side effect of another medication.

Prescription—A written or verbal order for a specific medication, to be dispensed to a patient by a licensed pharmacist.

Present illness—The symptoms, or what the patient considers to be the cause of the symptoms. Addressed by identifying the specific characteristics and details during examination such as prior health problems or conditions, treatments or medications that have been taken associated with the complaint, a list of current medications, and any allergies the patient may have.

Primary care provider (PCP)—A physician who coordinates all medical care for an individual and provides referrals to specialists.

Problem-oriented interview—A focused patient interview or health history that addresses a specific concern.

Proctitis—Inflammation of the rectum.

Proctologist—A medical specialist who studies the lower digestive tract.

Prodromal stage—The infectious disease stage between the initial symptoms and the symptoms that show a disease process is occurring.

Product—The amount obtained by multiplying two or more numbers.

Professional development—The skills and knowledge attained for both personal development and career advancement.

Professionalism—Status, methods, character, or standards of a person in his or her field.

Prolactin—A hormone produced by the pituitary gland that promotes breast development and the production of milk in the mammary glands.

Prone position—An examination position in which the patient lays face down on the examination table.

Proper fraction—A fraction that has a value that is always less than 1.

Prophylactic agent—Any drug that prevents a disease or illness from occurring.

Prophylaxis—The treatment given before an event or exposure to prevent a disease or symptom.

Proportion—An equation that states two ratios are equal.

Prostate—A gland that surrounds the top of the urethra in men and produces prostatic fluid.

Prostate cancer—A malignancy of the prostate.

Prostatectomy—The surgical removal of the prostate.

Prostate-specific antigen (PSA)—A protein produced by the prostate; used as a measure of prostate function.

Protected health information (PHI)—A term used under HIPAA for patients' personal health information protected under a covered entity except when used for treatment, payment, or healthcare operations.

Protein—A macronutrient that is composed of amino acids.

Proteinuria—Protein in the urine.

Protocol—The policies and procedures set by a practice.

Protussive—A product that changes the consistency of mucus, allowing it to be more easily expelled with a cough; also called an expectorant.

Proximal—The anatomic directional term that describes toward or nearest the trunk or the point of origin of a part.

Pruritis—Itchiness.

Psoriais—A chronic inflammatory condition of the skin characterized by dark red lesions covered in thick, silvery scales.

Ptyalin—An enzyme in saliva that breaks down polysaccharides; also called amylase.

Pulmonary circulation—The part of the circulatory system that transports blood between the lungs and the heart so gas exchange can occur.

Pulmonary embolism (PE)—An embolism that travels to the lungs.

Pulmonary function test—A group of tests used to measure respiratory function and measure lung volumes and gas exchange.

Pulmonary valve—One of four valves in the heart; separates the right ventricle and the pulmonary artery.

Pulmonology—The medical specialty that studies acute and chronic disorders of the lungs.

Pulse—The pressure that is felt through arteries near the skin that is created by the contraction and relaxation of the heart.

Pulse oximetry—A noninvasive test to measure the oxygenation of the blood.

Pulse rate—The number of heartbeats in one minute.

Pustule—Small, pus-filled lesions on the skin.

Pyelonephritis—An inflammation of the kidney and renal pelvis.

Pyloric sphincter—The muscle that controls the opening at the end of the stomach.

Pyrexia—An elevated body temperature; also called febrile.

Pyuria—Pus in the urine.

Q

Quotient—The amount obtained when dividing numbers.

R

Range of motion (ROM)—The total amount of movement allowed by a joint.

Ratio—The relationship between two like quantities.

Receiver—A person receiving a message in communication. To interpret the message being sent, the receiver must listen to and concentrate on the message, aware not only of what is being spoken but also the tone, pitch, and rate of speech.

Reconstitution—The addition of a diluent to a vial of powder.

Rectum—The portion of the colon that collects solid waste products of digestion.

Recumbent length—An assessment of height obtained while an infant or child is lying supine on an examination table and measured from head to feet.

Reduction—Relocation or realignment of a bone or joint.

Reference—An endorsement of a person's work ethic, skills, qualities, and ability to excel in a job.

Registered medical assistant (RMA)—A medical assistant who becomes registered through the AMT. RMAs have similar education backgrounds to CMAs (AAMA) and have formal education through an ABHES or CAHEEP accredited program.

Registered nurse (RN)—A graduate of a school of nursing, and in most scenarios, will have an associate degree. Most work in hospitals or clinics but they may also work alongside other healthcare professionals in ambulatory settings, research, education, and home health.

Rehabilitation medicine—The discipline within medicine that uses physical and mechanical agents to diagnose, treat, and prevent bodily disease and injury.

Reimbursement—The monetary compensation for medical care provided.

Renal calculi—The formation of stones or calculi in the kidney or urinary bladder; also called kidney stones or nephrolithiasis.

Renal corpuscle—A portion of the nephron; consists of the glomerulus and Bowman's capsule.

Renal cortex—The outer layer of the kidney.

Renal failure—A condition in which the kidneys are not able to function normally.

Renal medulla—The inner layer of the kidney.

Renal system—A body system composed of two kidneys, two ureters, one bladder, and one urethra.

Renal tubule—A portion of the nephron; the site of reabsorption.

Reproductive system—A body system that ensures survival of the species. It has four main functions: to produce egg and sperm cells, transport these cells, develop offspring, and produce hormones.

Reservoir—The place where a microorganism can thrive and reproduce.

Respiration—The process of exchanging oxygen for carbon dioxide; consists of inspiration and expiration.

Respiratory rate—The number of breaths completed in one minute.

Respiratory syncytial virus (RSV)—An infectious respiratory organism that can produce a life-threatening infection in infants.

Respiratory system—A body system composed of the nose and nasal cavities, pharynx, larynx, trachea, bronchial tree, and lungs. It works with the circulatory system to provide oxygen and to remove the waste products of metabolism. It also helps to regulate pH of the blood.

Respondeat superior—Describes a situation in which physicians are legally responsible for the actions of an employee or agent to whom the physician has delegated tasks.

Résumé—A document that summarizes one's job qualifications.

Retina—The light-sensitive layer of tissue at the back of the eye that contains the nerve endings that transmit electrical impulses to the brain.

Retinal detachment—A disorder in which the retina is separated from its underlying tissue.

Review of systems (ROS)—Occurs during the physician examination. When conducting the ROS, the physician asks systematic questions and checks all organs and body parts that are essential to make a diagnosis.

Rheumatoid arthritis (RA)—A chronic, inflammatory autoimmune disease.

Rhinorrhea—A runny nose.

RICE protocol—A method of using rest, ice, compression, and elevation to treat strains and sprains.

Rickettsiae—Intracellular parasites that depend completely on their host for survival.

Right atrium—One of two collecting chambers in the heart; receives blood from systemic circulation.

Right ventricle—One of two distributing chambers of the heart; pumps blood to pulmonary circulation.

Risk management—The study of medical liability and the prevention of malpractice.

Role model—A person who another may watch and try to emulate.

Route of administration—How the medication is to be administered.

Rugae—Folds in the mucous membrane of the inner lining of the stomach.

Rule of nines—An estimation of body-surface area.

Ruptured disk—A condition in which the gel between the vertebral disks of the spine is forced outside the disk; also known as a herniated disk.

S

Sagittal plane (lateral plane)—A vertical plane running from front to back that divides the body or any of its parts into right and left sides.

Saliva—Liquid produced by the salivary glands that contains mucus and digestive enzymes.

Salivary glands—Three sets of glands located in the mouth that produce saliva.

Salpingectomy—The removal of the fallopian tubes.

Saturated fatty acid—A fatty acid in which each carbon atom is connected to as many hydrogen atoms as possible.

Scabies—An infection caused by the external parasite *Sarcoptes scabiei*.

Schwann cells—Any of the cells that cover the axons in the peripheral nervous system and form the myelin sheath.

Sclera—The white outer wall of the eye.

Scoliosis—A sideways or lateral curvature of the spine.

Scoop method—A one-handed technique for recapping a needle that reduces the risk of injury or needlestick.

Scope of practice—A boundary that determines what a medical professional may and may not do based on his or her training, experience, and competency.

Screening interview—A phone interview in which the employer may simply want to assess your demeanor and personality, asking some general introductory questions to see if they should schedule you for a face-to-face interview in the future.

Scribe—Someone who writes down verbatim all information communicated during an examination either for later transcription or using a device such as an electronic tablet to make notations in the electronic health record.

Scrotum—A muscular sac that suspends from the perineum and holds the testes.

Sebaceous glands—Glands located in the dermis that produce sebum.

Seborrheic keratosis—A benign skin tumor.

Sebum—An oily substance produced by the sebaceous glands that lubricates the skin, retains water, and helps keep skin and hair soft and supple.

Second-degree burn—A burn that extends through the epidermis and dermis, causing blisters.

Seizures—An abnormal, sudden, excessive firing of a small number of neurons, which interferes with normal brain functioning.

Semen—Sperm and seminal fluid that is expelled from the body during ejaculation.

Seminal fluid—A thick secretion that provides nourishment and mobility for sperm.

Seminal vesicles—Muscular tubes that produce seminal fluid.

Seminiferous tubules—Tubes inside the testes where spermatogenesis takes place.

Sender—The person involved in the first part of the communication cycle. The sender begins by creating or encoding whatever message is being sent.

Septum—The muscle that divides the heart into right and left sections.

Sertoli cells—Cells in the testes that produce male sex hormones.

Sesamoid bones—Small, round bones that are embedded within a tendon.

Sexually transmitted diseases (STDs)—An infectious pathogen spread by sexual contact.

Sharps—Objects that can penetrate the skin, such as needles, scalpels, glass, and capillary tubes.

Shingles—*See* herpes zoster.

Short bones—Small bones that are made of cancellous bone and allow for greater flexibility than long bones.

Short-term goals—Plans or goals for the immediate future.

Side effect—The effect of a drug in addition to its intended effect.

Sigmoid colon—The S-shaped portion of the colon located in the pelvic cavity.

Sign—An objective identifier of a disease or condition.

Sims' position—An examination position in which the patient lays on his or her left side; also called lateral position.

Sinoatrial (SA) node—The area of the heart that generates the electrical impulse that initiates contraction; also known as the heart's pacemaker.

Sinus cavities—Hollow, air-filled pockets in the skull.

Sinusitis—An inflammation of the lining of the sinus cavities.

Site director—The person responsible for your assignment at the externship site as well the person who acts as your manager throughout your externship.

Skeletal muscle—The muscle attached to bones that holds the skeleton together and allows for voluntary movements. Also called striated muscle.

Skeleton—The bones that make up the body's frame and provide protection to internal organs.

Skull—The bones that encase the brain and support the face.

Slander—A defamatory statement that is spoken in words, intended to damage a person's reputation, profession, or means of living.

Small intestine—The tube that receives chyme from the stomach and completes the processes of digestion and absorption.

Smoking cessation—The process of quitting smoking.

Smooth muscle—Involuntary muscle found in the walls of the stomach and intestines and the walls of blood vessels; also called visceral muscle.

Snellen chart—A chart for testing visual acuity, usually consisting of letters, numbers, or pictures printed in lines of decreasing size, which a patient is asked to read or identify at a fixed distance.

SOAP method—A method of formatting in medical records that records the patient's examination or progress notes based on a problem-oriented format.

Social history—Documentation that includes the patient's status (married/single), sexual habits, occupations, hobbies, alcohol use, tobacco use, the use of drugs or any chemical substances, and home environment. This information is typically gathered when the patient first becomes affiliated with the physician and practice.

Somatic nervous system—The part of the peripheral nervous system that controls all the skeletal muscles in the body.

Specific gravity—The characteristic of how concentrated or dilute urine is, related to distilled water.

Sperm—The male gamete.

Spermatogenesis—The production of sperm.

Spirometry—A pulmonary function test that measures the breathing capacity of the lungs.

Splenic flexure—The point at which the transverse colon bends to form the descending colon; located near the spleen.

Spongy bone—One of two types of bone; soft, porous, and resembles a sponge; also called trabecular bone or cancellous bone.

Sprain—A tear in the ligaments surrounding a joint.

Sputum—Mucus of the lower respiratory tract.

Sputum culture—A test to determine bacterial growth in the lungs.

Squamous cell carcinoma (SCC)—The second most common type of skin cancer; exhibits rapid growth and the ability to metastasize.

Squamous epithelial cells—Flat, scalelike cells in the epidermis, or thin, outermost layer of skin.

Standard precautions—The minimum level of infection-control practices recommended by the CDC that should be used by all healthcare professionals all of the time when caring for people.

Statute of limitations—The time limit in which a person can file a claim of medical malpractice in most states.

Sterile—The absence of infection-causing organisms.

Sterility—The inability to reproduce.

Stomach—The saclike structure that stores and digests large particles of food.

Stool—Solid waste that is eliminated from the body through defecation; also called feces.

Strabismus—Also known as crossed eye. A condition in which one eye deviates from the other.

Strain—The overstretching or overuse of a tendon or muscle.

Stratum corneum—The outermost layer of the epidermis.

Stress test—A test used to assess how the circulatory system responds to physiological changes.

Striated muscle—Muscle that attaches to the skeleton and controls voluntary movement; also called skeletal muscle.

Stroke—The interruption in oxygen supply to an area of the brain; also known as a cerebrovascular accident.

Stye—A painful red bump inside the eyelid or at the base of an eyelash. A stye results from an infection of the glands of the eyelids that occurs after the glands have become clogged or from an infected hair follicle at the base of an eyelash.

Subarachnoid space—The space between the arachnoid and the pia mater.

Subcutaneous (subQ)—A route of administration by which a parenteral product is injected under the skin.

Subcutaneous tissue—The innermost layer of skin.

Subdural space—The space between the dura mater and the arachnoid.

Subjective information—Something a patient tells you that cannot be easily quantified or measured.

Subluxation—A partial or incomplete dislocation.

Subtraction—The process of subtracting numbers to find their difference.

Suffix—A word part that is found at the end of the medical term.

Sum—The amount obtained when adding numbers.

Superior (cranial)—The anatomic directional term that means toward the head of the body or upper.

Superior vena cava—Part of the largest vein in the body, which collects blood from the head and arms.

Supine position—An examination position in which the patient lays flat on his or her back; also called horizontal recumbent position.

Surgical asepsis—Procedures or techniques used to maintain sterile conditions during invasive procedures.

Sweat—A fluid produced by the sweat glands in response to elevated body temperatures that cools the body.

Sweat glands—The glands located in the dermis that produce sweat.

Sympathetic nervous system—The part of the peripheral nervous system that accelerates activity in the smooth, involuntary muscles of the body's organs.

Symptom—A subjective experience that a patient feels.

Synarthrosis—A joint that allows no movement between the bones it connects; also called a fibrous joint or fixed joint.

Syncope—Loss of consciousness.

Synergistic effect—When the effect of two substances (drugs) together is more than one drug alone.

Synovial cavity—The cavity that separates two bones in a synovial joint.

Synovial fluid—Fluid secreted by the synovial membrane that lubricates a synovial joint.

Synovial joint—A joint that allows for free movement of the bones it connects; also called a diarthrosis.

Synovial membrane—The membrane that encapsulates the joint cavity and secretes synovial fluid.

Syphilis—An STD caused by *Treponema pallidum*.

Syringe—A calibrated medical instrument that is used to accurately prepare, measure, or administer medication.

Systemic circulation—The part of the circulatory system that transports blood between the heart and the rest of the body so the exchange of nutrients, metabolites, and hormones can occur.

Systemic effect—When the effect of a drug is on the entire body.

Systemic lupus erythematosus (SLE)—An autoimmune disease of connective tissue.

Systole—The contraction phase of the heart; the greatest amount of blood pressure.

Systolic blood pressure—The pressure on the arteries during systole.

Systolic dysfunction—Any condition that reduces the contraction of the heart muscle.

T

Tachycardia—Increased heart rate.

Target—The tissue or organ that hormones affect.

Targeted résumé—Best used when focus is needed on a clear, specific job target. The targeted résumé should contain a career objective, which is a statement that gives the reader a quick idea as to what type of job the professional is seeking.

Taste buds—The sensory receptors for taste.

Temporal artery thermometer—A thermometer that measures body temperature of the skin surface of the forehead.

Temporal lobe—The part of the cerebrum that plays an important role in organizing sensory input, auditory perception, and language and speech production.

Tendinosis—Degeneration of the tendon.

Tendon—A cordlike structure of connective tissue that connects muscle to bone.

Tendonitis—Inflammation of a tendon.

Testes—The male gonads of the scrotum that produce sperm.

Testicular cancer—A malignancy of the testicles.

Testicular self-examination (TSE)—A self-examination of the testicles to identify early signs of testicular cancer.

Tetany—Muscle excitability or tremors that often result from a calcium deficiency.

Thalamus—The part of the brain that lies between the cerebrum and the midbrain. It is involved in sensory perception and regulation of motor functions. The thalamus controls sleep and awake states of consciousness.

Therapeutic agent—Any drug that relieves symptoms of a disease, stops or delays disease, or maintains health.

Therapeutic communication—In therapeutic communication, the healthcare provider shows empathy, giving the patient a sense of comfort when faced with frightening news or when feeling apprehensive about the healthcare information being relayed.

Therapeutic effect—The desired effect of a drug on the body, either to treat a disease or to relieve symptoms.

Thermotherapy—Therapy using heat.

Third-degree burn—A burn that extends through all three layers of skin.

Thoracentesis—A procedure to remove fluid from the space between the lining of the outside of the lungs (pleura) and the wall of the chest.

Thoracic cage—The bones that surround the organs and soft tissues of the chest.

Thoracic cavity—Closed system that contains the lungs and is protected and supported by the ribs.

Thoracic surgeon—A surgeon who performs surgical procedures on the heart, lungs, esophagus, and other organs in the chest.

Throat culture—A method for removing tissue or material from the pharynx to determine bacterial growth.

Thrombus—A blood clot.

Thrush—A fungal infection in the mouth caused by *Candida albicans*.

Thymus—An endocrine gland located in the mediastinum that stimulates the development of the immune system.

Thyroglobulin—The form of thyroxine stored by the thyroid gland.

Thyroid gland—The gland located anteriorly at the base of the neck.

Thyroid-stimulating hormone (TSH)—A hormone produced by the pituitary gland that increases the production of thyroid hormones in the thyroid; also called thyrotropin.

Thyrotoxicosis—Thyroid activity that is above normal; also called hyperthyroidism.

Thyrotropin—A hormone produced by the pituitary gland that increases the production of thyroid hormones in the thyroid; also called thyroid-stimulating hormone (TSH).

Thyroxine (T4)—One of the thyroid hormones produced by the thyroid gland; accounts for nearly all of the thyroid hormones in the body.

Tinea barbae—A fungal infection of the beard and mustache.

Tinea capitis—A fungal infection of the head and scalp.

Tinea corporis—A fungal infection of the trunk and extremities.

Tinea cruris—A fungal infection of the thighs and buttocks.

Tinea manuum—A fungal infection of the palm of the hand.

Tinea pedis—A fungal infection of the feet.

Tinea unguium—A fungal infection of the nail.

Tonsillitis—An inflammation of the tonsils.

Tonsils—Lymphatic tissue located in the pharynx that prevents infectious agents from entering the body through the upper respiratory tract.

Tophi—Uric acid crystals that collect in joints affected by gout.

Tort—A civil wrong or a wrongful act. It can be intentional or accidental (unintentional) when an injury occurs to another person.

Total lung capacity—The total volume of air present in the lungs.

Total peripheral resistance—The sum of the entire resistance in the blood vessels of systemic circulation.

Touch—Refers to touching a patient to communicate in many different ways that cannot be expressed in words.

Tourniquet—A device that is applied above the collection area during a venipuncture to slow blood flow and allow the vein to fill with excess blood.

Trabecular bone—One of two types of bone; soft, porous, and resembles a sponge; also called cancellous bone or spongy bone.

Trace elements—Minerals that are required in minute quantities.

Trachea—A major organ of the respiratory tract; connects the pharynx to the bronchi.

Traditional interview questions—Questions asked to determine how the candidate would behave in certain circumstances.

Transdermal patch—A dosage form in which the medication is in a patch to be applied to the skin.

Trans fats—Trans unsaturated fatty acids that are produced by hydrogenation.

Transient ischemic attack (TIA)—A brief period of decreased oxygen delivery to an area of the brain.

Transverse colon—The portion of the colon that extends across the abdomen from the hepatic flexure to the splenic flexure.

Treason—An attempt to overthrow the nation's government or, in the case of high treason, an attempt or involvement in a plan to assassinate the president of the United States.

Trendelenburg position—A position in which a patient lays in a supine position and the head of the table or bed is lowered.

TRICARE—A program administered by the Department of Defense that provides medical coverage for active and retired military personnel and their dependents.

Tricuspid valve—One of two atrioventricular valves in the heart; separates the right atrium from the right ventricle.

Triglycerides—A type of lipid found in the body that is synthesized from carbohydrates and releases free fatty acids into the body.

Triiodothyronine (T3)—One of the thyroid hormones produced by the thyroid gland; accounts for roughly 5 percent of all the thyroid hormones in the body.

Trimester—A 13-week period in pregnancy.

Tuberculosis (TB)—A contagious bacterial infection in the lining of the lungs.

Tuning fork—An instrument used to assess hearing.

Tympanic thermometer—A thermometer that measures body temperature in the ear canal.

Type 1 diabetes mellitus (DM)—An autoimmune disorder in which the body does not produce insulin.

Type 2 diabetes mellitus (DM)—A condition in which the body's cells cannot use insulin.

U

UB-04—The claims form used by a facility to seek reimbursement for services.

Ulcerative colitis (UC)—A type of IBD characterized by lesions in the rectum and colon.

Ultrasound therapy—A therapeutic modality that uses high-frequency sound waves to heat deep tissues.

Unauthorized disclosure—The unauthorized use of protected health information that compromises the security and privacy of the patient's health information.

Unbundling—The fraudulent practice of reporting multiple codes when only one is appropriate.

Undernutrition—A type of malnutrition characterized by inadequate nutrient intake.

Unintentional tort—A civil tort. An example of an unintentional tort would be when a physician did not use a standard of care that others in the profession would have, known as negligence.

Universal precautions—A set of precautions from the CDC designed to prevent transmission of blood-borne infections, such as HIV/AIDS, hepatitis B, and hepatitis C.

Unsaturated fatty acid—A fatty acid in which some of the carbon atoms are not attached to as many hydrogen atoms as possible.

Upcoding—The fraudulent practice of assigning additional codes that do not match patient documentation.

Upper respiratory tract—Filters, warms, and humidifies inspired air; consists of the nose, sinus cavities, and pharynx.

Ureter—The tube that drains urine from the renal pelvis to the urinary bladder.

Ureteritis—An inflammation of the ureter.

Urethra—The tube that drains urine from the bladder.

Urinalysis—A test that provides chemical and physical information about the quality of urine.

Urinary bladder—A muscular sac that holds urine.

Urinary catheterization—A procedure in which a small, sterile, flexible tube is inserted into the urethra and threaded to the bladder.

Urinary tract infection (UTI)—An infection of any part of the urinary tract.

Urine—The liquid produced by the kidney that contains waste products to be eliminated from the body.

Urologist—The medical specialist who studies the male urinary and reproductive systems.

Urticaria—An acute allergic reaction of the dermis; also known as hives.

Uterine cancer—A malignancy of the uterus.

Uterine leiomyomas—Benign tumors of the muscle cells of the uterus; also called fibroids.

Uterus—A hollow organ that functions as the womb during pregnancy.

V

Vaccine information statement (VIS)—A detailed explanation about a vaccine and its side effects.

Vagina—A muscular tube that connects the uterus to the vulva.

Vascular surgeon—A surgeon who performs surgical procedures involving the blood vessels of the circulatory system.

Vas deferens—A tube that delivers sperm from the epididymis to the urethra.

Vasectomy—A procedure in which a portion of the vas deferens is removed, preventing sperm from leaving the body.

Vasoconstriction—A decrease in the internal diameter of blood vessels.

Vastus lateralis—The muscle of the upper leg; an injection site for IM injections in infants and children.

Vector transmission—Transmission of an infection indirectly via a disease-carrying insect.

Veins—The vessels that carry deoxygenated blood from the body back to the heart.

Vena cava—The largest vein in the body.

Venipuncture—The practice of collecting blood samples from a vein.

Venous thromboembolism (VTE)—An abnormal clot formation in the venous circulation.

Ventilation—The process of moving air in and out of the lungs.

Ventrogluteal—The muscle located at the hip. It is a preferred site for larger dose medication injections.

Venules—The smallest vessel in the venous system.

Verbal communication—Takes place when a message is spoken in communication.

Vermiform appendix—A small, fingerlike projection connected to the cecum.

Verrucae—A viral infection of the skin; also known as warts.

Vertebral column—The bones of the spinal column.

Vertigo—A type of dizziness in which an individual feels a sense of motion even when still.

Viability—The ability of a fetus to grow and develop after birth.

Videonystagmograph—A special examination that measures eye movements. It is used to evaluate balance.

Villi—Microscopic projections covering the inner lining of the small intestine.

Viruses—The smallest of all the microorganisms that require a living host cell to replicate.

Visceral muscle—Muscle that lines hollow organs and controls involuntary movement; also called smooth muscle.

Vitamin—An organic molecule that regulates metabolic processes in the body.

Vulva—External female genitalia.

W

Walker—An assistive device that provides maximum support and stability for ambulation.

Warts—*See* verrucae.

Water-soluble vitamins—Vitamins that are present in extracellular fluid and excreted by the kidneys.

Wheelchair—An assistive device for people who are not able to ambulate.

White-coat syndrome—The phenomenon in which people experience fear or apprehension when visiting a physician's office that leads to inaccurate blood-pressure measurements.

Whole numbers—Counting numbers (0, 1, 2, 3 …).

Word root—A word part that does not have a combining form vowel attached.

X

X-ray—A diagnostic procedure that allows for visualization of the skeleton.

Z

Z-track method—A technique for administering IM injections that minimizes leakage of medication into the skin and subcutaneous tissue.

Zygote—The one-celled union of one male and one female gamete.

References

Chapter 1

About AANP. (2012). *American Association of Nurse Practitioners*. Retrieved November 5, 2012, from http://www.aanp.org/about-aanp

Accreditation. (2012). *Merriam-Webster*. Retrieved October 30, 2012, from http://www.merriam-webster.com/dictionary/accredit

Autonomy. (2012). *FindLaw Legal Dictionary*. Retrieved November 5, 2012, from http://dictionary.findlaw.com/definition/autonomy.html

Balasa, Donald A., JD, MBA. (2009). Certification and Licensure: Facts you should know. *American Association of Medical Assistants*. Retrieved October 30, 2012, from http://www.aama-ntl.org/resources/library/CMAandRMA.pdf

Basic Cardiac Life Support. (2012). *American Heart Association*. Retrieved October 30, 2012, from http://www.heart.org/HEARTORG/CPRAndECC/HealthcareTraining/BasicLifeSupportBLS/Basic-Life-Support-BLS_UCM_001281_SubHomePage.jsp

Booth, K., Whicker, L., Wyman, T., Pugh, D., & Thompson, S. (2009). *Medical Assisting: Administrative and Clinical Procedures Including Anatomy and Physiology, 3rd Edition*. New York, NY: McGraw-Hill Publishing Companies, Inc.

Buppert, C. (2008, November 3). Understanding Medical Assistant Practice Liability Issues. *MedScape News Today*. Retrieved November 5, 2012, from http://www.medscape.com/viewarticle/580647

Certified Medical Assistant (CMA-AAMA). (n.d.). *The American Association of Medical Assistants*. Retrieved October 30, 2012, from http://www.aama-ntl.org/medassisting/caahep_prgs.aspx

Consent. (2012). *FindLaw Legal Dictionary*. Retrieved October 30, 2012, from http://dictionary.findlaw.com/definition/consent.html

Contract. (2012). *FindLaw Legal Dictionary*. Retrieved October 30, 2012, from http://dictionary.findlaw.com/definition/contract.html

Damages. (2012). *The Free Dictionary*. Retrieved October 30, 2012, from http://encyclopedia.thefreedictionary.com/Damages

Emergency. (2012). *Merriam-Webster*. Retrieved October 30, 2012, from http://www.merriam-webster.com/dictionary/emergency

Ethics in Medicine. (2008). *University of Washington School of Medicine*. Retrieved October 30, 2012, from http://depts.washington.edu/bioethx/topics/law.html

Good Samaritan Law. (n.d.). *US Legal*. Retrieved October 30, 2012, from http://definitions.uslegal.com/g/good-samaritans/

Graves, Jada A. (2012, February 27). The Best Jobs of 2012. *U.S. News and World Report*. Retrieved October 30, 2012, from http://money.usnews.com/money/careers/articles/2012/02/27/the-best-jobs-of-2012

HIPAA. *United States Department of Health and Human Services, Office of Civil Rights*. Retrieved November 5, 2012, from http://www.hhs.gov/ocr/office/index.html

The History of the Medical Assistant. (n.d.). *Wake Technical Community College*. Retrieved October 30, 2012, from http://medicalassisting.waketech.edu/index.php?page=history

Larson, A. (2003, October). Assault and Battery. *Expert Law*. Retrieved November 5, 2012, from http://www.expertlaw.com/library/personal_injury/assault_battery.html

Libel. (2012). *Merriam Webster*. Retrieved October 30, 2012, from http://www.merriam-webster.com/dictionary/libel

Licensed Practiced and Licensed Vocational Nurses. (2012). *U.S. Department of Labor, Occupational Outlook Handbook, 2012–2013 Edition*. Bureau of Labor Statistics. Retrieved November 5, 2012, from http://www.bls.gov/ooh/healthcare/licensed-practical-and-licensed-vocational-nurses.htm

Lindh, W., Pooler, M., Tamparo, C., & Dahl, B. (2009). *Delmar's Medical Assisting: Administrative & Clinical Competencies, 4th Edition*. Clifton Park, NY: Delmar Publishing.

Medical Assistants. (2012). *U.S. Department of Labor, Occupational Outlook Handbook, 2012–2013 Edition*. Bureau of Labor Statistics. Retrieved November 4, 2012, from http://www.bls.gov/ooh/Healthcare/Medical-assistants.htm

Negligent. (2012). *The Free Dictionary*. Retrieved October 30, 2012, from http://encyclopedia.thefreedictionary.com/Negligent

Nonmaleficence. (2012). *The Free Dictionary*. Retrieved October 30, 2012, from http://encyclopedia.thefreedictionary.com/Nonmaleficence

Overton, Philip R. (1957, March 9). Rule of "Respondeat Superior." *The Journal of the American Medical Association*, 163(10): 847–52.

Patient Confidentiality. (2012). *The Free Dictionary*. Retrieved October 30, 2012, from http://medical-dictionary.thefreedictionary.com/Patient+confidentiality

Physician Assistants. (2012). *U.S. Department of Labor, Occupational Outlook Handbook, 2012–2013 Edition*. Bureau of Labor Statistics. Retrieved November 5, 2012, from http://www.bls.gov/oco/ocos081.htm

Questions & Answers. (n.d.). *United States Drug Enforcement Agency, Office of Diversion Control*. Retrieved October 30, 2012, from http://www.deadiversion.usdoj.gov/faq/general.htm

Recognition. (n.d.). Accrediting Bureau of Health Education Schools. *ABHES*. Retrieved October 30, 2012, from http://www.abhes.org/recognition

Registered Nurses. (2012). *U.S. Department of Labor, Occupational Outlook Handbook, 2012–2013 Edition*. Bureau of Labor Statistics. Retrieved November 5, 2012, from http://www.bls.gov/ooh/Healthcare/Registered-nurses.htm

Richards, E., JD, MPH. (2009, April 9). Criminal Law. *Law, Science & Public Health Program Site*. LSU Law Center. Retrieved October 30, 2012, from http://biotech.law.lsu.edu/map/CriminalLaw.html

42 USC § 17921—Definitions. (n.d.). Cornell University Law School, Legal Information Institute. Retrieved November 5, 2012, from http://www.law.cornell.edu/uscode/text/42/17921

What are the Basic Principles of Medical Ethics? (n.d.). *Stanford University*. Retrieved October 30, 2012, from http://www.stanford.edu/class/siw198q/websites/reprotech/New%20Ways%20of%20Making%20Babies/EthicVoc.htm

Chapter 2

Ansel, H. C., & Stoklosa, M. J. (2001). *Pharmaceutical Calculations, 11th ed*. Philadelphia, PA: Lippincott, William & Wilkins.

Shah, B., Gibson, J. L., & Tex, N. L. (2013). *The 21st Century Pharmacy Technician*. Burlington, MA: Jones & Bartlett Learning.

Chapter 3

Agur, A. M. R., & Lee, M. J. (1999). *Grant's Atlas of Anatomy*. Philadelphia, PA: Lippincott Williams & Wilkins.

Anatomy. (2012). *MedlinePlus*. Retrieved May 7, 2012, from http://www.nlm.nih.gov/medlineplus/anatomy.html

Anatomy Terms. (2011). *HealthPages.org*. Retrieved May 9, 2012, from http://healthpages.org/anatomy-function/anatomy-terms/

Animal Systems. (n.d.). *Biology4kids.com*. Retrieved May 7, 2012, from http://www.biology4kids.com/files/systems_main.html

Ansel, H. C., & Stoklosa, M. J. (2001). *Pharmaceutical Calculations, 11th ed*. Philadelphia, PA: Lippincott, William & Wilkins.

Atkinson, A. J., Daniels, C. E., & Dedrick, R. (2001). *Principles in Clinical Pharmacology*. San Diego, CA: Academic Press.

Bailey, R. (n.d.). Anatomic Directional Terms and Body Planes. *About.com*. Retrieved May 9, 2012, from http://biology.about.com/od/anatomy/a/aa072007a.htm

Bailey, R. (n.d.). Organ Systems. *About.com*. Retrieved May 9, 2012, from http://biology.about.com/od/organsystems/a/aa031706a.htm

Blesi, M., Wise, B., & Kelley-Arney, C. (2012). *Medical Assisting Administrative & Clinical Competencies, 7th ed*. Clifton Park, NY: Delmar Cengage Learning.

Brunton, L., John L., & Keith, P. (2005). *Goodman and Gillman's the Pharmacologic Basis of Therapeutics, 11th ed*. Elmsford, NY: McGraw-Hill.

DiPiro, J. T., Talbert, R. L., Yee, G. C., Matzke, G. R., Wells, B. G., & Posey, L. M. (2008). *Pharmacotherapy: A Pathophysiologic Approach, 7th ed*. New York, NY: McGraw-Hill Medical.

Dugdale III, D. C. (2011). Conjunctiva. *MedlinePlus*. Retrieved May 7, 2012, from http://www.nlm.nih.gov/medlineplus/ency/article/002326.htm

Dugdale III, D. C. (2011). Retina. *MedlinePlus*. Retrieved May 7, 2012, from http://www.nlm.nih.gov/medlineplus/ency/article/002291.htm

Dugdale III, D. C. (2011). Sclera. *MedlinePlus*. Retrieved May 7, 2012, from http://www.nlm.nih.gov/medlineplus/ency/article/002295.htm

Ehrlich A. (2009). *Medical Terminology for Health Professions, 6th ed*. Clifton Park, NY: Delmar Cengage Learning.

Facts About The Cornea and Corneal Disease. (n.d.). *National Eye Institute*. Retrieved May 7, 2012, from http://www.nei.nih.gov/health/cornealdisease/#0

Kasper, D., Braunwald, E., Fauci, A. S., Hauser, S. L., Longo, D. L., & Jameson, J. L. (2005). *Harrison's Principles of Internal Medicine, 16th ed*. New York, NY: McGraw-Hill Medical.

Medical Plurals. (n.d.). *Meditec*. Retrieved May 9, 2012, from http://www.meditec.com/resourcestools/medical-words/medical-plurals/

Medical Plurals. (n.d.). *MTWorld.com*. Retrieved May 9, 2012, from http://www.mtworld.com/tools_resources/medical_plurals.html

Medical Terminology. (2012). *Global RPh*. Retrieved May 11, 2012, from http://www.globalrph.com/medterm.htm

MedTerms Medical Dictionary. (n.d.). Retrieved May 7, 2012, from http://www.medterms.com

MedWord Resources. (n.d.). Retrieved May 9, 2012, from http://www.medword.com/combos.html

Physiology. (n.d.). *The Free Dictionary*. Retrieved May 7, 2012, from http://medical-dictionary.thefreediction-ary.com/physiology

Rhoades, R., & Pflanzer, R. (2003). *Human Physiology, 4th ed.* Pacific Grove, CA: Thomson Learning.

Shah, B., Gibson, J. L., & Tex, N. L. (2013). *The 21st Century Pharmacy Technician*. Burlington, MA: Jones & Bartlett Learning.

Spelling Tip: Latin and Greek Plurals. (n.d.). *Biomedical Editor*. Retrieved May 7, 2012, from http://www.bio-medicaleditor.com/spelling-tip-latin.html

Stedman's. (1997). *Stedman's Concise Medical Dictionary for Health Professionals, 3rd ed.* Baltimore, MD: Lippincott Williams & Wilkins.

Thibodeau, G., & Patton, K. (2007). *Structure and Function of the Body, 13th ed.* St Louis, MO: Mosby.

Chapter 4

Balasa, Donald A., JD, MBA. (2008). New Roles for the Certified Medical Assistant to Enhance Quality and Effectiveness of Care. *Journal of Medical Practice Management American Association of Medical Assistants*, March/April 2008. Retrieved November 2, 2012, from http://www.aama-ntl.org/resources/library/JMPM_New_Roles_CMAs.pdf

Blesi, M., Kelly-Arney, C., & Wise, B. (2012). *Medical Assisting: Administrative and Clinical Competencies, 7th Edition.* Clifton Park, NY: Delmar Publishing Companies, Inc.

Booth, K., Whicker, L., Wyman, T., Pugh, D., & Thompson, S. (2009). *Medical Assisting: Administrative and Clinical Procedures Including Anatomy and Physiology, 3rd Edition.* New York, NY: McGraw-Hill Publishing Companies, Inc.

Certification Commission for Healthcare Information Technology (CCHIT). (2010). *SearchHealthIT*. Retrieved November 2, 2012, from http://searchhealthit.techtarget.com/definition/CCHIT

Consulta, G. (2008). "Therapeutic Communications Skills: A Guide for Medical Assisting Students." June 19, 2008. Retrieved November 2, 2012, from http://www.slideshare.net/consgp/therapeutic-communications-skills

Culture. (2012). *Merriam Webster*. Retrieved November 2, 2012, from http://www.merriam-webster.com/medical/culture

Dictate. (2012). *The Free Dictionary*. Retrieved November 2, 2012, from http://www.thefreedictionary.com/dictate

Documentation. (2012). *The Free Dictionary*. Retrieved November 2, 2012, from http://www.thefreedictionary.com/documentation

Egede, Leonard E., MD, MS. (2006). Race, Ethnicity, Culture, and Disparities in Health Care. *Journal of General Internal Medicine, June 2006 21(6):667–669.*

Retrieved November 2, 2012, from http://www.ncbi.nlm.nih.gov/pmc/articles/PMC1924616/

HIPAA. (n.d.). *United States Department of Health and Human Services, Office of Civil Rights*. Retrieved November 2, 2012, from http://www.hhs.gov/ocr/privacy/index.html

Hudelson, P. (2004). Improving Patient-Provider Communication: Insights from Interpreters. *Oxford Journals Family Practice*, Volume 24, Issue 3, pp. 311–316. Retrieved November 2, 2012, from http://fampra.oxfordjournals.org/content/22/3/311.full

Lindh, B., Pooler, M., Tamparo, C., & Dahl, B. (2009). *Comprehensive Medical Assisting: Administrative and Clinical Competencies*. Clifton Park, NY: Delmar/Cengage Learning, Inc.

Nonverbal Communication. (2009). *Encyclopedia.com*. Retrieved November 2, 2012, from http://www.encyclopedia.com/topic/Nonverbal_communication

Penalties Under HIPAA. (2012). *UCD Davis Health Systems*. Retrieved November 2, 2012 from http://www.ucdmc.ucdavis.edu/compliance/guidance/privacy/penalties.html

Reid, John E. and associates. (n.d.). The Role of Eye Contact During Interpersonal Communication. *Police Link*. Retrieved November 2, 2012, from http://policelink.monster.com/training/articles/1951-the-role-of-eye-contact-during-interpersonal-communication

SOAP. (2012). *The Free Dictionary*. Retrieved November 2, 2012, from http://medical-dictionary.thefreediction-ary.com/SOAP

University of Massachusetts Medical School Office of Community Programs. (2004)."Physician Toolkit and Curriculum." Retrieved November 2, 2012 from http://minorityhealth.hhs.gov/assets/pdf/checked/1/toolkit.pdf

Chapter 5

AIDS. (n.d.). *Avert.org*. Retrieved May 20, 2012, from http://www.avert.org/aids.htm

Ansel, H. C., & Stoklosa, M. J. (2001). *Pharmaceutical Calculations, 11th ed.* Philadelphia, PA: Lippincott, William & Wilkins.

Atkinson, A. J., Daniels, C. E., & Dedrick, R. (2001). *Principles in Clinical Pharmacology*. San Diego, CA: Academic Press.

Amniocentesis. (2012). *MedlinePlus*. Retrieved May 16, 2012, from http://www.nlm.nih.gov/medlineplus/ency/article/003921.htm

Anthrax. (2012). *A.D.A.M. Medical Encyclopedia*. Retrieved May 15, 2012, from http://www.ncbi.nlm.nih.gov/pubmedhealth/PMH0002301/

Bacterial Infections. (2012). *MedlinePlus*. Retrieved May 16, 2012, from http://www.nlm.nih.gov/medlineplus/bacterialinfections.html

Basic Infection Control and Prevention Plan for Outpatient Oncology Settings. (2011). *Centers for Disease*

Control and Prevention. Retrieved May 15, 2012, from http://www.cdc.gov/HAI/settings/outpatient/basic-infection-control-prevention-plan-2011/transmission-based-Precautions.html

Basic Information about HIV and AIDS. (2012). *Centers for Disease Control and Prevention*. Retrieved May 26, 2012, from http://www.cdc.gov/hiv/topics/basic/index.htm

Blesi, M., Wise, B., & Kelley-Arney, C. (2012). *Medical Assisting Administrative & Clinical Competencies, 7th ed.* Clifton Park, NY: Delmar Cengage Learning.

Bloodborne Infectious Diseases: HIV/AIDS, Hepatitis B, Hepatitis C. (2011). *Centers for Disease Control and Prevention*. Retrieved May 15, 2012, from http://www.cdc.gov/niosh/topics/bbp/sharps.html

Brunton, L., John L., & Keith, P. (2005). *Goodman and Gillman's the Pharmacologic Basis of Therapeutics, 11th ed.* Elmsford, NY: McGraw-Hill.

Chlamydia. (2010). *A.D.A.M. Medical Encyclopedia*. Retrieved May 25, 2012, from http://www.ncbi.nlm.nih.gov/pubmedhealth/PMH0002321/

DiPiro, J. T., Talbert, R. L., Yee, G. C., Matzke, G. R., Wells, B. G., & Posey, L. M. (2008). *Pharmacotherapy: A Pathophysiologic Approach, 7th ed.* New York, NY: McGraw-Hill Medical.

Dugdale III, D. C., & Hadjiliadis, D. (2010). Thoracentesis. *MedlinePlus*. Retrieved May 16, 2012, from http://www.nlm.nih.gov/medlineplus/ency/article/003420.htm

E. coli. (2012). *Centers for Disease Control and Prevention*. Retrieved May 15, 2012, from http://www.cdc.gov/ecoli/

Epstein-Barr Virus and Infectious Mononucleosis. (2006). *Centers for Disease Control and Prevention*. Retrieved May 15, 2012, from http://www.cdc.gov/ncidod/diseases/ebv.htm

Fairfax, R. (2009). Letter to Teika Tanksley. Standard Interpretations: 1910:1030. *Occupation Safety and Health Administration*. Retrieved May 15, 2012, from http://www.osha.gov/pls/oshaweb/owadisp.show_document?p_table=INTERPRETATIONS&p_id=27092

Fungus. (2011). *Medicine.net*. Retrieved May 16, 2012, from http://www.medterms.com/script/main/art.asp?articlekey=3527

Garner J. S., Jarvis W. R., Emori, T. G., Horan, T. C., & Hughes, J. M. (1996). "CDC Definitions of Nosocomial Infections." In: Olmsted, R. N., (Ed.), APIC Infection Control and Applied Epidemiology: Principles and Practice. St. Louis, MO: Mosby. Retrieved May 25, 2012, from http://health.utah.gov/epi/diseases/legionella/plan/cdcdefsnosocomial%20infection.pdf

Genital Herpes–CDC Fact Sheet. (2012). *Centers for Disease Control and Prevention*. Retrieved May 15, 2012, from http://www.cdc.gov/std/herpes/stdfact-herpes.htm

Genital HPV Infection—Fact Sheet. (2012). *Centers for Disease Control and Prevention*. Retrieved May 15, 2012, from http://www.cdc.gov/std/hpv/stdfact-hpv.htm

Genital Warts. (2011). *A.D.A.M. Medical Encyclopedia*. Retrieved May 15, 2012, from http://www.ncbi.nlm.nih.gov/pubmedhealth/PMH0001889/

Gonorrhea. (2011). *A.D.A.M. Medical Encyclopedia*. Retrieved May 15, 2012, from http://www.ncbi.nlm.nih.gov/pubmedhealth/PMH0004526/

Guidance for the Selection and Use of Personal Protective Equipment (PPE) in the Healthcare Settings. (n.d.). *Centers for Disease Control and Prevention*. Retrieved June 1, 2012, from http://www.cdc.gov/HAI/pdfs/ppe/PPEslides6-29-04.pdf

Guidelines for Environmental Infection Control in Health-Care Facilities. (2003). *Centers for Disease Control and Prevention*. Retrieved May 15, 2012, from http://www.cdc.gov/hicpac/pdf/guidelines/eic_in_HCF_03.pdf

Guide to Infection Prevention for Outpatient Settings: Minimum Expectations for Safe Care. (2011). *Centers for Disease Control and Prevention*. Retrieved May 15, 2012, from http://www.cdc.gov/HAI/settings/outpatient/outpatient-care-gl-standard-Precautions.html

Health Care Wide Hazards: (Lack of) Universal Precautions. (n.d.). *Occupational Safety and Health Administration*. Retrieved May 15, 2012, from http://www.osha.gov/SLTC/etools/hospital/hazards/univprec/univ.html

Hepatitis A. (2011). *A.D.A.M. Medical Encyclopedia*. Retrieved May 25, 2012, from http://www.ncbi.nlm.nih.gov/pubmedhealth/PMH0001323/

Hepatitis C. (2011). *A.D.A.M. Medical Encyclopedia*. Retrieved May 25, 2012, from http://www.ncbi.nlm.nih.gov/pubmedhealth/PMH0001329/

How to Handrub? (2009). *World Health Organization*. Retrieved June 1, 2012, from http://www.who.int/gpsc/5may/How_To_HandRub_Poster.pdf

How to Handwash? (2009). *World Health Organization*. Retrieved June 1, 2012, from http://www.who.int/gpsc/5may/How_To_HandWash_Poster.pdf

Kasper, D., Braunwald, E., Fauci, A. S., Hauser, S. L., Longo, D. L., & Jameson, J. L. (2005). *Harrison's Principles of Internal Medicine, 16th ed.* New York, NY: McGraw-Hill Medical.

Morbidity and Mortality Weekly Report: Guideline for Hand Hygiene in Health-Care Settings. (2012). *Centers for Disease Control and Prevention*. Retrieved May 15, 2012, from http://www.cdc.gov/mmwr/PDF/rr/rr5116.pdf

Morbidity and Mortality Weekly Report: Summary of Notifiable Diseases United States, 2009. (2011). *Centers for Disease Control and Prevention*. Retrieved May 15, 2012, from http://www.cdc.gov/mmwr/preview/mmwrhtml/mm5853a1.htm?s_cid=mm5853a1_w

Needlesticks: Frequently Asked Questions. (n.d.). *Occupational Safety and Health Administration*. Retrieved May 15, 2012, from http://www.osha.gov/needlesticks/needlefaq.html

Occupational HIV Transmission and Prevention Among Health Care Workers. (2011). *Centers for Disease Control and Prevention*. Retrieved May 15, 2012, from http://www.cdc.gov/hiv/resources/factsheets/hcwprev.htm

OSHA Fact Sheet: Bloodborne Pathogen Exposure Incidents. *Occupational Safety and Health Administration*. Retrieved June 15, 2012, from http://www.osha.gov/OshDoc/data_BloodborneFacts/bbfact04.pdf

OSHA Fact Sheet: Protecting Yourself When Handling Contaminated Sharps. *Occupational Safety and Health Administration*. Retrieved May 25, 2012, from http://www.osha.gov/OshDoc/data_BloodborneFacts/bbfact02.pdf

Preventing Needlestick Injuries in Health Care Settings. (1999). *National Institute for Occupational Safety and Health*. Retrieved June 12, 2012, from http://www.cdc.gov/niosh/docs/2000-108/pdfs/2000-108.pdf

Pulmonary Tuberculosis. (2011). *A.D.A.M. Medical Encyclopedia*. Retrieved May 25, 2012, from http://www.ncbi.nlm.nih.gov/pubmedhealth/PMH0001141/

Schoenstadt, A. (2006). Polio Transmission. *eMedTV*. Retrieved May 15, 2012, from http://polio.emedtv.com/polio/polio-transmission.html

Shah, B., Gibson, J. L., & Tex, N. L. (2013). *The 21st Century Pharmacy Technician*. Burlington, MA: Jones & Bartlett Learning.

Standard Precautions. (2010). *Minnesota Department of Health*. Retrieved May 24, 2012, from http://www.health.state.mn.us/divs/idepc/dtopics/infectioncontrol/pre/standard.html

Standard Precautions in Health Care. (2007). *World Health Organization*. Retrieved May 15, 2012, from http://www.who.int/csr/resources/publications/EPR_AM2_E7.pdf

Stedman's. (1997). *Stedman's Concise Medical Dictionary for Health Professionals, 3rd ed.* Baltimore, MD: Lippincott Williams & Wilkins.

Syphilis. (2012). *Centers for Disease Control and Prevention*. Retrieved May 15, 2012, from http://www.cdc.gov/std/syphilis/

Tetanus. (2011). *A.D.A.M. Medical Encyclopedia*. Retrieved May 25, 2012, from http://www.ncbi.nlm.nih.gov/pubmedhealth/PMH0001640/

Travelers' Health: Infectious Diseases Related to Travel. (2011). *Centers for Disease Control and Prevention*. Retrieved May 15, 2012, from http://wwwnc.cdc.gov/travel/yellowbook/2012/chapter-3-infectious-diseases-related-to-travel/measles-rubeola.htm

Vaccines and Preventable Diseases: Rubella Disease In-Short (German Measles). (2011). *Centers for Disease Control and Prevention*. Retrieved May 15, 2012, from http://www.cdc.gov/vaccines/vpd-vac/rubella/in-short-adult.htm

Viral Infections. (2012). *MedlinePlus*. Retrieved May 16, 2012, from http://www.nlm.nih.gov/medlineplus/viralinfections.html

Chapter 6

Ansel, H. C., & Stoklosa, M. J. (2001). *Pharmaceutical Calculations, 11th ed.* Philadelphia, PA: Lippincott, Williams & Wilkins.

Ballington, D. A., & Anderson, R. J. (2010). *Pharmacy Practice for Technicians: Mastering Community and Hospital Competencies, 4th ed.* St. Paul, MN: Paradigm Publishing.

Bernard, D. (1999). *Clinical Medical Assistant Training Program: Workbook*. Albany, NY: Delmar.

Blesi, M., Wise, B., & Kelley-Arney, C. (2012). *Medical Assisting: Administrative & Clinical Competencies, 7th ed.* Clifton Park, NY: Delmar.

Brasin, G. A., & Dahl, B. M. (2010). *Workbook to Accompany Delmar's Clinical Medical Assisting, 4th ed.* Clifton Park, NY: Delmar.

DiPiro, J. T., Talbert, R. L., Yee, G. C., Matzke, G. R., Wells, B. G., & Posey, L. M. (2008). *Pharmacotherapy: A Pathophysiologic Approach, 7th ed.* New York, NY: McGraw-Hill Medical.

Fremgen, B. F. (1997). *Medical Terminology*. Upper Saddle River, NJ: Prentice-Hall.

Hayward, M. L. (1999). *Clinical Medical Assistant Training Program*. Albany, NY: Delmar.

Lacy, C. F., Armstrong, L., Goldman, M., & Lance, L. (2009). *Drug Information Handbook*. Washington, DC: American Pharmacists Association.

Lindh, W. Q., Pooler, M. S., Tamparo, C. D., & Dahl, B. M. (2010). *Clinical Medical Assisting, 4th ed.* Clifton Park, NY: Delmar.

Ostchega, Y., Dillon, C., Prineas, R. J., McDowell, M., & Carroll, M. (2006). Tables for the Selection of Correct Blood Pressure Cuff Size Based on Self-Reported Height and Weight and Estimating Equations for Mid-Arm Circumference: Data from the US National Health and Nutrition Examination Survey. *Journal of Human Hypertension, 20*(1):15–22.

Pickering, T. G., Hall, J. E., & Appel, L. J. (2005). Recommendations for Blood Pressure Measurement in Humans and Experimental Animals: Part 1: Blood Pressure Measurement in Humans: A Statement for Professionals from the Subcommittee of Professional and Public Education of the American Heart Association Council on High Blood Pressure Research. *Circulation, 111*(5):697–716.

Shah, B., Gibson, J. L., & Tex, N. L. (2013). *The 21st Century Pharmacy Technician*. Burlington, MA: Jones & Bartlett Learning.

Sparks, J., & McCartney, L. (2010). *Pharmacy Labs for Technicians: Building Skills in Pharmacy Practice.* St. Paul, MN: Paradigm Publishing.

Chapter 7

Ansel, H. C., & Stoklosa, M. J. (2001). *Pharmaceutical Calculations, 11th ed.* Philadelphia, PA: Lippincott, William & Wilkins.

Atkinson, A. J., Daniels, C. E., & Dedrick, R. (2001). *Principles in Clinical Pharmacology.* San Diego, CA: Academic Press.

Blesi, M., Wise, B., & Kelley-Arney, C. (2012). *Medical Assisting Administrative & Clinical Competencies, 7th ed.* Clifton Park, NY: Delmar Cengage Learning.

DiPiro, J. T., Talbert, R. L., Yee, G. C., Matzke, G. R., Wells, B. G., & Posey, L. M. (2008). *Pharmacotherapy: A Pathophysiologic Approach, 7th ed.* New York, NY: McGraw-Hill Medical.

Kasper, D., Braunwald, E., Fauci, A. S., Hauser, S. L., Longo, D. L., & Jameson, J. L. (2005). *Harrison's Principles of Internal Medicine, 16th ed.* New York, NY: McGraw-Hill Medical.

Lindh, W. Q., Pooler, M. S., Tamparo, C. D., & Dahl, B. M. (2010). *Delmar's Clinical Medical Assisting, 4th ed.* Clifton Park, NY: Delmar Cengage Learning.

Shah, B., Gibson, J. L., & Tex, N. L. (2013). *The 21st Century Pharmacy Technician.* Burlington, MA: Jones & Bartlett Learning.

Chapter 8

Acne. (2011). *A.D.A.M. Medical Encyclopedia.* Retrieved March 25, 2012, from http://www.ncbi.nlm.nih.gov/pubmedhealth/PMH0001876/

Agur, A. M. R., & Lee, M. J. (1999). *Grant's Atlas of Anatomy.* Philadelphia, PA: Lippincott, Williams & Wilkins.

Ansel, H. C., & Stoklosa, M. J. (2001). *Pharmaceutical Calculations, 11th ed.* Philadelphia, PA: Lippincott, Williams & Wilkins.

Basal Cell Carcinoma. (2011). *A.D.A.M. Medical Encyclopedia.* Retrieved March 25, 2012, from http://www.ncbi.nlm.nih.gov/pubmedhealth/PMH0001827/

Berardi, R. R., Ferreri, S. P., Hume, A. L., Kroon, L. A., Newton, G. D. et al. (2002). *Handbook of Nonprescription Drugs: An Interactive Approach to Self-Care, 13th ed.* Washington, DC: American Pharmacists Association.

Bickley, L. S. (2003). *Bates' Guide to Physical Examination and History Taking, 8th ed.* Philadelphia, PA: Lippincott, Williams, & Wilkins.

Cellulitis. (2011). *A.D.A.M. Medical Encyclopedia.* Retrieved March 25, 2012, from http://www.ncbi.nlm.nih.gov/pubmedhealth/PMH0001858/

Cutaneous candidiasis. (2010). *A.D.A.M. Medical Encyclopedia.* Retrieved March 25, 2012, from http://www.ncbi.nlm.nih.gov/pubmedhealth/PMH0001883/

DiPiro, J. T., Talbert, R. L., Yee, G. C., Matzke, G. R., Wells, B. G., & Posey, L. M. (2008). *Pharmacotherapy: A Pathophysiologic Approach, 7th ed.* New York, NY: McGraw-Hill Medical.

Folliculitis. (2010). *A.D.A.M. Medical Encyclopedia.* Retrieved March 25, 2012, from http://www.ncbi.nlm.nih.gov/pubmedhealth/PMH0001826/

Fremgen, B. F. (1997). *Medical Terminology.* Upper Saddle River, NJ: Prentice-Hall.

Herpes–Oral. (2012). *A.D.A.M. Medical Encyclopedia.* Retrieved March 25, 2012, from http://www.ncbi.nlm.nih.gov/pubmedhealth/PMH0001631/

Hives (Urticaria). (2011). *A.D.A.M. Medical Encyclopedia.* Retrieved March 25, 2012, from http://www.ncbi.nlm.nih.gov/pubmedhealth/PMH0001848/

Impetigo. (2010). *A.D.A.M. Medical Encyclopedia.* Retrieved March 25, 2012, from http://www.ncbi.nlm.nih.gov/pubmedhealth/PMH0001863/

Keir, L., Wise, B., Krebs, C., & Kelley-Arney, C. (2007). *Medical Assisting: Administrative and Clinical Competencies, 6th ed.* Clifton Park, NY: Delmar.

Lacy, C. F., Armstrong, L., Goldman, M., & Lance, L. (2009). *Drug Information Handbook.* Washington, DC: American Pharmacists Association.

Lindh, W. Q., Pooler, M. S., Tamparo, C. D., & Dahl, B. M. (2010). *Clinical Medical Assisting, 4th ed.* Clifton Park, NY: Delmar.

Melanoma. (2012). *A.D.A.M. Medical Encyclopedia.* Retrieved March 25, 2012, from http://www.ncbi.nlm.nih.gov/pubmedhealth/PMH0001853/

Psoriasis. (2012). *A.D.A.M. Medical Encyclopedia.* Retrieved March 25, 2012, from http://www.ncbi.nlm.nih.gov/pubmedhealth/PMH0001470/

Ringworm. (2011). *A.D.A.M. Medical Encyclopedia.* Retrieved March 25, 2012, from http://www.ncbi.nlm.nih.gov/pubmedhealth/PMH0002411/

Scabies. (2010). *A.D.A.M. Medical Encyclopedia.* Retrieved March 25, 2012, from http://www.ncbi.nlm.nih.gov/pubmedhealth/PMH0001833/

Shah, B., Gibson, J. L., & Tex, N. L. (2013). *The 21st Century Pharmacy Technician.* Burlington, MA: Jones & Bartlett Learning.

Shingles. (2012). *A.D.A.M. Medical Encyclopedia.* Retrieved March 25, 2012, from http://www.ncbi.nlm.nih.gov/pubmedhealth/PMH0001861/

Squamous Cell Carcinoma. (2011). *A.D.A.M. Medical Encyclopedia.* Retrieved March 25, 2012, from http://www.ncbi.nlm.nih.gov/pubmedhealth/PMH0001832/

Thompson, J. E. (1998). *A Practical Guide to Contemporary Pharmacy Practice.* Baltimore, MD: Lippincott, Williams & Wilkins.

Warts. (2011). *A.D.A.M. Medical Encyclopedia.* Retrieved March 25, 2012, from http://www.ncbi.nlm.nih.gov/pubmedhealth/PMH0001888/

Chapter 9

Agur, A. M. R., & Lee, M. J. (1999). *Grant's Atlas of Anatomy*. Philadelphia, PA: Lippincott, Williams & Wilkins.

Ansel, H. C., Allen, L. V., Jr., & Popovich, N. G. (1999). *Pharmaceutical Dosage Forms and Drug Delivery Systems, 7th ed.* Philadelphia, PA: Lippincott, Williams & Wilkins.

Ansel, H. C., & Stoklosa, M. J. (2001). *Pharmaceutical Calculations, 11th ed.* Philadelphia, PA: Lippincott, Williams & Wilkins.

Berardi, R. R., Ferreri, S. P., Hume, A. L., Kroon, L. A., Newton, G. D. et al., eds. (2002). *Handbook of Nonprescription Drugs: An Interactive Approach to Self-Care, 13th ed.* Washington, DC: American Pharmacists Association.

Bickley, L. S. (2003). *Bates' Guide to Physical Examination and History Taking, 8th ed.* Philadelphia, PA: Lippincott, Williams, & Wilkins.

Blesi, M., Wise, B., & Kelley-Arney, C. (2012). *Medical Assisting: Administrative & Clinical Competencies, 7th ed.* Clifton Park, NY: Delmar.

Centers for Disease Control and Prevention. *The National Health and Nutrition Examination Survey III: Spirometry Manual.* (1988). Rockville, MD: Westat, Inc. Retrieved April 12, 2012, from http://www.cdc.gov/nchs/data/nhanes/nhanes3/cdrom/nchs/manuals/spiro.pdf

Chronic Obstructive Pulmonary Disease. (2011). *A.D.A.M. Medical Encyclopedia.* Retrieved April 9, 2012, from http://www.ncbi.nlm.nih.gov/pubmedhealth/PMH0001153/

Cystic Fibrosis. (2012). *A.D.A.M. Medical Encyclopedia.* Retrieved April 9, 2011, from http://www.ncbi.nlm.nih.gov/pubmedhealth/PMH0001167/

DiPiro, J. T., Talbert, R. L., Yee, G. C., Matzke, G. R., Wells, B. G., & Posey, L. M. (2008). *Pharmacotherapy: A Pathophysiologic Approach, 7th ed.* New York, NY: McGraw-Hill Medical.

Fremgen, B. F. (1997). *Medical Terminology.* Upper Saddle River, NJ: Prentice-Hall.

Keir, L., Wise, B., Krebs, C., & Kelley-Arney, C. (2007). *Medical Assisting: Administrative and Clinical Competencies, 6th ed.* Clifton Park, NY: Delmar.

Lacy, C. F., Armstrong, L., Goldman, M., & Lance, L. (2009). *Drug Information Handbook.* Washington, DC: American Pharmacists Association.

Nebulizer Treatments. (2008). *Children's Hospitals and Clinics of Minnesota.* Retrieved April 12, 2012, from http://www.childrensmn.org/Manuals/PFS/HomeCare/018703.pdf

Pneumonia. (2012). *A.D.A.M. Medical Encyclopedia.* Retrieved April 9, 2012, from http://www.ncbi.nlm.nih.gov/pubmedhealth/PMH0001200/

Respiratory Syncitial Virus. (2011). *A.D.A.M. Medical Encyclopedia.* Retrieved April 10, 2012, from http://www.ncbi.nlm.nih.gov/pubmedhealth/PMH0002531/

Shah, B., Gibson, J. L., & Tex, N. L. (2013). *The 21st Century Pharmacy Technician.* Burlington, MA: Jones & Bartlett Learning.

Smoking & Tobacco Use. (2011). *Centers for Disease Control and Prevention.* Retrieved April 10, 2012, from http://www.cdc.gov/tobacco/data_statistics/fact_sheets/cessation/quitting/index.htm

Stop Smoking. (2012). *American Lung Association.* Retrieved April 10, 2012, from www.lung.org/stop-smoking/

Thompson, J. E. (1998). *A Practical Guide to Contemporary Pharmacy Practice.* Baltimore, MD: Lippincott, Williams & Wilkins.

Zieve, D., & Hadjiliadis, D. (2012). Metered Dose Inhaler Use. *MedLinePlus.* Retrieved April 12, 2012, from http://www.nlm.nih.gov/medlineplus/ency/presentations/100200_1.htm

Chapter 10

Agur, A. M. R., & Lee, M. J. (1999). *Grant's Atlas of Anatomy.* Philadelphia, PA: Lippincott Williams & Wilkins.

Allen, L. V., Popovich, N. G., & Ansel, H. C. (2010). *Ansel's Pharmaceutical Dosage Forms and Drug Delivery System, 9th ed.* Philadelphia, PA: Lippincott, Williams & Wilkins.

Ansel, H. C., & Stoklosa, M. J. (2001). *Pharmaceutical Calculations, 11th ed.* Philadelphia, PA: Lippincott, William & Wilkins.

Atkinson, A. J., Daniels, C. E., & Dedrick, R. (2001). *Principles in Clinical Pharmacology.* San Diego, CA: Academic Press.

Blesi, M., Wise, B., & Kelley-Arney, C. (2012). *Medical Assisting Administrative & Clinical Competencies, 7th ed.* Clifton Park, NY: Delmar Cengage Learning.

Brunton, L., John L., & Keith, P. (2005). *Goodman and Gillman's the Pharmacologic Basis of Therapeutics, 11th ed.* Elmsford, NY: McGraw-Hill.

DiPiro, J. T., Talbert, R. L., Yee, G. C., Matzke, G. R., Wells, B. G., & Posey, L. M. (2008). *Pharmacotherapy: A Pathophysiologic Approach, 7th ed.* New York, NY: McGraw-Hill Medical.

Drug Enforcement Administration. (2011). Drugs of Abuse 2011 Edition DEA Resource Guide. Retrieved June 27, 2012, from http://www.justice.gov/dea/pubs/drugs_of_abuse.pdf

Ehrlich A. (2009). *Medical Terminology for Health Professions, 6th ed.* Clifton Park, NY: Delmar Cengage Learning.

The Joint Commission. (2004). Facts About the Official "Do Not Use" List. Retrieved June 28, 2012, from http://www.jointcommission.org/assets/1/18/Do_Not_Use_List.pdf

Kasper, D., Braunwald, E., Fauci, A. S., Hauser, S. L., Longo, D. L., & Jameson, J. L. (2005). *Harrison's*

Principles of Internal Medicine, 16th ed. New York, NY: McGraw-Hill Medical.

Kumar, S. (2010). Crash Cart. *Emergency Medicine MIMS.* Retrieved June 27, 2012, from http://www.emergencymedicinemims.com/articles_details.php?id=16

Lindh, W. Q., Pooler, M. S., Tamparo, C. D., & Dahl, B. M. (2010). *Delmar's Clinical Medical Assisting, 4th ed.* Clifton Park, NY: Delmar Cengage Learning.

Medical Terminology. (2012). *Global RPh.* Retrieved May 11, 2012, from http://www.globalrph.com/medterm.htm

MedTerms Medical Dictionary. (2012). *MedicineNet.com.* Retrieved June 27, 2012, from http://www.medterms.com

Office of Diversion Control, Drug Enforcement Administration. (n.d.). Title 21 United States Code (USC) Controlled Substances Act. Retrieved June 28, 2012, from http://www.deadiversion.usdoj.gov/21cfr/21usc/index.html

Patrick, G. L., & Spencer, J. (2009). *An Introduction to Medicinal Chemistry.* New York: NY: Oxford University Press.

Shah, B., Gibson, J. L., & Tex, N. L. (2013). *The 21st Century Pharmacy Technician.* Burlington, MA: Jones & Bartlett Learning.

Stedman's. (1997). *Stedman's Concise Medical Dictionary for Health Professionals, 3rd ed.* Baltimore, MD: Lippincott Williams & Wilkins.

Thibodeau, G., & Patton, K. (2007). *Structure and Function of the Body, 13th ed.* St Louis, MO: Mosby.

The United States Pharmacopeial Convention. (2009). Pharmaceutical Dosage Forms. Retrieved June 28, 2012, from http://www.usp.org/sites/default/files/usp_pdf/EN/USPNF/pharmaceuticalDosageForms.pdf

Zieve, D., & Hadjiliadis, D. (2012). Metered Dose Inhaler Use. *MedLinePlus.* Retrieved June 27, 2012, from http://www.nlm.nih.gov/medlineplus/ency/presentations/100200_1.htm

Chapter 11

Ansel, H. C., Allen, L. V., & Popovich, N. G. (1999). *Pharmaceutical Dosage Forms and Drug Delivery Systems, 7th ed.* Philadelphia, PA: Lippincott, Williams & Wilkins.

Ansel, H. C., & Stoklosa, M. J. (2001). *Pharmaceutical Calculations, 11th ed.* Philadelphia, PA: Lippincott, Williams & Wilkins.

Ballington, D. A., & Anderson, R. J. (2010). *Pharmacy Practice for Technicians: Mastering Community and Hospital Competencies, 4th ed.* St. Paul, MN: Paradigm Publishing.

Bernard, D. (1999). *Clinical Medical Assistant Training Program: Workbook.* Albany, NY: Delmar.

Blesi, M., Wise, B., & Kelley-Arney, C. (2012). *Medical Assisting: Administrative & Clinical Competencies, 7th ed.* Clifton Park, NY: Delmar.

Brasin, G. A., & Dahl, B. M. (2010). *Workbook to Accompany Delmar's Clinical Medical Assisting, 4th ed.* Clifton Park, NY: Delmar.

Hayward, M. L. (1999). *Clinical Medical Assistant Training Program.* Albany, NY: Delmar.

Lacy, C. F., Armstrong, L., Goldman, M., & Lance, L. (2009). *Drug Information Handbook.* Washington, DC: American Pharmacists Association.

Lindh, W. Q., Pooler, M. S., Tamparo, C. D., & Dahl, B. M. (2010). *Clinical Medical Assisting, 4th ed.* Clifton Park, NY: Delmar.

McCartney, L. (2011). *Sterile Compounding and Aseptic Technique: Concepts, Training, and Assessment for Pharmacy Technicians.* St. Paul, MN: Paradigm Publishing.

Needlestick. (n.d.). Retrieved April 22, 2012, from http://needlestick.com/index.html

Rhinehart, E., & Friedman, M. M. (1999). *Infection Control in Home Care.* Gaithersburg, MD: Aspen Publishers.

Sabon, R. L., Cheng, E. Y., Stommel, K. A., & Hennen, C. R. (1989). Glass Particle Contamination: Influence of Aspiration Methods and Ampule Type. *Anesthesiology, 70*(5):859–62.

Safety and Health Topics: Bloodborne Pathogens and Needlestick Prevention. (n.d.). *Occupational Safety and Health Administration.* Retrieved April 22, 2012, from http://www.osha.gov/SLTC/bloodbornepathogens/

Shah, B., Gibson, J. L., & Tex, N. L. (2013). *The 21st Century Pharmacy Technician.* Burlington, MA: Jones & Bartlett Learning.

Shargel, L., & Yu, A. B. C. (1999). *Applied Biopharmaceutics and Pharmacokinetics, 4th ed.* New York, NY: McGraw-Hill.

Sparks, J., & McCartney, L. (2010). *Pharmacy Labs for Technicians: Building Skills in Pharmacy Practice.* St. Paul, MN: Paradigm Publishing.

Thompson, J. E. (1998). *A Practical Guide to Contemporary Pharmacy Practice.* Baltimore, MD: Lippincott, Williams & Wilkins.

Waller, D. G., & George, C. F. (1986). Ampoules, Infusions, and Filters. *British Medical Journal, 292*:714–5.

Chapter 12

Ansel, H. C., Allen, L. V., & Popovich, N. G. (1999). *Pharmaceutical Dosage Forms and Drug Delivery Systems, 7th ed.* Philadelphia, PA: Lippincott, Williams & Wilkins.

Ansel, H. C., & Stoklosa, M. J. (2001). *Pharmaceutical Calculations, 11th ed.* Philadelphia, PA: Lippincott, Williams & Wilkins.

Arthroscopy. (2010). *OrthoInfo.* American Academy of Orthopaedic Surgeons. Retrieved May 5, 2012, from http://orthoinfo.aaos.org/topic.cfm?topic=a00109

Ballington, D. A., & Anderson, R. J. (2010). *Pharmacy Practice for Technicians: Mastering Community and Hospital Competencies, 4th ed.* St. Paul, MN: Paradigm Publishing.

Bernard, D. (1999). *Clinical Medical Assistant Training Program: Workbook.* Albany, NY: Delmar.

Blesi, M., Wise, B., & Kelley-Arney, C. (2012). *Medical Assisting: Administrative & Clinical Competencies, 7th ed.* Clifton Park, NY: Delmar.

Brasin, G.A., & Dahl, B. M. (2010). *Workbook to Accompany Delmar's Clinical Medical Assisting, 4th ed.* Clifton Park, NY: Delmar.

Broken bone. (2009). *A.D.A.M. Medical Encyclopedia.* Retrieved May 5, 2012, from http://www.ncbi.nlm.nih.gov/pubmedhealth/PMH0001072/

Bursitis. (2010). *A.D.A.M. Medical Encyclopedia.* Retrieved May 5, 2012, from http://www.ncbi.nlm.nih.gov/pubmedhealth/PMH0001456/

Care of Casts and Splints. (2011). *OrthoInfo.* American Academy of Orthopaedic Surgeons. Retrieved May 6, 2012, from http://orthoinfo.aaos.org/topic.cfm?topic=a00095

Cast Types and Maintenance Instructions. (2012). *Lucile Packard Children's Hospital at Stanford.* Retrieved May 5, 2012, from http://www.lpch.org/diseasehealthinfo/healthlibrary/orthopaedics/casts.html

Fitch, M. T., Nicks, B. A., Pariyadath, M., McGinnis, H. D., & Manthey, D. E. (2008). Basic Splinting Techniques. *The New England Journal of Medicine, 359*(26):e32.

Gout. (2011). *A.D.A.M. Medical Encyclopedia.* Retrieved May 5, 2012, from http://www.ncbi.nlm.nih.gov/pubmedhealth/PMH0001459/

Hayward, M. L. (1999). *Clinical Medical Assistant Training Program.* Albany, NY: Delmar.

Herniated Disk. (2007). *OrthoInfo.* American Academy of Orthopaedic Surgeons. Retrieved May 5, 2012, from http://orthoinfo.aaos.org/topic.cfm?topic=a00334

How to Use Crutches, Canes, and Walkers. (2007). *OrthoInfo.* American Academy of Orthopaedic Surgeons. Retrieved May 5, 2012, from http://orthoinfo.aaos.org/topic.cfm?topic=a00181

Idiopathic Scoliosis in Children and Adolescents. (2010). *OrthoInfo.* American Academy of Orthopaedic Surgeons. Retrieved May 5, 2012, from http://orthoinfo.aaos.org/topic.cfm?topic=A00353

Kyphosis (Roundback) of the Spine. (2007). *OrthoInfo.* American Academy of Orthopaedic Surgeons. Retrieved May 5, 2012, from http://orthoinfo.aaos.org/topic.cfm?topic=A00423

Lacy, C. F., Armstrong, L., Goldman, M., & Lance, L. (2009). *Drug Information Handbook.* Washington, DC: American Pharmacists Association.

Lindh, W. Q., Pooler, M. S., Tamparo, C. D., & Dahl, B. M. (2010). *Clinical Medical Assisting, 4th ed.* Clifton Park, NY: Delmar.

McCartney, L. (2011). *Sterile Compounding and Aseptic Technique: Concepts, Training, and Assessment for Pharmacy Technicians.* St. Paul, MN: Paradigm Publishing.

Osteoporosis. (2012). *A.D.A.M. Medical Encyclopedia.* Retrieved May 5, 2012, from http://www.ncbi.nlm.nih.gov/pubmedhealth/PMH0001400/

Rheumatoid Arthritis. (2012). *A.D.A.M. Medical Encyclopedia.* Retrieved May 5, 2012, from http://www.ncbi.nlm.nih.gov/pubmedhealth/PMH0001467/

Shah, B., Gibson, J. L., & Tex, N. L. (2013). *The 21st Century Pharmacy Technician.* Burlington, MA: Jones & Bartlett Learning.

Sparks, J., & McCartney, L. (2010). *Pharmacy Labs for Technicians: Building Skills in Pharmacy Practice.* St. Paul, MN: Paradigm Publishing.

Systemic Lupus Erythematosus. (2011). *A.D.A.M. Medical Encyclopedia.* Retrieved May 5, 2012, from http://www.ncbi.nlm.nih.gov/pubmedhealth/PMH0001471/

Tendinitis. (2012). *A.D.A.M. Medical Encyclopedia.* Retrieved May 5, 2012, from http://www.ncbi.nlm.nih.gov/pubmedhealth/PMH0002209/

Thompson, J. E. (1998). *A Practical Guide to Contemporary Pharmacy Practice.* Baltimore, MD: Lippincott, Williams & Wilkins.

X-Rays, CT Scans, and MRIs. (2007). *OrthoInfo.* American Academy of Orthopaedic Surgeons. Retrieved May 5, 2012, from http://orthoinfo.aaos.org/topic.cfm?topic=A00188

Chapter 13

Ansel, H. C., & Stoklosa, M. J. (2001). *Pharmaceutical Calculations, 11th ed.* Philadelphia, PA: Lippincott, Williams & Wilkins.

Ballington, D. A., & Anderson, R. J. (2010). *Pharmacy Practice for Technicians: Mastering Community and Hospital Competencies, 4th ed.* St. Paul, MN: Paradigm Publishing.

Bernard, D. (1999). *Clinical Medical Assistant Training Program: Workbook.* Albany, NY: Delmar.

Blesi, M., Wise, B., & Kelley-Arney, C. (2012). *Medical Assisting: Administrative & Clinical Competencies, 7th ed.* Clifton Park, NY: Delmar.

Botvinivk, E. H. (2009). Current Methods of Pharmacological Stress Testing and the Potential Advantages of New Agents. *Journal of Nuclear Medicine Technology, 37*:14–25.

Brasin, G. A., & Dahl, B. M. (2010). *Workbook to Accompany Delmar's Clinical Medical Assisting, 4th ed.* Clifton Park, NY: Delmar.

DiPiro, J. T., Talbert, R. L., Yee, G. C., Matzke, G. R., Wells, B. G., & Posey, L. M. (2008). *Pharmacotherapy: A Pathophysiologic Approach, 7th ed.* New York, NY: McGraw-Hill Medical.

Fremgen, B. F. (1997). *Medical Terminology.* Upper Saddle River, NJ: Prentice-Hall.

Hayward, M. L. (1999). *Clinical Medical Assistant Training Program*. Albany, NY: Delmar.

Lacy, C. F., Armstrong, L., Goldman, M., & Lance, L. (2009). *Drug Information Handbook*. Washington, DC: American Pharmacists Association.

Lindh, W. Q., Pooler, M. S., Tamparo, C. D., & Dahl, B. M. (2010). *Clinical Medical Assisting, 4th ed.* Clifton Park, NY: Delmar.

Shah, B., Gibson, J. L., & Tex, N. L. (2013). *The 21st Century Pharmacy Technician*. Burlington, MA: Jones & Bartlett Learning.

Sparks, J., & McCartney, L. (2010). *Pharmacy Labs for Technicians: Building Skills in Pharmacy Practice*. St. Paul, MN: Paradigm Publishing.

Thompson, J. E. (1998). *A Practical Guide to Contemporary Pharmacy Practice*. Baltimore, MD: Lippincott, Williams & Wilkins.

Chapter 14

Amyotrophic Lateral Sclerosis. (2010). *A.D.A.M. Medical Encyclopedia*. Retrieved July 14, 2012, from http://www.ncbi.nlm.nih.gov/pubmedhealth/PMH0001708/

Ansel, H. C., & Stoklosa, M. J. (2001). *Pharmaceutical Calculations, 11th ed.* Philadelphia, PA: Lippincott, William & Wilkins.

Atkinson, A. J., Daniels, C. E., & Dedrick, R. (2001). *Principles in Clinical Pharmacology*. San Diego, CA: Academic Press.

Bailey, R. (2012). Organ Systems. *About.com*. Retrieved July 19, 2012, from http://biology.about.com/od/organsystems/a/aa031706a.htm

Bekker, M. (2002). Eyedrop Instillation. *Healthline*. Retrieved July 15, 2012, from http://www.healthline.com/galecontent/eyedrop-instillation

Bell's Palsy. (2012). *A.D.A.M. Medical Encyclopedia*. Retrieved July 14, 2012, from http://www.ncbi.nlm.nih.gov/pubmedhealth/PMH0001777/

Blesi, M., Wise, B., & Kelley-Arney, C. (2012). *Medical Assisting Administrative & Clinical Competencies, 7th ed.* Clifton Park, NY: Delmar Cengage Learning.

Brunton, L., Lazo, J., & Parker, K. (2005). *Goodman and Gillman's the Pharmacological Basis of Therapeutics, 11th ed.* Elmsford, NY: McGraw-Hill.

DiPiro, J. T., Talbert, R. L., Yee, G. C., Matzke, G. R., Wells, B. G., & Posey, L. M. (2008). *Pharmacotherapy: A Pathophysiologic Approach, 7th ed.* New York, NY: McGraw-Hill Medical.

Dugdale III, D. C. (2011). Conjunctiva. *MedlinePlus*. Retrieved July 7, 2012, from http://www.nlm.nih.gov/medlineplus/ency/article/002326.htm

Dugdale III, D. C. (2011). Retina. *MedlinePlus*. Retrieved July 7, 2012, from http://www.nlm.nih.gov/medlineplus/ency/article/002291.htm

Dugdale III, D. C. (2011). Sclera. *MedlinePlus*. Retrieved July 7, 2012, from http://www.nlm.nih.gov/medlineplus/ency/article/002295.htm

Ehrlich A. (2009). *Medical Terminology for Health Professions, 6th ed.* Clifton Park, NY: Delmar Cengage Learning.

Encephalitis. (2012). *A.D.A.M. Medical Encyclopedia*. Retrieved July 14, 2012, from http://www.ncbi.nlm.nih.gov/pubmedhealth/PMH0002388/

Facts About The Cornea and Corneal Disease. (n.d.). *National Eye Institute*. Retrieved May 7, 2012, from http://www.nei.nih.gov/health/cornealdisease/#0

Kasper, D., Braunwald, E., Fauci, A. S., Hauser, S. L., Longo, D. L., & Jameson, J. L. (2005). *Harrison's Principles of Internal Medicine, 16th ed.* New York, NY: McGraw-Hill Medical.

Lindh, W. Q., Pooler, M. S., Tamparo, C. D., & Dahl, B. M. (2010). *Delmar's Clinical Medical Assisting, 4th ed.* Clifton Park, NY: Delmar Cengage Learning.

Medical Terminology. (2012). *Global RPh*. Retrieved July 11, 2012, from http://www.globalrph.com/medterm.htm

MedTerms Medical Dictionary. (2012). *MedicineNet.com*. Retrieved July 7, 2102, from http://www.medterms.com

MedWord Resources. Retrieved July 9, 2012, from http://www.medword.com/combos.html

Meningitis. (2010). *A.D.A.M. Medical Encyclopedia*. Retrieved July 14, 2012, from http://www.ncbi.nlm.nih.gov/pubmedhealth/PMH0001700/

Rhoades, R., & Pflanzer, R. (2003). *Human Physiology, 4th ed.* Pacific Grove, CA: Thomson Learning.

Segre, L. (2011). The Eye Chart and 20/20 Vision. Retrieved July 14, 2012, from http://www.allaboutvision.com/eye-test

Stedman's. (1997). *Stedman's Concise Medical Dictionary for Health Professionals, 3rd ed.* Baltimore, MD: Lippincott Williams & Wilkins.

Stroke. (2011). *A.D.A.M. Medical Encyclopedia*. Retrieved July 14, 2012, from http://www.ncbi.nlm.nih.gov/pubmedhealth/PMH0001740/

Thibodeau, G., & Patton, K. (2007). *Structure and Function of the Body, 13th ed.* St Louis, MO: Mosby.

Wolff, R. (2008). Eye Irrigation Techniques. *ISHN Magazine*. Retrieved July 15, 2012, from http://www.ishn.com/articles/eye-irrigation-techniques

Chapter 15

Ansel, H. C., & Stoklosa, M. J. (2001). *Pharmaceutical Calculations, 11th ed.* Philadelphia, PA: Lippincott, Williams & Wilkins.

Ballington, D. A., & Anderson, R. J. (2010). *Pharmacy Practice for Technicians: Mastering Community and Hospital Competencies, 4th ed.* St. Paul, MN: Paradigm Publishing.

Bernard, D. (1999). *Clinical Medical Assistant Training Program: Workbook*. Albany, NY: Delmar.

Blesi, M., Wise, B., & Kelley-Arney, C. (2012). *Medical Assisting: Administrative & Clinical Competencies, 7th ed.* Clifton Park, NY: Delmar.

Blonde, L. (2011). Improving Care for Patients with Type 2 Diabetes: Applying Management Guidelines and Algorithms, and a Review of New Evidence for Incretin Agents and Lifestyle Intervention. *American Journal of Managed Care, Suppl. 14*:S368–76.

Brasin, G. A., & Dahl, B. M. (2010). *Workbook to Accompany Delmar's Clinical Medical Assisting, 4th ed.* Clifton Park, NY: Delmar.

Carter, P., Khunti, K., & Davies, M. J. (2012). Dietary Recommendations for the Prevention of Type 2 Diabetes: What Are They Based On? *Journal of Nutrition and Metabolism*, Epub January 19, 2012.

DiPiro, J. T., Talbert, R. L., Yee, G. C., Matzke, G. R., Wells, B. G., & Posey, L. M. (2008). *Pharmacotherapy: A Pathophysiologic Approach, 7th ed.* New York, NY: McGraw-Hill Medical.

Fremgen, B. F. (1997). *Medical Terminology*. Upper Saddle River, NJ: Prentice-Hall.

Guaraldi, F., & Salvatori, R. (2012). Cushing Syndrome: Maybe Not So Uncommon of an Endocrine Disease. *Journal of the American Board of Family Medicine, 25*(2):199–208.

Hayward, M. L. (1999). *Clinical Medical Assistant Training Program*. Albany, NY: Delmar.

Hypogonadism. (2010). *A.D.A.M. Medical Encyclopedia*. Retrieved June 12, 2012, from http://www.ncbi.nlm.nih.gov/pubmedhealth/PMH0002175/

Lacy, C. F., Armstrong, L., Goldman, M., & Lance, L. (2009). *Drug Information Handbook*. Washington, DC: American Pharmacists Association.

Lindh, W. Q., Pooler, M. S., Tamparo, C. D., & Dahl, B. M. (2010). *Clinical Medical Assisting, 4th ed.* Clifton Park, NY: Delmar.

Mazzola, N. (2012). Review of Current and Emerging Therapies in Type 2 Diabetes Mellitus. *The American Journal of Managed Care, 18*(Supplement 1):17supp–26.

Shah, B., Gibson, J. L., & Tex, N. L. (2013). *The 21st Century Pharmacy Technician*. Burlington, MA: Jones & Bartlett Learning.

Sparks, J., & McCartney, L. (2010). *Pharmacy Labs for Technicians: Building Skills in Pharmacy Practice*. St. Paul, MN: Paradigm Publishing.

Thompson, J. E. (1998). *A Practical Guide to Contemporary Pharmacy Practice*. Baltimore, MD: Lippincott, Williams & Wilkins.

Tsang, M. W. (2012). The Management of Type 2 Diabetic Patients with Hypoglycemic Agents. *ISRN Endocrinol*, Epub May 7, 2012.

Chapter 16

Ansel, H. C., & Stoklosa, M. J. (2001). *Pharmaceutical Calculations, 11th ed.* Philadelphia, PA: Lippincott, Williams & Wilkins.

Ballington, D. A., & Anderson, R. J. (2010). *Pharmacy Practice for Technicians: Mastering Community and Hospital Competencies, 4th ed.* St. Paul, MN: Paradigm Publishing.

Bernard, D. (1999). *Clinical Medical Assistant Training Program: Workbook*. Albany, NY: Delmar.

Blesi, M., Wise, B., & Kelley-Arney, C. (2012). *Medical Assisting: Administrative & Clinical Competencies, 7th ed.* Clifton Park, NY: Delmar.

Bope, E. T., & Kellerman, R. D., eds. (2012). *Conn's Current Therapy*. Philadelphia, PA: Elsevier Saunders.

Brasin, G. A., & Dahl, B. M. (2010). *Workbook to Accompany Delmar's Clinical Medical Assisting, 4th ed.* Clifton Park, NY: Delmar.

Colonoscopy (NIH Publication No. 10–4331). (2012). National Institute of Diabetes and Digestive and Kidney Diseases. Bethesda, MD: National Digestive Diseases Information Clearinghouse. Retrieved July 2, 2012, from http://digestive.niddk.nih.gov/ddiseases/pubs/colonoscopy/

DiPiro, J. T., Talbert, R. L., Yee, G. C., Matzke, G. R., Wells, B. G., & Posey, L. M. (2008). *Pharmacotherapy: A Pathophysiologic Approach, 7th ed.* New York, NY: McGraw-Hill Medical.

Fremgen, B. F. (1997). *Medical Terminology*. Upper Saddle River, NJ: Prentice-Hall.

Hayward, M. L. (1999). *Clinical Medical Assistant Training Program*. Albany, NY: Delmar.

Kyle, G. (2007). Bowel Care. Part 3: Obtaining a Stool Sample. *Nursing Times, 103*(44):24–5.

Lacy, C. F., Armstrong, L., Goldman, M., & Lance, L. (2009). *Drug Information Handbook*. Washington, DC: American Pharmacists Association.

Lindh, W. Q., Pooler, M. S., Tamparo, C. D., & Dahl, B. M. (2010). *Clinical Medical Assisting, 4th ed.* Clifton Park, NY: Delmar.

Lower GI Series (NIH Publication No. 10–4334). (2012). National Institute of Diabetes and Digestive and Kidney Diseases. Bethesda, MD: National Digestive Diseases Information Clearinghouse. Retrieved July 2, 2012, from http://digestive.niddk.nih.gov/ddiseases/pubs/lowergi/

Shah, B., Gibson, J. L., & Tex, N. L. (2013). *The 21st Century Pharmacy Technician*. Burlington, MA: Jones & Bartlett Learning.

Sparks, J., & McCartney, L. (2010). *Pharmacy Labs for Technicians: Building Skills in Pharmacy Practice*. St. Paul, MN: Paradigm Publishing.

Thompson, J. E. (1998). *A Practical Guide to Contemporary Pharmacy Practice*. Baltimore, MD: Lippincott, Williams & Wilkins.

Upper GI Series (NIH Publication No. 10–4335). (2012). National Institute of Diabetes and Digestive and Kidney Diseases. Bethesda, MD: National Digestive Diseases Information Clearinghouse. Retrieved July 2, 2012, from http://digestive.niddk.nih.gov/ddiseases/pubs/uppergi/index.aspx

Chapter 17

Ansel, H. C., & Stoklosa, M. J. (2001). *Pharmaceutical Calculations, 11th ed.* Philadelphia, PA: Lippincott, Williams & Wilkins.

Badura-Lotter, G. (2012). Sexually Transmitted Diseases: Reflections on Metaphors and Ethics. *Methods in Molecular Biology, 903*:419–35.

Ballington, D. A., & Anderson, R. J. (2010). *Pharmacy Practice for Technicians: Mastering Community and Hospital Competencies, 4th ed.* St. Paul, MN: Paradigm Publishing.

Bernard, D. (1999). *Clinical Medical Assistant Training Program: Workbook.* Albany, NY: Delmar.

Blesi, M., Wise, B., & Kelley-Arney, C. (2012). *Medical Assisting: Administrative & Clinical Competencies, 7th ed.* Clifton Park, NY: Delmar.

Bope, E. T., & Kellerman, R. D., eds. (2012). *Conn's Current Therapy.* Philadelphia, PA: Elsevier Saunders.

Brasin, G. A., & Dahl, B. M. (2010). *Workbook to Accompany Delmar's Clinical Medical Assisting, 4th ed.* Clifton Park, NY: Delmar.

Chlamydia–CDC Fact Sheet. (2012). *Centers for Disease Control and Prevention.* Retrieved July 16, 2012, from http://www.cdc.gov/std/chlamydia/STDFact-Chlamydia.htm

Crenner, C. (2012). The Tuskegee Syphilis Study and the Scientific Concept of Racial Nervous Resistance. *Journal of the History of Medicine and Allied Sciences, 67*(2):244–80.

Dialysis. (2012). *National Kidney Foundation.* Retrieved July 14, 2012, from http://www.kidney.org/atoz/content/dialysisinfo.cfm

Dipiro, J. T., Talbert, R. L., Yee, G. C., Matzke, G. R., Wells, B. G., & Posey, L. M. (2008). *Pharmacotherapy: A Pathophysiologic Approach, 7th ed.* New York, NY: McGraw-Hill Medical.

Eaton, D. K., Kann, L., Kinchen, S., Shanklin, S., Flint, K., Hawkins, J., et al., (2012). Youth Risk Behavior Surveillance–United States, 2011. *Morbidity and Mortality Weekly Report Surveillance Summary, 61*(4):1–162.

Elghany, N. A., Schumacher, M. C., Slattery, M. L., West, D. W., & Lee, J. S. (1990). Occupation, Cadmium Exposure, and Prostate Cancer. *Epidemiology, 1*(2):107–15.

Etter, D. J., Zimet, G. D., & Rickert, V. I. (2012). Human Papillomavirus Vaccine in Adolescent Women: A 2012 Update. *Current Opinion in Obstetrics and Gynecology, 24*(5):305–10.

Fremgen, B. F. (1997). *Medical Terminology.* Upper Saddle River, NJ: Prentice-Hall.

Genital Herpes–CDC Fact Sheet. (2012). *Centers for Disease Control and Prevention.* Retrieved July 16, 2012, from http://www.cdc.gov/std/Herpes/STDFact-Herpes.htm

Hayward, M. L. (1999). *Clinical Medical Assistant Training Program.* Albany, NY: Delmar.

Kasawara, K. T., Nascimento, S. L., Costa M. L, Surita, F. G., & Silva, J. L. P. (2012). Exercise and Physical Activity in the Prevention of Preeclampsia: Systematic Review. *Acta Obstetrica Gynecologica Scandinavica, 91*(10):1147–51.

Lacy, C. F., Armstrong, L., Goldman, M., & Lance, L. (2009). *Drug Information Handbook.* Washington, DC: American Pharmacists Association.

Lindh, W. Q., Pooler, M. S., Tamparo, C. D., & Dahl, B. M. (2010). *Clinical Medical Assisting, 4th ed.* Clifton Park, NY: Delmar.

MacKay, A. P., Berg, C. J., & Atrash, H. K. (2001). Pregnancy-Related Mortality from Preeclampsia and Eclampsia. *Obstetrics and Gynecology, 97*(4):533–8.

Prostate Cancer. (2011). *A.D.A.M. Medical Encyclopedia.* Retrieved July 14, 2012, from http://www.ncbi.nlm.nih.gov/pubmedhealth/PMH0001418/

Reiter, P. L., McRee A. L., Pepper, J. K., Chantala, K., & Brewer, N. T. (2012). Improving Human Papillomavirus Vaccine Delivery: A National Study of Parents and Their Adolescent Sons. *Journal of Adolescent Health, 51*(1):32–7.

Roberts, J. R. (2007). Urine Dipstick Testing: Everything You Need to Know. *Emergency Medicine News, 29*(6):24–27.

Shah, B., Gibson, J. L., & Tex, N. L. (2013). *The 21st Century Pharmacy Technician.* Burlington, MA: Jones & Bartlett Learning.

Sparks, J., & McCartney, L. (2010). *Pharmacy Labs for Technicians: Building Skills in Pharmacy Practice.* St. Paul, MN: Paradigm Publishing.

Syphilis–CDC Fact Sheet. (2012). *Centers for Disease Control and Prevention.* Retrieved July 16, 2012, from http://www.cdc.gov/std/syphilis/stdfact-syphilis.htm

Testicular Cancer. (2012). *A.D.A.M. Medical Encyclopedia.* Retrieved July 14, 2012, from http://www.ncbi.nlm.nih.gov/pubmedhealth/PMH0002266/

Thompson, J. E. (1998). *A Practical Guide to Contemporary Pharmacy Practice.* Baltimore, MD: Lippincott, Williams & Wilkins.

Turner, R. (2012). Strategies to Prevent Gonorrhea Reinfection in Men. *Nursing Standard, 26*(30):35–9.

Vorvick, L. (2012). Secondary Amennorhea. *MedlinePlus.* Retrieved July 16, 2012, from http://www.nlm.nih.gov/medlineplus/ency/article/001219.htm

Vorvick, L. (2012). Urinary Catheters. *MedlinePlus.* Retrieved July 14, 2012, from http://www.nlm.nih.gov/medlineplus/ency/article/003981.htm

Waalkes, M. P. (2000). Cadmium Carcinogenesis in Review. *Journal of Inorganic Biochemistry, 79*(1–4):241–4.

Yawn, B. P., Dietrich, A. J., Wollan, P., Bertram, S., Graham, D., Huff, J. et al. (2012). TRIPPD: A Practice-Based Network Effectiveness Study of Postpartum Depression Screening and Management. *Annals of Family Medicine, 10*:320–9.

Chapter 18

Bernard, D. (1999). *Clinical Medical Assistant Training Program: Workbook.* Albany, NY: Delmar.

Blesi, M., Wise, B., & Kelley-Arney, C. (2012). *Medical Assisting: Administrative & Clinical Competencies, 7th ed.* Clifton Park, NY: Delmar.

Brasin, G. A., & Dahl, B. M. (2010). *Workbook to Accompany Delmar's Clinical Medical Assisting, 4th ed.* Clifton Park, NY: Delmar.

Diagnosis and Procedure Codes: Abbreviated and Full Code Titles. (2012). *Centers for Medicare and Medicaid Services.* Retrieved July 21, 2012, from http://www.cms.gov/Medicare/Coding/ICD9Provider DiagnosticCodes/codes.html

Hayward, M. L. (1999). *Clinical Medical Assistant Training Program.* Albany, NY: Delmar.

Health Information Privacy. (2012). *U.S. Department of Health and Human Services.* Retrieved July 21, 2012, from http://www.hhs.gov/ocr/privacy/

ICD-10-CM Official Guidelines for Coding and Reporting. (2012). *Centers for Disease Control and Prevention.* Retrieved July 21, 2012, from http://www.cdc.gov/nchs/data/icd10/10cmguidelines2012.pdf

ICD-10 Implementation Timelines. (2012). *Centers for Medicare and Medicaid Services.* Retrieved July 21, 2012, from http://www.cms.gov/Medicare/Coding/ICD10/ICD-10ImplementationTimelines.html

Iglehart, J. K. (2012). Primary Care Update–Light at the End of the Tunnel. *New England Journal of Medicine, 366*(23):2144–6.

Lindh, W. Q., Pooler, M. S., Tamparo, C. D., & Dahl, B. M. (2010). *Clinical Medical Assisting, 4th ed.* Clifton Park, NY: Delmar.

McCarthy, R. L., & Schafermeyer, K. W. (2001). *Introduction to Health Care Delivery: A Primer for Pharmacists, 2nd ed.* Gaithersburg, MD: Aspen Publishers, Inc.

Medicare Program. (2012). Changes to the Medicare Advantage and the Medicare Prescription Drug Benefit Programs for Contract Year 2013 and Other Changes; Final Rule. Department of Health and Human Services. 77 Federal Register 7. April 12, 2012.

Napier, R. H. (2008). Insurance Billing and Coding. *Dental Clinics of North America, 52*(3):507–27.

Patient Protection and Affordable Care Act. (2012). Establishment of Exchanges and Qualified Health Plans; Exchange Standards for Employers; Final Rule and Interim Final Rule. Department of Health and Human Services. 77 Federal Register 59. March 27, 2012.

Pipes, S. (2012). The End of Private Health Insurance in America. *Forbes.* March 19, 2012.

Sade, R. M. (2012). Why Physicians Should Not Lie for Their Patients. *American Journal of Bioethics, 12*(3):17–9.

Shah, B., Gibson, J. L., & Tex, N. L. (2013). *The 21st Century Pharmacy Technician.* Burlington, MA: Jones & Bartlett Learning.

Chapter 19

The American Geriatrics Society 2012 Beers Criteria Update Expert Panel. (2012). American Geriatrics Society Updated Beers Criteria for Potentially Inappropriate Medication Use in Older Adults. *Journal of the American Geriatrics Society, 60*(4):616–31.

Ansel, H. C., & Stoklosa, M. J. (2001). *Pharmaceutical Calculations, 11th ed.* Philadelphia, PA: Lippincott, Williams & Wilkins.

Ballington, D. A., & Anderson, R. J. (2010). *Pharmacy Practice for Technicians: Mastering Community and Hospital Competencies, 4th ed.* St. Paul, MN: Paradigm Publishing.

Barba, B. E., Hu, J., & Efird, J. (2012). Quality Geriatric Care as Perceived by Nurses in Long-Term and Acute Care Settings. *Journal of Clinical Nursing, 21*(5–6):833–40.

Berkman, B. J. (2011). Seizing Interdisciplinary Opportunities in the Changing Landscape of Health and Aging: a Social Work Perspective. *Gerontologist, 51*(4):433–40.

Bernard, D. (1999). *Clinical Medical Assistant Training Program: Workbook.* Albany, NY: Delmar.

Blesi, M., Wise, B., & Kelley-Arney, C. (2012). *Medical Assisting: Administrative & Clinical Competencies, 7th ed.* Clifton Park, NY: Delmar.

Brasin, G. A., & Dahl, B. M. (2010). *Workbook to Accompany Delmar's Clinical Medical Assisting, 4th ed.* Clifton Park, NY: Delmar.

DiPiro, J. T., Talbert, R. L., Yee, G. C., Matzke, G. R., Wells, B. G., & Posey, L. M. (2008). *Pharmacotherapy: A Pathophysiologic Approach, 7th ed.* New York, NY: McGraw-Hill Medical.

Fremgen, B. F. (1997). *Medical Terminology.* Upper Saddle River, NJ: Prentice-Hall.

Hayward, M. L. (1999). *Clinical Medical Assistant Training Program.* Albany, NY: Delmar.

Healey, W. E., Broers, K. B., Nelson, J., & Huber, G. (2012). Physical therapists' health promotion activities for older adults. *Journal of Geriatric Physical Therapy, 35*(1):35–48.

Kliegman, R. M., Stanton, B. F., St. Geme, J. W., Schor, N. F., & Behrman, R. E. (2011). *Nelson Textbook of Pediatrics, 19th ed.* Philadelphia, PA: Elsevier Saunders.

Lacy, C. F., Armstrong, L., Goldman, M., & Lance, L. (2009). *Drug Information Handbook.* Washington, DC: American Pharmacists Association.

Lindh, W. Q., Pooler, M. S., Tamparo, C. D., & Dahl, B. M. (2010). *Clinical Medical Assisting, 4th ed.* Clifton Park, NY: Delmar.

Locatelli, C., Piselli, P., Cicerchia, M., & Repetto, L. (2012). Physician's Age and Sex Influence Breaking Bad News to Elderly Cancer Patients. Beliefs and Practices of 50 Italian Oncologists: the G.I.O. Ger Study. *Psychooncology*, Epub June 7, 2012.

McLean, A. J., & LeCouteur, D. G. (2004). Aging Biology and Geriatric Clinical Pharmacology. *Pharmacological Review, 56*(2):163–84.

Price, B. (2011). Making Better Use of Older People's Narratives. *Nursing Older People, 23*(6):31–7.

Retraction–Ileal-Lymphoid-Nodular Hyperplasia, Non-Specific Colitis, and Pervasive Developmental Disorder in Children. (2010). *The Lancet, 675*(9713):445.

Scott, I. A., Gray, L. C., Martine, J. H., & Mitchell, C. A. (2012). Effects of a Drug Minimization Guide on Prescribing Intentions in Elderly Persons with Polypharmacy. *Drugs & Aging, 29*(8):659–67.

Shah, B., Gibson, J. L, & Tex, N. L. (2013). *The 21st Century Pharmacy Technician.* Burlington, MA: Jones & Bartlett Learning.

Sheppard, J. P., Singh, S, Fletcher, K., McManus, R. J., & Mant, J. (2012). Impact of Age and Sex on Primary Preventive Treatment for Cardiovascular Disease in the West Midlands, UK: Cross Sectional Study. *BMJ 2012, 345*:e4535.

Sparks, J., & McCartney, L. (2010). *Pharmacy Labs for Technicians: Building Skills in Pharmacy Practice.* St. Paul, MN: Paradigm Publishing.

Tschudy, M. M., & Arcara, K. M., eds. (2012). *The Harriet Lane Handbook, 19th ed.* Philadelphia, PA: Elsevier Mosby.

Turner, M. D., & Ship, J. A. (2007). Dry Mouth and Its Effects on the Oral Health of Elderly People. *Journal of the American Dental Association, 138*(Supplement 1):155–205.

Turnheim, K. (1998). Drug Dosage in the Elderly. Is It Rational? *Drugs & Aging, 13*(5):357–79.

Wolstenholme, B. (2011). Medication-Related Problems in Geriatric Pharmacology. *Aging Well, 4*(3):8.

Zager, B. S., & Yancy, M. (2011). A Call to Improve Practice Concerning Cultural Sensitivity in Advance Directives: A Review of the Literature. *Worldviews on Evidence-Based Nursing, 8*(4):202–11.

Chapter 20

10 Things to Leave Off Your Résumé. (2011). *CareerBuilder.com.* Retrieved November 4, 2102, from http://www.careerbuilder.com/Article/CB-1479-Resumes-Cover-Letters-10-Things-to-Leave-Off-Your-R%C3%A9sum%C3%A9/

Blesi, M., Kelly-Arney, C., & Wise, B. (2012). *Medical Assisting: Administrative and Clinical Competencies, 7th Edition.* Clifton Park, NY: Delmar Publishing Companies, Inc.

Booth, K., Whicker, L., Wyman, T., Pugh, D., & Thompson, S. (2009). *Medical Assisting: Administrative and Clinical Procedures Including Anatomy and Physiology, 3rd Edition.* New York, NY: McGraw-Hill Publishing Companies, Inc.

Constructive Criticism. (n.d.). *Dictionary.com's 21st Century Lexicon.* Retrieved November 4, 2012, from http://dictionary.reference.com/browse/constructive+criticism

Employment Agency. (n.d.). *The Free Dictionary.* Retrieved November 4, 2012, from http://www.thefreedictionary.com/employment+agency

Employment Screening. (n.d.). *The Free Dictionary.* Retrieved November 4, 2012, from http://encyclopedia.thefreedictionary.com/employment+screening

Full-Time Employment. (n.d.). *The Business Dictionary.* Retrieved November 4, 2012, from http://www.businessdictionary.com/definition/full-time-employment.html

Global Digital Communication: Texting, Social Networking Popular Worldwide. (2011). *Pew Research Center.* Retrieved November 4, 2012, from http://www.pewglobal.org/files/2011/12/Pew-Global-Attitudes-Technology-Report-FINAL-December-20-20111.pdf

Lindh, B., Pooler, M., Tamparo, C., & Dahl, B. (2009). *Comprehensive Medical Assisting: Administrative and Clinical Competencies, 4th Edition.* Clifton Park, NY: Delmar/Cengage Learning, Inc.

Networking. (2011). *Crew Career Center.* Retrieved November 4, 2012, from http://www.crew.cc/Services/Networking

Portfolio. (n.d.). *The Free Dictionary.* Retrieved November 4, 2012, from http://www.thefreedictionary.com/portfolio

Preceptor. (n.d.). *The Free Dictionary.* Retrieved November 4, 2012, from http://www.thefreedictionary.com/preceptor

Professional Development. (n.d.). *The Free Dictionary.* Retrieved November 4, 2012, from http://encyclopedia.thefreedictionary.com/professional+development

Sample Career Objectives—Examples for Resumes. (n.d.). *Job Interview and Career Guide.* Retrieved November 4, 2012, from http://www.job-interview-site.com/sample-career-objectives-examples-for-resumes.html

Index